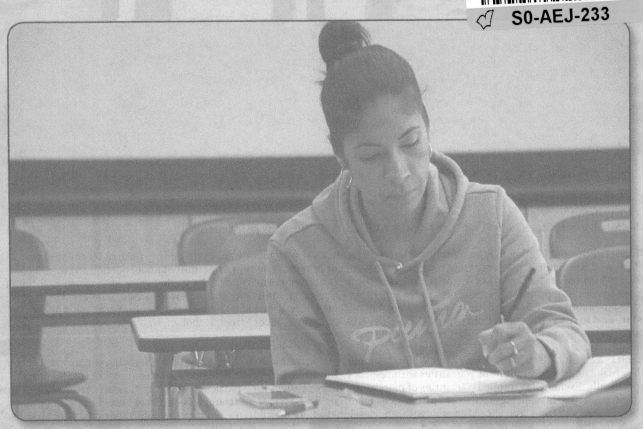

FOUNDATIONS FOR COMMUNITY HEALTH WORKERS

SECOND EDITION

Tim Berthold, Editor

JB JOSSEY-BASS™

A Wiley Brand

Published by Jossey-Bass
A Wiley Brand
One Montgomery Street, Suite 1000, San Francisco, CA 94104-4594—*www.josseybass.com*

Library of Congress Cataloging-in-Publication Data

Names: Berthold, Tim, editor.
Title: Foundations for community health workers / [edited by]
  Timothy Berthold.
Description: 2nd edition. | San Francisco, CA : Jossey-Bass & Pfeiffer
  Imprints, Wiley, [2016] | Includes bibliographical references and index.
Identifiers: LCCN 2015046271 (print) | LCCN 2015047137 (ebook) | ISBN
  9781119060819 (pbk.) | ISBN 9781119060673 (epdf) | ISBN 9781119060734 (epub)
Subjects: | MESH: Community Health Workers | Community Health Services |
  Vocational Guidance
Classification: LCC RA427 (print) | LCC RA427 (ebook) | NLM W 21.5 |
  DDC 362.12—dc23
LC record available at http://lccn.loc.gov/2015046271

Cover design: Wiley
Cover images: © City College of San Francisco

Printed in the United States of America

SECOND EDITION

PB Printing   SKY10026432_042121

CONTENTS

Acknowledgments

We wish to acknowledge and thank the faculty who have taught in the CHW Certificate Program and collaborated with students and community-based organizations to develop the curriculum that informs this book. These faculty include Alma Avila, Carol Badran, Tim Berthold, Carol Chao-Herring, Dayo Diggs, Amie Fishman, Susana Hennessy-Lavery, Tandy Iles, Vicki Legion, Melissa Jones, Obiel Leyva, Joani Marinoff, Ida McCray, Marcellina Ogbu, Abby Rincón, Janey Skinner, Darouny Somsanith, Jill Tregor, Darlene Weide, and Donna Willmott.

We are deeply grateful to all the students and CHWs who contributed to the book through their interviews, photographs, and participation in educational videos, including Veronica Aburto, Juanita Alvarado, Jill Armour, Kathleen Banks, Ramona Benson, John Boler, Anthony Brooks, Rene Celiz, Esther Chavez, Andrew Ciscel, Phuong An Doan-Billings, Tomasa Bulux, Cameron Dunkley, Ariann Harrison, Darnell Farr, Tracy Reed Foster, Durrell Fox, Thomas Ganger, Lee Jackson, Sandra Johnson, Yudith Larez, Rose Letulle, Michael Levato, Phyllis Lui, Sergio Matos, Jermila McCoy, Richard Medina, Francis Julian Montgomery, Alvaro Morales, David Pheng, Kent Rodriguez, Romelia Rodriguez, LaTonya Rogers, Ron Sanders, Martha Shearer, Somnang Sin, Jerry Smart, Letida Sot, Charlie Starr, Jason Stanford, Adrieann Lo, Lexon Lo, Manith Thaing, Michelle Vail, Alma Vasquez, and Emory Wilson.

The educational videos linked throughout the book were codirected by Tim Berthold and Jill Tregor. Matt Luotto and Amy Hill served as videographers. The digital stories featured in this Introduction and Chapter 15 were produced by the Center for Digital Storytelling (with the leadership of Amy Hill and Matt Luotto). Several City College staff and faculty were instrumental to the development of the videos including Carol Cheng, Amie Fishman, Janey Skinner, and Emily Marinelli.

Ernest Kirkwood, Matt Luotto, Sam Wolson, and Len Finocchio took photographs for the second edition of this textbook along with graduates of the CHW Program: Juanita Alvarado, Tracy Reed Foster, and Ron Sanders. Some photos were taken for the first edition by Ramona Benson, Phuong An Doan Billings, Lee Jackson, Alvaro Morales, and Cindy Tsai.

Pamela DeCarlo, Amie Fishman, Mike Kometani, and Emily Marinelli supported the development of the *Foundations* textbook by reviewing early drafts of chapters, conducting research, verifying citations, securing permissions, coordinating photo shoots, selecting photographs, and managing photo and video releases. Maureen Forys and the team at Happenstance Type-O-Rama created the design for the second edition of the book (and the *companion Training Guide*). Jill Tregor, Tim Berthold, and Mickey Ellinger conducted qualitative interviews with CHWs to develop the quotes that are included throughout the book. We also acknowledge the leadership and support provided by several CCSF colleagues: Carol Cheng, administrative coordinator of the Health Education Department; Terry Hall, dean of the School of Health and Physical Education; and Kirstin Hershbell-Charles, dean of Grants & Resource Development. We would like to thank proposal reviewers Juliana Anastasoff, Karen Winkler, Michele Montecalvo, and Kaysie Schmidt, who provided valuable feedback on the original book proposal.

This book would not have been possible without the leadership of Mary Beth Love and Vicki Legion. Mary Beth is the chair of the Health Education Department at San Francisco State University (SFSU) and founder of Community Health Works, a unique and enduring partnership between the Health Education Departments at SFSU and City College of San Francisco (CCSF) (*www.communityhealthworks.org*). This partnership established the CHW Certificate Program at CCSF. Vicki Legion served as the first coordinator and created the model CHW program that serves as the basis for this book.

The development of the second edition and all educational videos was made possible through a grant from the Centers for Medicare and Medicaid Innovations (CMMI). This grant was a partnership with the national

Transitions Clinic Network (TCN), an expanding group of clinics across the United States and in Puerto Rico that provide primary health care to patients coming home from prison (*http://transitionsclinic.org/*). We owe a special debt of gratitude to the CHWs employed by the Transitions Clinic Network who participated in online training and provided feedback about our curriculum: Precious Bedell, Karim Butler, Joe Calderon, Monique Carter, Donna Hylton, Arlinda Love, Richard Medina, Felix Medina, Marc Narcisse, Matt Pedragon, Tracy Reed Foster, Martha Shearer, and Jerry Smart.

The project was supported by Grant Number 1CMS331071-01-00 and 1C1CMS331300-01-00 from the U.S. Department of Health and Human Services, Centers for Medicare & Medicaid Services. Disclaimer: The contents of this publication are solely the responsibility of the authors and do not necessary represent the official view of the U.S. Department of Health and Human Services or any of its agencies.

We are grateful for the support and editorial guidance provided by Seth Schwartz from Jossey-Bass.

Most importantly, this book acknowledges and is dedicated to community health workers past, present, and future.

About the Authors

Abby M. Rincón, MPH   Abby M. Rincón is the Assistant Dean for Graduate Diversity with the University of California, Berkeley. She's been in the public health field for over 28 years and has worked with diverse populations, in a variety of settings addressing a multitude of topics domestically and internationally.

Alma Avila, MPH   Alma Avila is the coordinator of the community health worker (CHW) program at the City College of San Francisco. Alma has a master's degree in public health and has been involved with community health worker programs and *promotora* programs for more than 20 years.

Amber Straus, MEd   Amber Straus teaches academic literacy at the City College of San Francisco. She loves working with and learning from students. Amber sees education as a vital tool for ending cycles of oppression and creating social justice.

Craig Wenzl, BA   Craig Wenzl is associate director of drug and alcohol studies at the City College of San Francisco. Prior to City College, Craig worked for 10 years as the director of programs at the Monterey County AIDS Project in Seaside and Salinas, California. In addition to program coordinating, Craig also worked as a community health outreach worker, HIV testing counselor, and group facilitator, with a focus on sexual risk and substance use.

Darlene Weide, MPH, MSW   Darlene Weide is a faculty member in the Health Education Department at the City College of San Francisco and the executive director of Community Boards, the nation's longest-running community-based dispute-resolution organization.

Darouny Somsanith, MPH   Darouny Somsanith is an instructor at City College of San Francisco with the Health Education Department and has taught for the Community Health Worker (CHW) and the Health Care Interpreter Certificate programs. She started her public health career as a CHW, and for nearly 15 years has worked on issues of workforce development and training for those wanting to enter community health work.

David Spero, RN   David Spero is a nurse, health educator, and a health journalist. He is the author of three books on chronic illness, including *Diabetes: Sugar-Coated Crisis*. He was a trainer in Stanford's Chronic Disease Self-Management program, and writes and blogs for *Diabetes Self-Management* magazine.

Donna Willmott, MPH   Donna Willmott is a formerly incarcerated community organizer and advocate who has worked on issues of health and incarceration for 25 years. She is a retired member of the faculty of the Health Education Department of City College of San Francisco.

Edith Guillén-Núñez, JD, LMFT   Edith Guillén-Núñez is an attorney, and licensed marriage family therapist and the Associate Director of the Community Mental Health Worker Certificate Program at City College of San Francisco. Her therapy practice focuses on working with families and children in the areas of family violence, trauma, and substance abuse. She specializes in family law and consults in the area of ethical and legal issues to mental health agencies.

Ellen Wu, MPH   Ellen Wu is the Executive Director of Urban Habitat, and previously Executive Director of the California Pan-Ethnic Health Network (CPEHN). She has over 20 years of experience working to improve the health and well-being of California's low-income communities of color.

Emily Marinelli, MFT   Emily Marinelli is the program manager for the Infectious Disease Prevention in Priority Populations Certificate in the Health Education Department at CCSF. Emily has over 15 years' experience working in HIV prevention and with lesbian, gay, bisexual, transgender, and queer communities. Emily is also a marriage and family therapist who provides sliding scale mental health services in San Francisco.

Janey Skinner, MPH   Janey Skinner is a faculty member with the Health Education Department at City College of San Francisco. She has worked for decades with diverse communities, focused on grassroots leadership, workforce development, violence prevention, and community action.

Jeni Miller, PhD   Jeni Miller is communications manager and codirector of Partnership for the Public's Health, a project of the Public Health Institute.

Jill R. Tregor, MPH   Jill Tregor is an adjunct instructor with the Community Health Worker, Alcohol & Drug Counselor, and HIV/Infectious Disease Prevention certificate programs at City College of San Francisco. She has many years of experience working with community-based organizations addressing hate-motivated violence, women's health, and domestic violence.

Joani Marinoff, MPH   Joani Marinoff is the coordinator of HIV/STI Prevention Studies in the Health Education Department at City College of San Francisco. She has more than 35 years of experience in health care and education, participatory learning, and organizing strategies for addressing health disparities through reflection and community action. She is also a longtime meditator and teaches restorative yoga.

E. Lee Rosenthal, PhD, MS, MPH   E. Lee Rosenthal is a researcher and advocate for the CHW workforce with more than 25 years' experience of CHW collaborative-inquiry at the local and national level. She serves as a faculty member at the Texas Tech University Health Sciences Center, Paul L. Foster School of Medicine in El Paso. Lee is also a cofounder and Research Affiliate of the University of Texas Institute for Health Policy's Project on CHW Policy and Practice.

Len Finocchio, DrPH   Len Finocchio was part of Governor Jerry Brown's team that implemented the Affordable Care Act in California. He is currently an independent policy consultant. Len taught courses for many years on the health care system and health policy at San Francisco State University and City College of San Francisco.

Mele Lau-Smith, MPH   Mele Lau-Smith is Executive Director of Family Engagement and School Partnerships for the Student, Family, Community Support Department of the San Francisco Unified School District. Prior to this position she worked with the San Francisco Department of Health's Tobacco Free Project and provided technical assistance and training to community based organizations implementing the Community Action Model.

Mickey Ellinger, PhD   Mickey Ellinger interviewed community health workers and wrote early drafts of some chapters of the textbook. She was part of the team that produced Community Health Works' *Asthma Toolkit—Managing Children's Asthma*.

J. Nell Brownstein, PhD   J. Nell Brownstein is a researcher and consultant with a specialty in chronic disease management. She worked on CHW programs and related sustainability issues in her 25 years of service (1990–2015) at the Centers for Disease Control and Prevention. Dr. Brownstein serves as an adjunct Associate Professor at the Rollins School of Public Health at Emory University, an affiliation she has had since 1992.

Philip Colgan, PhD   Philip Colgan is a psychologist in private practice in San Francisco, specializing in the treatment of attachment disorders in close relationships, including problems with addiction, communication, and sexuality.

Rhonella C. Owens, MEd, PhD   Rhonella C. Owens has been a counselor and instructor at the City College of San Francisco for 30 years. Rhonella is also the author of *The Journey of Your Life* (life coaching workbook) and *Turn Your Dreams into Reality* (goal setting and achievement).

Sal Núñez, PhD, LMFT   Sal Núñez is a licensed psychologist and marriage and family therapist. He is the Director of the Community Mental Health Certificate program at the Health Education Department and has been teaching at CCSF since 2000.

Sharon Turner, MPH, EdD   Sharon Turner is currently the Director of the SB 1070 Southwest Pathways Consortium and Codirector of AB 86, both statewide grants which aim to help the transition of high school and adult school students in Career and Technical Education programs into community college. Prior to this, Sharon worked at City College of San Francisco for seven years teaching a variety of courses in the Health Education Department.

Susana Hennessey Lavery, MPH   Susana Hennessey Lavery teaches in the Community Health Worker Certificate Program at CCSF and is a health educator with the San Francisco Department of Public Health. In that capacity she codesigns and implements comprehensive health promotion plans, including design and implementation of the CAM (Community Action Model for policy development). Previously, she was the Community Health Education supervisor at La Clinica De La Raza.

Tim Berthold, MPH   Tim Berthold is a faculty member with the Health Education Department at the City College of San Francisco. He has 25 years' experience working with diverse communities in the United States and internationally, and as a trainer of community health and human rights workers.

Introduction

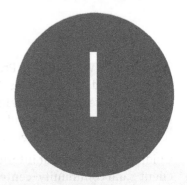

This book is based on the Community Health Worker Certificate Program established at City College of San Francisco (CCSF) in 1992 (*www.ccsf.edu/hlthed/chw*). The program was developed by Community Health Works, a partnership between CCSF and San Francisco State University (SFSU). It was informed by research on the roles and core competencies of community health workers (CHWs) undertaken by Mary Beth Love and colleagues (*www.communityhealthworks.org*).

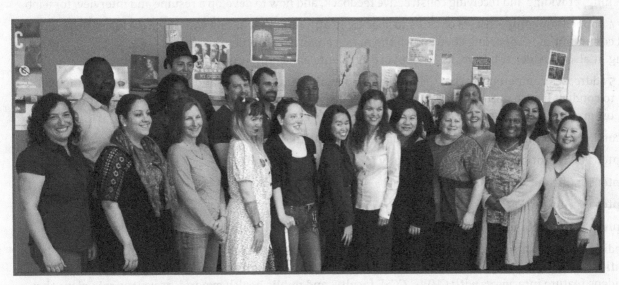

CHW students and faculty at City College of San Francisco.

When the CHW Certificate Program began, the faculty were unable to find an existing curriculum that addressed core roles and competencies. Over the past 20 years the faculty at CCSF have collaborated with students, internship preceptors, working CHWs, and their employers to develop, evaluate, and revise a curriculum that is responsive to the field of public health and the emerging roles of CHWs. Over time, the idea emerged to write a textbook that could be used in our classrooms. We published the first edition of this book in 2009.

Guiding principles that inform this book include a commitment to social justice, cultural humility, and client- and community-centered practice that respects the experience, wisdom, and autonomy of CHWs and the communities they serve. The book is also inspired by the ideas of popular education and the works of Paolo Freire, who believed that education should be a process of political awakening and liberation.

The book is designed for CHWs in training, and is divided into five sections as detailed in the Table of Contents:

- Part 1 provides information about the broad context that informs the work of CHWs, including an introduction to the role and history of CHWs, the discipline of public health, health inequalities, the U.S. health care system, and the public policy process.

- Part 2 addresses the core competencies or skills that most CHWs rely upon day to day, including cultural humility, ethics, how to conduct initial interviews with new clients and provide ongoing client-centered counseling or coaching and care management services, and how to conduct home visits.

- Part 3 addresses key professional skills for career success including stress management, conflict resolution, code switching, providing and receiving constructive feedback, and how to develop a resume and interview for a job.

- Part 4 applies key competencies or skills to specific health topics including working with formerly incarcerated communities, supporting clients with the management of chronic conditions, healthy eating, and active living. It also provides frameworks for supporting clients and communities in their recovery from trauma.

- Part 5 addresses competencies that CHWs use when working at the group and community levels, including how to conduct health outreach and a community diagnosis, and how to facilitate educational trainings, support groups, and community organizing and advocacy efforts.

This second edition of *Foundations* includes four new chapters in Part 4:

- Chapter 15: Promoting the Health of Formerly Incarcerated People

- Chapter 16: Chronic Conditions Management

- Chapter 17: Healthy Eating and Active Living

- Chapter 18: Understanding Trauma and Supporting the Recovery of Survivors

In this edition we have also included short educational videos (URLs or Web addresses are provided in the hard copy edition of the book, and direct links in the e-book version) highlighting key CHW concepts and skills. These videos feature interviews with CHWs, CCSF faculty, and public health experts, as well as role plays that show CHWs working with clients. The role plays are designed to demonstrate key CHW skills. We have also included "counter" role plays that highlight common mistakes or approaches that we wouldn't recommend for CHWs. We use these videos to generate discussion in our classrooms and to engage students in applying key concepts for working effectively with clients. An index to all educational videos included in this edition is provided at the end of the book.

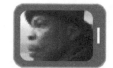

CHW DIGITAL STORY: ROBERT'S STORY

http://youtu.be/ Acaf7cKFGyo

If you wish, please watch the following two videos ▶, which were created by students who graduated from the City College CHW Certificate Program. These are called "digital stories" and they briefly describe what motivated each video maker to become a CHW.

One book cannot possibly address all the knowledge and skills required of CHWs. Our intention is to provide an introduction to the competencies most commonly required of CHWs. This textbook does not attempt to provide information about the specific health issues that CHWs will address in the field. CHWs work in such a wide variety of settings, addressing a broad range of health issues, that it wouldn't be possible to address them satisfactorily in one book. Health knowledge also changes rapidly as new research findings are released, and many reputable health organizations provide regularly updated information online. Instead our approach is to cover the key skills that CHWs provide in the field, and to let employers take the lead for providing additional training on any specific health topics and issues that the CHWs will focus on in the course of their work.

We acknowledge that the topics addressed in each chapter (such as public health, care management or group facilitation) could form the basis of an entire book. We ask you to keep this in mind, and to remember that the process of becoming a CHW is ongoing. Your knowledge and skills will be influenced by a wide variety of factors, including your training, on-the-job experience, and guidance and support from experienced CHWs, supervisors, and other colleagues. Your own life experience, cultural identity, and personality also contribute to your development as a CHW. *Most importantly, please listen closely for the lessons that clients and communities have to teach you.*

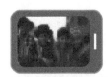

CHW DIGITAL STORY: LUCIANA'S STORY

http://youtu.be/ FS9leOmwACk

A companion *Training Guide to Foundations for Community Health Workers* is available for free at Jossey-Bass (*http://wileyactual.com/bertholdshowcase*). The Training Guide is designed as a resource for anyone who is training CHWs and includes step-by-step lesson plans and assessment resources corresponding to each chapter of the Foundations textbook. Additional educational videos are also provided at *http://wileyactual.com/bertholdshowcase*. Additional materials such as videos, podcasts, and readings can be found at *www.josseybasspublichealth.com*. Comments about this book are invited and can be sent to *publichealth@wiley.com*.

This book was created in collaboration with many people. Some contributors have experience working as CHWs. Some have experience training CHWs in college classrooms or community-based settings. Some have experience working in public health in other ways, and others have experience conducting research and advocating with and on behalf of CHWs. *All* of us have had the privilege of working closely with CHWs. We have witnessed the passion, commitment, skills, and creativity that CHWs bring to their work. Because the contributors have different life and professional experiences, we bring different writing styles and different opinions to this book. These differences echo those that exist in the field of public health and among CHWs.

CHWs contributed to this book in a variety of ways. Some chapters were written by CHWs or former CHWs. We recruited more than twenty working CHWs who graduated from the CCSF Program to contribute quotes and photographs, and to create educational videos that appear throughout the book.

We have written this book for CHWs and for the agencies and institutions that train CHWs. We understand that CHWs are trained in a variety of ways: by the agencies they work or volunteer for, by participating in workshops or training institutes in the community, and in college settings. While this book is based on our experience training CHWs at a community college, we support programs that provide high-quality training of CHWs in any setting. We are opposed to policy efforts that would require college-based training of CHWs or certification of CHWs that would discriminate against any community, such as communities who do not speak English, English Language Learners, undocumented residents, or formerly incarcerated communities. We address these issues in greater detail in Chapters 1 and 2 of the book.

This book is rooted in a deep hope for a world characterized by social justice and equal access to the basic resources—including education, employment, food, housing, safety, health care, and human rights—that everyone needs in order to be healthy. CHWs play a vital role in helping to create such a world. They partner with clients and communities and support them to take action to bring this hope closer to reality.

We welcome your responses to this book and your suggestions for how to improve it, should we have that opportunity. Your comments may be sent to us at

The CHW Program

Health Education Department

City College of San Francisco

50 Phelan Avenue, MUB 353

San Francisco, CA 94112

COMMUNITY HEALTH WORK: THE BIG PICTURE

PART 1

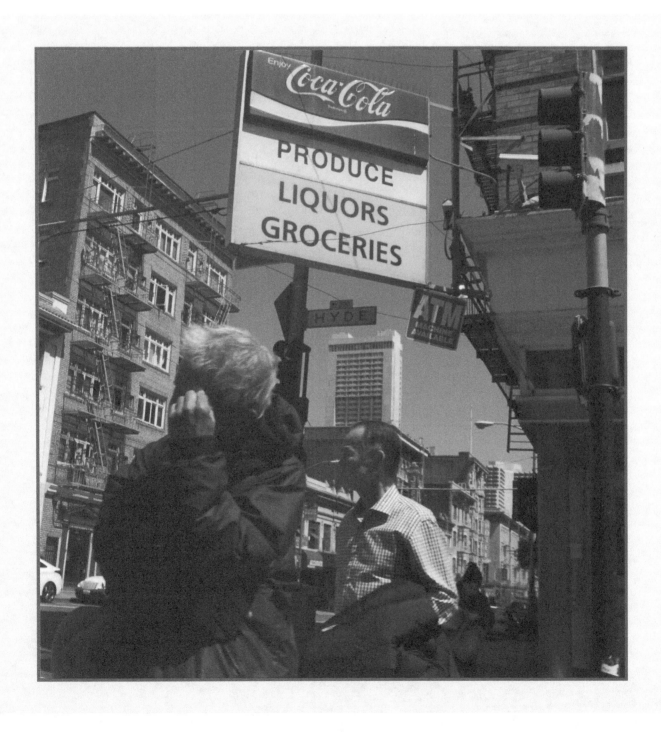

The Role of Community Health Workers

1

Darouny Somsanith and Janey Skinner

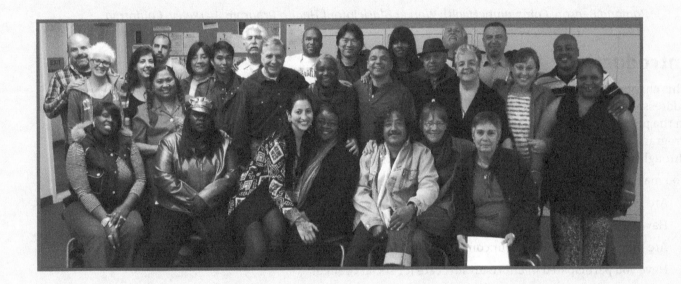

I was homeless, living in a shelter with my daughter. There was a nurse practitioner who provided prenatal care at the shelter two days a week. When a pregnant woman came in, sometimes they came in the middle of the night, so I would give them a short presentation about the prenatal services at the shelter, and tell them when the nurse practitioner lady was coming in.

I didn't know why I was doing it, I just was doing it. I got housing after three months of being at the shelter. While I was there, I was interacting with the nurse practitioner. And when I got ready to move into my housing, she asked me did I want to become a community health worker for her. I'm like, "Sure, but what is a community health worker?" I was the second CHW with her organization. She had just started this organization called the Homeless Prenatal Program, and she and a part-time social worker took me on the streets to show me what a CHW does. I learned the ropes and I used my life experience, and the part-time social worker showed me what to do in the community, and then I just took off from there. That's how I became a CHW.

—*Ramona Benson, Community Health Worker Black Infant Health Program, Berkeley, California*

Introduction

This chapter introduces you to the key roles and competencies of community health workers (CHWs) and addresses common qualities and values of successful CHWs. It will also introduce you to the four CHWs pictured in the photograph that appears on page 22 in this chapter. They are each graduates of the CHW Certificate Program at City College of San Francisco, on which this book is based. Their quotes and photographs appear throughout the book, providing examples of the work they do to promote community health.

You may already possess some of the qualities, knowledge, and skills common among CHWs.

- Are you a trusted member of your community?
- Have you ever assisted a family member or friend to obtain health care services?
- Are there things harming your community's health that you feel passionate about changing?
- Have you participated in efforts to advocate for social change?
- Do you hope that, in your work, you can work with your community members to become healthy, strong, and in charge of their lives?

If you answered yes to any of these questions, you have some of the characteristics of a successful CHW.

WHAT YOU WILL LEARN

By studying the information in this chapter, you will be able to:

- Describe CHWs and what they do
- Identify where CHWs work, the populations they work with, and the health issues they address
- Explain the core roles that CHWs play in the health and social services fields
- Discuss the core competencies that CHWs use to assist individuals and communities
- Describe personal qualities and attributes that are common among successful CHWs
- Discuss emerging models of care and opportunities for CHWs

WORDS TO KNOW

Advocate (noun and verb)

Capitation

Credentialing

Health Inequalities

Social Justice

1.1 Who Are CHWs and What Do They Do?

CHWs help individuals, families, and communities to enhance their health, access services, and to improve the conditions for health, especially in low-income communities. CHWs generally come from the communities they serve and are uniquely prepared to provide culturally and linguistically appropriate services (HRSA, 2007; Rosenthal, Wiggins, Brownstein, Rael, & Johnson, 1998; Rosenthal et al., 2010). They work with diverse and often disadvantaged communities at high risk of illness, disability, and death.

CHWs provide a wide range of services, including outreach, home visits, health education, and client-centered counseling and care management. They support clients in accessing high-quality health and social services programs. They facilitate support groups and workshops and support communities to organize and **advocate** (to actively speak up and support a client, community, or policy change) for social change to advance the community's health and welfare. CHWs also work with health care and social services agencies to enhance their capacity to provide culturally sensitive services that truly respect the diverse identities, strengths, and needs of the clients and communities they serve.

As a result of the work of CHWs, clients and communities learn new information and skills, increase their confidence, and enhance their ability to successfully advocate for themselves. Most important, the work that CHWs do reduces persistent **health inequalities** or differences in the rates of illness, disability, and death (or mortality) among different communities, in particular those differences that are preventable, unfair, and unjust (Hurtado et al., 2014).

The American Public Health Association adopted an official definition for CHWs during their annual meeting in 2009, a definition developed by CHWs along with researchers and advocates:

> *A Community Health Worker (CHW) is a frontline public health worker who is a trusted member of and/or has an unusually close understanding of the community served. This trusting relationship enables the CHW to serve as a liaison/link/intermediary between health/social services and the community to facilitate access to services and improve the quality and cultural competence of service delivery. A CHW also builds individual and community capacity by increasing health knowledge and self-sufficiency through a range of activities such as outreach, community education, informal counseling, social support and advocacy. (APHA, 2009)*

The Bureau of Labor Statistics adapted this definition to establish a standard occupational classification (SOC) for CHWs in 2010, for the first time distinguishing CHWs as a profession in standard employment statistics. Prior to this, CHWs were included in the broad category of "social and human service assistants."

The U.S. Bureau of Labor Statistics forecasts a 25 percent growth rate for CHWs over the 10-year period 2012–2022, so while official recognition of the CHW profession is recent, interest in employing CHWs is widespread. This growth rate is faster than average, when compared to other occupations (BLS, 2014). Health departments, community-based organizations, hospitals and clinics, foundations, and researchers value the important contributions of CHWs to promoting the health and well-being of low-income and at-risk communities.

You might know a CHW already. You might be one. CHWs work under a wide range of professional titles. Some of the most popular are listed in Table 1.1.

Table 1.1 Common Titles for CHWs

Case manager/Case worker	Health educator
Community health advocate	Health worker
Community health outreach worker	Lay health advisor
Community health worker	Public health aide
Community outreach worker	Patient navigator
Community liaison	Peer counselor
Community organizer	Peer educator
Enrollment specialist	Promotor/a
Health ambassador	

• *Can you think of other titles for CHWs?*

Please watch this video interview about becoming a CHW. The interview features two CHWs, both graduates of the City College of San Francisco CHW Certificate program.

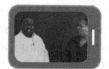

BECOMING A CHW: CHW INTERVIEW

http://youtu.be/ BASkvuq1epw

The term *community health worker* describes both volunteers who work informally to improve their community's health and those who are paid for providing these services. Regardless of compensation, they serve as "frontline" health and social service workers and are often the first contact a community member has with a health or social service agency. CHWs typically are trusted members of the community they serve, having deep knowledge of the resources, relationships, and needs of that community.

Community health workers are motivated by compassion and the desire to assist those in need, leading CHWs to work for equality and **social justice** or equal access to essential health resources such as housing, food, education, employment, health care, and civil rights. Many CHWs take on this work because they have experienced discrimination and poverty themselves and can relate to the situations of those they are working with. Others simply see a need and want to improve conditions in their communities. Regardless of how the CHW comes to the work, every CHW is an **advocate**—someone who speaks up for a cause or policy or on someone else's behalf—working to promote health and improve the conditions that support wellness in local communities.

Esther Chavez: The reason I got into community health work was because of the immediate need in my community. There was a lack of education among youth with regard to safer sex and sexually transmitted diseases. It didn't seem to be an important topic for other community-based organizations and the need was great. So my colleague and I started an organization that provided sex education and peer support around health issues for youth in our community.

Because CHWs work under so many different job titles and perform a wide variety of duties, it has been difficult to determine how many people are working in the field in the United States, and what types of jobs they hold. One recent national study attempted to do this. A study of the CHW field was completed in 2007 by the U.S. Department of Health and Human Services and the University of Texas in San Antonio. The study was called the Community Health Worker National Workforce Study (HRSA, 2007) and to date is the most accurate national estimate of the workforce. There have been more recent studies of the workforce—notably the 2010 and 2014 National Community Health Worker Advocacy Surveys (NCHWAS)—but none that estimate its total size and composition. The following data are drawn from the 2007 study, with a few additions from the 2014 NCHWAS survey or other sources (as noted).

OVERALL NUMBER, GENDER, AND ETHNICITY

• In 2000, there were approximately 86,000 CHWs working in the United States (with California and New York having the most workers) (HRSA, 2007).

• The majority of CHWs were female (82 percent) between the ages of 30 and 50. One-fourth of the workforce was younger than 30 and one-fourth was older than 50 years old (HRSA, 2007).

• CHWs were Hispanic (35 percent) or Non-Hispanic Whites (39 percent); African Americans made up 15.5 percent of the workforce, followed by Native Americans (5 percent), and Asian and Pacific Islanders (4.6 percent) (HRSA, 2007).

• The Centers for Disease Control and Prevention (CDC) more recently has estimated the CHW workforce in the United States at over 100,000 (CDC, 2014c).

EDUCATION AND WAGES

- Thirty-five percent of CHWs had high school diplomas, 20 percent had completed some type of college, and 31 percent had at least a four-year college degree, as shown in the 2007 report (HRSA). The 2014 survey showed a shift toward greater educational attainment. For example, in 2014, 33 percent of CHWs responding had completed some college, and 35 percent had a college degree (NCHWAS).

- In the 2007 HRSA study, the majority of experienced CHWs (70 percent) received an hourly wage of $13 or more, and about half received $15 or more

- In the 2014 NCHWAS survey of CHWs, almost a third of respondents made between $25,000 and $35,000 annually, while about a third made less than that and about a third made more. The most common sites of employment for CHWs were community-based organizations (37 percent), Federally Qualified Community Health Centers and other clinics (27 percent), hospitals (14 percent), and local health departments (12 percent).

POPULATIONS SERVED

- CHWs provided services to all racial and ethnic communities: Hispanic/Latino (78 percent), Black/African American (68 percent), and Non-Hispanic White (64 percent). One-third of CHWs surveyed reported services to Asian/Pacific Islander (34 percent) and American Indian/Alaska Natives (32 percent) (HRSA, 2007).

- The majority of the clients served were females and adults ages 18 to 49. Other populations served included the uninsured (71 percent), immigrants (49 percent), homeless individuals (41 percent), isolated rural and migrant workers (31 percent each), and colonial or community residents (9 percent) (HRSA, 2007).

- Programs serving immigrants, migrant workers, and the uninsured were more likely to have volunteer CHWs (HRSA, 2007).

- CHWs work primarily with low-income communities. They work with children, youth and their families, adults and seniors, men and women, and people of all sexual orientations and gender identities (HRSA, 2007).

- The 2014 NCHWAS survey had especially strong participation from CHWs working in states that border Mexico, so it is not surprising that 65 percent reported working primarily with the Latino/a population. The next most common group worked with was African Americans (41 percent), non-Hispanic White (38 percent), Native Americans (16 percent), and Asian/Pacific Islander (12 percent). Both the 2007 study and the 2014 survey demonstrate that CHWs work with a highly diverse population.

HEALTH ISSUES AND ACTIVITIES

- The top health areas that CHWs were found to work in were women's health and nutrition, child health and pregnancy/prenatal care, immunizations, and sexual behaviors (HRSA, 2007).

- The most common specific illnesses CHWs were working to address, according to the 2007 report, included HIV/AIDS (39 percent), diabetes (38 percent), high blood pressure (31 percent), cancer (27 percent), cardiovascular diseases (26 percent), and heart disease (23 percent) (HRSA, 2007). The 2014 NCHWAS survey reported the top five health issues that CHWs work on as prevention (including nutrition and/or physical activity) (36 percent), accessing health services (36 percent), diabetes (34 percent), chronic disease prevention (31 percent), and behavioral health/mental health (24 percent).

- Specific work activities highlighted in the 2007 report included culturally appropriate health promotion and education (82 percent), assistance in accessing medical and nonmedical services and programs (84 percent and 72 percent, respectively), translating (36 percent), interpreting (34 percent), counseling (31 percent), mentoring (21 percent), social support (46 percent), and transportation (36 percent) (HRSA, 2007).

- Related to the work activities listed, specific CHWs duties included case management, risk identification, patient navigation, and providing direct services such as blood pressure screening (HRSA, 2007).

Because most CHWs work within the field of public health (see Chapter 3) and primarily with low-income communities, they address a wide range of health issues, including homelessness, violence, environmental health, mental health, recovery, and civil and human rights issues, as well as more traditional health issues (cancer prevention, asthma, HIV disease). They work with children, youth and their families, adults and seniors, men and women, and people of all sexual orientations and gender identities. CHWs are flexible, and can work with individual clients and families, with groups, and at the community level.

MODELS OF CARE

The 2007 CHW National Workforce Study further identified five "models of care" that incorporated CHWs within them. These models continue to be common in both clinical and community settings, as of the writing of this chapter:

1. *Member of a care delivery team:* CHWs work with other providers (for example, doctors, nurses, or social workers) to care for individual patients.

2. *Navigator:* CHWs are called upon to use their extensive knowledge of the complex health care system to assist individuals and patients in accessing the services they need and gaining greater confidence in interacting with their providers.

3. *Screening and health education provider:* CHWs administer basic health screening (for example, pregnancy tests, blood pressure checks, and rapid HIV antibody tests), and provide prevention education on basic health topics.

4. *Outreach/enrolling/informing agent:* CHWs go into the community to reach and inform individuals and families about the services they qualify for, and to encourage them to enroll in the programs.

5. *Organizer:* CHWs work with other community members to advocate for change on a specific issue or cause. Often their work aids community members to become stronger advocates for themselves.

- *When did you first become aware of CHWs?*

- *Are there CHWs working in your community?*

- *Do some or all of these five models of care reflect your experience of how CHWs serve the community?*

What Do YOU? Think!

CHWs AROUND THE WORLD

CHWs are working throughout the world, on every continent and in every country. Some examples of these workers are Latin American *promotoras de salud*, Bangladesh Rural Advancement Committee (BRAC) outreach workers, *accompagnateurs* in Haiti, doulas in the United States, and community health representatives in Alaska and the southwestern United States, and, a few decades ago, the "barefoot doctors" of rural China. While their roles, duties, and even titles are flexible, what is the common thread in their work is their ability to adapt to the needs of the communities they serve. This responsiveness to the needs of the communities and clients is what makes CHWs so important to the health of populations, especially for the one billion people living on less than $1.25 a day (World Bank, 2014).

Around the world, government officials and doctors are now recognizing the important role CHWs can play in providing critically needed primary care to communities living in poverty. A recent example of this was the "One Million Community Health Workers Campaign" launched in Tanzania in 2013 (see sidebar). This first of its kind conference and training workshop was part of a greater agenda to train more lay health workers and improve the health conditions of Africa's most vulnerable populations. Similarly, the Frontline Health Workers Coalition, led by noted international health organizations such as Save the Children, formed in 2012 to "urge greater and more strategic U.S. investment in frontline health workers in developing countries as a cost-effective way to save lives and foster a healthier, safer and more prosperous world" (Frontline Health Workers Coalition, n.d.).

While campaigns to expand health programs that feature CHWs demonstrate growing recognition and respect for the profession, it should come as no surprise—after all, CHWs have proven highly effective at bringing basic, life-saving care and prevention services directly to people's homes. CHWs have been a key element of global efforts that successfully reduced new cases of HIV/AIDS around the world by 33 percent and reduced new cases of malaria by 25 percent between 2000 and 2012 (Frontline Health Workers Coalition, 2014a, 2014b). How much more could be achieved, if enough CHWs were trained and employed in every community with outstanding needs?

In October 2007, a peer-reviewed journal published by the Public Library of Science asked renowned public health leaders this question: "Which single intervention would do the most to improve the health of those living on less than $1 per day?" Dr. Paul Farmer, founding director of Partners in Health and Presley Professor of Medical Anthropology, at Harvard Medical School, Boston, provided the following answer:

> Hire community health workers to serve them [emphasis added]. *In my experience in the rural reaches of Africa and Haiti, and among the urban poor too, the problem with so many funded health programs is that they never go the extra mile: resources (money, people, plans, services) get hung up in cities and towns. If we train village health workers, and make sure they're compensated, then the resources intended for the world's poorest—from vaccines, to bed nets, to prenatal care, and to care for chronic diseases like AIDS and tuberculosis—would reach the intended beneficiaries. Training and paying village health workers also creates jobs among the very poorest. (Yamey, 2007)*

One Million CHWs Campaign

In the United States and Canada, CHWs often work as part of a clinical team, alongside health care providers with a higher level of clinical training. In less-developed countries where health resources are much scarcer, CHWs are often the frontline provider of a complex set of health care services. In these settings, clinical supervision of CHWs may be available only intermittently, when a doctor, nurse, or physician's assistant visits the village or the CHW attends a regional training. CHWs in less-developed countries around the world, despite little access to medications, technology, and diagnostic tests, nonetheless have made significant positive impacts on community health. The 2014 Ebola crisis in Western Africa brought world attention to a reality that has long affected both rural village and growing urban slums in poorer parts of the world—many residents lack access to medical care, or even the most basic hygiene supplies and medications. In Liberia, for example, there is only one physician for every 100,000 people (World Bank, 2010). In this context, CHWs are of paramount importance in helping to bridge the enormous gaps in the medical system and to facilitate access to health information and services for the majority of the population.

While CHWs are already having an impact around the world, there are not enough trained CHWs available, nor do they always have the best tools and supervision possible. The One Million Community Health Worker campaign seeks to change that, with a particular focus on Sub-Saharan Africa. This campaign, launched by the UN Sustainable Development Solutions Network, seeks to recruit and train one million CHWs and link them to a network of health care providers who will provide remote supervision and supply appropriate technologies. For example, a smart phone can be used to report on medication availability, to consult with a nurse or doctor, and to submit test results for TB or HIV tests. A growing number of medical tests can be safely and accurately conducted by CHWs visiting patients in their homes or workplaces. The One Million Community Health Worker Campaign also focuses on training and engaging national and regional health systems that may not be well coordinated with CHW efforts. Where existing CHW programs are having success, the campaign seeks to expand and network these programs.

A driving motivation for the One Million CHW campaign has been the eight Millennium Development Goals (MDGs) set by the United Nations in 2000 with a target year of 2015. The MDGs sought to cut poverty worldwide in half, reduce child mortality, improve maternal health, ensure universal primary education, increase gender equality, and combat infectious diseases such as HIV/AIDS and malaria, among other things. Increasingly, both governments and nongovernmental organizations (nonprofits) recognize that the health-related MDGs will be impossible to reach by the target year of 2015 without the help of a much larger CHW workforce. For example, the Deputy Minister of Health and Social Welfare of Tanzania stated at the first international workshop sponsored by the One Million CHW Campaign, "We have to recognize that advances toward the Millennium Development Goals can be greatly accelerated by urgently expanding primary health care delivery capacity across Sub-Saharan Africa. Community Health Workers are foundational to this strategy" (One Million Community Health Workers Campaign, 2013). CHWs not only supplement health care services, they are often the main component of health care delivery and prevention efforts in low-resource settings.

1.2 CHWs and Public Health

CHWs often work within the field of public health (see Chapter 3). Unlike medicine, public health works to promote the health of entire communities and populations. Public health understands the primary causes of illness and health to be more than just access to health care, but also whether or not people have equal access to basic resources and rights, including food, housing, education, employment with safe working conditions and a living wage, transportation, clean air and water, and civil rights—understanding that people's social and physical environments play a huge role in their health and wellness. Collectively, the conditions that shape health are called the "social determinants of health."

The field of public health not only provides services to prevent illness and improve care, it also influences the social determinants of health by advocating for policies to assure basic resources and rights for all people. CHWs share in this advocacy work. For example, one of the core values listed on the website of the Community Health Worker Network of New York City (n.d.) states, "Community health workers are agents of change who pursue social justice through work with individuals and communities to improve social conditions." CHWs also play a key role in strengthening the social fabric of communities, which can enhance the health of community residents.

To achieve the goal of eliminating health disparities among racial and ethnic minorities, attention must shift to the social determinants of health. Included in the list of social determinants of health are social support, social cohesion, and universal access to medical care. Social support refers to support on the individual level when resources are provided by others, and social cohesion refers to support on a community level when the trust and respect between different sections of society result in cherishing people and their health. Community health workers (CHWs) impact these social determinants of health as they build supportive relationships with community members and community groups to promote access to resources and to health care (McCloskey, Tollestrup, & Sanders, 2011).

1.3 Roles and Competencies of CHWs

The roles of CHWs, and the competencies that are required to fulfill those roles, continue to evolve in response to changing health care delivery models and public health strategies. CHWs have proven to be an effective— as well as a cost-effective—component of programs focused on prevention, chronic condition management, healthy maternity, and health care access or enrollment (CHWA, 2013; CDC, 2011; Rosenthal et al., 2010). CHWs help to ensure that services are culturally and linguistically appropriate, especially when they are involved in designing those services. As more CHWs are employed in health care and public health, and as new mechanisms for funding and institutionalizing CHW positions emerge, the demand for greater clarity in defining CHW roles and competencies also increases. In this section we examine the CHW roles and competencies that have served as a benchmark for almost two decades, as well as noting where additional roles have been identified by efforts in several states to define CHW's scope of practice.

It should be noted that defining what a CHW does is not without controversy. Other health professionals may raise concerns when they see overlap between their profession and that of a CHW in areas such as health education, counseling, systems navigation, and case management. Even some CHWs, since they serve in so many different capacities and models of care in both volunteer and paid positions, worry that too narrow a definition of the CHW role could leave out some valuable CHW practices. Yet many CHWs and others who work with them have advocated for a clearer definition of the CHW role and scope of practice. A *scope of practice* refers to the range of services and duties that a category of worker, such as CHWs, is competent to provide. While many CHWs express mixed feelings about how formalized the field should be, all agree that the work they do deserves more recognition from government and other professionals, and increased funding.

A step towards national recognition is to be officially classified by the U.S. Department of Labor, Bureau of Labor Statistics. In 2010, the Department of Labor approved a standard occupational code—21-1094—and definition for CHWs as professionals who:

> *Assist individuals and communities to adopt healthy behaviors. Conduct outreach for medical personnel or health organizations to implement programs in the community that promote, maintain, and improve individual and community health. May provide information on available resources, provide social support and informal counseling, advocate for individuals and community health needs, and provide services such as first aid and blood pressure screening. May collect data to help identify community health needs. (Bureau of Labor Statistics, 2010)*

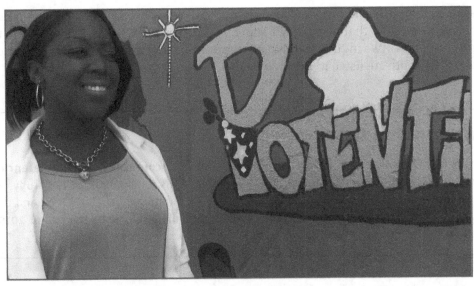

CHWs take on many different roles and provide a wide range of services to clients and communities.

This official recognition of the CHW occupation may speed the development of more stable mechanisms for the financing of CHW services from state and federal programs such as Medicaid and Medicare. Reimbursement of CHW services under Medicaid was formally allowed under the Affordable Care Act of 2010 (the ACA, also known as "Obamacare"), and each state has the option to establish policies to do this. In fact, even before the ACA passed, states could seek a Medicaid waiver to allow "fee for service" reimbursement of certain CHW services. Minnesota was the first state to do so in 2007, and Minnesota also supports CHW services through other non-Medicaid funds (National Healthcare for the Homeless Council, 2011). Reimbursement for CHW services through large public insurance programs like Medicaid means a more sustained and stable funding stream for CHW jobs, instead of a reliance on grants that come and go. As discussed in Chapter 2, reimbursement or "fee for service" payments is just one of many mechanisms for financing the CHW profession. Formal recognition of the occupation also makes other avenues of financing CHW jobs more feasible.

- *What do you think of this definition of the CHW field? What does it include and what does it leave out?*

- *How would it affect your family and community if CHW services were more widely available?*

What Are Core Roles and Competencies?

Core roles are the major functions a person commonly performs on the job. For example, the core roles of a farmer include clearing fields, planting, and harvesting crops. The core roles of CHWs include providing outreach, health education, client-centered informal counselling, case management, community organizing, and advocacy.

Core competencies are the knowledge and skills a person needs in order to do his or her job well. Again, a farmer must be able to operate equipment, assess timing for planting, and prepare the soil. Core competencies for CHWs include knowledge of public health, behavior change, ethics, and community resources and the ability to provide health information, facilitate groups, resolve conflicts, and conduct an initial client interview or assessment. CHW educational programs seek to strengthen CHW competencies or skills.

A landmark study that defined CHW work was published in 1998 by the University of Arizona (Rosenthal, Wiggins, Brownstein, Rael, & Johnson, 1998). As one of the first major studies of the CHW profession, it documented the duties that CHWs perform and identified core CHW roles and skill sets, and discussed the values or personal characteristics that many CHWs share. Identifying CHW competencies allows trainers and employers to better support CHWs in their work. In all, the study identified seven core roles and eight core competencies for a CHW (both are listed in Table 1.2 below).

The CHW Common Core Project

As we are writing this chapter, a new comprehensive review of CHW **core roles and competencies** is underway. The Community Health Worker Common Core (3C) project aims to update the 1998 study, reviewing CHW work and training in six states and consulting directly with a national panel of CHWs and those who work closely with CHWs. The results of the 3C project will be broadly available by the end of 2015. For more information about the 3C project, please see *www.chrllc.net/*.

The 1998 study of CHWs continues to be an important reference for the profession nationally. In recent years, especially as CHW coalitions and public health advocates have worked to develop mechanisms for greater employment of CHWs and reimbursement of CHW services under the ACA, different states have defined CHW roles differently. While there has been substantial overlap with the roles and competencies identified in the 1998 study, some roles have been added or defined in more detail (such as outreach and participatory research). New terms, such as system navigation and care coordination, have gained popularity, and more sophisticated methods of providing these services have been developed by CHWs and other health professionals. Table 1.2 compares roles identified in the 1998 CHW study with those from state CHW networks in Minnesota and New York (other states have already or may soon create their own definition of the CHW roles). These lists do not contradict one another and, when combined, provide a more complete picture of the many roles CHWs fulfill (Minnesota Community Health Worker Alliance, 2013; New York State Community Health Worker Initiative, 2011).

Table 1.2 Personal Qualities of Successful CHWs

1998 CHW WORKFORCE STUDY	NEW YORK STATE CHW INITIATIVE	MINNESOTA CHW ALLIANCE
Cultural mediation between community and health system	Outreach and community mobilization	Bridge the gap between communities and the health and social service systems
Informal counseling and social support	Community/cultural liaison	Navigate the health and human services system
Providing direct services and referrals	Case management and care coordination	Advocate for individual and community needs
Providing culturally appropriate health education	Home-based support	Provide direct services
Advocating for individual and community needs	Health promotion and health coaching	Build individual and community capacity
Assuring people get the services they need	System navigation	
Building individual and community capacity	Participatory research	

We provide greater detail below on the seven core roles and eight core competencies identified in the 1998 CHW study. While we address all of these roles and competencies in later chapters of this book, the book (and our curriculum at CCSF) is not structured around them explicitly. Instead, we focus most on specific skill sets, such as client-centered counseling (Chapter 9), care management (Chapter 10), outreach (Chapter 19), home visits (Chapter 11), and community organizing and advocacy (Chapter 23).

CORE CHW ROLES

1. **Cultural mediation between communities and the health and social services systems**: Intimate knowledge of the communities they work with permits CHWs to serve as cultural brokers between their clients and health and social services systems. By being a bridge that links community members to essential services, CHWs ensure that the clients receive culturally appropriate quality care.

Letida Sot: As a CHW, I work regularly with doctors to assist them to communicate with our Cambodian patients. Because the Cambodian community is so small, sometimes patients have to wait many hours to speak to someone at a clinic who can understand them. By me working at the clinic, the patient doesn't get lost in the system—they can easily come to me for what they need. Besides not understanding English, some of our patients don't read or write well and have a hard time understanding their medications. One of the patients I worked with suffered from hypertension, diabetes, and heart disease. She thought that she needed to finish one type of medicine first before she can start on another, even though sometimes she needed to take 15 different medications a month. Because of this, her diabetes was out of control and the doctor asked me to aid in the arrangement of her daily medication schedule. When I explained to her that she could take the medications simultaneously, she was shocked because she had been doing what she thought was right for 10 years.

2. **Informal counseling and social support:** CHWs provide client-centered counseling to support clients to live healthier and better lives. A CHW may help clients to set health-related goals and may use techniques such as motivational interviewing (see Chapter 9) to support clients in reducing health-related risk behaviors.

Tina Diep: Smoking within the Asian community, especially with men, is very integrated into the cultures. Many men know about some of the health hazards of smoking for themselves but don't really know about second-hand smoke or the other health impacts of smoking on their families. Because it is so hard for them to quit, the doctors refer them to me to get smoking cessation counselling. Of course not everyone is ready to quit or even wants to quit, but for those who are, I assist them in creating a plan to reduce or stop smoking, give them some education on the harmful effects of cigarettes, and just provide support and encouragement. In every session, I talk with them about their smoking experience and explore their ambivalence to quitting. Sometimes just talking will get those who were not ready to quit at least thinking about the possibility of it, and this can lead to another appointment and another opportunity to make a plan to quit.

3. **Providing direct services and referrals:** Some CHWs provide direct care to clients through the services they are trained and qualified to provide, such as blood pressure monitoring, reproductive health counseling or HIV-antibody test counseling. They may also provide case management services or otherwise link clients to services by knowing what services exist and referring clients appropriately.

Somnang Sin: When I can't provide the services for a patient, I refer them to services at another program or agency. It is important as a CHW to know what resources are available in the community. Part of my job is to make sure the patient gets the right care—I'll walk them to their appointment or to another agency if the patient needs me to.

4. **Providing culturally appropriate health education:** Because CHWs usually come from the communities they serve, they are familiar with the cultures of the clients they work with (for example, language, values, customs, sexual orientation, and so on) and are better prepared to provide health information in ways that the community will understand and accept. Health education can be provided one-on-one, in small groups, or through large presentations.

David Pheng: I am a CHW at a clinic in Oakland [California]. I see and give presentations to patients who are young adults ages 14 to 20. I find that during my presentations, I have to ditch lecture-based teaching and make it as entertaining as possible. But the entertainment is also speaking to the youth and relating to their everyday experiences—not from a textbook but from the radio, Internet, music, and the everyday words they use. Being culturally appropriate isn't just knowing their language but relating to them as youth, not talking down to them, and respecting their space so they feel comfortable and willing to ask questions. I find the more the youth laugh, the more they pick up on ideas and information that deal with safer sex practices and access to clinical services.

5. **Advocating for individual and community needs:** CHWs speak out with and on behalf of clients and communities. They advocate—with the community whenever possible—to make sure that clients are treated respectfully and given access to the basic resources that they need in order to live healthy lives.

Jinyoung Chun: For a couple of years now, I've taken my clients to Sacramento [California] for Immigrant Day. I think it is important that they understand how our government works and that they can have a chance to talk directly to their legislators. The clients also get to see and connect with community members from other cultures who are there for the same cause. They see that they are not alone and that people can come together and make a difference. At the legislative meetings, the clients talk about issues that impact their lives and their community while I interpret. We do a lot of preparation together before the day so they understand the process and decide what they want to say. After the meeting, they feel so empowered and heard! Many of the clients I work with now also attend and speak at local Board of Supervisors' meetings, as well as other community events on issues that they are passionate about.

6. **Assuring people get the services they need:** A CHW often is the first person many clients interact with, whether through an outreach encounter, or when a client arrives at an agency or clinic. It is the job of the CHW to ensure that these clients get the services they need. CHWs often assist clients in navigating health and social service systems, which can be confusing and overwhelming in the best of times, let alone when someone may be suffering from illness, and may or may not speak the language, read fluently, have identification, or be able to pay for services.

David Pheng: We are usually the first ones to receive questions—and complaints—from the patients. It's fun but challenging work, because the routine is never the same. Once patients come in, I find out what services they need and assist them to get these services. I try to empower the patients to seek the services themselves, but if they need it, I'll assist in guiding them through the clinical side of checking in, seeing a doctor and offering additional resources. I see what else they might need and try to find an organization in the community that can assist them, like with food or legal issues.

7. **Building individual and community capacity:** CHWs support clients and community members to develop the skills and the confidence to promote and advocate for their own health and well-being. Often this work is done with individual clients, or clients and their family members. Other times, CHWs work with groups and community networks, to build the capacity to speak out and take action in their own lives and communities.

Alvaro Morales: One of the most important ways that I know that I am doing a good job is when my clients no longer need me, or need me as much. Everything I do is based on supporting the client not to be dependent on me anymore. I want to support them to take charge of their own health, to negotiate healthy relationships, to navigate the health care system, to communicate with health care providers to get the treatment they want and deserve. And sometimes I get to work with communities and to support them to speak out for policy changes. Instead of me testifying before the Board of County Supervisors or City Council on behalf of the communities I work with, I want to support them to testify and speak out for themselves. They are the experts about what they need and want, and their voices are the voices that need to be heard.

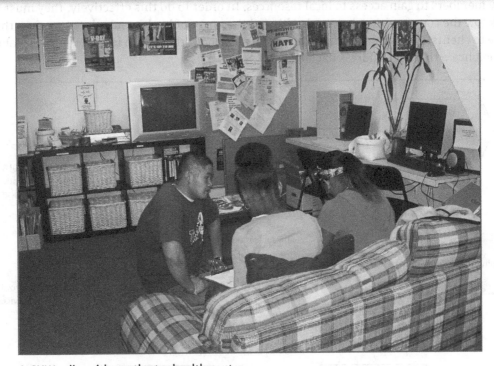

A CHW talks with youth at a health center.

- *Have you ever taken on any of these CHWs' roles?*

- *What were some of the challenges that you faced in performing the role?*

- *Can you think of other roles that a CHW might play?*

EIGHT CORE COMPETENCIES FOR CHWs

Core competencies are the skills and knowledge that enable CHWs to carry out their roles. There are some core competencies that all CHWs use—communication skills, interpersonal skills, organizational skills, and a knowledge base relevant to the CHW's community and types of services provided. Other core competencies are commonly used by many CHWs, but the extent to which they are used may depend on the role that the CHW fulfills. These include skills for teaching, service coordination, capacity building, and advocacy.

The eight core competencies that are highlighted here were identified in the 1998 CHW study mentioned above. Additional tasks and skills have been identified in subsequent reviews of the CHW workforce at the state level, such as that carried out by the New York State CHW Initiative. The 3C project mentioned above will release a national review of CHW competencies in late 2015. For example, CHW tasks and skills include family engagement, problem solving, treatment adherence promotion, harm reduction, translation and interpretation, leading support groups, and documentation, among others. Many of these duties fit within the eight broad competencies discussed in this chapter (for example, documentation can be considered an organizational skill).

The eight broad competencies, as well as many more specific duties and tasks, are addressed in subsequent parts and chapters of this book. Part 1 is focused on building understanding of the broader context in which CHWs work including concepts of public health, health systems, equality, and cultural humility (part of the "knowledge base" competency listed below).

1. **Communication skills:** CHWs must be good listeners in order to learn about their clients' experiences, behaviors, strengths, and needs, and to provide health information and client-centered counseling or coaching. Group communications skills become important for leading group health education and community advocacy.

2. **Interpersonal skills:** CHWs work with diverse groups of people and must be able to develop positive relationships with clients, community members, supervisors, doctors, nurses, social workers, and policymakers. This includes the ability to provide and receive constructive feedback, and to resolve conflict.

3. **Knowledge base about the community, health issues, and available services:** CHWs often support community members to gain access to local resources. In order to do this effectively, they must spend time getting to know the communities they work with and the range of health and related services that may be available to clients. CHWs must also be knowledgeable about the health issues—such as diabetes or domestic violence—that they address day to day.

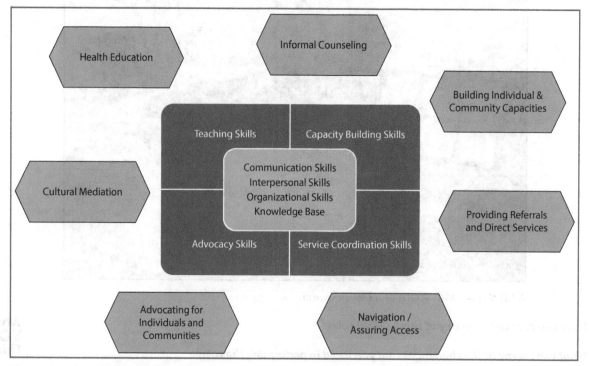

Figure 1.1 The relationship between CHW core competencies and roles

4. **Service coordination skills:** The health care and social service systems are complex, not very well integrated, and sometimes difficult to access. CHWs sometimes work as care managers and frequently work with clients to access available services and to create and follow realistic plans to improve their health, despite the complexity of the systems.

5. **Capacity-building skills:** CHWs do not want clients and communities to become dependent upon them or other service providers. They teach and support clients and communities to develop new skills and confidence to promote their own health, including, for example, communication skills, risk reduction behaviors, chronic disease management, and community organizing and advocacy skills.

6. **Advocacy skills:** CHWs sometimes speak up on behalf of their clients and their communities within their own agencies, with other service providers, and to support changes in public policies. More important, CHWs support clients and communities in raising their own voices to create meaningful changes—including changes in public policies—that influence their health and well-being.

7. **Teaching skills:** CHWs educate clients about how to prevent and manage health conditions. CHWs teach about healthy behaviors and support clients in developing healthier habits. They also teach community members how to advocate for social change.

8. **Organizational skills:** CHWs support individuals, families, and communities in getting the services they need. The work is demanding, with many details to keep track of and document, not only for oneself but also for one's clients. Being organized ensures that CHWs are able to properly follow up with clients and accurately document data for their employers.

- *What other skills are important for CHWs to have?*

- *Do you already have some of the skills identified?*

- *Which skills do you want to learn or improve?*

1.4 Personal Qualities and Attributes of CHWs

All of us bring unique life experiences to our work. These experiences, along with our individual personalities, shape our value systems and how we see the world around us. The work of a CHW depends upon their ability to build and maintain positive interpersonal relationships with people of diverse backgrounds and identities. Without the capacity to build relationships based on trust, CHWs cannot do their job effectively. The qualities that enable this capacity can be strengthened through practice and self-reflection. We highlight several desirable personal qualities and attributes in Table 1.3, adapted from work of the International Training and Education Center on HIV in Zimbabwe (International Training and Education Center on HIV, 2004). With these qualities and attributes, CHWs inspire confidence and trust and build positive professional relationships with clients and communities.

Table 1.3 Personal Qualities of Successful CHWs

PERSONAL QUALITIES	DEFINITIONS
1. Interpersonal warmth	The ability to listen and respond to clients and communities with compassion and kindness
2. Trustworthiness	Being honest, allowing others to confide in you, maintaining confidentiality, and upholding professional ethics
3. Open-mindedness	The willingness to embrace others' differences, including their flaws, and be non-judgmental in your interactions with them

(continues)

Table 1.3 (*Continued*)

PERSONAL QUALITIES	DEFINITIONS
4. Objectivity	Striving to work with and view clients and their circumstances without the influence of personal prejudice or bias
5. Sensitivity	To be aware of and truly respect the experience, culture, feelings, and opinions of others
6. Competence	Developing the knowledge and skills required to provide quality services to all the clients and communities you work with
7. Commitment to social justice	The commitment and heart to fight injustice and to advocate for social changes that promote the health and well-being of clients and communities
8. Good psychological health	Having the mental and emotional capacity to perform your work professionally, without doing harm to clients, colleagues, or yourself
9. Self-awareness and understanding	Being willing and able to reflect upon and analyze your own experiences, biases, and prejudices, to ensure that they do not negatively affect your interactions with clients and colleagues

- *What other personal qualities and values should CHWs have?*

- *What personal qualities and values do you bring to this work?*

- *What qualities do you want to build and enhance?*

What Do YOU Think?

The last quality in the list above has special importance: self-awareness serves as a foundation that assists CHWs to cultivate other key qualities and skills. Developing awareness of our own personal biases helps ensure that we do not harm a client or the community by judging them based on our own experiences, values, and beliefs. This is an ethical obligation for all CHWs and is essential for three key principles of CHW practice: client-centered practice, community-centered practice, and cultural humility.

Throughout this book you will find questions directed to you as a person who is training to become a CHW or to enhance your CHW skills. Some of the questions invite you to take time to reflect and to cultivate self-awareness. The questions also invite you to bring your own experience, insights, ideas, and wisdom into the conversation. Your life experience, whatever it may be, is an important foundation for the work you will do as a CHW.

The challenges of developing self-awareness and using it to inform your work as a CHW is a theme that runs throughout this book. It is addressed in greater detail in Chapters 6 and 7.

1.5 The Role of CHWs in the Management of Chronic Conditions

As CHWs become more recognized and respected, their professional role within the health and social services fields is expanding, especially in the area of primary health care and chronic disease management. Earlier in this chapter we talked about five models of care, one of which features a CHW as a "member of a care delivery team."

There is considerable interest in expanding the use of CHWs in care delivery teams, and many hospitals and clinics are already doing so. A study at the University of Utah found that CHWs were typically employed as members of a care delivery team or as part of a health care continuum, coordinating CHW services with health care providers, both nationally and within the state of Utah (McCormick, Glaubitz, McIlvenne & Mader, 2012). A report from the Urban Institute also notes that rising levels of poverty and increased immigration create an incentive for health care organizations to hire CHWs, to help bridge cultural gaps and meet the needs of communities with high levels of chronic disease (Bovbjerg, Eyster, Ormond, Anderson, & Richardson, 2013).

The ACA has provided additional incentives to employ CHWs and strategies to finance them, in particular to assist with managing chronic conditions (the ACA is discussed at greater length in Chapter 5). The ACA promotes what's known as the "triple aim"—improve the patient's experience of health care, reduce the costs, and improve the health of individuals and populations. CHWs have a key role to play in helping health care organizations attain the triple aim. The California Health Workforce Alliance, for example, has released recommendations for scaling up the use of CHWs and *promotores de salud* (a term common in Spanish-speaking communities for community health workers who work at the grassroots, often as volunteers), specifically to help health care organizations achieve the triple aim (CHWA, 2013). The ACA not only opens up the door to Medicaid reimbursement (discussed elsewhere in this chapter and in Chapter 5, but also provides grants to eligible organizations "to promote positive health behaviors and outcomes for populations in medically underserved communities through the use of community health workers"—an important recognition of the role CHWs play. CHWs are being embraced not only as a means to conduct outreach or enrollment, but also in promoting "positive health behaviors and discouraging risky health behaviors" (CDC, 2011).

CHRONIC DISEASE: THE DOMINANT TYPE OF ILLNESS IN THE UNITED STATES

Today, chronic conditions—such as cardiovascular disease (primarily heart disease and stroke), cancer, lung diseases and diabetes—are the most common, costly, and preventable of all health problems in the United States. Data from the CDC show that:

- About half of all adults—117 million—live with chronic illness, with one of four of these adults having two or more chronic health conditions (CDC, 2014b).

- More people die of chronic conditions in the United States than from all other causes combined. Heart disease and cancer alone account for almost half of all deaths annually in the United States (CDC, 2014b).

- The costs of medical care for people with chronic diseases account for more than 84 percent of the nation's $2.7 trillion total health care expenditures (CDC, 2014a; Robert Wood Johnson Foundation, 2010).

- Chronic diseases not only cause the majority of deaths in the United States, with many of those deaths occurring well before the patient reaches his or her full life expectancy—the prolonged illness and disability from chronic diseases such as diabetes and arthritis also result in extended pain and suffering and decreased quality of life for millions of Americans (CDC, 2014b).

- Health inequalities in chronic disease are pervasive, with higher rates of death and illness among low-income communities and among communities of color in the United States (CDC, 2013).

- Close to 40 percent of deaths from the five leading causes of death in the United States (four of which are chronic diseases—heart disease, cancer, chronic lung diseases, and stroke—plus unintentional injuries) are considered preventable (Yoon, Bastian, Anderson, Collins & Jaffe, 2014).

In March 2011, the CDC published a report about CHWs and their role in supporting patients to manage chronic disease. The report highlights

> the unique role of CHWs as culturally competent mediators (health brokers) between providers of health services and the members of diverse communities and the effectiveness of CHWs in promoting the use of primary and follow-up care for preventing and managing disease have been extensively documented and recognized for a variety of health care concerns, including asthma, hypertension, diabetes, cancer, immunizations, maternal and child health, nutrition, tuberculosis, and HIV and AIDS. (CDC, 2011, p. 2)

One of the ways to do this is to integrate CHWs into the health care team, discussed below. You will also read more about health care teams and chronic conditions management in Chapter 16.

CHWS WITHIN THE HEALTH CARE DELIVERY TEAM

Many clinics and hospitals now employ CHWs as members of a care delivery team for patients with chronic diseases. Typically in the team model, CHWs work with a medical provider (a doctor, a nurse practitioner or physician's assistant), a nurse, a medical assistant, and sometimes other health professionals (such as a social worker or a respiratory therapist). The team works together consistently to manage the care of patients. The health care delivery team may combine social support (provided by CHWs) and clinical care (provided by doctors and nurses) to assist patients to more effectively manage and control their illnesses. Team-based care developed as a strategy to improve quality, access, and patient centeredness; reduce health care costs for high-cost patients; and strengthen health care delivery teams. Within this model, CHWs are trained to educate, counsel, and work with patients to improve their health through one-on-one and group sessions. CHWs may also provide home visits. Some of the chronic conditions that CHWs address in their work include diabetes, high blood pressure, HIV/AIDS, and cancer (Bodenheimer & Laing, 2007; Martinez, Ro, Villa, Powell, & Knickman, 2011).

The financing of health care under the ACA creates new incentives for health care teams, and rewards clinics and hospitals for achieving positive health outcomes. One of the important ways the ACA does this is through capitation. **Capitation** means that the health care organization receives a set amount of funding to serve each patient, instead of reimbursement for each appointment, test, or treatment provided. This creates a financial incentive to keep all people in that group as healthy as possible—so they won't need more frequent or more expensive treatment. CHWs, because of their strong links to communities, can help clients get into care early, access the appropriate level of care (for example, a primary care clinic instead of the emergency department at a hospital), overcome barriers to chronic conditions management, and help the rest of the health care team understand the patients' needs and resources more completely. This can translate into lower health care costs. Under capitation, there is the potential for some of those health care savings to be redirected to create permanent jobs for CHWs as members of the health care team.

Community health workers can play a vital role in helping clinics and hospitals attain the Triple Aim, in a variety of ways (Bodenheimer, 2015; CHWA, 2013; Findley, Matos, Hicks, Chang & Reich, 2014; Martinez et al., 2011). Some of benefits of hiring CHWs as part of a care delivery team include:

- Improve health outcomes for individuals and populations
  - Improving access to health care and insurance is a key component of improving health outcomes. If people cannot access affordable primary care, screening tests, and prevention services, they are more likely to show up for care with advanced diseases that are much more difficult and expensive to treat. CHWs play an important role in expanding access to care. They have signed up thousands of people for health insurance. They conduct outreach and build community awareness of services. They identify cases (people with a disease or at high risk) and help them to access the appropriate services.
  - Beyond access, CHWs help patients stay in treatment and achieve better health outcomes by providing health education and peer counseling, health coaching, systems navigation, and advocacy. These services have been shown to have a real impact on health outcomes, for example, reducing the need for hospitalization (CDC, 2011).

- Reduce health care costs
  - CHWs provide clients with the health education, social support, and follow-up required to manage their chronic health conditions. Successful self-management of the condition will mean fewer complications, thereby decreasing the chances of a patient ending up in the emergency room or hospitalized, where care is more expensive.
  - The contributions of CHWs may free doctors, nurses, and other clinicians to invest their time providing the services that only they can provide. CHWs reinforce the work of doctors, nurses, and others—for example, by reviewing the doctor's instructions with the client, or by making the medical provider aware of the patient's concerns.

- Improve patient-centeredness and the patient's experience of health care
  - CHWs speak the languages of their patients and can connect them to culturally appropriate health and social services resources. By being a cultural bridge between their community and the service providers, CHWs ensure that clients receive better care.
  - CHWs can also help other members of the health care team to understand the patient's perspective and adapt to the patient's needs.

As our society grows and diversifies, and as poorly treated chronic conditions become an increasing strain on the health care system, employing CHWs is a cost effective and culturally appropriate solution to improving the health and wellness of all community members. Not incidentally, this approach also has a strong potential to reduce health inequalities.

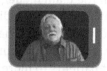

THE EMERGING ROLES OF CHWs: INTERVIEW

Please watch this video interview ▶ with Dr. Carl Rush.   ⬩ *http://youtu.be/SnaaAUKK640*

1.6 Professionalizing the CHW Field

The CHW field is growing and transforming. You will learn more about this in Chapter 2. There are disagreements among CHWs, CHW supporters, researchers, educators, employers, and other health professions about how best to professionalize the field. Some people advocate for **credentialing** (CHWs would need certification from an educational institution, professional association, or employer in order to work—see Chapter 2 for more details) and greater integration into the health care field. As of 2012, 15 states and the District of Columbia had issued one law or regulation regarding CHWs, and at least five states (Massachusetts, Minnesota, Ohio, Oregon, and Texas) have developed credentialing procedures (Miller, Bates, & Katzen, 2014). Others worry that credentialing may harm or diminish the connection that CHWs have to local communities and their commitment to social justice. Everyone, however, seems to agree that the field deserves greater recognition, respect, and funding.

Strategies that are being used to advance the CHW field include:

- Conducting research about the field to further clarify what CHWs do and how effective they are
- Founding national and regional CHW organizations as a way for CHWs to have a collective voice in determining the development of their profession, and to advocate on behalf of the communities they serve
- Developing appropriate ways to credential or certify the work of CHWs
- Developing training programs and materials that teach the core competencies required for success as a CHWs
- Advocating for policy changes that will result in more stable funding for CHWs
- Developing regulations and procedures to take advantage of the funding opportunities in the ACA

- *What do you see as the key opportunities and challenges for CHWs as the field becomes more professionalized?*

An Inherent Tension

Sergio Matos, longtime CHW and current (2015) Chair of the Education and Capacitación Committee of the CHW Section of the American Public Health Association, discusses issues that arise as the role of CHWs within the health and social services systems expands.

"There is tension between our community's needs and desires, and the programs that pay CHWs—they often have conflicting goals and objectives. There is a big risk that CHWs will just get co-opted by the service industry. It's attractive—it provides salaries, it provides benefits, it provides a lot of stuff. But it betrays much of our tradition and history.

"Our society has become a service economy and in order to keep it going you need clients to sell your service to. We often don't even think about it, but we continuously label people in a way that oppresses them so that they are dependent on our services. So, for example, people are no longer people but they're diabetics, or they are handicapped or disabled, they're homeless, they're poverty stricken, or underprivileged. All these labels that we put on people—and once we get you to accept that label we say, 'Oh, but fear not, we have a service for you!'

"The work of CHWs is directly opposed to that—directly and fundamentally opposed to that. A CHW is successful when the person they work with no longer needs us. That's our true measure of success—when we've helped somebody develop self-sufficiency and independence so that they no longer need us or our services."

1.7 Introducing Four CHWs

Throughout this book, you will find quotes from CHWs who have firsthand knowledge, experience, and information to share. Quotes and photographs from four CHWs appear frequently throughout the entire book. The CHWs are **Ramona Benson, Phuong An Doan-Billings, Lee Jackson,** and **Alvaro Morales.** They each graduated from the CHW Certificate Program at City College of San Francisco and contributed to the development of this book by participating in extensive interviews and taking photographs that represent their work. In this section, each of them is introduced. Through the rest of the book, you'll see an icon every time we include a quote from a CHW.

Ramona Benson journeyed from being a client at a San Francisco homeless shelter to becoming a CHW with the Homeless Prenatal Program in San Francisco in 1990. She completed her CHW certificate from City College of San Francisco in 1994 and trained CHWs at the Homeless Prenatal Program until 2000. She was the supervisor of supportive services at San Francisco's Tenderloin Housing Clinic from 2000 to 2001, when she became the CHW at the Black Infant Health Program in Berkeley, California. In 2008, she became the coordinator of the Black Infant Health program at Berkeley's Department of Public Health. She completed her Bachelor's degree in Liberal Studies with a minor in Health Education, and is considering applying for a Master's program.

Ramona Benson: You have to have a variety of skills to be effective as a CHW. There are going to be some long hours that you're not going to get paid for. You have to be committed and passionate and you have to be a team player: we can't do it all by ourselves. My reward is seeing my community become healthy, becoming empowered. That's how I measure my success, by watching those who I've worked with overcome barriers. They may have had 10 barriers and they overcame two of them—but that's success, for me.

In my career, I've worked as both a CHW and a supervisor. I'm a coordinator now, but I'm still doing CHW work because it's in me. When I was at Homeless Prenatal and Tenderloin Housing, as rewarding as it was to be promoted as a supervisor, being in that role for a good amount of time, I began missing providing services hands on. I wanted to get back into a CHW role because that's where my passion is. I came to Black Infant Health as their first CHW. Now as a coordinator there, I wear multiple hats. I do the CHW work as well as the coordinator work and supervision.

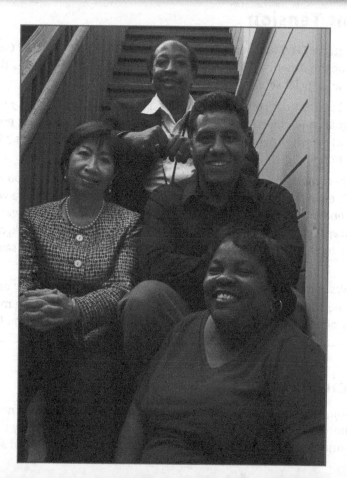

Four graduates of the CCSF CHW training program. From top clockwise: Lee Jackson, Alvaro Morales, Ramona Benson, Phuong An Doan-Billings.

Born in Vietnam, Phuong An Doan-Billings holds a BA degree in English from Saigon University (1979). She taught French and English in Vietnam until she came to the United States in 1990. She started working for Asian Health Services (AHS) in Oakland in 1992 as a health care interpreter and CHW. In 2005, Phuong An became the supervisor of the AHS Community Liaison Unit, which reaches out to Asian communities for health education services and health care advocacy. She also contributes her in-depth language skills to the AHS Language Culture Access Program, which provides training for hundreds of health care interpreters in the Bay Area. Since 2012 she has been the Healthy Nail Salon Program Coordinator.

Phuong An Doan-Billings: A lot of what I do with the Healthy Nail Salon program is coordinating the members, the nail salon workers and owners, organizing, holding them together. We just graduated our second group of core leaders. We train them in public speaking and outreach, so they can take the role of advocacy for their own industry. We build awareness of the hazards of the products they use that are notoriously toxic. Advocacy requires a little public speaking, something that Vietnamese women are definitely not trained for over the generations. It's a very big challenge for them. I know the culture, the community. I use my own personality so people get involved. In our culture, we appeal to personal relationships. When they see you are committed to helping, they trust you. It's like what I did in the clinic, before. It's holding the relationship with them, facilitating their participation in programs, educating and motivating them.

Lee Jackson has seven certificates from City College of San Francisco, including Drug and Alcohol Studies, HIV/STI Outreach, Case Management, Group Facilitation, Infectious Disease Prevention in Priority Populations, Diversity and Social Justice, and Community Health Worker and Post-Prison Health Worker; he completed the CHW certificate in 2004. Originally from Texas, Lee moved to Los Angeles in 1979 and San Francisco in 1987. He has worked as a CHW at several nonprofits including the South Beach Resource Center, Walden House, and PlaneTree, and currently works for San Francisco Department of Public Health's Early Intervention Program at Southeast Health Center. Lee works with clients who are HIV positive, multiply diagnosed, or struggling with substance abuse. Lee has completed an A.S. degree in Health Education.

Lee Jackson: As a CHW, you have to work from the heart and give your all to do what's best for your client. Some of my clients are really sick and I go wherever I have to find them. I visit them on the streets and in their apartments, in detox and residential drug recovery programs, in jail and at the General Hospital. I even accompany them to court when they have legal problems. In this work, you have to learn how to take care of yourself, too. I'm really into jazz, so I listen to music a lot. What keeps me going is my strong lease on my spirituality. The only way you are going to remain relevant in this changing field is to stay up-to-date, so it's important to me to take classes, get these certificates and attend conferences, workshops and seminars.

Alvaro Morales: I am originally from Guatemala, where I got an accounting degree. I started out working here in the United States as a cook for a big hotel in San Francisco. But that isn't what I wanted to do. I started volunteering for an AIDS hotline, answering questions, talking to people over the phone. Someone told me about the CHW training program at City College. I started the program, and for my internship I went to a community health center and worked with their outreach worker. We went out on the streets, to the parks, and to different agencies, talking to people about HIV, passing out condoms, telling people about the health center and about how to get tested for HIV. It was a great training because I learned to work with all kinds of people, to talk with people about all kinds of topics, including things like relationships and sex and drug use and to work in both Spanish and English. When the outreach worker quit, they offered me the job.

Then I started doing HIV antibody test counselling at the clinic. It was a great chance to learn how to do client-centered counselling, how to assist people to reduce their risks for HIV, and how to work with people

(continues)

(continued)

that were HIV positive to stay healthy. I listened a lot, and provided emotional support and a safe place for people to talk about things that are private, or that they were scared of. I had great supervisors who really taught me a lot about this work.

Since then, I worked all around the [San Francisco] Bay Area. I managed a mobile HIV testing project for a local health department. I did Healthy Families (SCHIP) outreach and enrollment, assisting low-income families in getting health insurance and primary health care for their children. I worked at a drop-in center for the homeless. I worked for the San Francisco Department of Public Health, doing environmental health work for day laborers and restaurant workers.

I have benefited from every experience working as a CHW and everyone I ever worked with. I think, as a CHW, you learn a lot from your colleagues, but you learn the most from your clients. I try to keep them in mind, to remember the things they have taught me, and to put that to use in the work I am doing today. But I also know that I don't know it all. I'm a person who likes to keep learning. Not just for my job, but for myself, too, and my family.

About 10 years after I finished the CHW certificate at City College, I went back to school. In December 2007, I completed my BA in Humanities with an emphasis on Social Change and Activism. In 2010, I completed a master's degree program in public health at San Francisco State University. I always wanted to work in Alameda County, and I found a job as a clinic manager at a school-based health center. From there, I was hired in 2014 as Director of Administrative Affairs and Outreach/Eligibility Assistance for the Alameda County Public Health Nursing Unit, and I'm really happy there. Among other things, I get to work with our eight outreach workers, providing training, also involving them not only in program implementation but in the ideas, the evaluation. I am taking the same approach I have taken in other positions—equal participation and team decision-making approach. I feel fortunate to have been given the opportunity to share my experiences and to work with CHWs, and together we will be planning, developing, implementing, and evaluating effective strategies to better serve the residents of Alameda County. We just got started, stay tuned!

Chapter Review

1. Which communities or populations do CHWs most commonly work with? What experiences (if any) have you had with CHWs in your own community?

2. If you were to tell someone how you got interested in community health work, like Ramona Benson's story at the start of this chapter, what would you say?

3. What health issues do CHWs commonly address in their work? Which health issues most motivate you as you train to work as a CHW?

4. How would you explain the relationship between roles and competencies? Review the quotes from the four CHWs profiled in the preceding section. What examples of the core CHW roles do you see in their biographies?

5. Which of the seven core roles are you most comfortable fulfilling? Which do you know the least about?

6. Explain the eight core competencies of CHWs, and provide an example of each. Have you had the opportunity to develop and practice any of these skills? Which of these skills are you currently least prepared to put into practice?

7. Describe personal qualities and attributes that are common among successful CHWs. Which of these qualities will you bring to the work? What additional qualities, attributes, or values will you bring?

8. Think about a chronic condition that you or a family member lives with. How could you imagine a CHW supporting you or your family in managing this chronic condition, as part of a clinical team?

9. As the profession grows, what are some of the challenges you see CHWs encountering? What new opportunities or recognition would you like to see CHWs gain?

References

American Public Health Association. (2009). *Policy statement 20091.* Retrieved from *www.apha. org/policies-and-advocacy/public-health-policy-statements/policy-database/2014/07/09/14/19/ support-for-community-health-workers-to-increase-health-access-and-to-reduce-health-inequities*

Bovbjerg, R. R., Eyster, L., Ormond, B. A., Anderson, T., & Richardson, E. (2013). *The evolution, expansiveness, and effectiveness of community health workers.* Washington, DC: Urban Institute. Retrieved from *www.urban.org/ UploadedPDF/413072-Evolution-Expansion-and-Effectiveness-of-Community-Health-Workers.pdf*

Bodenheimer, T. (2015). Unlicensed health care personnel and patient outcomes. *Journal of General Internal Medicine.* doi:10.1007/s11606-015-3274-x

Bodenheimer, T., & Laing, B. Y. (2007). The teamlet model of primary care. *Annals of Family Medicine, 5,* 457–461.

Bureau of Labor Statistics. (2010). *Standard occupational classification: 21-1094 community health workers.* Retrieved from *www.bls.gov/soc/2010/soc211094.htm*

Bureau of Labor Statistics. (2014). *Occupational Outlook Handbook: Health educators and community health workers.* Retrieved from *www.bls.gov/ooh/community-and-social-service/health-educators.htm#tab-6*

Centers for Disease Control and Prevention. (2011). *Addressing chronic disease through community health workers: A policy and systems-level approach.* Retrieved from *www.cdc.gov/dhdsp/docs/chw_brief.pdf*

Centers for Disease Control and Prevention. (2013). *About CDC's office of minority health and health equity.* Retrieved from *www.cdc.gov/minorityhealth/OMHHE.html*

Centers for Disease Control and Prevention. (2014a). *Faststats: Health expenditures.* Retrieved from *www.cdc.gov/ nchs/fastats/health-expenditures.htm*

Centers for Disease Control and Prevention. (2014b). *Chronic disease prevention and health promotion.* Retrieved from *www.cdc.gov/chronicdisease/overview/*

Centers for Disease Control and Prevention. (2014c). *Technical assistance guide: States implementing community health worker strategies.* Retrieved from *www.cdc.gov/dhdsp/programs/spha/docs/1305_ta_guide_chws.pdf*

California Health Workforce Alliance. (2013). *Taking innovation to scale: Community health workers, promotores, and the triple aim.* Retrieved from *www.michwa.org/wp-content/uploads/2013_CHWA_Taking-innovation-to-scale- community-health-workers-promotores-and-the-triple-aim.pdf*

Community Health Worker Network of New York City. (n.d.). *Core values.* Retrieved from *www.chwnetwork.org/ about-chwnyc/core-values/*

Findley, S., Matos, S., Hicks, A., Chang, J., & Reich, D. (2014). Community health worker integration into the health care team accomplishes the triple aim in a patient-centered medical home: A Bronx tale. *Journal of Ambulatory Care Management, 37,* 82–91. doi: 10.1097/JAC.0000000000000011

Frontline Health Workers Coalition. (2014a). *Frontline health workers: Reducing the burden of HIV/AIDS.* Retrieved from *http://frontlinehealthworkers.org/wp-content/uploads/2014/04/FLHW-HIV-Fact-Sheet.pdf*

Frontline Health Workers Coalition. (2014b). *Frontline health workers: Reducing the burden of malaria.* Retrieved from *http://frontlinehealthworkers.org/wp-content/uploads/2014/04/FLHW_Malaria-Factsheet-4.24.2014-v2.pdf*

Frontline Health Workers Coalition. (n.d.). *Our mission: Urging U.S. investment in frontline health workers.* Retrieved from *http://frontlinehealthworkers.org/about-the-coalition/our-mission/*

Health Resources and Services Administration, Bureau of Health Professions. (2007). *Community health worker national workforce study.* Washington, DC: U.S. Department of Health and Human Services. Retrieved from *http://bhpr.hrsa.gov/healthworkforce/reports/chwstudy2007.pdf*

Hurtado, M., Spinner, J. R., Yang, M., Evensen, C., Windham, A., Ortiz, G., . . . Ivy, E. D. (2014). Knowledge and behavioral effects in cardiovascular health: Community Health Worker Health Disparities Initiative, 2007– 2010. *Preventing Chronic Disease, 11,* 130250. Retrieved from *www.cdc.gov/pcd/issues/2014/13_0250.htm*

International Training and Education Center on HIV (I-TECH) and the Zimbabwe Ministry of Health. (2004). *Integrated counseling for HIV and AIDS prevention and care: Primary care counselor training: Trainer's guide.* Unpublished. Seattle and San Francisco: I-TECH.

Martinez, J., Ro, M., Villa, N. W., Powell, W., & Knickman, J. R. (2011). Transforming the delivery of care in the post-health reform era: What role will community health workers play? *American Journal of Public Health, 101,* e1–e5. doi:10.2105/AJPH.2011.300335

McCloskey, J., Tollestrup, K., & Sanders, M. (2011). A community integration approach to social determinants of health in New Mexico. *Family and Community Health, 34,* S79–S91. Retrieved from *www.nursingcenter.com/lnc/ journalarticle?Article_ID=1109823*

McCormick, S., Glaubitz, K., McIlvenne, & M., Mader, E. (2012). *Community health workers in Utah: an assessment of the role of CHWs in Utah and the national health care system.* Salt Lake City (UT): University of Utah, Center for Public Policy and Administration. Retrieved from *www.choosehealth.utah.gov/documents/pdfs/chw/UDOH_ CHW_final_report.pdf*

Miller, P., Bates, T., & Katzen, A. (2014). *Community health worker credentialing: State approaches.* Cambridge, MA: Harvard Law School, Center for Health Law and Policy Innovation. Retrieved from *www.chlpi.org/wp-content/ uploads/2014/06/CHW-Credentialing-Paper.pdf*

Minnesota Community Health Worker Alliance. (2013). Who are CHWs: Roles. Retrieved from *http:// mnchwalliance.org/who-are-chws/roles/*

National Healthcare for the Homeless Council. (2011). Community health workers: Financing and administration. [Policy brief.] Retrieved from *www.nhchc.org/wp-content/uploads/2011/10/CHW-Policy-Brief.pdf*

National Community Health Worker Advocacy Survey (NCHWAS). (2014). 2014 Preliminary Data Report for the United States and Territories. Tucson, Arizona: Arizona Prevention Research Center, Zuckerman College of Public Health, University of Arizona.

New York State Community Health Worker Initiative. (2011). *Paving a path to advance the community health worker workforce in New York State: A new summary report and recommendations.* Retrieved from *http://nyshealthfounda- tion.org/uploads/resources/paving-path-advance-community-health-worker-october-2011.pdf*

One Million Community Health Workers Campaign. (2013). Tanzania hosts global "one million health workers campaign" forum. [Blog]. Retrieved from *http://1millionhealthworkers.org/2013/04/15/ tanzania-hosts-global-one-million-community-health-workers-campaign-forum/*

Robert Wood Johnson Foundation. (2010). *Chronic care: Making the case for ongoing care.* Retrieved from *www.rwjf. org/content/dam/farm/reports/reports/2010/rwjf54583*

Rosenthal, E. L., Brownstein, J. N., Rush, C. H., Hirsch, G. R., Willaert, A. M., Scott, J. R., . . . Fox, D. J. (2010). Community health workers: Part of the solution. *Health Affairs, 29,* 1338–1342. doi:10.1377/hlthaff.2010.0081

Rosenthal, E. L., Wiggins, N., Brownstein, J. N., Rael, R., & Johnson, S. (1998). *The Final Report of the National Community Health Advisor Study: Weaving the Future.* Tucson: University of Arizona. Retrieved from *http://crh. arizona.edu/sites/default/files/pdf/publications/CAHsummaryALL.pdf*

World Bank. (2010). *Data: Physicians (per 1000 people).* Retrieved from *http://data.worldbank.org/indicator/SH.MED. PHYS.ZS*

World Bank. (2014). *Poverty overview.* Retrieved from *www.worldbank.org/en/topic/poverty/overview*

Yamey G, on Behalf of the Interviewees. (2007). Which single intervention would do the most to improve the health of those living on less than $1 per day? *PLoS Medicine, 4,* e303. doi:10.1371/journal.pmed.0040303

Yoon, P. W., Bastian, B., Anderson, R. N., Collins, J. L., & Jaffe, H. W. (2014). Potentially preventable deaths from the five leading causes of death—United States, 2008–2010. *Morbidity and Mortality Weekly Report, 63*(17), 369–374.

Additional Resources

American Public Health Association. (n.d). Community health workers section. Retrieved from *www.apha.org/ apha-communities/member-sections/community-health-workers*

Bureau of Labor Statistics. (2014). *Occupational employment statistics: 21-1094 community health workers.* Retrieved from *www.bls.gov/oes/current/oes211094.htm*

City College of San Francisco Health Education Department. (n.d.). Retrieved from *www.ccsf.edu/healthed*

Community Health Worker Network of New York City. (n.d.). Retrieved from *www.chwnetwork.org/*

Community Health Worker Project of the Urban Institute. (n.d.). Retrieved from *www.urban.org/careworks/*

Community Health Workers Health Disparities Initiative of the National Institutes of Health. (n.d.). *Medicaid will allow reimbursement for community health worker preventative services.* Retrieved from *www.abcardio.org/articles/cms_rule.html*

Community Health Works: A Partnership of San Francisco State University and City College of San Francisco. (n.d.). Retrieved from *http://communityhealthworks.org*

Massachusetts Association of Community Health Workers. (n.d.). Retrieved from *www.machw.org*

Sinai Urban Health Institute. (2014). Best practice guidelines for implementing and evaluating community health worker programs in health care settings. Retrieved from *www.sinai.org/sites/default/files/SUHI%20Best%20Practice%20Guidelines%20for%20CHW%20Programs.pdf*

University of Southern Mississippi Center for Sustainable Health Outreach. (n.d.). Retrieved from *www.usm.edu/health/center-sustainable-health-outreach*

Vision Y Compromiso. (n.d.). Retrieved from *www.visionycompromiso.org*

CHW Network in your state or region: _____

The Evolution of the Community Health Worker Field in the United States

2

The Shoulders We Stand On

E. Lee Rosenthal and J. Nell Brownstein

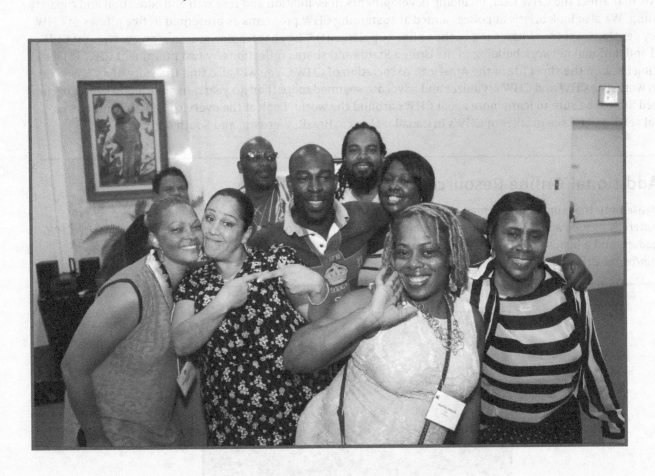

A great river always begins somewhere. Often it starts as a tiny spring bubbling up from a crack in the soil, just like the little stream in my family's land (in Ihithe), which starts where the roots of the fig tree broke though the rocks beneath the ground. But for the stream to grow into a river, it must meet other tributaries and join them as it heads for a lake or the sea . . .

—*Wangari Maathai, Unbowed: A Memoir (2006)*

Introduction

There are many Community Health Workers (CHWs) throughout the United States and the world. In all communities, we see natural helping and aid-giving networks that may include CHWs; however, formal CHW programs and services, including both paid and volunteer CHWs, are not found in all the communities. In the United States, CHWs are not yet a routine part of health and human service systems, but they are becoming increasingly common, often being added to service systems in both clinical and community settings. CHWs are seen by many as invaluable members of the safety net for communities, and they can be an important force for improving the health of individuals, families, and communities.

The focus of this chapter is the growth and development of CHWs in the United States, including ongoing efforts to define CHW roles or "scope of practice" (what CHWs are allowed to do). As a part of looking at the documented history of CHWs, we will look at the early origins of the field in the United States and various trends that affect the CHW field, including developments in evaluation and research and education and capacity building. We also look briefly at polices aimed at sustaining CHW programs as presented in five phases of CHW policy development (see Phases 1–4 in the online supplement). The chapter also presents an overview of CHW local and national network building in the United States and shares reflections by two prominent CHW leaders looking back on the short life of the American Association of CHWs. You will also find the story of a CHW whose life's work as a CHW and CHW organizer and advocate spanned more than 40 years. In addition to CHWs in the United States, be sure to learn more about CHWs around the world. Look at the overview of CHWs in international settings and see profiles of CHWs in Canada, Mexico, Brazil, Vietnam, and South Africa.

Additional Online Resources

Please note that supplemental materials for this chapter will be posted on the publisher's website. These materials include additional information about the work of CHWs around the world, and interviews with CHW leaders, and a history of key policy decisions that have influenced the CHW profession. (*http://wileyactual. com/bertholdshowcase*).

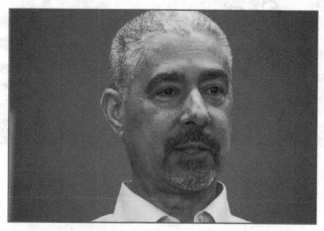

CHWs have a long history of promoting the health of vulnerable communities.

The history of the CHW field in the United States includes the contributions of many individuals and organizations working together to establish culturally tailored and community-specific ways to promote the health of our most vulnerable communities. CHWs and their allies understand that CHWs support families and communities by enabling them to take greater control over their own lives and health and to better access and use formal health care systems.

As we begin this review of the CHW journey in the United States, take a moment to ask yourself, "Where have I made my contributions?" If you are new to CHW work, ask yourself, "Where will I fit into this history?" Think about your role in assisting people, such as your neighbors and friends, one by one, and any role you have played in making your community healthier. You already have, or one day will have, an important story to tell about your contributions as a CHW.

WHAT YOU WILL LEARN

By studying the material presented in this chapter, you will be able to:

- Describe the contributions of CHWs in promoting the health of individuals and communities in the United States and around the world
- Identify and discuss major trends and debates that have impacted the development of the CHW field in the United States
- Discuss the role that CHWs have played in advocating for greater recognition and respect for their field
- Consider what place you want to have in the CHW field

WORDS TO KNOW

Natural Helping System

Self-Determination

Author's Note to the Second Edition

E. Lee Rosenthal, PhD, MS, MPH: At the time of this writing (2015) the CHW workforce in the United States appears to be making a shift. CHWs are becoming increasingly recognized and valued in medical care settings, especially as they find their place on health care home teams. CHWs also continue to make a difference in community development and play a pivotal role in addressing social determinants of health and promoting health equity. In this light, it is interesting to update the history chapter of this ground-breaking textbook. Our perspective on the past changes more than I first realized when I agreed to revise this short chapter.

Given the challenges of the task and the opportunity, I am excited that in this updated version of the history chapter I have had the opportunity to work with a number of esteemed colleagues. I am happy that Carl H. Rush, Sergio Matos, and Durrell Fox each accepted the invitation to contribute to this chapter by writing brief pieces on health policy and national association development among CHWs. I am also pleased to have had Noelle Wiggins update her piece on CHWs in international settings. In addition to Dr. Wiggins's viewpoint on CHWs around the globe, I am excited to share short pieces on CHWs in different countries led by my colleagues Sara Torres (Canada), Hector Balcazar (United States/Mexico), Rosemary Blake (South Africa), Nguyen Thi Thanh Ha (Vietnam), and Estelle Dutra Prado (Brazil). Finally, I am truly grateful and pleased to have my longtime colleague Dr. J. Nell Brownstein join me as a coauthor of the chapter.

It takes many voices to tell the Community Health Worker story. We cannot capture all the history that has gone before but I hope together we have begun to unravel the cloth so we can see each thread and its rich color, which together make a whole and strong tapestry.

Why Study History?

Some say the past predicts the future or creates the present, so looking at history helps us to understand the world we live in today. As you study and work as a CHW you are becoming part of something bigger—a world shared with your peers—other CHWs known by many names including *promotores*, Community Health Representatives, and peer health educators. At times CHWs and their allies would describe this field as part of a movement—one dedicated to health equity, social justice, and to economic development. Learning about how the CHW field has grown in the United States since the 1950s can give you insights into your work today, the people you serve, and about the relationships CHWs have with others working throughout the nation to promote health and deliver medical care.

A Note on Writing Down Histories

E. Lee Rosenthal: Sometimes, when people met my mother, Betty Clark Rosenthal, she would tell them about her life and the work she did, and they would say, "You should write down your story." And she would say, "I am too busy living my life and doing my work to stop and write it down." Just because something is published in a book or article does not mean that it is the only story or the best story. Research can tell us only about what has been documented in some way, especially in the articles published in scientific journals. These research articles are a valuable source of history. Yet our experiences are also valuable sources of information. As someone who has played a role in the U.S. CHW field for many years, I have been honored to contribute to its history. I am pleased to have a chance to share some of what I have witnessed and learned. I also understand that, even with the literature to help me, I am able to shed light on only a small piece of the much bigger and richer CHW story.

Please reflect on your own story as a CHW and the story of the communities you come from.

What Do YOU Think?

- *When did you start working or volunteering as a CHW?*

- *How has your work as a CHW impacted individual clients or families?*

- *How has your work as a CHW impacted the communities you serve?*

- *How have you helped to build the CHW field (or how would you like to help develop the CHW field)?*

2.1 Neighbor Assisting Neighbor

The history of CHWs began when neighbors first aided each other to take care of their health. Over time those seeking to promote wellness saw the promise of building on these *natural* helping systems to establish more formal approaches. The many programs and CHW services we see today include both paid CHWs and volunteer "lay" aid programs and networks. The informal assistance-giving tradition still continues today; CHWs extend that tradition.

What Is a "Natural Helping System"?

A **natural helping system** is a naturally occurring community network through which family, friends, neighbors, and others, connected by shared experience (in the same geographic setting or shared experience), watch out for one another and reach out with assistance on a regular basis and in times of crisis.

What natural helping networks do you rely on?

2.2 CHW Names, Definitions, and Scope of Practice

MANY NAMES FOR CHWs

As the CHW field has evolved, no one definition for a CHW has been adopted. In this textbook we use the term *community health worker* to include the volunteer and paid health practitioners known nationally and internationally by many different names or titles. The National Community Health Advisor Study (NCHAS) identified more than 60 titles for CHWs, including lay health advocate, *promotor,* outreach educator, Community Health Representative, peer health promoter, and of course, CHW (Rosenthal et al., 1998); other sources state that more than 100 names for CHWs have been identified (CHW Initiative of Sonoma County, n.d.). This last term, CHW, is used by the World Health Organization and is the title most commonly used in international settings. It is also used by the American Public Health Association CHW Section.

Having many titles reflects the diversity of the field but it can make it hard for CHWs to identify one another and find the support they need for training, improving practice, and their own professional development.

Durrel Fox: During a series of meetings in the mid 1990s of diverse leaders in the CHW movement in the United States, it was decided that we needed a unifying, umbrella term for the many titles under which CHWs fall. CHW was the agreed-upon, common, unifying term to help the movement for sustainability of our CHW workforce to progress, especially to help inform policy development.

—Durrell Fox served on the Executive Board of American Public Health Association from 2011–2015

DEFINING CHWs

Because CHWs work in so many communities, under a wide variety of titles, and provide such a wide variety of services, the field and the occupation have not been well defined. As part of a movement for greater recognition and respect for the work that CHWs do, several groups have been advocating for a formal definition of CHW. In the early 2000s, a newly formed Policy Committee for the American Public Health Association (APHA) CHW Special Interest Group (SPIG, later a Section of APHA) took the lead in developing such a definition. As a part of this effort, the Center for Sustainable Health Outreach (CSHO) collected definitions from CHWs and CHW networks across the United States and from other sources.

In 2006, the APHA CHW SPIG submitted a definition of CHWs to the U.S. Department of Labor and Statistics (DOL) for consideration. Other groups have also submitted definitions for consideration. In March of 2009, the U.S. Department of Labor (DOL) approved a separate occupational (work-related) category—21-1094—for CHWs (U.S. Bureau of Labor Statistics, 2009). The Department of Labor's new definition was used in collecting U.S. Census data in 2010, but given the newness of the established definition, counts in this first federal census are not widely cited. In 2014, CHWs and their supporters, with leadership once again from the Policy Committee of the CHW Section of APHA, have advocated for an updated definition that better reflects the community-based nature of CHWs.

In the past several years, many local and state CHW networks have adopted the APHA CHW definition as a part of campaign to create greater unity in the field. The updated (2009) definition is:

A Community Health Worker (CHW) is a frontline public health worker who is a trusted member of and/or has an unusually close understanding of the community served. This trusting relationship enables the CHW to serve as a liaison/link/intermediary between health/social services and the community to facilitate access to services and improve the quality and cultural competence of service delivery. A CHW also builds individual and community capacity by increasing health knowledge and self-sufficiency through a range of activities such as outreach, community education, informal counseling, social support and advocacy. (APHA, 2009)

The APHA CHW Section and many others are urging the DOL to update its definition to be more in alignment with the APHA definition and to ensure the definition includes reference to CHWs having close affiliation to the communities they serve; something the current definition lacks.

At the time of this writing, the DOL has just finished a review period in which they were accepting public comments and feedback on the CHW occupational category.

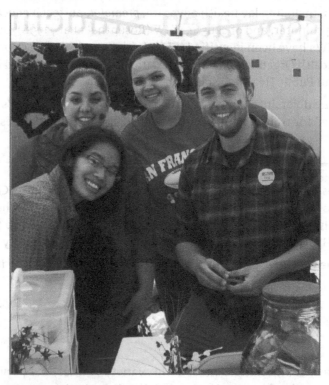

CHWs conducting outreach.

What Is a "Scope of Practice"?

A Federation of State Medical Boards (2005) report defined scope of practice as the "Definition of the rules, the regulations, and the boundaries within which a fully qualified practitioner with substantial and appropriate training, knowledge, and experience may practice in a defined field. Such practice is also governed by requirements for continuing education and professional accountability."

Within the CHW field we use the term *scope of practice* more broadly (outside the context of granting a license to CHWs) to talk about the breadth and depth of CHW roles or functions that allow you to do your work. A scope of practice for CHWs may be found in various places, including CHW job descriptions or within state legislation.

The concept of scope of practice is described in greater detail in Chapter 7.

IDENTIFYING WHAT CHWs DO: CHW ROLES AND COMPETENCIES

There is no official agreement about the definition of CHWs, likewise there is no official agreement about core CHW roles or competencies. This is in part due to the lack of leadership from any single independent national CHW network or association (see the discussion of CHW networks later in this chapter and in Chapter 1). In the absence of official roles and competencies, many have looked to the National Community Health Advisor Study conducted from 1994–1998 NCHAS, 1998). Notably, roles and competencies identified in the Study (Wiggins and Borbón, 1998) were not formally endorsed by the field, but they were adopted in 2000 by the American Public Health Association. Though not formally identified as standards, the NCHAS roles and competencies have influenced many CHW job descriptions, training curricula, and state-level guidance on roles and scope of practice and training standards.

Given the continual use of the NCHAS roles and competencies and the absence of national standards, beginning in 2014, a team of researchers including CHWs and CHW allies joined together in a 2014–2015 study known as the CHW Core Consensus (C3) Project. The aim of the study is to revisit the roles and competencies identified in the 1994–1998 NCHAS and compare them with more current role and competency documents that reflect current scope of practice and CHW competencies.

In summer 2015, at the time of this writing, the C3 project team is releasing its findings to U.S. CHW network leaders. These networks are invited to review the findings and to give input on them to create a field-driven list of roles and competencies. Following the network's review, the C3 project team will release the findings more widely. The short-term goal of the project is to build national awareness of CHW roles and competencies and the long-term goal is the use and endorsement of the identified roles and competencies by local, state, and national organizations seeking to initiate and/or support existing CHW education, practice, and policies.

AN EMERGING WORKFORCE

Generally, health professions have become recognized by defining themselves and helping others to understand what they do to improve health. At times, health professionals have faced conflicts with other competing professions, and have had to struggle for respect and legitimacy. This has been true for many health professions groups such as nurse practitioners, midwives, home health aides, and CHWs (Rosenthal, 2003). For the past few decades, U.S. CHWs are actively organizing on local, state, and national levels to ensure that their knowledge, skills, and contributions are valued, respected, and integrated into health and public health systems.

SELF-DETERMINATION BY CHWs ABOUT CHW PRACTICE

With the many elements of the CHW field being defined and refined, one key is to place CHWs themselves in charge of that process. CHWs' self-determination about their practice and the policies that impact it is actively promoted by many CHWs and CHW allies. In 2014, the APHA passed a resolution entitled "Support for Community Health Worker Leadership in Determining Workforce Standards for Training and Credentialing" that called CHWs to be 50 percent of participants in all efforts aimed at defining or regulating CHWs (APHA, 2014). Two of the four action steps of the resolution directly reference this important topic:

1. Urges state governments and other entities considering creating policies regarding CHW training standards and credentialing to engage in collaborative CHW-led efforts with local CHWs and/or CHW professional groups. If CHWs and other entities partner in order to pursue policy development on these topics, a working group comprised of at least 50 percent self-identified CHWs should be established.

2. Encourages state governments and any other entity drafting new policy regarding CHW training standards and credentialing to include in the policy the creation of a governing board comprised of at least half CHWs. This board should, to the extent possible, minimize barriers to participation and ensure a representation of CHWs that is diverse in terms of language preference, disability status volunteer versus paid status, past source of training received, and CHW roles.

2.3 The International Roots of CHWs

CHWs throughout History and around the World

As a CHW you are part of a worldwide community with historical roots that go back hundreds of years. In this section of the chapter, I explain three of the historical roots that produced CHW programs outside the United States.

(continues)

CHWs throughout History and around the World

(continued)

In nearly all human communities, people have been recognized for their skill in preserving and restoring health. These informal healers have gone by many names: *curanderos*, shamans, elders, and *sobadores*, among others. At a certain point in history, these informal healers began to be seen as different from the more formal healers who practiced health care as a profession. But in many places around the world, especially in rural areas, there were not enough formal healers to go around, and community members were trained to fill the gap. For example, in seventeenth-century Russia, laypeople called *feldshers* were trained for one year so that they could care for the health of civilians and soldiers. *Feldshers* are still part of the health care system in many parts of the Russian-speaking world. Three centuries later, Chinese leader Mao Tse-Tung promised that he would increase access to health care in the rural areas. Initially, he sent doctors from the cities to serve rural communities. But the urban doctors didn't want to stay, so the Chinese government began to train villagers to treat common illnesses, promote sanitation, and give immunizations. They were called "barefoot doctors" because many were so poor they could not afford shoes. Similarly, in the 1960s and 1970s, newly independent Tanzania in East Africa and Zimbabwe in southern Africa developed programs of community health promoters. People with some formal education were trained for a relatively brief time— six months was common—to improve access to health services. These early programs were staffed by locally supported volunteers or, in the case of China, as part of the revolutionary division of labor.

Another important factor that led to the creation of CHW programs was the desire to create more just and equitable societies. In many colonial societies, and among colonized communities of color in the United States, health care and education had been systematically denied to keep people under control.

Popular movements for social justice throughout the world influenced or supported the development of CHW programs. For example, CHWs or *promotores de salud* throughout Latin America became active in promoting the health of poor communities, often supporting these communities to organize and advocate for greater access to basic rights and resources. In many parts of Latin America, such as El Salvador, CHWs were targeted for intimidation, violence, and death by right-wing governments and affiliated paramilitary groups and death squads simply because they worked with and on behalf of poor communities or were associated with organizations, including the Catholic Church, that had been labeled "subversive."

The final root of CHW programs outside the United States is the effort to provide primary health care for all. In 1978, at a conference in Alma Ata, Russia, the World Health Organization adopted the concept of primary health care (PHC) as its main strategy for achieving "health for all by the year 2000." An important part of this strategy was "community participation in health," which meant involving community members to iden- tify health problems and participate in their solution. The WHO said that "village health workers" (VHWs) were the best strategy for achieving community participation in health. This formal recognition and support led in the 1970s and 1980s to large-scale government-sponsored CHW programs in developing countries such as Indonesia, Costa Rica, and Colombia.

A variety of historical situations have produced CHW programs in many parts of the world. However, none of these programs could have been created if community members were not motivated to aid other commu- nity members achieve more control over their lives and their health. This is, in the final analysis, the most important root of CHW programs.

Additional information from Noelle Wiggins about the international roots of CHWs, including a participatory Radio Play, has been posted on the *Foundations* for CHWs site (*http://wileyactual.com/bertholdshowcase*).

Source: Noelle Wiggins, MSPH, founder and manager, Community Capacitación Center, Multnomah County Health Department, Oregon.

PROFILES OF CHWS ACROSS THE GLOBE

CHWs are found across the world. Their important contributions to health systems have been widely documented and recognized by the World Health Organization (Lehmann, Friedman, & Sanders, 2004). In each country CHW services reflect the system and health needs of their country. CHWs educational and employment needs change and evolve just as individual, family, and environmental health issues change. Health system reforms also impact the organization of CHW services. In this next section, CHW allies share a brief snapshot of the history and work of CHWs in their countries.

The following profiles highlight the work of CHWs in Brazil, Canada, Mexico, South Africa, and Vietnam. We have included a brief excerpt of each country profile here, with additional information posted on the *Foundations* website (*http://wileyactual.com/bertholdshowcase*).

Community Health Workers in Canada

Sara Torres—L'Université de Montréal:

In Canada, CHWs are primarily involved in health education and health promotion projects that include: prevention and management of chronic illnesses (diabetes, cancer) and infectious diseases (HIV/Aids, gonorrhea); prenatal and postnatal support; and access to health and social services. Generally, CHWs come from the communities they serve; they have developed close relationships with these communities, and share similar experiences to members of those communities (Torres, Labonté, Spitzer, Andrew, & Amaratunga, 2014). While many CHWs are selected through formal hiring processes, some are recruited because employers know of their work in the community. CHWs require many skills, but a key one is their ability to advocate with and/or for communities regarding access to health services, and social programs, such as housing, childcare, and food security. Many CHWs establish collaboration between communities and local systems and work to build community capacity by giving voice to clients (potential patients) and citizens who otherwise have no voice.

Community Health Workers—*Promotores* in Mexico

Hector G. Balcazar Ana Bertha Perez Lizaur, Ericka Escalante Izeta, Maria Angeles Villanueva—Universidad Ibero Americana:

The Health Promotion Operational Model developed in 2006 provides a platform from which the CHW model can be best examined in contemporary Mexico. Mexico, a country like many in the Americas, is burdened with an increase of chronic diseases such as obesity, diabetes, and cardiovascular disease. Mexico is responding to these challenges with strategies in public health, and medical care, and community outreach mobilization aimed at all levels of health promotion and disease prevention. The CHW model in Mexico has seen key developments, especially along the Mexico–U.S. border. Also, community-based participatory research which involves community members and CHWs is popular.

Brazil's Agentes Comunitários de Saúde

Estelle Regina Dutra Prado, MS—Seção de Assistência Nutricional/Coordenadoria de Saúde Ocupacional e Prevenção/Secretaria de Serviços Integrados de Saúde/Superior Tribunal de Justiça:

Lay health workers had been providing health education and basic care to poor communities in the Amazon and the Northeast of Brazil since the 1950s. In the 1980s, they carried out a Catholic Church—based program that taught basic hygiene and nutrition to poor women with children, thus contributing to a successful decrease in Brazilian infant mortality rate. But it was the need to reform a medical- and hospital-centered health model that led the Brazilian government to create the *Programa de Agentes Comunitários de Saúde* (*PACS*, Community Health Workers Program) in 1991. This federally funded program was incorporated to the *Estratégia de Saúde da Família* (*ESF*, Family Health Strategy) in 1994 (Morosini, Corbo, & Guimarães, 2007; Santos, Pierantoni, & Silva, 2010) and deploys CHWs to provide much-needed health education and social services to local households in communities throughout the country.

Village Health Workers in the Vietnam Health Care System

Nguyen Thi Thanh Ha, Institute of Population, Health, and Development, Vietnam:

It is reported that approximately 70 percent of Commune Health Stations (CHS) in Vietnam have a doctor and almost 80 percent are reported to have volunteer Village Health Workers (VHWs) (World Health Organization and Ministry of Health, 2012). Village Health Workers volunteers are members of the community who receive training from the provincial health service, often at the district level, to cope with the most common medical needs of the members of the village. During the past few years, the government has revived and promoted the Village Health Worker strategy of providing a minimum of health care to the people living in more remote areas. Village Health Workers are supposed to assist with immunizations, antenatal care, and family planning programs, advise about clean water and sanitation, and offer simple treatments to people in remote villages.

South Africa

Rosemary Blake, PhD Candidate—Department of Social Anthropology, University of Cape Town:

During apartheid the public health system in South Africa reflected the racist ideology of its government. When the African National Congress (ANC), led by Nelson Mandela, became the first democratically elected government in 1994, it inherited a health care system characterized by deep fragmentation and stark inequalities in health care access and the distribution of resources (Coovadia, Jewkes, Sanders, & McIntyre, 2009). On the new government's agenda was a plan to radically reform the health system, and

(continues)

(continued)

to this end they shifted the health system away from an emphasis on hospital-based, curative medicine that was accessible to only a minority toward a system focused on primary and preventative health care and accessible to all South Africans (through the decentralization of many services). Initially, CHWs were excluded from the new system. It was only in 2003, prompted by a severe human resource shortage, and in the grips of a massive HIV/AIDS and TB epidemic, that the Department of Health began to officially support CHW programs. In the mid-1990s there were only 5,600 CHWs working in South Africa, but by 2011 this number had risen dramatically to 72,839 (Malan, 2014). CHWs now provide a variety of services within the health system, but the vast majority of their work responds to the high burden of communicable diseases in South Africa, particularly HIV/AIDS and TB. They deliver essential services through their work as home-based caregiver lay counselors, antiretroviral (ART) adherence counselors, and directly observed therapy (DOT) supporters for patients with tuberculosis.

2.4 CHWs in the United States

CHWs have an important role to play in the United States that is increasingly being recognized. In both health care and in community-based settings, CHWs work in partnerships with community members and other health and human services providers with the goal of improving health and access to systems of care. CHWs carry out many or all of the roles described at the start of this chapter (and textbook) to do this work. For example, in their role of cultural mediator, they can help make health and social service systems more culturally competent. Often the communities they represent have traditional healing systems that were developed long before Western medicine developed. Now the two systems coexist, with individuals and families integrating what they consider the best from both systems to maintain or improve their health. These systems take many forms. For example, in American Indian communities, traditional healers such as medicine men were and are an important part of health networks (Mohatt & Eagle Elk, 2000). In Latino communities, *curanderos* assist in promoting health in the community (Brown & Fee, 2002; Gonzalez and Ortiz, 2004; Reyes-Ortiz, Rodriguez, & Markides, 2009; Rothpletz-Puglia, Jones, Storm, Parrott, & O'Brien, 2013). CHWs help to bridge these worlds. They help to increase the two-way flow of information so that both providers and those they serve can identify ways to best support health gains and use formal medical and social prevention and treatment services. CHWs do the same to increase understanding of other social, political, and economic issues. This bridging role of CHWs is just one of the many ways CHWs help those whom they serve and ultimately help address health equity and improve health.

Many different groups recognize the potential and importance of CHWs in health promotion and disease prevention. Public health and other health professionals recruit and partner with individuals who are connected to the natural helping networks in their communities (Eng & Young, 1992; Gilkey, Garcia, & Rush, 2011) supporting them in developing skills as a formal CHW. CHWs address many health and social issues, sometimes prioritized by community members themselves, as well as issues identified by those serving communities. Health care systems and community-based agencies are increasingly hiring and integrating CHWs to serve within teams in public health departments, hospitals, community clinics, or other sites. Other CHWs contribute on a volunteer basis in these settings and in community centers and social and faith-based organizations. In these cases, programs often provide incentives such as educational credits or modest financial stipends to CHWs to support their participation. About one-third of formal CHW programs are volunteer based, while the rest are paid CHW programs (Rosenthal et al., 1998; U.S. Department of Health and Human Services, Human Resources and Services Administration, 2007).

CHWs' FORMAL EARLY HISTORY IN THE UNITED STATES: 1950–2000

In the 1950 and 1960s, the first documented volunteer and paid CHW programs established in the United States emerged. During this period, Native American tribes and migrant farmworkers became the best-known programs (Giblin, 1989; Gould & Lomax, 1993; Hoff, 1969; Meister, Warrick, de Zapien, & Wood, 1992). Strong CHW programs still serve these communities today.

The Federal Migrant Act of 1962 required federally qualified migrant clinics to conduct outreach in migrant labor camps. CHWs were hired to provide this outreach, a move that established many CHW programs. This outreach built on the *promotor(a)* tradition common in Mexico and throughout Latin America, where many farmworkers were raised or have family ties (Mahler, 1978).

The largest program of that period (and still the largest today) got its official start in the late 1960s; the Community Health Representative (CHR) Program. It was established by the Indian Health Services (IHS) with support from the Office of Economic Opportunity in collaboration with American Indian tribes (Indian Health Service, n.d.; Indian Health Service, 2006; Satterfield & Burd, 2002). The CHR program has stood the test of time, and there have been more than 1,600 CHRs serving more than 250 tribes for nearly 50 years. It is estimated that there are still over 1,400 CHRs serving today. Since the program began, many tribes have taken over their federal healthcare funding from I.H.S., and they now oversee and manage their tribe's health programs. In doing this they have also made decisions about whether to keep their CHR programs and then manage them directly. Like all CHWs, CHRs address many health issues including maternal and child health, asthma, diabetes, and other chronic disease management. In all CHR programs, tribal leaders select the issues they will prioritize and the roles CHRs will play. Due to great distances in rural reservation communities, CHRs also often assist families with transportation to health care providers.

In the 1960s and 1970s, new CHW programs continued to develop throughout U.S. rural and urban communities. CHW programs addressed important public health issues, and at the same time they were often credited with creating valuable employment opportunities for people who had a hard time entering the paid workforce (Domke & Coffey, 1966). The Office of Economic Opportunity invested in CHWs in many urban areas (Meister, 1997). CHWs and other community-based workers were seen as critical to the reorganization of the human services system (Pearl & Reissman, 1965). CHWs were recognized for their connection to the community and their unique insight into the individuals they served (Withorn, 1984).

In this period, opportunities for paid and volunteer CHWs and *promotores* increased and were hailed as contributing to the reorganization of health and human services delivery systems (Pynoos, Hade-Kaplan, & Fleisher, 1984; Service & Salber, 1977). CHWs were paid to work across a range of health projects and programs targeting different issues and populations (Hoff, 1969; Potts & Miller, 1964; Wilkinson, 1992). In this era, groups like the Black Panther Party and the Young Lords advocated for the government to provide free health care, including prevention services, and accessible services to treat drug addiction for African American, Latino, and all oppressed peoples. The Black Panthers also created free breakfast programs for schoolchildren and free medical clinics for their communities (Black Panther Party Research Project, 2009; Brand & Burt, 2006).

CHWs were an important part of the early years of Community Health Centers (CHC) (Northwest Regional Primary Care Association, 2015) beginning in the mid 1960s, helping to first establish these clinics and tie them to communities. Today, many CHCs integrate CHWs into their health promotion and other community programming where they help to assure that CHC achieve their mission of delivery culturally competent and community-centered services (NACHC, 2010; Spiro, Marable, & Collins, 2012).

In the 1970s, Service and Salber (1977) started to use the term "lay health advisors" (LHAs) and called attention to the important community roles of LHAs, such as health promotion, social support, mediation (helping two sides reach an agreement), and community empowerment (Salber, 1979).

In the 1980s, funding for job creation programs slowed, and the number of paid CHWs participating in forums such as the American Public Health Association declined. At the same time, a number of CHW programs expanded their roles. Programs for migrants grew with funding from private and government sources (Booker, Grube-Robinson, Kay, Najjera, & Stewart, 2004; Harlan, Eng, & Watkins, 1992; Meister, Warrick, de Zapien, & Wood, 1992). The number of CHWs making home visits to aid mothers and infants increased (Julnes, Konefal, Pindur, & Kim, 1994; Larson, McGuire, Watkins, & Mountain, 1992; McFarlane & Fehir, 1994; Poland, Giblin, Waller, & Hankin, 1992). The federal Healthy Start program began to rely on outreach workers to address inequalities in infant mortality rates, especially in cities among African Americans mothers and infants. CHWs also started supporting community members at risk for chronic conditions or diseases (for example, high blood pressure, cancer, diabetes) to maintain better control, keep appointments with and talk to their doctors, check their blood pressure and blood sugar levels, and know the signs of serious illness (Brandeis University, 2003; Brownstein et al., 2005; Norris, Chowdhury, & Van Le, 2006).

In this same period the emergency of HIV-AIDS challenged and motivated activists to organize and advocate for civil rights protections and investment in community health outreach, education, and testing programs, research into treatments, and access to quality health care. Perhaps the best-known activist organization was the AIDS Coalition to Unleash Power (ACT UP), founded in 1987. ACT UP built on the protest traditions that came out of the civil rights movement and opposition to the Vietnam War (Klitzman, 1997). Activists were successful in building strategic alliances with health and public health professionals, in drawing public attention to HIV/AIDS, in advocating for changes to public policies and the creation of new public health programs and research on treatments for HIV disease. As a result, local health departments and community-based organizations began to hire CHWs to conduct outreach and provide client-centered education, counseling, and HIV-antibody-testing services. CHWs conducted home and hospital visits, facilitated support groups, trained physicians and other providers in providing culturally competent care, initiated syringe exchange programs, and much more. With the development of the AIDS epidemic in the United States "a disease [became] the basis of a political movement" (Klitzman, 1997). The success of CHWs in aiding to address the HIV epidemic in turn influenced the development of the CHW field.

In the 1990s, CHWs gained increased recognition for their important contributions to health and job creation (Rosenthal et al., 1998; Witmer, Seifer, Finocchio, Leslie, & O'Neil, 1995). Jobs creation was pushed by Welfare Reform, which brought with it renewed federal attention and resources. Welfare-to-work programs explored CHW jobs as an important option for individuals newly entering or re-entering the paid workforce. CHW program coordinators reminded all involved of the importance of looking for individuals who were already known to be natural aides in their communities when recruiting CHWs (Aguirre & Palacio-Waters, 1997).

From 2000 on, workforce studies, articles, and reports about CHWs became more common (Love et al., 2004; Proulx, 2000a, 2000b; Matos, Findley, Hicks, Legendre, & Do Canto, 2011). At the same time, public and private grant funding for CHW programs continued to grow, focusing on assisting individuals in managing health conditions such as HIV disease, diabetes (Norris, Chowdhury, & Van Le, 2006; Tang et al., 2014) high blood pressure (Allen, Dennison, Himmelfarb, Szanton, & Frick, 2013; Brownstein et al., 2007; CDC, 2015a), cancer, and asthma (Margellos-Anast et al., 2012; Prezio, Pagán, Shuval, & Culica, 2014) and other health areas (Guide to Community Preventive Services, 2015).

During this period, we began to learn more about the work of CHWs and the evidence base grew. A colorectal cancer navigation program designed for Hispanic men showed an increase in life expectancy by six months for participant as compared to nonparticipants with a health care savings of $1,148 per program participant (Wilson, Villareal, Stimpson, & Pagan, 2015). Interventions incorporating CHWs have been found to be effective for improving knowledge about cancer screening, as well as screening outcomes for both cervical and breast cancer (Viswanathan et al., 2007). Integrating CHWs into multidisciplinary health teams has emerged as an effective strategy for improving the control of asthma, diabetes, and high blood pressure among high-risk populations, along with cost savings (CDC, 2015a). With this growing evidence base showing the impact that CHWs make, interest in developing the CHW workforce has continued to grow.

2.5 Interview with CHW Yvonne Lacey

FROM THE FRONT DOOR TO THE HEAD OF THE TABLE

After nearly 40 years of formal service as a CHW beginning in the 1970s, Yvonne Lacey retired as coordinator of the City of Berkeley, California, Black Infant Health Program in 2007. She played a key role in the development of the CHW Certificate Program at City College of San Francisco where she was a frequent guest lecturer and trainer during the first two years of the program. She served as the CHW cochair of the National Community Health Advisor study from 1994–1998 and led a group of CHWs and their allies within the American Public Health Association at the turn of the century. From 2004–2006 she again cochaired a national project with CHW Durrell Fox that looked at key considerations for CHW education in community colleges (chw-nec.org).

It was a pleasure to work with Yvonne in these last three roles, supporting her in helping to increase understanding and recognition of the CHW field. The following is an excerpt from an interview with Yvonne conducted in the spring 2008; thanks to CCSF staffer Mickey Ellinger for making this possible (www.ccsf.edu).

"I've Been Doing This Work All My Life"

Yvonne Lacey: As I think back over my history, I realize that I've been doing this work all my life. I live by this old song I heard in church as a child: "If I can help somebody as I pass along, then my living shall not be in vain."

Back when I was a dressmaker, friends would come to my shop so I could help fix a zipper or a hem, and we'd end up talking about daily problems and relationships and all that. There wasn't a week that went by that I didn't have women in there helping each other get through our daily lives.

In October 1970, I was sewing out of my home. A friend called and said, "I saw the perfect job for you!" I finally went down to the City of Berkeley's Department of Public Health and got hired as a CHW for maternal and child health. My life has never been the same.

The Maternity and Infant Care Program provided prenatal care to low-income women. It was one of the most comprehensive programs that I have ever seen up to today. There was a social worker, two CHWs, a public health nurse, a nurse practitioner, and doctors who took rotation in our clinics. That's where I learned the team concept of delivering health services. That's when I began to love this community health work. I began to really see what we could do in the community to make a difference.

Although I began the work knowing my community, I gained years of experience and training on the streets of Berkeley. I also got an education from a cherished mentor public health nurse in the department—although we fought constantly.

In the early 1990s, City College of San Francisco was planning a course for CHWs and they recruited CHWs to be on the planning committee. We were planning the curriculum and trying to see the benefits of having a course, and what CHWs would get from it. In 1993, I contributed as a guest lecturer and trainer for the first groups of CHW students. I did that for two years.

After that experience I really got involved with building the CHW profession. Many of us worked so hard to get more recognition for CHWs (through the American Public Health Association. When I first started attending APHA meetings in 1996, CHWs were called the "New Professionals." In 2000, we convinced APHA to change the group's name to the CHW Special Primary Interest Group (SPIG). I chaired that group for three years. It is my opinion that the chair of any CHW group has to be a CHW, not an advocate for CHWs.

From 1994 to 1998, we worked on the National Community Health Advisor Study. I was the cochair of the 36-member advisory committee that included a large group of experienced CHWs. We are the only ones who really know the work that we do. With our voices we can make sure that the value of the work is known and recognized and with our voices we can lead the way to more investment in our communities.

In 2004, I was asked to cochair the CHW National Education Collaborative (CHW NEC; Proulx, Rosenthal, Fox, & Lacey, 2008). C). It was trying to bring community colleges together to have a standard competency-based training that covers the basic things that all CHWs need to know. We also helped colleges understand that CHWs have to be at the table at every stage of developing our profession. CHWs have to help plan the trainings and be involved in the teaching. Maybe having a mentorship program built into that training. I wouldn't want CHWs to lose touch with their own communities, or lose the fire and passion they have just because they earn a degree. Also, we want these colleges to understand they are training CHW leaders.

It was such rewarding work—the work I did in my 37 years at the Berkeley Health Department and at the national level. You don't always see the results of the work right away. But I've gone to get gas and somebody's come up to me and said, "You're Miss Lacey, aren't you? You helped me during such and such." Or, "If it hadn't been for you I wouldn't have gone back to school." Or, "I only had that one baby, Miss Lacey, because you told me . . . " And sometime around the country I have had that same kind of confirmation from CHWs that somehow, I have touched their lives. That has made it all worthwhile. "I did touch somebody's life here." And to me that has been worth the whole thing.

2.6 Trends in the CHW Field: Growing Strong in the New Millennium

The CHW field has been increasingly recognized in the United States as evidenced by the development of public policy related to CHWs in numerous states (CDC, 2013; State Reform, 2015), activities in federal agencies in support of CHWs (CDC, 2014; Office of Minority Health, 2015), and attention to CHWs in peer review literature, in the press, and on social media (Goldfield, Rosenthal, & Macinko, 2011). With the nation's focus in health care on the often-cited "triple aim" of improved health outcomes, improved experience of care, and efficiency related to costs, interest in CHWs is not surprising. CHW services have sought to address all three aims with promising impacts documented (Findley et al., 2014). The Patient Protection and Affordable Care Act passed by the Obama Administration in 2010 also brings increased attention to CHWs and the roles they have in improving access to care and in the delivery of prevention services. Related new regulations has begun to open up more opportunities for the sustainability of CHW services (Witgert et al., 2014).

With this promising horizon in place for CHWs, let's explore what trends are influencing development in the field in this period.

RESEARCH: BUILDING THE EVIDENCE BASE ABOUT THE WORK OF CHWs

Through the 1990s, researchers conducted a number of regional and national studies of CHWs. Together, these studies demonstrated the power, value, and importance of the work that CHWs have been doing in the United States in a form that could be understood by the fields of public health and medicine.

As noted earlier, the NCHAS (Rosenthal et al., 1998) was carried out in collaboration with many partners including CHWs. The NCHAS was a participatory research project, meaning the group being studied participated in designing the study, and in analyzing and interpreting findings. CHWs comprised the majority of the NCHAS advisory council members, and the council alone was responsible for making recommendations based on the data for the field. Many of the actions recommended by the 36 council members are now being implemented throughout the United States. These include increased access to CHW educational programs that offer college credit, and the controversial recommendation to credential CHWs.

In addition to identifying the core roles and competencies of CHWs, the study also identified the many community and clinical settings where CHWs work, including homes, schools, clinics, and hospitals. The settings in which CHWs work clearly influence the activities of CHWs. According to the California Workforce Initiative, CHWs working in clinics are more likely to perform duties focused on traditional patient care, whereas CHWs working door to door act more in the roles associated with social workers and community organizers (Keane, Nielsen, & Dower, 2004).

Early workforce studies in the San Francisco Bay Area (Love, Gardener, & Legion, 1997) inspired other regions and states to conduct similar assessments to determine the extent and roles of CHWs in local labor markets. The Annie E. Casey Foundation funded another study of the CHW workforce, looking at the potential of worker-owned CHW cooperatives (Rico, 1997). More recently, the federal government funded and coordinated the CHW National Workforce Study (HRSA, 2007). The study explored the roles and functions of CHWs in different settings and estimated that there were 120,000 CHWs throughout the United States in 2005.

In 1995, a commentary entitled "Community Health Workers: Integral Members of the Health Care Work Force" appeared in the *American Journal of Public Health* (Witmer, Seifer, Finocchio, Leslie, & O'Neil, 1995). The article's title alone stimulated attention to the field. The Institute of Medicine's landmark book, *Unequal Treatment: Confronting Racial and Ethnic Disparities in Health Care*, talked about the importance of CHWs in reducing health inequalities (Smedley, Stith, & Nelson, 2002). A study funded by the Centers for Medicare and Medicaid Services (CMS) on approaches to cancer prevention among elders of color found that CHWs were the "primary mechanism for cultural tailoring" (Brandeis University, 2003).

Over the years, research has continued to document the evidence of the effectiveness of CHWs in promoting health outcomes (Giblin, 1989; HRSA, 2007; Nemcek & Sabatier, 2003; Swider, 2002). In 2007, CHWs, researchers, and other stakeholders met to develop a CHW Research Agenda by and for the field (Rosenthal, De Heer,

Rush, & Holderby, 2008). At this two-day conference led by Carl Rush, conference participants identified the most important areas for additional research (complete findings may be accessed online at www.famhealth.org/researchagenda.htm):

- CHW cost-effectiveness or return on investment
- CHW impact on health status
- Building CHW capacity and sustaining CHWs on the job
- Funding options
- CHWs as capacity builders
- CHWs promoting real access to care

Practitioners, policy makers, and researchers continue to examine the workforce. Minnesota and Massachusetts have taken comprehensive approaches to the development of policy regarding CHWs and conducted studies of their workforce to guide their thinking. The accomplishments of these two states in implementing systems changes to build capacity for an integrated and sustainable CHW workforce serve as models for the nation (Rosenthal et al., 2011).

In 2010, an influential report by the Massachusetts Department of Public Health was released entitled the "Community Health Workers in Massachusetts: Improving Health Care and Public Health" (Massachusetts Department of Public Health, 2009). The report presented strong evidence that the state's nearly 3,000 CHWs have improved access to health care as well as the quality of that care. It also presented 34 recommendations for further integrating CHWs into health care and public health services in the state. It suggested that state policy changes—including workforce development and training, occupational regulation, guidelines for research and evaluation, and sustainable financing—are needed to promote and sustain CHWs services. CHWs have also been included in the State CHW Certification Act of 2010, and a regulatory process for certifying individual CHWs and approving CHW training programs is being developed at the state's Department of Public Health. CHWs are part of a priority program strategy in Massachusetts for strengthening clinical-community linkages to improve chronic disease outcomes (Mason et al., 2011).

Minnesota initiated studies to better understand their CHW workforce (Willaert, 2005). Support from the Minnesota Community Health Worker Alliance, coupled with widespread recognition of the cost-effective care provided by CHWs, resulted in the development of state legislation in 2008 that authorizes hourly reimbursement for CHWs. As a result, CHWs who have graduated from the standardized curriculum and received a certificate are eligible to enroll under the Minnesota Health Care Plans and can provide services—supervised by a physician, advanced practice nurse, dentist, or public health nurse—that are billable to Medicaid. Mental health providers have also been added to this list.

In 2013, the U.S. Centers for Disease Control and Prevention identified 15 states and the District of Columbia that had laws addressing CHW infrastructure, professional identity, workforce development, and financing (CDC, 2013). Of these 15 states, six had advisory boards working to investigate the impact of CHWs on health care savings and health disparities, eight had created a CHW scope of practice, seven had laws authorizing Medicaid payments for some CHW services, and seven had created laws that encouraged the integration of CHWs into team-based care models for select health care organizations and services. Alaska, Minnesota, and, most recently, New Mexico, support CHW services with Medicaid financing.

Additionally, states and organizations (e.g., CHW Network of New York, California, Virginia, Community Health Foundations, Foundations for Health Generations, American Association of Diabetes Educators) have developed reports on a variety of CHW issues such as scope of practice, training, financing, and cost effectiveness. These and other states continue to explore options for supporting CHW integration and sustainability. New research studies on workforce issues help inform those who are trying to integrate CHWs into health care teams and sustain their employment (O'Brien, 2009; Volkman & Castanares, 2011).

A new 2014 ruling by the Center for Medicare & Medicaid Services (CMS) allows states to develop payment systems for preventive services by unlicensed individuals such as CHWs. The new ruling helps improve people's access to preventive services, aids the partnerships between health care providers and advocates for CHWs, increases access to CHWs, reduces program costs, and has the potential for CHWs to be reimbursed under

Medicaid. States must include a summary of the qualifications of CHWs, their required training, education, experience, and credentialing or registration. Credentialing of CHWs is not required by CMS (CDC, 2015b, 2015c).

The Centers for Medicare and Medicaid Services Innovation Center (CMMI) funded projects from 2013–2016 to work on models that reduce costs, improve care for populations with special needs, test approaches to transform clinic models, and improve the health of populations by focusing, for example, on diabetes or hypertension prevention programs that go beyond clinics. Many of the funded projects center on CHWs. For example, Oregon was given a grant to test the effects of its Coordinated Care Organizations (CCOs) and new payment model on health outcomes and costs. All of the CCOs have integrated CHWs into their care teams (Foundation for Health Generation, 2013).

Research on the work of CHWs is key to making the case for bringing more resources to the field. Furthermore, an emerging role for CHWs is to participate in conducting research, for, with, and about the communities they serve. Durrell Fox observes that CHWs have an important role to play in conducting research; he observed that that CHWs have already informed research and public health theories and science for decades (Rosenthal, De Heer, Rush, & Holderby, 2008) and will continue to do so.

A Look at How Research Can Influence Policy

J. Nell Brownstein

Taking a close look a the evolution of research on a single health topic: A snapshot about CHWs helping people control high blood pressure.

During my work at the Centers for Disease Control and Prevention (CDC), I learned of several research studies focused on CHWs' efforts in helping people control high blood pressure (also called hypertension). Uncontrolled high blood pressure is a major risk factor for stroke and heart and kidney disease. Most of the existing studies were carried out by researchers at Johns Hopkins University. I invited those researchers to join me in writing a paper (Brownstein et al., 2005) in which we gave a summary of the research involving CHW work and made recommendations for future research and practice. We recommended that CHWs be included in health care teams and in community-based research to allow CHWs to play an important role in helping to reduce disparities in heart disease and stroke. We noted that what was needed was sustainable funding and reimbursement for CHW services, better use of CHW skills, improved CHW supervision, training and career development, policy changes, ongoing education, and a reporting of CHW program costs. Since then, other researchers, agencies, program developers, evaluators, practitioners, and other CHW stakeholders have addressed these issues through meetings, reports, and new studies. A new tool from CDC can help inform people about the strengths and limitations of the CHW policies. www.cdc.gov/dhdsp/pubs/docs/chw__evidence_assessment_report.pdf

In 2007, I was the lead author of a team that conducted a systematic literature review of the effectiveness of CHWs in the care of persons with high blood pressure. Our review showed that most of the patients had significant improvements in blood pressure because CHWs helped people keep medical appointments and stay on their prescribed medicines.

This paper influenced the 2010 Institute of the Medicine Report (A Population-Based Approach to Prevent and Control Hypertension) that recommended that the CDC work with state partners to bring about policy and systems changes that result in trained CHWs ". . . deployed in high-risk communities to help support health living strategies that include a focus on hypertension."

In 2013, the CDC gave states the opportunity to work on (a) integrating CHWs into health care teams to support self-management and ongoing support for adults with high blood pressure and diabetes, (b) having

(continues)

A Look at How Research Can Influence Policy

(continued)

CHWs lead or support diabetes self-management classes, and (c) having CHWs promote linkages between health systems and community resources for adults with high blood pressure and diabetes.

In 2015, the CDC's Community Preventive Task Force released the results of its systematic review of 23 CHW hypertension studies. It recommends "interventions that engage community health workers to prevent cardiovascular disease (CVD). There is strong evidence of effectiveness for interventions that engage community health workers in a team-based care model to improve blood pressure and cholesterol in patients at increased risk for CVD. There is sufficient evidence of effectiveness for interventions that engage community health workers for health education, and as outreach, enrollment, and information agents to increase self-reported health behaviors (physical activity, healthful eating habits, smoking cessation) in patients at increased risk for CVD."

I have developed and supported others to develop resources to support CHWs, including technical assistance and a heart disease and stroke prevention training, and *fotonovelas* about blood pressure and sodium and cholesterol in English and Spanish (www.cdc.gov/dhdsp/pubs/chw-toolkit.htm). Additional trainings can be found at www.nhlbi.nih.gov/health/healthdisp/aa.htm.

2.7 Capacity Building and Education

Capacity building refers to strengthening the knowledge, skills, and confidence of individuals—like CHWs—or communities. CHWs learn from many sources and in many settings, and these keep changing over time.

CHW TRAINING GUIDES AND CURRICULA

Many training guides and educational curricula have been developed for CHWs. Some educational resources are shared freely, while other training materials are proprietary and are not made available by the individuals and organizations that developed them. Publicly and privately developed curricula address specific health issues, such as diabetes, heart health, cancer, HIV/AIDS, and prenatal health. In the early 1990s, the National Commission for Infant Mortality developed a curriculum for maternal and child CHW programs that included a training manual, a CHW pocket manual, and even a community guide to starting CHW programs. Though issue specific curricula are still very common, there appears to be a shift to curriculum that develops core or foundational CHWs skills. In Minnesota, a core curriculum on CHWs was developed collaboratively by educators, employers, and CHWs in that state (Willaert, 2005); that curriculum was designated as a required curriculum for CHWs seeking reimbursement by the state. As states have begun to formalize regulations for CHWs, some have considered the option of a single curriculum but more have chosen to identify core competencies and play a role in approving a range of curricula (Miller, Bates, & Katzen, 2014) to address these areas. As of 2015, no single CHW curriculum, book, or textbook for CHWs has been adopted throughout the United States, but some resources have been widely used. *Helping Health Workers Learn*, developed by the Hesperian Foundation, has been popular, especially in international settings (Werner & Bower, 1982). The City College of San Francisco developed the textbook you are now using. This is the first textbook specifically developed for use by CHWs in classroom settings. It was first released in 2009 and now this second edition is being updated in 2014–2015. *The book itself is of historic significance, especially for the U.S. CHW field.*

ON-THE-JOB LEARNING

On-the-job learning (also known as on-the-job training) has been a mainstay of CHW education (HRSA, 2007). In the early days of the field in the U.S., CHW program coordinators often developed CHW trainings in their own organizations (Rosenthal et al., 1998). These trainings were accessible to working CHWs, and employers covered the costs. It meant that CHWs could be selected directly from communities due to the qualities that would make them good CHWs versus their prior formal learning (Jennings, 1990). This meant high access to the field for CHW candidates. At the same time, training on the job requires significant resources from each employer. CHWs also reported that on-the-job training was a barrier to career development, because it is not recognized when they moved from one job to another (Rosenthal et al., 1998). Additionally, some CHWs and administrators reported that on-the-job training was too limited and even off-base (Love et al., 2004).

Today it appears to be increasingly common for CHWs to come into a paid CHW position having completed their core training from a community college or in a CHW training center or program (Rosenthal et al., 2011). In this way, employers are largely freed from covering CHW educational costs. In some cases, however, employers sponsor their CHWs to go through these educational programs. Also, many employers take responsibility for CHW continuing education, scheduling trainings and covering the time and costs associated with participation for their staff or volunteers. In the state of Massachusetts, organizations receiving public funds for CHW services are required to support ongoing training and CHW networking opportunities.

APPRENTICESHIPS FOR CHWs, IN THE CLASSROOM AND ON THE JOB

On-the-job learning is closely related to the skills development approaches that are found in professions where training is based on an apprenticeship model, in which a professional called a "journeyman" (or woman) mentors an apprentice. In the United States, the Department of Labor runs a formal system of Registered Apprenticeships (http://www.dol.gov/apprenticeship/). The apprenticeship model has certain standards and blends a required classroom component with a significant on-the-job learning component. It also requires that apprentices be paid and provides an incentive for increased pay during the apprenticeship training period. Due to collaborative efforts in the state of Texas, in 2011, the Department of Labor officially accepted the CHWs workforce as eligible for apprenticeship opportunities. Find out more through the Department of Labor (n.d.). Texas did a pilot test of the model with a small number of apprentices in rural Texas under the coordination of the Coastal AHEC. At the time of this writing, several states including Wisconsin and Rhode Island are actively exploring developing CHW apprenticeship programs.

CENTER-BASED AND COLLEGE-BASED CHW EDUCATIONAL APPROACHES

In the 1990s, there was a move toward center-based trainings (rather than on-the-job training), as well as college-supported educational programs for CHWs. An early example of center-based training comes from Boston's Community Health Education Center, developed by the City of Boston to respond to a citywide need for CHW capacity building. Since the 1990s, the center has provided core initial training to CHWs. It has also been a resource center for training and other materials and has served as a gathering place for CHWs, hosting activities like job-sharing luncheons.

Early in their history, efforts were made in some areas to assist CHWs to gain access to academic pathways and credit within college programs. Early reports of CHWs in academic settings showed that there were challenges in the college setting; some CHWs felt their competence gained through life experience and experience on the job were undervalued (Sainer, Ruiz, & Wilder, 1975).

City College of San Francisco started a CHW Certificate Program in the early 1990s. The program, designed to address some of these challenges and barriers, offered the first full-scale college credit–earning educational opportunity for CHWs (Love et al., 2004). Building on this model and other emerging programs, Project Jump Start at the University of Arizona (1998–2002) focused on creating credit-bearing training for CHWs through four Arizona community colleges predominately serving rural communities (Proulx, 2000b). During 2004–2008, CHWs, allies, and representatives of 22 CHW college-based educational programs formed the CHW National Education Collaborative (CHW NEC) to advise college-based CHW programs about best practices for such programs (Proulx, Rosenthal, Fox, Lacey, & CHW NEC, 2008). The project saw CHW leadership as imperative, and its majority CHW Advisory Council and cochairs Lacey and Fox were important to the project. I (Lee Rosenthal) served as the project's codirector along with Director Don Proulx and Coordinator Nancy Collyer. In 2008, as the CHW NEC project came to an end, we generated a guidebook for the field, looking at ways colleges and other institutions can start and strengthen CHW educational and capacity-building programs.

HOW DOES THE ORGANIZATION OF CHW TRAINING AND EDUCATION IMPACT THE FIELD?

Many of the skills and personal qualities needed to excel as a CHW can be learned on the job and through life experience. The skills that lead to success in higher education do not, in themselves, translate into job effectiveness as a CHW. Veteran CHWs have often been suspicious of college-based training programs: the typical college classroom is not an avenue that is open to all community people. In addition, it is common in the health workforce that higher education credentials are set as a requirement for employment. This can limit access to employment for CHWs who are highly skilled but lack formal education. Specifically, *requirements* for college-based programs may present barriers to and adversely affect the very communities with the greatest potential to be outstanding CHWs, including low-income communities, communities of color, undocumented immigrant communities, and English language learners. At the same time, college credit and education are closely linked to employment outcomes, career advancement, and higher income. Well-designed educational programs that are accessible and that offer college credit to CHWs can provide these students with valuable opportunities for professional growth and advancement.

Many in the CHW field believe it is important to maintain multiple approaches to CHW education and training and to develop ways to recognize and credit the value of life and job experience. To the extent that college-based training becomes more widespread, it is important to ensure that these programs are accessible to CHWs financially and in their preferred teaching and learning approaches. See www.chw-nec.org to learn about "Key Considerations" for starting or strengthening CHW educational programs (Proulx, Rosenthal, Fox, Lacey, & CHW NEC, 2008). It is also important to make sure that employers continue to support and fund CHW training and education, which historically has been an important ingredient for success in the field, maintaining access to many CHWs who are, and who continue to become outstanding CHWs.

THE USE OF TECHNOLOGY AND ONLINE EDUCATION

The CHW field has some curricula and training resources that are offering online CHW education, both in real time and self-paced. Resources in the online environment come from both public and private sources. Some are offered at no cost, while others have associated fees and, in some cases, credits. No matter what the cost, online or distance education training means that there are more resources available for CHW learning that may be especially valuable for CHWs in geographically isolated communities. In using online training curricula it is important to consider how this high-tech approach may impact what we could call the "high touch" role of CHWs. Generating a hybrid plan for face-to-face learning time and online education still seems the best fit for CHWs.

CHW CREDENTIALING

Many health occupations use credentialing in some form, including certification and licensure, in an effort to assure that workers have the knowledge and skills necessary to do their jobs. Credentials may be administered by a public entity, such as a state health department, or by a free-standing organization led by members of the occupation itself, or by another interested organization. Credentialing may directly certify individuals (nurses, social workers, or CHWs) or may credential programs (agencies, clinics, training programs, institutions) and training curriculum. Trainers may also be certified. In some cases all of these strategies are used.

Credentialing has been a controversial issue in the CHW field (Keane, Nielsen, & Dower, 2004; National Human Services Assembly, 2006; Rosenthal et al., 1998). Some feel that credentialing will support the ongoing effort to increase recognition and respect for CHWs, and to create stable sources of funding for CHW positions. Others question or oppose credentialing because they feel that it may make the field too bureaucratic and weaken the strong ties and allegiance that CHWs have to the community. Others are concerned that it may keep people from becoming CHWs who would otherwise have the necessary commitment, knowledge, and skills. For example, many CHWs have had an experience, such as felony drug convictions, that would disqualify them from receiving a credential if the process is modeled after those of other professions. At the same time, individuals with this background may be the best fit for working with marginalized communities that could fall through the cracks without CHWs whose life experience provides a meaningful connection. There are also concerns that credentialing is driven by the norms of other health care professionals rather than a genuine understanding of CHW work and a desire to strengthen the field.

In spite of these concerns, it is increasingly common for states to pursue approaches to formally certify CHWs and/or the agencies where they work. Funds from the CDC for managing chronic diseases (CDC, 2015a) provide

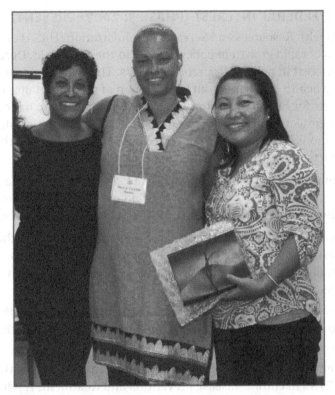

A CHW earns her certificate from City College of San Francisco.

states with the opportunity to address issues related to integrating CHWs into health care teams, having CHWs lead diabetes self-management courses, and having CHWs become critical links between health care systems and community resources. The first state to formally establish a CHW credentialing programs was Texas, in 2001. The credential is coordinated by the Department of Health Services with a committee that includes certified CHWs (Nichols, Berrios, & Samar, 2005). In 2003, Ohio adopted a credentialing program regulated by the state Board of Nursing. Groups in other states are considering credentialing at various levels, including credentialing individual CHWs, their trainers and/or curricula, and CHW programs.

Numerous other states have started or begun planning for ways to monitor CHWs. In some states, like Florida, a network of CHWs has taken the lead in creating and administering CHW certification, diminishing the role of the state in this process. Other states like Massachusetts are choosing voluntary certification in recognition that certification, in some cases, may prevent able CHWs from serving as CHWs. To learn more about what states are doing to establish credentialing and related processes see the following interactive maps:

National Academy for State Health Policy:

www.nashp.org/state-community-health-worker-models/

Association of State and Territorial State Health Officials:

www.astho.org/Public-Policy/Public-Health-Law/Scope-of-Practice/CHW-Certification-Standards/

2.8 CHW Policy Initiatives and Sustainability

Numerous policy changes over the past several decades have helped to shape the CHW field. To better understand these changes, CHW advocate Carl Rush has divided the history of CHW policy into five phases. See a description of the most recent phase below. To learn about the first four phases, please link to our online supplement.

Carl Rush has worked for and with community health workers for close to 20 years. He serves as a core team member of the Project on CHW Policy and Practice at the University of Texas' Institute for Health Policy, and has supported numerous state and national studies on CHW employment policy.

EXPLOSION OF STATE AND FEDERAL INTEREST (PHASE 5: 2007–PRESENT)

The publication by the U.S. Health Resources and Services Administration (HRSA) of the CHW National Workforce Study launched a period of rapid growth in policy activity in the CHW field. During this period, several trends helped to stimulate interest in policies favorable to CHWs. These include a new emphasis on increasing health equity (or reducing health disparities), an appreciation of the importance of "social determinants of health," and renewed efforts for health care reform or transformation at the national level, including the establishment of the Patient Protection and Affordable Care Act (ACA). The period also has seen more concerted efforts to integrate CHW positions into ongoing financing of public health and health care, to move away from short-term grants and contracts to finance paid CHW positions.

- In 2007, the State of Minnesota submitted a Medicaid State Plan Amendment to authorize reimbursement for CHW "self-management education" services to Medicaid recipients. The State specified completion of a standard training curriculum as a requirement for CHWs to be Medicaid "providers."

- In 2009, the Office of Management and Budget published a series of changes to the Standard Occupational Classification, used to classify employment data from employers and the Census. Effective in 2010, the system now includes "community health worker" as a distinct occupation (SOC 21-1094). The revision produced record numbers of comments, many from CHWs.

- Licensing was ruled out in three states as a means of credentialing CHWs. Licensing boards in New York, Massachusetts, and Virginia all declined to consider licensing of CHWs, finding that there is minimal risk of harm to the public from the work of CHWs.

- During this period, the Centers for Disease Control and Prevention (CDC) dramatically increased their emphasis on the role of CHWs in chronic disease prevention and treatment, funding numerous demonstration projects and the creation of specialty training curricula for CHWs in fields like diabetes and heart disease. The CDC's National Center for Chronic Disease Prevention and Health Promotion included in their strategic priorities encouraging policy and system change to increase employment of CHWs, and published several policy briefs and reports related to evidence-based policy.

- State legislation calling for task forces to recommend CHW policies was passed in Massachusetts in 2010 (creating a CHW Board of Certification), and rapidly passed in early 2014 in New Mexico, Illinois, and Maryland. Many other states created CHW policy initiatives during the period, most of these with active sponsorship and/or participation by state government officials. By mid-2015 almost all states had some form of CHW policy initiative underway.

- Several states have created new policy initiatives involving CHWs, such as Oregon's "Coordinated Care Organizations" and a pilot of Medicaid funding of CHWs in 14 primary care practices in South Carolina.

- Federal interest in CHWs led to the development of numerous committees and work groups:

  - The Office of Minority Health convened a committee in 2010 to examine the role of CHWs or *promotores* among Hispanic residents of the United States; the U.S.-Mexico Border Health Commission helped to convene that group.

  - The Centers for Disease Control and Prevention established a CHW Work Group in 2011 (CDC, 2014).

  - In 2011, the U.S. Department of Health and Human Services (HHS) Office of Minority Health convened staff to support the National Promotores Initiative by promoting *promotores de salud* and recognizing their efforts in strengthening underserved Hispanic communities. A *promotores de salud* steering committee (with 15 *promotores* members) was to provide feedback and guidance on support for *promotores*. This work group and its steering committee are still active.

  - The HHS Interagency CHW Work Group grew out of the *promotores* workgroup in 2014. HHS staff share information and resources to keep Work Group members informed about CHW programs, projects, and trends so they can better serve states, grantees, and others. Work Group members helped plan and presented at the 2014 Unity Meeting.

- This period has been capped (2014) by a Medicaid rule change allowing payment for preventive services by "nonlicensed" individuals. At this writing many states are considering how to use this provision to authorize more sustainable employment for CHWs under Medicaid.

To see more CHW Policy History (Phases 1–4) adapted from the CHW National Workforce Study (2007), see the online supplements to the *Foundations for CHWs* textbook at http://wileyactual.com/bertholdshowcase.

2.9 Convening CHWs: Networks and Conferences

CHWs have organized local, state, and national networks out of the belief that they must have a strong voice in shaping the field as it evolves and to provide mutual support, mentoring, and peer learning.

Durrell Fox, Founder of the Massachusetts Association of CHWs

In 2001 there was a crisis in public health funding in my state [Massachusetts] that deeply impacted CHWs. We had emergency budget cuts. Our state had new and long-standing outreach and prevention programs with evidence of effectiveness. Some programs that had a full year of funding were notified that funding was cut in half. Some programs were notified on a Wednesday that by Friday they would have no more funding. They had to close and lay off staff, including CHWs. We began to see a pattern where CHWs were the first to go and last to know.

Since some CHWs were already connected through training and networking we got together and said, "We've got to do something." We created the Massachusetts Association of CHWs (MACHW) to build strength, support, independence, and sustainability for CHWs. At the time, CHWs were not paid well, were disenfranchised and disconnected. We had maternal child health outreach workers, HIV outreach workers funded by different agencies and not communicating with each other. You could be in a housing development stepping over other outreach workers who might be dealing with some of the same families yet have no communication or coordination with them. This was crazy and inefficient. We didn't have enough resources to have six CHWs serving one family. So MACHW brought CHWs together to learn about what each other was doing and what communities they served. We began to do strategic planning to help CHWs be more efficient and effective.

MACHW linked up with a couple of training programs, one in Boston (CHEC) and in Worcester (Outreach Worker Training Institute [OWTI] in Worcester), and that's where we developed a way to have CHWs coming together from across the state to network, support, and learn from each other.

NATIONAL AND REGIONAL NETWORKS

There are many national groups in the United States that assist in regularly convening CHWs. The names of the groups, and their size and capacity, have varied with funding over the years, but each group works to provide leadership and opportunities for CHW networking and sharing.

The APHA CHW Special Primary Interest Group (CHW SPIG)

In 1970, 500 CHWs and their supporters joined together within the American Public Health Association in what was then called the New Professionals Special Primary Interest Group (SPIG). The name, the "New Professionals," was chosen in protest against the many terms used to describe them, including *nonprofessional, subprofessional, aide, auxiliary,* and *paraprofessional* (Bellin, Killen, & Mazeika, 1967; D'Onofrio, 1970; Murphy, 1972). In the year of their formation, the New Professionals wrote:

> For too long, non-degreed health workers have been left out of the mainstream of planning for the delivery of health services and [have] gone without recognition and reward. . . . It is our hope that the National New Professional Health Workers will be able to change the status of workers across the country and thereby improve the health of the nation. (American Public Health Association, 1970)

In the 1980s, membership and activity in the SPIG declined. In the 1990s, the SPIG membership was small, and it was held together by long-time CHW member and SPIG leader Ruth Scarborough. At that stage, those working in the field across the country were looking for a way to stay connected, and in the early 1990s we began to rebuild the SPIG. Many CHWs and allies played a role in this effort in the 1990s, and the group grew strong once again. We worked together to create a visible niche within APHA for CHWs. Many CHW allies (including the authors of this chapter) and CHWs worked together to build the SPIG. Yvonne Lacye, a CHW leader in the late 1990s, pushed for the New Professional SPIG to become the CHW SPIG. A few years later, with another push under the leadership of Sergio Matos and Lisa Renee Holderby Fox, the CHW SPIG became the CHW Section, which meant we now had a greater number of members and were a bigger part of APHA.

Moving forward since the new millennium, the CHW SPIG once again grew and as of early 2015, we are few hundred short of 1,000 members. With growth of the Section its committees have become stronger and taken on important tasks of working on issues impacting CHWs both inside and outside APHA.

The National Association of Community Health Representatives

The National Association of Community Health Representatives (NACHR and pronounced "nature") is a network of CHRs and CHR coordinators across the country. It was established in the 1970s to be the voice of what is now more than 1,700 CHRs serving their tribal communities. This association has twelve service areas. Their leadership structure includes having lead representatives from each of these 12 health service regions. They coordinate the activities of NACHR in collaboration with the Indian Health Service. For many years NACHR held its national meetings once every three years, when more than 1,000 CHRs gathered to learn about other health issues and programs as well as to honor leadership and longevity in the CHR program. Currently, meetings are less frequent, but NACHR regional leaders work together to connect CHRs across the country, and national meetings are still being held. Some of the 12 regional CHR networks meet regularly to explore issues in their area. Find out more at www.nachr.net.

The Center for Sustainable Health Outreach and the Unity Conference

Beginning in 2000, CHWs began meeting under the auspices of the National Center for Sustainable Health Outreach (CSHO), a partnership between Southern Mississippi University ("CSHO south") and Georgetown University Law School in Washington, D.C. ("CSHO north"). After nearly a decade of collaboration, the CSHO partnership ended, but the Unity Conference lives on bringing together CHWs every one to two years in various cities across the U.S. Dr. Susan Mayfield Johnson continues to coordinate the meetings with funding from various sources.

In the past, several other CHW groups were active, including the following:

The National Association of Hispanic CHWs

The National Association of Hispanic CHWs grew out of the CHW National Network Association, based in Yuma, Arizona, at the regional Western Area Health Education Center. The association was established in Arizona for the southwestern states in 1992; it grew to include people from other regions, including the Midwest and New England, eventually becoming a national network. The annual conference was held primarily in Spanish along with simultaneous translation of selected sessions. In 2007, the organization announced that it would officially focus on Hispanic promoters while maintaining its interest in all CHWs. At the time of this writing it is no longer active, but its legacy lives on with many *promotores* actively networking at the state level and participating in national meetings on behalf of CHWs.

The American Association of CHWs

CHWs and allies came together in 2006 to explore development of a national CHW leadership organization. The CSHO (noted above) staff team played an important role in supporting this strategic network development meeting and Unity meetings provided an important networking forum. The meeting led to the development the American Association of Community Health Workers (AACHWs). Though the network's efforts were not sustained long term, many important lessons can be learned from its efforts and can inform any future efforts to develop or restart other regional and national networks. The group left the legacy of a Code of Ethics that it established (referenced in Chapter 7). Over its few years of collaboration the association focused on organizing issues generally and around providing support for regional and national efforts to promote CHW sustainability.

To learn more about AACHW, read the thoughts of two CHWs, Durrell Fox and Sergio Matos, that follow. Both were among the group of committed CHWs who were active in AACHW when it was active.

A Look Back at the Rise and Decline of the American Association of Community Health Workers (AACHW)

Durrell Fox and Sergio Matos:

In honor of the *Foundation for Community Health Workers* textbook, two well-known leaders of the U.S. CHW field, Durrell Fox and Sergio Matos, share their reflections on the rise and decline of the first broad-based multicultural national association for and by CHWs. Their reflections were written in response to a series of questions about the strengths and challenges that AACHW faced during its several years of active development. The majority of their response can be found in the online supplement to the Foundations for CHWs textbook. Below you will find comments by Fox and Matos to give you an understanding of AACHW.

To put these critical reflections in context, Durrell Fox, who led AACHW for several years and who helped found the Massachusetts Association of CHWs, shares a brief overview of the early hopes of those involved in the creation of the CHWs' association.

Durrell Fox, Responding to the Question: What Was the AACHW?

The American Association of Community Health Workers (AACHW) is currently dormant but not forgotten, and there is a possibility to revisit what it stood for to make sure it fits today's climate. AACHW was a concept and a hope, some might say a dream that grew out of over six years of CHW-led dialogs and organizing meetings during a range of national meetings, including the Unity Conference (for CHWs) and American Public Health Association (APHA) as well as during some local and statewide CHW meetings. Over those six years, approximately 200 CHWs alongside approximately 50 allies and partners, talked about the need for a unified CHW-led national association that could lead national CHW workforce development and sustainability efforts, while connecting the many state and local CHWs networks and associations to advance national advocacy and policy development in an equitable way. One of the driving forces behind developing a CHW-led national association was a belief in the importance of CHW self-determination. This need was identified in a time when some cities and states were moving forward with CHW workforce development and credentialing without CHW participation or leadership in decision making.

For many years, I was honored to coordinate and facilitate some of the CHW national organizing meetings. Other CHW leaders volunteered their time as well since we had no funding support, but we did receive some in-kind contributed support from several agencies in the form of meeting space. Extensive notes were taken during the meetings and shared widely across the country. These notes included consensus agreements on proposed structure, leadership, and governance for a diverse, independent, CHW-led national association.

In 2006 the Harrison Institute for Public Law at the Georgetown University Law Center and the Center for Sustainable Health in Mississippi were able to use some of the information from the CHW national organizing meetings to successfully apply for Foundation funding to support staff who could dedicate time to advance efforts to develop a CHW national association. The inaugural meeting of AACHW was convened in September 2006 in Potomac, Maryland. Over 50 CHWs, allies, and partners from more than one dozen states developed a steering committee, an interim leadership structure, proposed governance structure, and plans to appoint and advisory board. A decision was made to move forward with a CHW steering committee made up entirely of CHWs and plan to activate an advisory board. Within a few months of the meeting, there was drop-off in participation for various reasons, including participants losing employment, leaving the field, and being busy working on critical local and statewide CHW organizing and workforce development issues. One year after the inaugural AACHW meeting, less than 50 percent of the original steering committee members were still fully engaged and active.

(continues)

A Look Back at the Rise and Decline of the American Association of Community Health Workers (AACHW)

(continued)

Participation continued to dwindle in AACHW over a few years and allies would check in but after several years it became clear that AACHW was not able to survive as an organization at that time. Given that, we look back now at lessons learned from AACHW, some of which may serve the CHW field today.

Reflections on AACHW from Sergio Matos, Active in the AACHW Leadership and a Lead in the New York City CHW Association, on the Road Ahead:

The climate for advancing the CHW workforce is much different today from what it was in 2006 and 2007. Early local and regional organizing has progressed in the absence of a national AACHW. Numerous states have developed and implemented workforce standards and regulatory processes—often in the absence of CHW leadership. The Affordable Care Act and its mandates for improved outcomes at lower cost have piqued interest in the CHW workforce. The recent ruling by the Centers for Medicare and Medicaid Services (CMS) to allow reimbursement for preventive services delivered by nonlicensed staff has also driven much activity at the state level to establish workforce standards for the CHW practice. Increasing attention to the importance of addressing the social determinants of health, especially in emerging health reform innovations such as Patient-Centered Medical Homes, health homes, and Accountable Care Organizations, has also fueled interest in the CHW workforce. In short, the issues of importance today are different from what they were in 2006. Today we are more concerned with regulatory oversight of our practice and preserving the integrity of our work. As health care and state systems gain interest in our work, they also venture to define and govern our practice. Although this is a completely unprofessional approach, it is not uncommon for people and organizations in power. In addition to being unprofessional, it is quite illogical for the very systems that have failed to achieve the triple aim to govern our practice and its integration with inter-professional health care teams. A small number of states in which CHWs have, in fact, surrendered their self-determination provide valuable lessons learned and strategies to avoid.

Fortunately, CHWs have been able to advance a policy agenda and continue the battle for self-determination through activities at the APHA CHW Section. We have gained consensus on a national definition and issued policy statement with APHA supporting that definition. We have gained our own unique standard occupational classification with the U.S. Department of Labor. We have issued numerous policy positions though APHA in support of the CHW workforce and CHW self-governance. The scientific evidence supporting our work has exploded over the past five years. Much more evidence exists supporting our scope of practice, our impact on improved outcomes, and the business case for CHW interventions.

In spite of these advances, the need for an independent professional association is greater now than it has ever been. Forces beyond our control stand poised to co-opt our practice for their own purposes. Our principal challenge in the coming years will be to preserve the integrity of our work. Only a self-governing association can accomplish that goal.

REGIONAL AND STATE NETWORKS

There are numerous CHW regional, state, and city-level CHW networks throughout the United States.

One group that has focused at the state level has recently seen itself as providing networking activities at the regional level. That group is *Vision y Compromiso,* a California-based network. The network works to bring together *promotores* and networks of *promotores* for annual conferences, assuring language access in Spanish at those meetings. Their annual conference is well attended. Additionally, within California they work with regional partners to develop a well-connected network. At their 2014 annual conference, four state networks of *promotores* and Community Health Workers explored some ways in which their networks can come together. The participating networks represent large communities of *promotores* and Community Health Workers; working or volunteers, affiliated with or independents with local, regional, and state organizations that support

Spanish-speaking families in rural and urban communities. They currently represent the states of Washington, Nevada, Arizona, and Colorado. *Vision y Compromiso* plans to support these networks with leadership, training, and advocacy activities.

As noted in the discussion of national networks, tribal Community Health Representatives are part of regional networks across 12 Indian Health Service regions. Some regions are more active than others and all connect back to their larger national association, NACHR. Working at the regional level, tribes can exchange insights about more local issues and examine how they are participating in their various states in other CHW organizing activities. For example in the New Mexico/outer Colorado region CHRs are sharing about CHRs' role in New Mexico's state policy developments and can see how that may impact their practice and anticipate such activities in Colorado through their exchange.

Much of the networking activity in the CHW field takes place in state-level networks. The first statewide network of U.S. CHWs was formed in the early 1990s in New Mexico as the New Mexico Community Health Worker Association. About the same time, the Oregon Public Health Association formed a committee on CHWs that was chaired by CHWs. This committee provided leadership at the state level and nationally by working as a part of the Oregon Public Health Association.

Over several decades CHW networks have formed in many states including Arizona, California, Florida, Maryland, Massachusetts, Minnesota, Mississippi, New York, Texas, and Virginia, to name a few. In some states, regional and issue-specific networks have been established so a number of states have more than one network, with Texas currently having eleven small regional networks.

Some cites also have networks of CHWs such as the CHW Network of NYC. At the time of this writing there are close to 50 state and regional CHW networks in the United States. In 2015, discussion about again forming a national association made up of those networks is again underway (see the Fox and Matos reflections on the rise and decline of the American Association of CHWs that formally began its launch in 2006). Networks clearly have a role to play in helping the field develop.

THE VALUE OF CHW NETWORKS

By joining together in regional, state, and national networks and associations, CHWs are taking leadership in the development of the field, defining their roles, establishing new standards, research priorities, educational and training models, and advocating for greater recognition and increased funding to support the valuable contributions of CHWs. Visit the website of the American Public Health Association Community Health Worker Section to help you find local, regional, and national contacts: www.apha.org/apha-communities/member-sections/community-health-workers.

If you cannot find a contact at the website, reach out to other colleagues to be sure there is not a newly forming group or a longstanding one in need of your energy and input.

If there really is not a network of CHWs in your area, maybe it is time for you to start one!

Chapter Review

1. Why is it so hard to develop a common definition of CHWs and CHW roles and competencies?

2. How could a common definition of roles and competencies benefit the CHW field?

3. What has been the role of CHW leaders in defining and developing the CHW field?

4. Why is academic research about CHWs important to developing the CHW field? What are research priorities for the CHW field?

5. How are developments in CHW training, education, and credentialing shaping the CHW field? Why are these developments controversial?

6. How do CHW networks develop and why are they important to the future of CHWs in the United States?

7. Are there CHW networks in your city, county, or state? How can you get involved?

References

Aguirre, A., & Palacios-Waters, A. (1997). El Rio Colorado border vision. *Fronterieza*. Video. San Luis, AZ.

Allen, J., Dennison, C., Himmelfarb, D., Szanton, S., & Frick, K. (2013). Cost-effectiveness of nurse practitioner/community health worker care to reduce cardiovascular health disparities. *Journal of Cardiovascular Nursing, 29*(4), 1–7.

American Public Health Association. (1970). *Minutes.* New Professionals Special Primary Interest Group. Washington, DC: American Public Health Association.

American Public Health Association. (2009). *Support for community health workers to increase health access and to reduce health inequalities.* Policy 20091. Retrieved from www.apha.org/policies-and-advocacy/public-health-policy-statements/policy-database/2014/07/09/14/19/support-for-community-health-workers-to-increase-health-access-and-to-reduce-health-inequities

American Public Health Association. (2014). *Support for community health worker leadership in determining workforce standards for training and credentialing.* Retrieved from www.apha.org/policies-and-advocacy/public-health-policy-statements/policy-database/2015/01/28/14/15/support-for-community-health-worker-leadership

Bellin, L. Killen, E. M., & Mazeika, J. J. (1967). Preparing public health subprofessionals recruited from the poverty group lessons from an OEO work-study program. *American Journal of Public Health, 57,* 242–252.

Black Panther Party Research Project. (2009). Stanford University. Retrieved from http://web.stanford.edu/group/blackpanthers/

Booker, V., Grube-Robinson, J., Kay, B., Najjera, L. G., & Stewart, G. (2004). *Camp health aide program overview.* Working paper. Saline, MI: Migrant Health Promotion 5.

Brand, W., & Burt, C. (2006, October 8). A legacy of activism: Behind fury, black panthers laid course for social programs. *Oakland Tribune.*

Brandeis University. (2003). *Evidence report and evidence-based recommendations: Cancer prevention and treatment demonstration for ethnic and racial minorities.* Retrieved from www.cms.gov/Medicare/Demonstration-Projects/DemoProjectsEvalRpts/downloads/cptd_brandeis_report.pdf

Brown, T. M., & Fee, E. (2002). Voice from the past: Sidney Kark and John Cassel: Social medicine pioneers and South African emigrés. *American Journal of Public Health, 92*(11), 1744–1745.

Brownstein, J. N., Bone, L. R., Dennison, C. R., Hill, M. N., Kim, M. T., & Levine, D. M. (2005). Community health workers as interventionists in the prevention and control of heart disease and stroke. *American Journal of Preventive Medicine, 29*(5S1), 128–133.

Brownstein, J. N., Chowdhury, F. M., Norris, S. L., Horsley, T., Jack, L., Zhang, X., & Satterfield, D. (2007). Effectiveness of community health workers in the care of people with hypertension. *American Journal of Preventive Medicine, 32*(5), 435–447.

Centers for Disease Control and Prevention. (2013). *State law fact sheet: a summary of state community health worker laws.* Retrieved from http://www.cdc.gov/dhdsp/pubs/docs/chw_state_laws.pdf

Centers for Disease Control and Prevention. (2014). *How the Centers for Disease Control and Prevention (CDC) Supports Community Health Workers in Chronic Disease Prevention and Health Promotion.* Retrieved from www.cdc.gov/dhdsp/programs/spha/docs/chw_summary.pdf

Centers for Disease Control and Prevention. (2015a). *Addressing chronic disease through community health workers: A policy and systems-level approach.* Retrieved from www.cdc.gov/dhdsp/docs/chw_brief.pdf

Centers for Disease Control and Prevention. (2015b). *Technical assistance guide: States implementing community health worker strategies.* Retrieved from www.cdc.gov/dhdsp/programs/spha/docs/1305_ta_guide_chws.pdf

Centers for Disease Control and Prevention. (2015c). *Community health worker toolkit.* Retrieved from www.cdc.gov/dhdsp/pubs/chw-toolkit.htm

Community Health Worker Initiative of Sonoma County. (n.d.). *CHW job titles.* Retrieved from http://chwisc.org/CHW_Job_Titles.html

Coovadia, H., Jewkes, R., Sanders, D., & McIntyre, D. (2009). The health and health system of South Africa: Historical roots of current public health challenges. *The Lancet, 374*(9692), 817–834.

Department of Labor. (n.d.) *Apprenticeship USA.* Retrieved from *http://www.dol.gov/apprenticeship/*

Dieleman, M., Cuong, P. V., & Anh, L. V. (2003). *Identifying factors for job motivation of rural health workers in North Viet Nam.* doi: *10.1186/1478-4491-1-10.* Retrieved from *www.ncbi.nlm.nih.gov/pmc/articles/PMC280735/*

Domke, H. R., & Coffey, G. III. (1966). The neighborhood-based public health worker: Additional manpower for community health services. *American Journal of Public Health 56*, 603–608.

D'Onofrio, C. N. (1970). Aides—pain or panacea? *Public Health Reports 85*(9), 788–801.

Eng, E., & Young, R. 1992. Lay health advisors as community change agents. *Family and Community Health, 15*, 24–40.

Findley, S., Matos, S., Hicks, A., Chang, J., & Reich, D. (2014). Community health worker integration into the health care team accomplishes the triple aim in a patient-centered medical home: A Bronx tale. *The Journal of Ambulatory Care Management, 37*(1), 82–91.

Foundation for Health Generation. (2013). *Community Health White Paper: Report and Recommendations.* Retrieved from *www.healthygen.org/sites/default/files/2013%20Revised%20%20White%20Paper_Healthy%20Gen.pdf*

Giblin, P. T. (1989). Effective utilization and evaluation of indigenous health-care workers. *Public Health Reports, 104*, 361–368.

Gilkey, M., Garcia, C. C., & Rush, C. (2011). Professionalization and the experience-based expert: Strengthening partnerships between health educators and community health workers. *Health Promotion Practice, 12*(2), 178–182.

Goldfield, R., & Macinko, J. (Eds.). (2011). *The Journal of Ambulatory Care Management.* Special Issues on Community Health Workers. CHWs: Taking Their Place in Systems of Care (Vol. 34; No. 3) July-September 2011 & CHWs (Vol. 34; No. 4) October-December 2011.

Gonzalez Arizmendi, L., & Ortiz, L. (2004). Neighborhood and community organizing in Colonias: A case study in the development and use of *Promotoras. Journal of Community Practice, 12*(1/2), 23–35.

Gould, J., & Lomax, A. (1993). Evolution of peer education: Where do we go from here? *Journal of American College Health, 41*(6), 235–240.

Guide to Community Preventive Services. (2015). *Cardiovascular disease prevention and control: Interventions engaging community health workers.* Retrieved from *http://www.thecommunityguide.org/cvd/CHW.html*

Harlan, C., Eng, E., & Watkins, E. (1992, May 10–15). *Migrant lay health advisors: A strategy for health promotion.* Paper presented at the Third International Symposium: Issues in Health, Safety and Agriculture, Saskatchewan, Canada.

Hoff, W. (1969). Role of the community health aide in public health programs. *Public Health Reports, 84*(11), 998–1002.

Human Resources and Services Administration. (2007). *Community health worker national workforce study.* U.S. Health and Human Services Administration, Bureau of Health Professions. Retrieved from *http://bhpr.hrsa.gov/healthworkforce/supplydemand/publichealth/*

Indian Health Service. (n.d.). *General CHR background: History and background development of the program.* Retrieved from http://www.ihs.gov/chr/index.cfm?module=history

Indian Health Service. (2006). U.S. Department of Health and Human Services, Community Health Representative Program. Retrieved from *www.ihs.gov/chr/*

Jennings, W. (1990, October). Barriers to employment for public health assistance recipients. Presented at the American Public Health Association, New York.

Julnes, G., Konefal, M., Pindur, W., & Kim, P. (1994). Community-based perinatal care for disadvantaged adolescents: Evaluation of the Resource Mothers Program. *Journal of Community Health, 19*(1), 41–53.

Keane, D., Nielsen, C., & Dower, C. (2004). *Community health workers and promotores in California.* San Francisco, CA: Center for the Health Professions.

Klitzman, R. (1997). *Being positive: The lives of men and women with HIV.* Chicago, IL: Ivan R. D.

Larson, K., McGuire, J., Watkins, E., & Mountain, K. (1992). Maternal care coordination for migrant farmworker women: Program structure and evaluation of effects on use of prenatal care and birth outcome. *Journal of Rural Health, 8*(2), 128–133.

Lehmann, U., Friedman I., & Sanders, D. (2004). *Review of the utilisation and effectiveness of community-based health workers in Africa.* Working paper of the Joint Learning Initiative. Retrieved from *www.rmchsa.org/wp-content/resources/resources_by_theme/MNCWH%26NSystemsStrengthening/ReveiwUse%26Effectivenes-sOfCHWsInAfrica.pdf*

Love, M. B., Legion, V., Shim, J. K., Tsai, C., Quijano, V., & Davis, C. (2004). CHWs get credit: A ten-year history of the first college-credit certificate for community health workers in the United States. *Health Promotion Practice, 5,* 418–428.

Love, M. B., Gardener, K., & Legion, V. (1997). Community health workers: Who they are and what they do: A survey of eight counties in the San Francisco Bay Area. San Francisco Department of Health Education, San Francisco State University. *Health Education and Behavior, 24,* 510–522.

Maathai, W. (2006). *Unbowed: A memoir.* New York, NY: Knopf.

*Malan, M. (2014). Analysis: Why policy is failing community health workers. *Mail and Guardian.* Retrieved from *http://mg.co.za/article/2014-09-04-why-policy-is-failing-community-health-workers*

Margellos-Anast, H., Gutierrez, M. A., Whiteman, S. (2012). Improving asthma management among African-American children via a community health worker model: Findings from a Chicago-based pilot intervention. *Journal of Asthma, 49*(4), 380–389.

Mason, T., Wilkinson, G. W., Nannini, A., Martin, C. M., Fox, D. J., & Hirsch, G. (2011). Winning policy change to promote community health workers: Lessons from Massachusetts in the health reform era. *American Journal of Public Health, 101*(12), 2211–2216.

Matos, S., Findley, S., Hicks, A., Legendre, Y., & Do Canto, L. (2011). Paving a path to advance the community health worker workforce in New York state: A new summary report and recommendations. The New York State Community Health Worker Initiative. Retrieved from *http://nyshealthfoundation.org/uploads/resources/paving-path-advance-community-health-worker-october-2011.pdf*

Mahler, H. (1978). Promotion of PHC in member countries of WHO. *International Health, 93,* 107–113.

McFarlane, J., & Fehir, J. (1994). *De madres a madres:* A community, primary health care program based on empowerment. *Health Education Quarterly, 21*(2), 381–394.

Meister, J. S., Warrick, L. H., de Zapien, J. G., & Wood, A. H. (1992). Using lay health workers: Case study of a community-based prenatal intervention. *Journal of Community Health, 17,* 37–51.

Meister, J. S. (1997). Community outreach and community mobilization: Options for health at the U.S.-Mexico border. *Journal of Border Health, 2*(4), 32–38.

Miller, P., Bates, T., & Katzen, A. (2014). Community health worker credentialing: State approaches. Center for Health Policy and Innovation. Harvard Law School. Retrieved from www.chlpi.org/wp-content/uploads/2014/06/CHW-Credentialing-Paper.pdf

Mohatt, G., & Eagle Elk, J. (2000). *The price of a gift: A Lakota healer's story.* Lincoln: University of Nebraska Press.

Morosini, M. V., Corbo, A. D., & Guimarães, C. C. (2007). O agente comunitário de saúde no âmbito das políticas voltadas para a atenção básica: concepções do trabal he da formação profissional. *Trabalho, educação e saúde, 5*(2), 261–280.

Murphy, M. A. (1972). Improvement of community health services through the support of indigenous nonprofessional. *New York State Nurses Association, 3,* 29–33.

Massachusetts Department of Public Health. (2009). *Community health workers in Massachusetts: Improving health care and public health.* Retrieved from *www.mass.gov/eohhs/docs/dph/com-health/com-health-workers/legislature-report.pdf*

Ministry of Health of Vietnam. (2006). *Vietnam Health Report 2006.* Retrieved from: *http://jahr.org.vn/downloads/ Nghien%20cuu/Khac/Vietnam%20National%20Health%20Report%202006.pdf*

Ministry of Health of Vietnam. (2008). *Joint Annual Health Review 2007.* Retrieved from *http://jahr.org.vn/downloads/ JAHR2007-EN.pdf*

National Association of Community Health Centers. (2010). *Community health centers lead the primary care revolution.* Retrieved from *www.nachc.com/client/documents/Primary_Care_Revolution_Final_8_16.pdf*

National Human Services Assembly. (2006). *Community health workers: Closing the gap on family's health resources.* Family Strengthening Policy Center. Washington, DC: National Human Services Assembly.

Nemcek, M. A., & Sabatier, R. (2003). State of evaluation: Community health workers. *Public Health Nursing, 20,* 260–270.

Nichols, D. C., Berrios, C., & Samar, H. (2005, November). Texas's community health workforce: From state health promotion policy to community-level practice. *Preventing Chronic Disease 2* (special issue). Retrieved from *www.cdc.gov/pcd/issues/2005/nov/05_0059.htm*

Norris, S. L., Chowdhury, F. M., & Van Le, K. (2006). Effectiveness of community health workers in the care of persons with diabetes. *Diabetic Medicine, 23*(5), 544–556.

Northwest Regional Primary Care Association. (2015). *Celebrating 50 years in the American community health center movement. Our vision remains the same: A conversation with Dr. Jack Geiger.* Retrieved from *www.nwrpca. org/?page=chc50th_anniversary*

O'Brien, M. J., Squires, A. P., Bixby, R. A., & Larson, S. C. (2009). Role development of community health workers: An examination of selection and training processes in the intervention literature. *American Journal of Preventive Medicine, 37*(6 Suppl 1). S262–S269.

Office of Minority Health. (2015). Promotores de salud/Community health workers. Retrieved from *www.cdc.gov/ minorityhealth/promotores.html*

Pearl, A., & Riessmann, F. (1965). *New careers for the poor: Nonprofessionals in human service.* New York, NY: Free Press.

Poland, M. L., Giblin, P. T., Waller, J. B., & Hankin, J. (1992). Effects of a home visiting program on prenatal care and birthweight: A case comparison study. *Journal of Community Health, 17*(4), 224–229.

Potts, D., & Miller, C. W. (1964). Community health aide. *Nursing Outlook, 12,* 33–35.

Prezio, E. A., Pagán, J. A., Shuval, K., & Culica, D. (2014). The Community Diabetes Education (CoDE) program: Cost-effectiveness and health outcomes. *American journal of Preventive Medicine, 47*(6), 771–779.

Proulx, D. E. (2000a). Arizona's Project Jump Start: A community college/AHEC partnership. *National AHEC Bulletin 17*(Spring/Summer).

Proulx, D. E. (2000b). Project Jump Start: A community college and AHEC partnership initiative for community health worker education. *Texas Journal of Rural Health 18*(3), 6–16.

Proulx, D. E., Rosenthal, E. L., Fox, D., Lacey, Y., & Community Health Worker National Education Collaborative (CHW NEC) Contributors. (2008). *Key considerations for opening doors: Developing community health worker educational programs.* Tucson, AZ: University of Arizona. Retrieved from *www.chw-nec.org/pdf/Guidebook.pdf*

Pynoos, J., Hade-Kaplan, B., & Fleisher, D. (1984). Intergenerational neighborhood networks: A basis for aiding the frail elderly. *Gerontologist, 24,* 233–237.

Rico, C. (1997). *Community health advisors: Emerging opportunities in managed care.* Baltimore, MD: Annie E. Casey Foundation and Seedco—Partnerships for Community Development.

Reyes-Ortiz, C. A., Rodriguez, M., & Markides, K. S. (2009). The role of spirituality healing with perceptions of the medical encounter among Latinos. *Journal of General Internal Medicine, 24*(3), 542–547.

Rosenthal, E. L. (2003). *The sustainability dance: Lessons to learn for an emerging force in community health community.* Doctoral dissertation. Boston, MA: University of Massachusetts.

Rosenthal, E. L., De Heer, D., Rush, C. H., & Holderby, L. R. (2008). Focus on the future: A research agenda by and for the U.S. community health worker Field. *Progress in Community Health Partnerships: Research, Education, and Action, 2*(3), 225–235.

Rosenthal, E. L., Wiggins, N., Brownstein, J. N., Johnson, S., Borbon, I. A., Rael, R., . . . Blondet, L. (1998). *The final report of the national community health advisor study: Weaving the future.* Tucson: University of Arizona and Annie E. Casey Foundation. Retrieved from *http://crh.arizona.edu/publications/studies-reports/cha*

Rosenthal, L., Wiggins, N., Ingram, M., Mayfield Johnson, S., & Zapien, J. (2011). Community health workers then and now: An overview of national studies aimed at defining the field. *Journal of Ambulatory Care, 34*(3), 247–259.

Rothpletz-Puglia, P., Jones, V. M., Storm, D. S., Parrott, J. S., & O'Brien, K. A. (2013). Building social networks for health promotion: Shout-out health, New Jersey, 2011. *Preventing Chronic Disease.* doi:10:130018. Retrieved from *www.cdc.gov/pcd/issues/2013/13_0018.htm*

Sainer, E. A., Ruiz, P., & Wilder, J. F. (1975). Career escalation training. *American Journal of Public Health, 65,* 1208–1211.

Salber, E. J. (1979). Lay advisor as a community health resource. *Journal of Health Politics, Policy and Law, 3*(4), 469–478.

Santos, M. R., Pierantoni, C. R., & Silva, L. L. (2010). Agentes Comunitários d Saúde: experiências e modelos do Brasil. *Physis: Revista de Saúde Coletiva, 20,* 1165–1181.

Satterfield, D., & Burd, C. (2002). The "in-between people": Participation of community health representatives in diabetes prevention and care in American Indian and Alaska native communities. *Health Promotion Practice, 3*(2), 166–175.

Service, C., & Salber, E. J. (1977). *Community health education: The lay health advisor approach.* Durham, NC: Duke University.

Smedley, B., Stith, A., & Nelson, A. (2002). *Unequal treatment: What healthcare providers need to know about racial and ethnic disparities in healthcare.* Washington, DC: Institute of Medicine.

Spiro, A., Oo, S. A., Marable, D., & Collins, J. P. (2012). A unique model of the community health worker: The MGH Chelsea community health improvement team. *Family Community Health, 35*(2), 147–160.

State Reform. (2015). *State community health worker models.* Retrieved from *www.statereforum.org/state-community-health-worker-models*

Swider, S. M. (2002). Outcome effectiveness of community health workers: An integrative literature review. *Public Health Nursing, 19*(1), 11–20.

Tang, T. S., Funnell, M., Sinco, B., Piatt, G., Palmisano, G., Spencer, M. S., Kieffer, E. C., & Heisler, M. (2014). Comparative effectiveness of peer leaders and community health workers in diabetes self-management support: results of a randomized controlled trial. *Diabetes Care, 37*(6):1525–1534. doi: 10.2337/dc13-2161.

Torres, S., Labonté, R., Spitzer, D. L., Andrew, C., & Amaratunga, C. (2014). Improving health equity: The promising role of community health workers in Canada. *Healthcare Policy, 10*(1), s71–s83.

U.S. Bureau of Labor Statistics. (2009). *Standard occupational classification. Responses to comments on 2010 SOC, Multiple Dockets.* Retrieved from *www.bls.gov/soc/soc2010responses.htm*

U.S. Department of Health and Human Services, Health Resources and Services Administration. Bureau of Health Professions. 2007. *Community Health Worker National Workforce Study, Rockville, MD.* Retrieved from *http://bhpr.hrsa.gov/healthworkforce/reports/chwstudy2007.pdf*

Viswanathan, M., Kraschnewski, J., Nishikawa, B., Morgan, L. C., Thieda, P., Honeycutt, A., Lohr, K. N., & Jonas, D. (2007). *Outcomes of community health worker interventions.* Evidence Report/Technology Assessment No. 181 (Prepared by the RTI International—University of North Carolina Evidence-based Practice Center under Contract No. 290 2007 10056 I) AHRQ Publication No. 09-E014. Rockville, MD.

Volkman, K., & Castanares, T. (2011). Clinical community health workers: Linchpin of the medical home. *Journal of Ambulatory Care Management, 34*(3), 221–233.

Werner, D., & Bower, B. (1982). *Helping health workers learn: A book of methods, aids, and ideas for instructors at the village level.* Berkeley, CA: Hesperian Foundation.

Wiggins, N., & Borbón, A. (1998). Chapter 3: Core roles and competencies of community health advisors. In *The Final Report of the National Community Health Advisor Study: Weaving the Future* (pp. 15–49). Retrieved from *http://crh.arizona.edu/publications/studies-reports/cha*

Willaert, A. (2005). *Minnesota community health worker workforce analysis: Summary of findings for Minneapolis and St. Paul.* Mankato, MN: Healthcare Education Industry Partnership.

Wilkinson, D. Y. (1992). Indigenous community health workers in the 1960s and beyond. In R. L. Braithwaite & S. E. Taylor (Eds.), *Health issues in the Black community* (pp. 255–266). San Francisco, CA: Jossey-Bass.

Wilson, F. A., Villarreal, R., Stimpson, J. P., & Pagan, J. A. (2015). Cost-effectiveness analysis of a colonoscopy screening navigator program designed for Hispanic men. *Journal of Cancer Education, 30*(2), 260–267. doi:10.1007/s13187-014-0718-7

Witgert, K., Kinsler, S., Dolatshahi, J., & Hess, C. (2014). *Strategies for supporting expanded roles for nonclinicians on primary care team.* National Academy of State Health Policy.

Withorn, A. (1984). *Serving the people: Social services and social change.* New York, NY: Columbia University Press.

Witmer, A., Seifer, S. D., Finocchio, L., Leslie, J., & O'Neil, E. H. (1995). Community health workers: Integral members of the health care work force. *American Journal of Public Health, 85,* 1055–1058.

World Health Organization and Ministry of Health of Viet Nam. (2012). *Health Service Delivery Profile, Viet Nam.* Retrieved from *www.wpro.who.int/health_services/service_delivery_profile_vietnam.pdf*

An Introduction to Public Health

3

Tim Berthold, Janey Skinner, and Sharon Turner

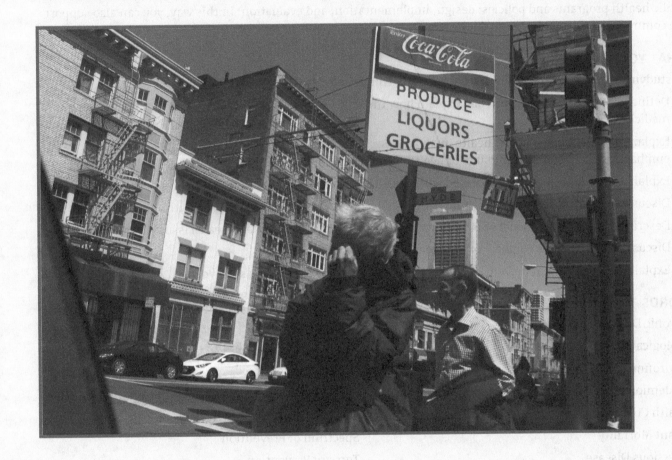

Health care matters to all of us some of the time; public health matters to all of us all of the time.

—*Former Surgeon General C. Everett Koop*

Introduction

This chapter provides a brief introduction to the complex field of public health. We focus on the concepts we believe are most essential to guiding your work as a CHW. If you are new to the practice of public health, you may not be familiar with some of the language used in the field. One of the goals of this textbook is to assist you in becoming more comfortable with public health concepts, so that you can actively participate in all phases of public health programs and policies: design, implementation, and evaluation. In this way, you can also support the communities you work with to do the same.

WHAT YOU WILL LEARN

By studying in the information in this chapter, you will be able to:

- Define health and public health and explain how the field of public health is different from the field of medicine
- Explain how the field of public health analyzes the causes of illness and health of populations and emphasizes the social determinants of health
- Explain why public health is concerned with health inequalities
- Discuss the relationship between promoting social justice and promoting public health
- Describe the ecological model of public health and apply it to specific public health issues
- Discuss public health's emphasis on prevention
- Explain the spectrum of prevention and provide examples for each of the six levels

WORDS TO KNOW

Chronic Disease	Prevalence
Ecological Model	Populations
Environmental Justice	Primary Prevention
Epidemiology	Secondary Prevention
Health Cobenefit	Social Determinants of Health
Infant Mortality	Spectrum of Prevention
Infectious Disease	Tertiary Prevention
Life Expectancy	

3.1 Defining Health

Public health promotes the health and well-being of all people. There are many definitions of *health*. The World Health Organization (WHO) defines *health* as "the complete state of physical, mental, and social well-being, not just the absence of disease" (1948). This widely used definition encourages us to think about health broadly and in positive terms. By including "social well-being," it suggests that an individual's health is linked to the health of his or her family and community. Other definitions of health emphasize additional dimensions, such as emotional, intellectual, occupational, environmental, political, and spiritual health.

- *How do you define health?*

The field of public health embraces the broadest definition of health. The discipline addresses a wide range of issues that influence human health including infections and chronic diseases and disability, as well as challenges such as homelessness, hunger and access to sufficient food, violence, and civil and human rights issues.

To increase health for all, the United States sets national health goals and objectives on a 10-year cycle. *Healthy People 2020* (USDHHS, 2015) establishes four overarching goals and dozens of focus areas. The goals are to:

1. Create higher quality, longer lives.
2. Eliminate health disparities.
3. Create social and physical environments that promote health.
4. Promote quality of life and healthy behaviors across all life stages.

- *What do you think about the public health goals established by the United States?*
- *What do you consider to be the most important public health issues facing the communities you live in and work with?*
- *How do the WHO definition and the Healthy People 2020 goals fit with how you think about health?*

3.2 Defining the Field of Public Health: Key Concepts

The World Health Organization (2015b) defines public health as follows:

> *Public health refers to all organized measures (ether public or private) to prevent disease, promote health, and prolong life among the population as a whole. Its activities aim to provide conditions in which people can be healthy and focus on entire populations, not on individual patients or diseases. Thus, public health is concerned with the total system and not only the eradication of a particular disease.*

To further define and describe the field of public health, this chapter discusses several key concepts.

PUBLIC HEALTH EMPHASIZES PREVENTION

The one word most strongly associated with public health is prevention. Public health focuses on preventing illness or injury before it starts, or as soon as possible in its development. This emphasis on prevention distinguishes public health from medicine, which is more strongly associated with treatment of a health condition after it is identified or diagnosed.

The "upstream story" is frequently used to illustrate this point.

The Upstream Story of Prevention

Four hikers beside a river heard cries for help and saw a man struggling against the current, trying to reach the shore. They managed to save him, but just as they were pulling him to safety, along came a boy in the river, slamming against the boulders. Before they pulled the boy out, two more people swept by: The hikers barely rescued them. Exhausted, they treated the victims. Then they heard another cry for help. One of the hikers said, "That's it—I'm going upstream to investigate." The others said, "You can't! More people will need to be rescued, and we can't do it without you. If you leave, someone might drown." The hiker replied, "I want to find out why they are falling in the river, so we can find a way to stop it!"

Just as the hiker moved upstream to see what could be done to prevent people from falling into the river, public health tries to intervene "upstream" to prevent epidemics from developing in the first place. Money spent on upstream programs and policies that promote social equality and equal access to basic resources will not only save lives; they will aid in preventing the expense of caring for people who would become ill. If we apply this example to the AIDS epidemic, public health emphasizes the importance of investing "upstream" in programs and policies that will prevent new HIV infections.

Primary, Secondary, and Tertiary Prevention

The public health model distinguishes among three different types of prevention. **Primary prevention** is defined as preventing the development of a disease (or other health condition) from occurring—before it starts. Primary prevention measures often are applied to the whole population. **Secondary prevention** involves the early diagnosis and treatment of illnesses or conditions before they become symptomatic or turn into something worse. Targeted prevention programs aimed at high-risk populations (those with serious risk factors or precursors of disease) are considered secondary prevention, too. **Tertiary prevention** involves services for those already living with illness or injury to delay further progression of disease, alleviate symptoms, prevent complications, and delay death. Tertiary prevention often involves treatment, and in this way it overlaps with the role of clinical medicine.

Applied to HIV disease, primary prevention might include comprehensive sex education in schools and safer sex media campaigns. Secondary prevention might include affordable and confidential HIV antibody-testing programs for the early diagnosis of HIV disease, as well as civil rights protections from discrimination in housing and employment and affordable health care for those newly diagnosed. Tertiary prevention might include access to free and low-cost antiretroviral medications (medications used to treat HIV disease) and supportive services (like housing or food) that can delay the progression of HIV disease. At each level of prevention, creating public policies to ensure access to information and services is a key public health function.

PUBLIC HEALTH IS POPULATION BASED

While the field of medicine focuses on the health of individual patients, the field of public health is concerned with the health of large groups of people or **populations**. These populations are usually defined by one or more factors, such as:

- Geographic and political boundaries (ZIP code, city, county, nation)
- Demographic characteristics such as ethnicity, gender, age, and immigration status
- Health-related data on groups with similar patterns of risk factors, illness, injury, disability, or mortality

For example, a population could be defined as women in the United States, Latina women in California, or pregnant Latina women under the age of 21 in the city of Oakland, California.

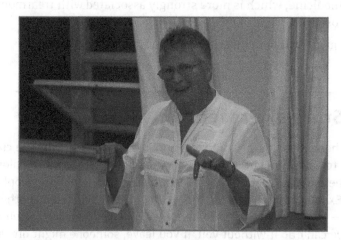

CHWs promote public health through their work with individuals, families, and groups, and at the community level.

- *What populations do you belong to?*

- *Which populations are you most interested in working with as a CHW?*

What Do YOU? Think ?

PUBLIC HEALTH IS ROOTED IN SCIENCE, ESPECIALLY THE SCIENCE OF EPIDEMIOLOGY

Public health is an **interdisciplinary** field. This means that it taps into a wide range of science, social science, and professional disciplines, including biology, anatomy, economics, demography, statistics, business, urban planning, law, anthropology, sociology, medicine, psychology, and political science.

Public health has also developed its own science of **epidemiology**, the study of the health and illness of populations.

Dr. John Snow is often called the father of modern epidemiology. He worked to stop a cholera epidemic in London in 1854. Cholera is a terrifying disease that causes extreme vomiting and diarrhea and can result in death from dehydration in a matter of hours. Today we know that disease can be spread from person to person by invisible microorganisms, such as the bacteria that cause cholera and viruses that cause the flu. The germ theory of disease, however, was not widely understood or believed before the 20th century. People were not certain what caused cholera or other communicable diseases like smallpox, measles, and diphtheria. Many people believed that disease was spread by *miasma,* or foul air identified with the conditions of poverty.

Snow had a theory that cholera was spread by contaminated water. He interviewed cholera patients and their surviving family members and studied death records. He plotted deaths from cholera on a map of London and observed that the death rate was much higher among families who got their water from the Broad Street Pump. Snow convinced local leaders to turn off the Broad Street Pump. Once the handle to the pump was removed, there was a sudden and dramatic decline in the number of local residents infected with and dying from cholera (Kukaswadia, 2013).

Mapping Cholera

Chapter 22, "Community Diagnosis," shows how Dr. Snow used a map to record cholera deaths in London. The chapter also demonstrates how CHWs can work in partnership with local communities to create similar maps of local health risks and resources.

The methods that John Snow used to investigate the cholera epidemic are still used today. They are used to study epidemics as varied as HIV/AIDS, tuberculosis, automobile accidents, and child malnutrition.

Today, public health applies a range of scientific methods, including epidemiology, in order to:

- Identify patterns of illness, injury, disability, and death within populations
- Analyze the causes of disease within populations
- Compare disease rates between different populations to identify those with the highest rates of illness and death
- Guide the development of public health programs and policies designed to promote the health of populations
- Evaluate the effectiveness of public health programs and policies
- Guide future investments, programs, and policies to methods that have been proven effective

Public health analyzes existing government data and gathers new information in order to analyze patterns of disease and death. In the United States, each state keeps a record of all deaths and their primary causes. These records are used to analyze the leading causes of death within a population, to compare changes in the causes of death over time, and to establish priorities for public health programs and policies. The National Center for Health Statistics, of the Centers for Disease Control and Prevention (CDC) (Hoyert & Xu, 2012), lists the leading causes of death in the United States for 2011 as follows:

- Heart disease: 596,339
- Cancer: 575,313
- Chronic lower respiratory diseases (such as emphysema): 143,342
- Stroke (cerebrovascular diseases): 128,931
- Accidents (unintentional injuries): 122,777
- Alzheimer's disease: 84,691
- Diabetes: 73,282
- Influenza and pneumonia: 53,667

- Kidney disease (nephritis, nephrotic syndrome, and nephrosis): 45,731
- Intentional self-harm (suicide): 38,285

The leading causes of death in the United States today are primarily chronic diseases such as heart disease, cancer, stroke, chronic lung diseases, and diabetes. A century ago, in 1900, the leading causes of death were infectious diseases such as tuberculosis, the flu, pneumonia, and diarrheal diseases. Injuries also cause a large number of deaths, and injuries (including many accidents, suicides, and homicides) and can be prevented.
A baby born in 1900 was expected to live only to age 47—while by the year 2000, that life expectancy had grown to age 77. People often assume that the dramatic change in the leading causes of death during the twentieth century must have been due to innovations in medicine; however, public health research shows the change was mainly a result of new public policies and public health actions. Certainly, reductions in infectious disease came about in part through actions we easily recognize as health-related, such as the development of vaccines and antibiotics. Still, much more of the shift away from infectious diseases and the 30-year increase in life expectancy came about through improved social conditions, such as universal schooling, safer work sites, improvements in sanitation, more access to clean water, the establishment of a minimum wage, and improved nutrition (CDC, 2013; House, Schoeni, Kaplan & Pollack, 2009).

Chronic versus Acute Disease

A **chronic disease** or condition lasts for at least three months (and may last for years or a lifetime). Chronic conditions are usually slow in developing (not sudden), often do not have a cure, and require ongoing management of symptoms (Please see Chapter 16 for more information). Common chronic diseases include heart disease, diabetes, asthma, cancer, arthritis, and lupus.

An acute disease or condition is one that develops quickly (usually), and may change quickly, leading to recovery, worsening, or death. It sometimes has a cure. Acute conditions often require quick and intensive interventions medically, over a relatively short period of time.

Infectious Versus Noninfectious Disease

Infectious diseases are caused by a pathogen or infectious agent (such as a virus, bacteria, or parasite) and can be passed from one person to another, or between humans and animals. Noninfectious diseases are not contagious and not caused by an infectious agent—they develop for other reasons.

Interactions

There is some cross-over and interaction between these categories of diseases and health conditions. In general, most chronic conditions are noninfectious, and most infectious diseases produce acute illness. However, some infections lead to chronic conditions—for example, Hepatitis B or C can become chronic. Some acute conditions are not infectious, for example, radiation sickness, which is caused by overexposure to radioactive material.

There are sometimes interactions between chronic and acute conditions. For example, sometimes an acute episode can happen in the midst of a chronic health condition—like a severe and acute asthma attack in someone who has a chronic asthma. Sometimes acute conditions that are not cured may contribute to the development of chronic conditions—certain strains of human papilloma virus (HPV), for example, can lead to cervical cancer.

Records of births and deaths are generally available for study, but it is not as easy to document the number of people living with a specific illness or disability, such as HIV disease. Epidemiology uses statistical research methods to gather information from a sample (a smaller but representative number) of the population and to make reliable estimates of the number and percentage of people with a particular illness, and how rapidly the illness or other health condition is increasing within the population. Statistical methods guide researchers in determining how to gather this information, whom to gather it from, and how many people must be sampled in order to provide a reliable estimate of the number or percentage of the population who are affected.

For example, the field of public health uses statistical methods to estimate the **prevalence** (or the percentage of a population with a specific health condition) of HIV in populations throughout the United States and around the world. In the United States, it is estimated that about 0.4 percent of people over the age of 13 are infected with HIV (CDC, 2014a; U.S. Census Bureau, 2014). In comparison, approximately 15 percent of people between the ages of 15 and 49 in Zimbabwe are infected with HIV (UNAIDS, 2014). That's roughly 38 times the rate of infection in the United States, or about one in eight adults.

Epidemiologists conduct research to estimate basic health indicators in order to describe the health of a population. These indicators are also used to compare the health status of different populations. The most widely used health indicators are infant mortality and life expectancy. **Infant mortality** is the estimated number of children, out of every 1,000 children born alive, who die before the age of one. **Life expectancy** is the estimated number of years that people will live. In 2013, infant mortality for the United States was estimated at 6 per 1,000 live births. In comparison, infant mortality for Zimbabwe was estimated in 2013 at 55 per 1,000 live births (World Bank, n.d.). In 2015, life expectancy in the United States was estimated at 76 years for males and 81 years for females. In comparison, life expectancy in Zimbabwe was estimated at 59 years for males and 61 years for females (United Nations, 2015a, 2015b). As a discipline, public health often starts with the statistical information in health indicators to raise new questions about what shapes our health, and what we can do about it.

- *Are you surprised by the large difference in infant mortality and life expectancy rates between the United States and Zimbabwe?*

- *What do these life expectancy and infant mortality rates tell you about the relative health of each nation?*

While CHWs are not expected to have an in-depth knowledge of epidemiology or statistics, the more you know, the better prepared you will be to participate in decisions about public health research, programs, and policies. You may wish to begin by locating and reviewing reports from your local health department on the health status of communities you belong to and are working with, such as reports on infant mortality, diabetes, or domestic violence. Many health departments now have websites where recent reports are posted. In San Francisco, for example, statistical information about health indicators can be found at the website, *sfhip.org*. Look up the website for your county or state's health department, and select a report to read or skim. Identify language or information that you don't fully understand, and talk about it with a colleague.

- *What type of health statistics do you most want to learn about?*

- *How can health data guide and support your work as a CHW?*

PUBLIC HEALTH IS CONCERNED WITH SOCIAL JUSTICE AND HEALTH INEQUALITIES

One of the most important public health issues of our time is the growing inequality in health among different populations. Health inequalities, also referred to as *health inequities* or *disparities*, occur when one group of people experience significantly higher rates of illness and death than others. As you will read in Chapter 4, epidemiological data documents these differences in health status between nations and between different communities within the United States.

Since the earliest days of public health research, the field has been concerned about health inequalities and specifically, the social injustices that underlie them. For example, in 1848 an early public health researcher, Rudolf Virchow, identified the lack of democracy as being one root cause of a typhus outbreak. More recently, public health scholars Krieger and Birn (1998) wrote:

> *To declare that social justice is the foundation of public health is to call upon and nurture that invincible human spirit that led so many of us to enter the field of public health in the first place: a spirit that has a compelling desire to make the world a better place, free of misery, inequity, and preventable suffering, a world in which we all can live, love, work, play, ail, and die with our dignity intact and our humanity cherished.*

An example of the health inequalities that strip away the opportunity of some populations to live and die in conditions of dignity is the dramatic inequality in HIV prevalence between the populations of the United States and Zimbabwe presented earlier. The data underscore the critical need facing the people of Zimbabwe, where about 15 percent of the population lives with HIV disease. Dr. Paul Farmer points out that the HIV epidemic follows patterns of class, race, and gender inequalities in which the health care needs of the poor are too often ignored (Farmer, 1999, 2013). In Zimbabwe, colonialism, unequal distribution of basic economic resources, political oppression, poverty, famine, and rigid gender roles set the stage for HIV/AIDS. Health cannot be separated from the social and economic conditions that shape human lives.

HIV disease is also unequally distributed among populations within the United States. For example, the chance of a woman being diagnosed with HIV in her lifetime is more than 15 times higher for African American women (1 in 32) compared to White women (1 in 526). For Latinas, the likelihood is more than 3 times higher (1 in 106) compared to White women. While African American women make up only 13 percent of the total population of women in the United States, they account for 64 percent of estimated AIDS cases among women. Although African American women are still disproportionately affected by HIV/AIDS, there was a promising 21 percent decrease in new infections among African American women between 2008 and 2010, yet another indication that health inequalities *can* be reduced with concerted effort (Henry J. Kaiser Family Foundation, 2014).

Health inequalities are not inevitable. They are the consequence of the way a society structures access to the basic resources, rights, and opportunities that all people require in order to live long and healthy lives. Eliminating health inequalities requires changing social policies that determine access to resources that all people need to be healthy such as housing, food, education, employment, health care, safety, and human rights.

Leading institutions in the United States and internationally—including the National Association of County and City Health Officials (NACCHO), CDC, the Institutes of Medicine (IOM), the Office of Minority Health (OMH), and the WHO—have recognized health inequalities as a public health priority. The Healthy People 2020 goals noted above, for example, put both the elimination of health inequalities and the creation of social and physical environments that promote health as two of the top priorities.

For many of us, working to eliminate health inequalities is the central challenge facing public health today. CHWs, working directly with communities that experience disproportionately high rates of illness and death, have a significant role to play in the movement to eliminate health inequalities. Indeed, several research studies have demonstrated how CHWs make a difference in the health of patients and the reduction of persistent health inequalities (CDC, 2011).

PUBLIC HEALTH EMPHASIZES THE SOCIAL DETERMINANTS OF HEALTH

The field of public health understands the factors that cause illness and death differently than the field of medicine does. Traditionally, medicine focuses on the causes of disease located within the individual patient. For example, physicians want to know if a patient is infected with a specific pathogen (or disease-causing agent) such as HIV. For a patient already diagnosed with HIV disease, medicine focuses on what the patient knew, believed, or did that caused or contributed to the infection or progression of disease: Did the patient understand how HIV is transmitted? Did the patient engage in unprotected sex? Is the patient taking her medications properly?

In contrast, public health investigates the factors that cause and contribute to patterns of illness and death in populations. Public health research has demonstrated that the most significant of these factors are located at the societal level. These **social determinants of health** include economic, social, and political policies and dynamics that influence whether or not people have access to resources and opportunities essential to good health. In general, populations with less access to resources experience higher rates of illness and death. These resources, rights, and opportunities include:

- Safe housing and public transportation
- Proper and sufficient nutrition
- Personal safety (from interpersonal violence and war, for example)
- Civil rights and protection from discrimination
- Employment, safe working conditions, and a living wage
- Clean water, air, and soil
- Quality education

- Recreational facilities and green space
- Cultural resources
- Affordable health care

All these factors affect health. Therefore, working to ensure that all people have access to these resources and opportunities *is* public health work.

- *What resources and opportunities do you consider to be essential for the health and wellness of communities or populations?*

Alvaro Morales: I worked for the environmental health program at a local department of public health. I investigated the health risks people are exposed to at work, at home, and in their communities. I visited families whose children have lead poisoning. These children were sick just because their families are poor, and they live in houses with lead paint. The parents are devastated. I was lucky to have a great job and health benefits in case I get sick, and when I went home at night, I knew that my children would have a good meal and a safe place to sleep. It's just so unfair. People are getting sick because they live and work in bad conditions. It doesn't need to be this way. That is what is so frustrating: All of this is preventable.

3.3 The Practice of Public Health

PUBLIC HEALTH IS PRACTICED BY DIVERSE INDIVIDUALS, GROUPS, AND ORGANIZATIONS

Public health is not a coordinated system, and is practiced by a large and diverse group of public (government) and private sector agencies, groups, and individuals, including:

- **International and intergovernmental organizations** such as the World Health Organization and the United Nations Children's Fund (UNICEF).
- **Local, state, tribal, and national government agencies**, such as the department of public health in your city or county, and national organizations such as the Department of Health and Human Services, the CDC, and the Office of Minority Health.
  - Which government agencies in your area are involved in the community's health?
- **Public and private clinics and hospitals**, particularly those that provide health care services to low-income and uninsured patients.
  - Which clinic or hospital, if any, provides services to low-income patients in your community?
- **Colleges and universities** with departments or schools of public health, health education, medicine, public policy, and social work that educate professionals and conduct research and advocacy related to public health.
  - *Is there a college or university close to where you live? Does it provide education and training or conduct research or advocacy related to public health?*
- **Many small and large private or nongovernmental organizations** that provide health and social services to promote the health of low-income and at-risk communities (communities with increased risks for illness, disability, injury, or premature death). These may include agencies that work with youth or seniors and address issues such as domestic violence, homelessness, or drug and alcohol use.
  - *Which agencies provide services in your community?*
- **Individuals, groups, and associations** work to promote the health and welfare of low-income and otherwise vulnerable communities. Individual activists lobby local governments to develop policies or fund programs to improve health. Informal groups of people come together to advocate on behalf of shared issues, for

example, public housing residents might advocate for the repair of hazardous living conditions. More formal associations are also active in public health and social justice. Labor unions, for example, have taken leadership in promoting occupational health.

○ *Can you identify individual activists, groups, or associations that are working to promote public health in your community?*

Though the practice of public health is largely invisible and not often publicized, our lives are affected by public health programs and policies every day. When you turn on the tap, do you drink clean water? Are you or your children immunized against infectious disease? Do you ride in a vehicle that has seatbelts and airbags? Each of these measures represents a very concrete gain in quality of life, achieved through public health efforts. *Can you think of other examples?*

Despite former Surgeon General C. Everett Koop's statement that "Health care matters to all of us some of the time, public health matters to all of us all of the time," public health agencies in the United States have been historically underfunded. Funding remains inadequate (Kinner & Pelligrini, 2009), despite increased public concern about reemerging infectious diseases and new threats to health, like terrorism and climate change. The vast majority of health-related funding is spent on expensive and relatively inefficient health care services (see Chapter 5). Public health professionals seek to change the balance of these investments and to increase government spending on effective public health programs and policies.

Policies that affect the public's health are largely determined by the decisions that our governments make, including the level of investment in essential resources such as education, housing, transportation, food, safe working conditions, and access to comprehensive health care. Every time your government makes a decision about where to invest public dollars, it has an impact on public health (Please note that everyone, regardless of citizenship status, pays taxes, including sales taxes, automobile, gasoline, and tobacco taxes). When governments enforce civil rights, raise the minimum wage, or build affordable housing, they are promoting public health. When international bodies negotiate a cease fire or treaty, or fail to, they are taking action that affects public health.

- *What decisions has your local government made in the past year that affects the health of the communities you work with?*

- *How could you and the communities you work with influence such decisions in ways that improve the community's health?*

THREE CORE FUNCTIONS OF PUBLIC HEALTH

As we have discussed, the field of public health is wide-reaching and varied. However, there are three core functions that help distinguish public health from other related fields. Every public health department carries out these three functions, in one way or another, to improve population health:

- Assessment
- Policy development
- Assurance

Assessment focuses on the need to understand a particular health-related issue or concern before taking action to do something about it. Assessment includes actions such as:

- Monitor health through regular reporting of the community's health status, such as the number of births, deaths, or flu cases.
- Investigate and diagnose the causes of a new outbreak of disease, or the risk factors associated with poor health or premature death.

Policy development is how we address a problem and promote a better health outcome. It means taking actions such as:

- Inform, educate, and empower clients and communities so they can do something about their own health and the health of their families.

- Mobilize community partnerships to change the conditions of health in the neighborhood or city or county. For example, a community task force on children's health might bring together schools, service providers, parents, and youth to take action to reduce health risks for children.

- Develop public policies to make lasting changes in health, for example, expanding the Special Supplemental Nutrition Program for Women, Infants, and Children (WIC), improving health insurance programs, or developing affordable housing.

Assurance means making sure that a policy, program or service is implemented properly. Assurance includes actions such as:

- Enforce the laws that protect our health, for example, inspecting restaurants for cleanliness, or making sure that the drinking water supply is kept clean.

- Link to and provide care to those who need it, by coordinating services in the best way possible.

- Assure that the workforce is highly skilled by providing training and education for people who work in public health, including CHWs.

- Evaluate programs and policies, and use that evidence to improve them.

To carry out these functions, every public health department (whether it's the CDC at a national level, a state health department, or a health department for a specific region, county or city) organizes itself into specialized units. For example, a health department might have units for infectious disease, chronic disease, maternal and child health, environmental health, public health nursing, nutrition, epidemiology, and health education.

PUBLIC HEALTH USES ECOLOGICAL MODELS TO UNDERSTAND AND PROMOTE HEALTH

Because the issues that public health tackles are so complex, it's important to be able to visualize and analyze the wide range of factors that influence health. Ecological models are frequently used in public health to examine risk factors that lead to disease, as well as to develop policies and programs to address them. Ecological models help us to better understand how smaller and larger environments influence health.

- *What do you see in your community that contributes to illness or injuries? What do you see that contributes to good health and well-being?*

- *Have you witnessed a community's health improve because a root cause or a risk factor was eliminated or reduced? For example, was a source of pollution cleaned up, or a dangerous corner made safer?*

Because **ecological models** emphasize the social and physical environment, they draw attention to the social determinants of health. These models guide CHWs and other public health practitioners to view the health status of individual clients within a larger context that includes the influence of their families, neighborhoods, and the broader society in which they live. While there are many different ecological models used in the field of public health, we refer throughout this book to the model presented as Figure 3.1.

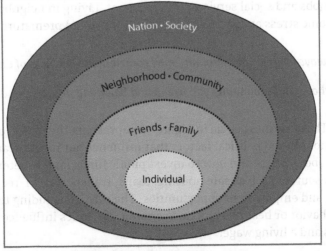

Figure 3.1 Ecological Model of Health

Figure 3.1 shows interconnected circles representing the individual; relationships with family and friends; the neighborhood or community in which people live, work, and go to school; and the broader society.

- **The individual:** The innermost circle represents the individual. A person's health status is influenced by their genes, values, beliefs, knowledge, and behaviors. In reference to HIV disease, how people think and feel about themselves (self-esteem), and their perception of risk (young people, for example, often feel invulnerable to HIV) influence rates of infection. So do individuals' acceptance of and comfort with their own sexuality and sexual orientation, their past experiences, including their record of accomplishments, whether or not they engage in sex and drug use, and whether or not they practice safer sex (such as the regular use of condoms).

  - *Can you think of other ways that individuals influence their own health?*

  - *How do you influence your health?*

- **Family and friends:** The next circle represents family and friends, who may influence health in many ways. In reference to HIV disease, families have not always provided effective education or guidance in order to understand and prevent the transmission of HIV. Some families have judged, alienated, and even disowned relatives who are lesbian, gay, bisexual, or transgender, who engage in sex with members of their own sex, who use drugs, or who are living with HIV. Other families are supportive of their relatives. While friends sometimes encourage healthy behaviors, they may also promote risk-taking, such as the use of drugs and unprotected sex. People who are in relationships, including marriage, are sometimes pressured or threatened into doing things that they don't want to do, such as having unprotected sex. People sometimes experience physical, sexual, and emotional abuse or assault from family members, and these traumatic experiences have been shown to influence their health status and risks for HIV disease.

  - *Can you think of other ways in which family and friends influence health status?*

  - *How do your family and friends influence your health?*

- **The community:** The next circle represents the neighborhood or community we live in. Our health is strongly influenced by whether or not we have a safe home to live in, safe working conditions, a living wage, or exposure to environmental hazards and violence. Neighborhoods and communities also influence whether people have access to recreational and cultural activities, public transportation to get back and forth from our homes to school, work, or grocery stores, and to visit with family and friends. In reference to HIV disease, some neighborhoods have community-based organizations that provide culturally appropriate outreach, education, HIV-antibody testing, and counseling services, while others do not. Some communities have safe places for youth to congregate, while others do not. Some neighborhoods have lots of billboards and stores that market and sell alcohol; others do not. Some communities have good schools and job training, with easy access to jobs and social services; others do not. Living in neighborhoods that lack these basic resources results in chronic stress and increased risks for illness and premature death (please see Chapter 4).

  - *Can you think of other ways in which a community may contribute to the risks of disease?*

  - *How does the neighborhood and community you live in and belong to influence your health?*

- **The nation or society:** The outermost circle in Figure 3.1 represents the nation or society we live in, and the social, cultural, economic, and political factors that influence our health status. The decisions that our governments make about where and how to invest public funds largely determines which populations have greater access to resources such as safe housing, loans, transportation, recreational facilities, quality schools, social services, and employment opportunities. The media, including television and the Internet, may encourage risky behavior or healthy choices. Economic dynamics influence access to jobs that provide safe working conditions and a living wage.

In reference to HIV disease, most governments, including the government of the United States, hesitated to acknowledge or take action to prevent HIV disease, often due to economic concerns (such as a negative impact on tourism) or prejudice against the populations who are most affected (such as injection drug users, communities of color, and gay men). Governments have not always provided accurate information about how to prevent HIV infections, access to HIV-antibody test counseling, medical care, and other services that people living with HIV need in order to live healthy and productive lives. People with HIV do not always have civil rights and protection from discrimination in housing, education, health care, and employment. Poverty rates also influence health status and risks for HIV. People who live in poverty often take risks just to survive and assist their families to survive, such as engaging in sex in exchange for food, shelter, or money. Incarceration has also been shown to facilitate HIV transmission, and the United States has the highest rate of imprisonment among industrialized nations (CDC, 2014b). HIV disease is much more prevalent among communities characterized by poverty, histories of discrimination, violence, inadequate housing, and poor access to other basic resources.

Whether CHWs work with individuals, families, or communities, an ecological perspective is essential to guide their efforts.

- *What would you add to the ecological model presented above?*

- *Can you think of other ways that our society and our government influence our health?*

DEVELOPING PROGRAMS AND POLICIES FOR PREVENTION

The spectrum of prevention provides a framework for understanding different "levels" of prevention activities. It is a useful tool to guide the development of public health programs in areas such as injury prevention, violence prevention, nutrition, HIV/AIDS, and fitness (Prevention Institute, 1999; n.d.).

We use the spectrum of prevention (Table 3.1) to teach CHWs about the range of public health interventions that they may participate in. An intervention is a public health program or activity aimed at producing a change. The spectrum is used in many agencies, and is sometimes modified to include additional levels, such as "mobilizing communities and neighborhoods" (Contra Costa Health Services, n.d.).

In Table 3.2, we provide an example of how CHWs can work at each level of the spectrum of prevention. The examples provided in Table 3.2 are drawn from the HIV/AIDS field. In the Chapter Review, you will have a chance to apply the spectrum of prevention to a different public health issue.

Table 3.1 The Spectrum of Prevention

SPECTRUM	DEFINITION
1. Strengthening individual knowledge and skills	Enhancing an individual's ability to prevent injury or illness and promote safety
2. Promoting community education	Reaching groups of people with information and resources to promote health and safety
3. Educating providers	Informing health providers who will transmit skills and knowledge to others
4. Fostering coalitions and networks	Bringing individuals and groups together to work for common goals with a greater impact
5. Changing organizational practices	Adopting regulations and shaping norms within organizations to improve health and safety
6. Influencing policy and legislation	Developing strategies to change laws and policies in order to influence health outcomes

Table 3.2 The Spectrum of Prevention, Examples

SPECTRUM	EXAMPLE
1. Strengthening individual knowledge and skills	CHWs work in a clinic and provide client-centered education and counseling to high-school-aged youth regarding how to prevent HIV and other sexually transmitted infections.
2. Promoting community education	CHWs visit local high schools and provide educational presentations designed to assist youth to reduce their risks for HIV infection.
3. Educating providers	CHWs facilitate trainings for the staff at a youth-serving agency on topics related to HIV prevention and how to work effectively with at-risk youth, including lesbian, gay, bisexual, and transgender youth.
4. Fostering coalitions and networks	CHWs facilitate the formation and planning process of a coalition of youth and youth-serving organizations interested in preventing HIV disease and providing increased access to prevention education and HIV antibody test counseling, especially in the populations most impacted by HIV.
5. Changing organizational practices	CHWs work with local youth networks and youth leaders to advocate with local schools or school districts to provide comprehensive sexuality education; to support civil rights protections for lesbian, gay, bisexual, and transgender students; or to implement condom availability programs.
6. Influencing policy and legislation	CHWs advocate with state policymakers on behalf of new policies, such as policies to prohibit discrimination of people living with HIV or those that support syringe exchange programs, living wages, and universal health care.

- *Have you participated as a volunteer or paid staff in programs that represented one or more levels of the spectrum of prevention?*

- *Which levels of the Spectrum of Prevention have you worked at?*

- *Which levels do you hope to work at over the course of your career as a CHW, and why?*

PUBLIC HEALTH PRACTICE IS EVIDENCE-BASED

The field of public health conducts research, gathering and analyzing data to identify the populations at greatest risk for illness and premature death, and to evaluate the effectiveness of public health programs and policies. This information is then used to guide future public health investments. Rather than investing money in programs or policies that we *think* will promote health outcomes among a specific population, public health encourages investments in programs and policies that have already proven to be successful with similar populations, or the adaptation and testing of similar models with different populations. As we noted earlier, public health is rooted in a scientific approach (using epidemiology and other disciplines), and using evidence to assess effective programs is another example of how science informs the practice of public health.

At the same time, it is important to acknowledge that political beliefs and goals sometimes undermine this process, and scientific evidence may be disregarded in the development of policies. For example, state and federal governments have at times deemphasized the use of condoms and focused on abstinence-only education despite overwhelming evidence that condoms are an effective means of preventing HIV and abstinence-only education is not (Underhill, Operario, & Montgomery, 2007).

As a CHW, you can benefit from keeping up-to-date with public health research about the issues you address in your work. You can learn from both successful and unsuccessful public health programs to find more effective ways to serve your clients and communities. The most useful research evidence will be drawn from program models and strategies that are very similar to your own, and with populations that are very similar to those you work with. For example, just because a diabetes management program was effective with Native American women in Arizona, a similar program may not be equally successful serving White men in New Hampshire. As we have tried to emphasize, the environment in which people live and the identities and culture of the community you serve need to be taken into consideration. Public health departments, research universities and the CDC are all good sources for evidence about model programs that have been demonstrated to work, at least in some settings. A few of these are listed in the Resources section at the end of this chapter.

Finally, as a CHW you may have opportunities to participate in public health research and will certainly have opportunities to participate in the evaluation of the programs and services you provide. We encourage you to talk with your colleagues about the programs you work with. How were they developed? Are they guided by existing research? Have they been evaluated? If so, what are the findings? If they haven't been evaluated, ask to participate in developing an evaluation method to learn if and how the programs are making a positive difference. Even if you are unfamiliar with research or evaluation methods, your experience as a CHW may be vital in identifying what information to gather from the community and how to gather it. Please refer to information provided in Chapter 22 for an introduction to some types of evaluation and assessment.

PUBLIC HEALTH ADVOCATES FOR SOCIAL JUSTICE

The factors that often have the biggest impact on human health are social determinants, including political decisions about where and how to invest public resources. It follows, therefore, that the most powerful strategy for promoting public health is to advocate for changes to public policies that will provide equal access to the resources and opportunities that are essential to health (education, housing, nutrition, safety, civil rights, and so on). If everyone, regardless of their educational background, income, ethnicity, immigration status, or other demographic characteristics, had access to these resources and opportunities, our society wouldn't experience such high rates of infectious or chronic disease, or such pronounced inequalities in illness, death, and wellness between different populations.

We define *social justice* as the equal access to these basic human resources, rights, and opportunities. Leading public health researchers and institutions such as the American Public Health Association, schools of public health at many universities, NACCHO, and the World Health Organization have articulated the connections between social justice and public health, and committed themselves to advocating for social justice as a best practice for promoting public health (Beauchamp, 1976; NACCHO, 2015; Northridge, 2014; Satcher, 2010; WHO, 2015a).

Anthony Iton (2006), former Medical Officer for the Alameda County Health Department in Oakland, California, says:

> *In virtually every public health area . . . be it immunizations, chronic disease, HIV/AIDS . . . or even disaster preparedness, local public health departments are confronted with the consequences of structural poverty, institutional racism and other forms of systemic injustice. By designing approaches that are specifically designed to identify existing assets and build social, political and economic power among residents of afflicted neighborhoods, local public health departments can begin to sustainability reduce and move towards eliminating health inequities in low-income communities of color. Additionally, local public health agencies must simultaneously seek opportunities to strategically partner with advocates for affordable housing, labor rights, education equity, environmental justice, transportation equity, prison reform. . . . Without such a focus, local health departments will most likely only succeed in tinkering around the edges of health disparities at a cost too great to justify. (p. 135)*

One of the primary roles of all public health practitioners, including CHWs, is to advocate for social justice on behalf of and in partnership with the clients and communities you serve. Only by doing so can we change and improve the conditions that have the biggest impact on health status.

Alvaro Morales: I've been working in public health for 14 years now. I've learned that if we could change things so that the communities I work with—mostly low-income communities of color and immigrant communities—if they had access to things like education, housing that isn't dangerous, a job with benefits for enough money to live on, good places for my children to go to school, then we could prevent most of the health problems I see on a daily basis. People's children wouldn't get lead poisoning, and there wouldn't be so many homeless people. The communities I work with wouldn't have a life expectancy that is so much lower than others. It all comes down to working for social justice, and I'm proud to be part of that.

Public Health Has Not Always Promoted Justice

Unfortunately, public health is sometimes practiced from the top down: professional "experts" develop and implement programs and policies they think will promote the health of a vulnerable community. This approach has sometimes resulted in significant harm to the community. For example, the Tuskegee Syphilis Trials, an infamous public health research project, withheld treatment from African American men who were being studied to learn more about syphilis. As a result, men enrolled in the study were disabled and died. (For more information about Tuskegee, see Chapter 6.) Unfortunately, public health history has many such examples.

- *Have your communities been harmed by public health programs or policies in the past?*

- *How do the communities you belong to view the government?*

What Do YOU Think?

PUBLIC HEALTH WORKS IN PARTNERSHIP WITH COMMUNITIES

At its best, public health is practiced in collaboration with the communities that have the most to gain or lose. One of the key roles of CHWs is to assist in flipping the top-down strategy described above, and to partner with community ,members to develop public health programs and policies that represent and benefit from the wisdom, creativity, skills, and leadership of affected communities. This is important for many reasons, including:

- *It is the right thing to do:* Communities with the most to gain or lose from a public health program or policy have the right to be consulted regarding its design, management, and evaluation. The right of a community to self-determination, and a voice in the decisions that affect them, is rooted in our most fundamental beliefs in democracy.

- *Long-term effectiveness:* Public health programs and policies come and go. Programs developed with leadership from the community are much more likely to be culturally relevant, and to result in significant and lasting changes.

- *Capacity building:* You may have heard the expression, "Give a person a fish and they will eat well for a day. Teach a person to fish, and they will eat well forever." A key dimension to enhancing the health of communities is to foster community leadership and skills that may be used to address other health concerns in the future.

The quality of your work as a CHW can be judged to great extent by the degree to which you establish and maintain respectful partnerships with the communities you work with and your ability to facilitate and support their leadership. For more information about community-centered practice and the role of the CHW, please see Part 5 of this textbook.

PUBLIC HEALTH PROMOTES THE HEALTH OF THE NATURAL ENVIRONMENT

Our ancestors understood that human health was dependent upon the health of the planet. Modern societies have largely forsaken this knowledge and often operate in ways that harm our planet, the air and atmosphere, our oceans, ground water, soil, plants, and animal species. The health of the planet and the health of human populations are integrally connected and mutually dependent, and increasingly, public health is beginning to promote both goals.

Our societies have concentrated industrial pollution in low-income areas. The branch of public health known as Environmental Health works to decrease exposures to pollution in communities and worksites. CHWs often serve as an invaluable bridge between researchers and communities in public health efforts to clean up pollution and protect health. Campaigns that address the inequalities that result from concentrating pollution in certain neighborhoods and communities are part of the broader **environmental justice** movement.

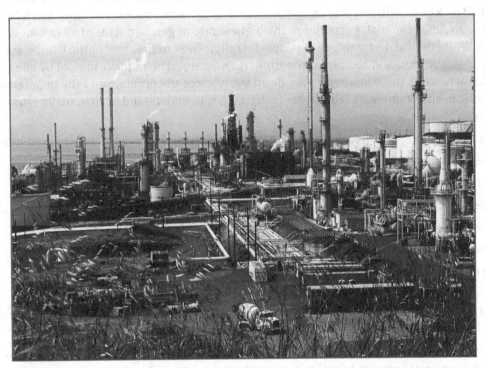

Refineries and other environmental hazards are more commonly located near low-income communities of color, harming their health. CHWs and other advocates are organizing to change this.

Increasingly, public health has turned its attention to global climate change. Public health practitioners have an important role in developing policies both to mitigate (slow down or reverse) climate change and to adapt to a changing world. Public health leaders in California, for example, have been key supporters of the response to climate change. They have supported laws to reduce the amount of carbon that goes into the atmosphere, while at the same time preparing for the worst (heat waves, fires, floods, etc.). See *www.climatechange.ca.gov/* for more examples. One creative contribution that public health makes to the policy discussions around climate change is an emphasis on the **health cobenefits**. A cobenefit is like a positive side effect; it's something that, in addressing climate change, also improves the health of the population—for example, building bike paths so that people can travel around cities on bicycle improves cardiovascular health at the same time that reduces the use of gasoline. When addressing climate change, just like any other major health threat, particular attention must be paid to health equality. While climate change affects all populations, the poorest and most marginalized are often at greatest risk and have the least resources to adapt. A strong public health infrastructure is essential to handling the ongoing effects of climate change, including heat waves, floods and natural disasters, food shortages, and changes in patterns of infectious disease.

Chapter Review

To review the concepts presented in this chapter, answer the following questions and apply the ecological model and the spectrum of prevention to the public health issue of gun violence.

GUN VIOLENCE IN AMERICA

The homicide rate in the United States, mostly death by firearms, peaked in 1993 and declined since, probably due to a combination of policy changes and demographic shifts (Goldstein, 2014). Even so, the United States still has a rate of death from gun violence that is 20 times higher than the average of all developed countries (Fisher, 2012). In the United States in 2013, 11,208 people lost their lives to a homicide by firearm, and 65 percent of those were children, youth, and young adults (under the age of 34). Racial inequalities in deaths by gun violence are also stark; in the most affected communities, funerals for victims of gun violence are still far too common. In 2013, African Americans were 8 times more likely, and Latinos were over twice as likely, than Whites to be killed by a gun. Within every community, males are more likely to die from a gun homicide than females, and African American males experience the highest rate of gun homicide of all (a rate 15 times higher than the rate for White males). In total, 33,636 people lost their lives to firearms in the United States in 2013, including homicides, suicides, and accidental shootings (CDC, 2015). The number injured by guns, but not killed, is many times higher. While these statistics provide an overview of the problem and the populations most affected, the public health framework requires us to dig deeper to understand what actually causes gun violence and what we can do about it.

1. Apply your understanding of the ecological model to the public health issue of gun-related homicides.
   - What types of individual factors might contribute to gun-related homicides?
   - How might family and friends contribute to gun-related homicides?
   - What types of community or neighborhood-level factors might contribute to gun-related homicides?
   - What types of societal factors contribute to gun-related homicides?

2. How would you explain that gun violence is considered a public health issue?

3. How might the three functions of public health—assessment, policy development, and assurance—be used to help prevent gun violence?

4. Imagine that you are going to work with a public health program focused on preventing gun violence in a large city. What type of public health statistics would you want to study?

5. Using the spectrum of prevention framework shown in Table 3.3, provide examples of public health strategies that CHWs can participate in, to assist in preventing gun homicides, or gun violence in general.

6. How would promoting social justice help to prevent gun violence in the United States?

Table 3.3 The Spectrum of Prevention Applied to Gun Violence in the United States

SPECTRUM	STRATEGY
1. Influencing policy and legislation	CHWs will
2. Changing organizational practices	CHWs will
3. Fostering coalitions and networks	CHWs will
4. Educating providers	CHWs will
5. Promoting community education	CHWs will
6. Strengthening individuals' knowledge and skills	CHWs will

References

Beauchamp, D. E. (1976). Public health as social justice. *Inquiry, 13*, 3–14.

Centers for Disease Control and Prevention. (2013, April 26). *Ten great public health achievements in the 20th century.* Retrieved from *www.cdc.gov/about/history/tengpha.htm*

Centers for Disease Control and Prevention (CDC). (2014a, November 10). *HIV/AIDS statistics overview.* Retrieved from *www.cdc.gov/hiv/statistics/basics/index.html*

Centers for Disease Control and Prevention. (2014b, February 20). *HIV among incarcerated populations.* Retrieved from *www.cdc.gov/hiv/risk/other/correctional.html*

Centers for Disease Control and Prevention, National Center for Chronic Disease Prevention and Health Promotion, Division of Health Disease and Stroke Prevention (2011). *Addressing chronic disease through community health workers: A policy and systems-level approach.* [Report]. Retrieved from *www.cdc.gov/dhdsp/docs/chw_brief.pdf*

Centers for Disease Control and Prevention, National Center for Health Statistics. (2015). Deaths: Final data for 2013. *National Vital Statistics Reports, 64* (2). Advance online publication.

Contra Costa Health Services. (n.d.). *The spectrum of prevention.* Retrieved from *http://cchealth.org/prevention/spectrum/*

Farmer, P. (1999). *Infections and inequalities: The modern plagues.* Berkeley, CA: University of California Press.

Farmer, P. (2013). Chronic infectious disease and the future of health care delivery. *New England Journal of Medicine, 369*, 2424–2436. doi:10.1056/NEJMsa1310472

Fisher, M. (2012, December 14). Chart: the US has far more gun-related killings than any other country. *The Washington Post.* Retrieved from *www.washingtonpost.com/blogs/worldviews/wp/2012/12/14/chart-the-u-s-has-far-more-gun-related-killings-than-any-other-developed-country/*

Goldstein, D. (2014, November 24). *Ten (not entirely crazy) theories explaining the great crime decline.* Retrieved from *www.themarshallproject.org/2014/11/24/10-not-entirely-crazy-theories-explaining-the-great-crime-decline*

The Henry J. Kaiser Family Foundation. (2014, March 6). *Women and HIV/AIDS in the United States.* Retrieved from *http://kff.org/hivaids/fact-sheet/women-and-hivaids-in-the-united-states/*

House, J. S., Schoeni, R. F., Kaplan, G. A., & Pollack, H. (2009). The health effects of social and economic policy: The promise and challenge for research and policy. *National Poverty Center Policy Brief 20.* Retrieved from *www.npc.umich.edu/publications/policy_briefs/brief20/policy_brief_20_web.pdf*

Hoyert, D. L., & Xu, J. Q. (2012). Deaths: Preliminary data for 2011. *National Vital Statistics Reports, 61*, 6. Hyattsville, MD: National Center for Health Statistics.

Iton, A. (2006). Tackling the root causes of health disparities through community capacity building. In R. Hofrichter (Ed.), *Tackling health inequities through public health practice: A handbook for action* (pp. 115–136). Washington, DC: National Association of County and City Health Officials.

Kinner, K., & Pelligrini, C. (2009). Expenditures for public health: Assessing historical and prospective trends. *American Journal of Public Health, 99*, 1780–1791. doi:10.2105/AJPH.2008.142422

Krieger, N., & Birn, A. E. (1998). A vision of social justice as the foundation of public health: Commemorating 150 years of the Spirit of 1848. *American Journal of Public Health, 88*, 1603–1606.

Kukaswadia, A. (2013, March 11). John Snow—The first epidemiologist [blog]. PLOSblogs, Public Health Perspectives. Retrieved from *http://blogs.plos.org/publichealth/2013/03/11/john-snow-the-first-epidemiologist/*

National Association of County and City Health Officials (NACCHO). (2015). *Health equity and social justice.* Retrieved from *www.naccho.org/topics/justice/*

Northridge, M. E. (2014). The social justice agenda. *American Journal of Public Health, 104*, 1576–1578. doi:10.2105/AJPH.2014.302127

Prevention Institute. (n.d.). *Creating effective strategies.* Retrieved from *www.preventioninstitute.org/tools/strategy-tools.html*

Prevention Institute. (1999). *The spectrum of prevention: Developing a comprehensive response to injury prevention.* Retrieved from *www.preventioninstitute.org/component/jlibrary/article/id-105/127.html*

Satcher, D. (2010). Include a social determinants of health approach to reduce health inequities, *Public Health Reports, 125*, S4, 6–7.

UNAIDS. (2014). *Gap report.* Retrieved from *www.unaids.org/sites/default/files/media_asset/UNAIDS_Gap_report_ en.pdf*

Underhill, K., Operario, D., & Montgomery, P. (2007). Abstinence-only programs for HIV infection prevention in high-income countries. *Cochrane Database of Systematic Reviews, 17*, CD005421. doi:10.1002/14651858. CD005421.pub2

United Nations. (2015a). *UN Data country profile: United States.* Retrieved from *http://data.un.org/CountryProfile. aspx?crName=United%20States%20of%20America#Social*

United Nations. (2015b). *UN Data country profile: Zimbabwe.* Retrieved from *http://data.un.org/CountryProfile. aspx?crName=ZIMBABWE#Social*

U.S. Census Bureau. (2014, December 3). *State and county quick facts.* Retrieved from *http://quickfacts.census.gov/ qfd/states/00000.html*

U.S. Department of Health and Human Services (USDHHS). (2015, January 29). *About Healthy People.* Retrieved from *www.healthypeople.gov/2020/About-Healthy-People*

World Bank. (n.d.) *Data: Mortality rate, infant, per 1000 live births.* Retrieved from *http://data.worldbank.org/ indicator/SP.DYN.IMRT.IN*

World Health Organization. (1948). *WHO definition of health.* Retrieved from *www.who.int/about/definition/en/ print.html*

World Health Organization (WHO). (2015a). *Social determinants of health.* Retrieved from *www.who.int/ social_determinants/en/*

World Health Organization (2015b). *WHO definition of public health.* Retrieved from *www.who.int/trade/glossary/ story076/en/#*

Additional Resources

American Public Health Association. (n.d.). Retrieved from *www.apha.org*

Centers for Disease Control and Prevention. (2013). *The U.S. Public Health Service syphilis study at Tuskegee.* Retrieved from *www.cdc.gov/tuskegee/index.html*

International Institute for Society and Health. (n.d.). Retrieved from *www.ucl.ac.uk/iish*

Office of Minority Health. (n.d). Retrieved from *http://minorityhealth.hhs.gov/*

Outbreak at Watersedge. [Interactive game]. (n.d.) Retrieved from *www.mclph.umn.edu/watersedge/*

Prevention Institute. (n.d). Retrieved from *http://preventioninstitute.org*

Public Health Online. (n.d). *A guide to public health careers.* Retrieved from *www.publichealthonline.org/careers/*

Robert Wood Johnson Foundation. (n.d). Retrieved from *www.rwjf.org*

United States Department of Health and Human Services. (n.d.). *Healthy People 2020. www.healthypeople.gov*

University of California, San Francisco. (n.d.). *Center for AIDS Prevention Studies. www.caps.ucsf.edu*

World Health Organization. (n.d). Retrieved from *www.who.int/en/*

World Health Organization. (2008). *Closing the gap in a generation: Health equity through action on the social determinants of health.* [Report]. Retrieved from *http://whqlibdoc.who.int/hq/2008/WHO_IER_CSDH_08.1_eng. pdf?ua=1*

Your State health department here: _____

Your local city or county health department here: _____

Health for All

Promoting Health Equality

Janey Skinner and Tim Berthold

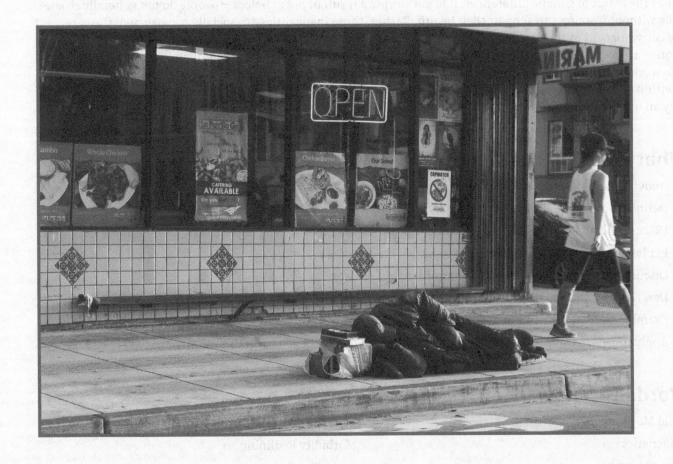

A toxic combination of poor social policies, unfair economic arrangements, and bad politics is responsible for most of the inequities we see in the world today, within and between countries. To be clear, those are the causes, and we need to address the fundamental causes.

—*Sir Michael Marmot (Marmot, 2009, p.1)*

Introduction

The United States and the world are characterized by dramatic inequalities in health. Bluntly stated, some populations get sick more often and die much earlier than others. These inequalities do not happen by mere chance, nor as the result of genetic differences. It is not simply a result of poor choices—people do not generally *choose* to be without resources to support their health. Rather, these inequalities are socially constructed: they are the consequences of the decisions we make about the allocation of basic resources and rights all people require in order to live healthy lives. These resources include human rights, safety, sufficient and proper nutrition, safe working conditions, a living wage, economic opportunity, quality housing, health care, and education. It is within our power to prevent communities from experiencing excess illness and premature death, and CHWs play an important role in these efforts.

What You Will Learn

By studying the information in this chapter, you will be able to:

- Define health inequalities
- Discuss and analyze the data that document health inequalities among populations
- Explain how social inequalities result in health inequalities
- Discuss how health inequalities are harmful to our society
- Describe and analyze how health inequalities are preventable
- Examine the role of CHWs in overcoming health inequalities and promoting social justice
- Apply the ideas from this chapter to issues of health equality in your own community

Words to Know

Child Mortality	Maternal Mortality
Epigenetics	Morbidity Redlining
Infant Mortality	Social Gradient
Life Expectancy	

4.1 Defining Health Inequality

Health inequalities, also referred to as "health disparities" and "health inequities," are differences in health status between populations that are avoidable and preventable. While some researchers draw a distinction between "health inequalities" and "health inequities," (e.g., World Health Organization [WHO]), we use both terms to refer to the same problem. The following definition of health inequalities comes from Richard Hofrichter (2007, p. 1) with the National Association of County and City Health Officials (NACCHO): "Differences in population health status and mortality rates that are systemic, patterned, unfair, unjust, and actionable, as opposed to random or caused by those who become ill."

Addressing and overcoming health inequality is a leading public health priority. In the United States, the national plan for health—Healthy People 2020—states the goal to: "Achieve health equity, eliminate disparities, and improve the health of all groups" (DHHS, n.d.). Fostering health equality is also a guiding principle for the World Health Organization, including the Millennium Development Goals (UNDP, n.d.) and the Commission on Social Determinants of Health (CSDH, 2008). Addressing the root causes of health inequalities is an "upstream" approach to transforming the conditions for health everywhere, and especially necessary in communities and populations experiencing the worst health outcomes.

Unnatural Causes

Since its premiere in 2008, the documentary series *Unnatural Causes* has been a leading resource to translate research on health inequalities into straightforward language and relatable stories. This series, produced by California Newsreel, explores the causes of health inequalities and highlights local efforts to promote health justice (Adelman, 2008). We strongly recommend viewing this series and reviewing the case studies, research, and educational materials posted on the Unnatural Causes website (www.unnaturalcauses.org). In 2015, the producers of Unnatural Causes released a second series on social inequality, this time focused on early childhood: The Raising of America (www.raisingofamerica.org). Both websites contain invaluable information for CHWs working for health equality.

The idea of health equality or "health for all" has deep roots in public health. Early public health researchers highlighted the connections between social conditions, democracy, and health (see Chapter 3). Through the WHO, the health ministries of 134 countries signed the Alma Ata Declaration in 1978, setting a goal of providing primary care for all by the year 2000 (a goal that was not met, although advancements were made). In 1998, the WHO's plan, "Health for All in the 21st Century" updated the Alma Ata declaration, including recognition of the importance of gender equality and participation of the nongovernmental sector (WHO, n.d.). More recently, the banner of Health for All has been carried forward by the People's Health Movement, an international network of organizations and governments to promote health equality and improved health outcomes for all people, especially those in less-developed countries. The People's Health Movement emphasizes the role of social conditions in shaping health along with the need for universal health care (www.phmovement.org/).

4.2 Evidence of Health Inequalities

It is no surprise to most CHWs that people who lack access to resources are more likely to experience higher rates of illness. In general, CHWs work with people who lack access to key resources, and often come from the same circumstances themselves. CHWs see the "wear and tear" that poverty, discrimination, and other hardships cause in the health and well-being of their clients. Yet even CHWs may be surprised to learn of the extent of health inequalities that persist today. And they may not be aware that health inequalities affect people up and down the socioeconomic ladder—not only the poorest or most disadvantaged communities.

HEALTH INEQUALITIES AMONG NATIONS

Table 4.1 documents significant differences in health status among nations. The table documents differences in **child mortality**, or the estimated number of children who die before the age of five out of every 100,000 live births; **maternal mortality**, or the estimated number of women who die as a result of pregnancy or childbirth per 100,000 live births; and **life expectancy**, or the average number of years that a population is expected to live, from birth. **Infant mortality** (not shown here) is another common measure of population health—infant mortality measures deaths before age one, while child mortality measures deaths before age five.

Table 4.1 International Comparison of Health Indicators

NATION	CHILD MORTALITY (2013) (DEATHS BEFORE AGE 5 PER 100,000 LIVE BIRTHS)	MATERNAL MORTALITY (2013) (MATERNAL DEATHS PER 100,000 LIVE BIRTHS)	LIFE EXPECTANCY (2012) (EXPECTED LIFE SPAN FROM BIRTH)
Japan	3	6	83
Sweden	3	3	82
United States	7	11	79
Nepal	40	190	68
Iraq	34	67	69
Afghanistan	97	400	61
Zimbabwe	89	470	58

Source: World Bank Databank, 2015.

The data reveal that children born in Afghanistan are 32 times more likely to die before the age of five than children born in Sweden or Japan (97 deaths per 100,000 compared to 3 per 100,000). Mothers in Nepal are 63 times more likely to die from complications related to pregnancy and childbirth than mothers in Sweden (190 deaths per 100,000 compared to 3 per 100,000). And people in Japan are estimated to live, on average, 25 years longer than people in Zimbabwe. These are not small or trivial differences or inequalities in health: they represent enormous loss to families, communities, and nations.

It is also worth noting that the gaps in health status between rich and poor countries have narrowed in recent years. Life expectancy has increased in many lower-income countries (faster than it has increased in wealthy countries), and the rates of maternal mortality and child mortality have declined. In Afghanistan, life expectancy increased 20 years (from 41 to 61) between 1980 and 2012. Over the same period of time, life expectancy in Iraq grew nine years (from 60 to 69), despite several wars. Child mortality in Nepal decreased by more than 500 percent between 1980 and 2013 (from 211 to 40 deaths per 100,000 live births). These numbers demonstrate that inequalities in health are not set in stone—they can change as conditions for health change. (For a demonstration of recent health improvements in less developed countries, visit http://gapminder.org.)

HEALTH STATUS IN THE UNITED STATES COMPARED TO OTHER WEALTHY NATIONS

As we discuss in Chapter 5, the United States spends significantly more money on health care than other industrialized nations yet ranks near the bottom in most leading health indicators. For example, in 2012, the United States spent approximately $8,895 per person on health care, compared to $51 in Afghanistan, $226 in Iraq, $5,319 in Sweden, and $4,752 in Japan (World Bank Databank, 2015). While the United States spent more money on health care than any other country, it only ranks 40th among nations in terms of life expectancy (2012 data), lower than Cuba, Lebanon, or Cyprus. The United States ranks 45th in terms of infant mortality (2013 data) (World Bank Databank, 2015). While there are many reasons why health in the United States is worse than in other wealthy nations, or even in many middle-income countries, the high level of inequality in the United States is a contributing factor (Wilkinson & Pickett, 2009; Rowlingson, 2011).

A SOCIAL GRADIENT IN HEALTH

In the United States, the United Kingdom, and in other nations in which health inequalities have been studied, there is a pronounced social gradient in health. A **social gradient** is a slope or a ladder, where for each step you go up or down in social status (for example, going up in income or educational level), there is a corresponding change in health. This means that it is not only the very poor who die earlier than the super-rich.

There is a steady and direct relationship between income and health: as annual income increases from under $10,000 to over $100,000, so too does life expectancy (Kawachi, Kennedy, Gupta, & Prothrow-Stith, 1999) and other measures of good health (Evans, Wolfe, & Adler, 2012). The working class lives longer than the poor; the middle class lives longer than the working class; and the wealthy live longer than the middle class (Kawachi, Kennedy, Gupta, & Prothrow-Stith, 1999). The same is true for educational level—people with college degrees tend to be healthier than high school graduates, and high school graduates tend to be healthier than those who don't finish high school. While we don't know yet all the mechanisms to explain how income or education or accumulated wealth affects health, we can clearly see that there *is* a relationship, because of these social gradients.

Health Inequality Is Bad for Everyone's Health

There is an association between high levels of inequality within a nation and a wide number of negative health outcomes. This does not affect only the poor or the middle class—it affects those in the top 10 percent, too. The wealthy in a highly unequal country like the United States experience higher rates of illness and lower life expectancy than wealthy people in a highly equal country like Sweden. While the connections between inequality and health are complex, there are clear population health benefits for everyone when greater equality is achieved (Wilkinson & Pickett, 2009; Rowlingson, 2011).

High levels of inequality also have economic impacts. One recent study found that almost one third of all medical expenditures for African Americans, Latinos, and Asians/Asian Americans were a direct result of health inequalities. The total direct and indirect costs of health inequalities in the United States are estimated to be about $309.3 billion annually. It is in everyone's interests, as an economic question as well as an ethical one, to work to eliminate health inequalities (LaVeist, Gaskin, & Richard, 2009).

HEALTH INEQUALITIES WITHIN THE UNITED STATES

Health inequalities exist among different populations in the United States based on race, ethnicity, income, education, gender, gender identity, disability, immigration status, sexual orientation, geographic location, and other factors. Of these, inequalities based on income and ethnicity have received the most attention and focused research.

RACE, ETHNICITY, AND HEALTH INEQUALITY

Despite the federal government's stated policy to eliminate health disparities, health inequalities based on race or ethnicity are significant and are increasing in the United States. According to the federal Office of Minority Health (OMH), "Compelling evidence indicates that race and ethnicity correlate with persistent and often increasing health disparities among U.S. populations . . . and demands national attention" (OMH, 2007).

As we discuss racial inequalities in health, it is important to understand that race is a social construct, not a biological one. There is much more genetic variation among people of any given race than there is between different races. While individuals who share a specific place of origin (say, Greek Americans or Laotian Americans) have certain genetic traits in common, the Greek American who is "white" may have no more genes in common with an Irish American than they do with a Japanese American. Likewise, Laotian Americans, Japanese Americans, and Pakistani Americans may all be considered "Asian/Pacific Islander"—but their genes are tremendously varied. Still, race remains is a socially meaningful term. Many people identify strongly as being a member of a particular race, and even if they don't, others may treat them in a certain way based on assumptions about their race. In a race-conscious (and racially stratified) country like the United States, there are some similarities of experience within any given race. For this reason, and it is still meaningful to discuss racial inequalities in health (American Anthropological Association, 2011; Kawachi, Daniels, & Robinson, 2005; Krieger, 2006).

The National Partnership for Action to End Health Disparities (U.S. Department of Health and Human Services, 2011) finds that Native Americans, Hispanics/Latinos, American Indians and Alaska Natives, Asian Americans, native Hawaiians and Pacific Islanders have higher rates of infant mortality, cardiovascular disease, diabetes, HIV/AIDS, cancer, and lower rates of immunizations and cancer screening than do Whites. While there is great variation in health within any racial or ethnic group, and on certain measures one group may be doing better than most—for example, the life expectancy for Asian American women is the highest of all groups reported in the United States (CDC, 2013b)—the overall picture is one of higher rates of illness and premature death among non-White populations in the United States.

Learning about Health Inequalities

When we present data on health inequalities in our classes at City College of San Francisco, students often experience anger, sorrow, and other powerful emotions. The authors of this book share these responses. We usually pair the evidence of deep inequalities in health with evidence that the rates of inequality have changed over time, and can be changed in the future by improving public policies that shape health. Our hope is that a growing awareness of health inequalities will inspire us to advocate for a more just world.

What are your reactions as you study the topic of health inequalities?

Table 4.2 Health Indicators for African Americans and White Americans

POPULATION	INFANT MORTALITY (2013) (PER 1,000 LIVE BIRTHS)	MATERNAL MORTALITY (2011) (PER 100,000 LIVE BIRTHS)	LIFE EXPECTANCY (2013) (LIFE SPAN EXPECTED AT BIRTH)
African Americans	11.22	42.8	75.5
White Americans	5.07	12.5	79.1

Source: National Center for Health Statistics (2014a), and Centers for Disease Control and Prevention (2014b).

Health inequalities between African Americans and White Americans have been most studied because they are the most extreme. African Americans of all ages die at higher rates than do Whites. The data presented in Table 4.2 show that African American infants are 2.2 times more likely to die before the age of one than are White infants born in the United States. African American mothers are still almost three and a half times more likely to die due to complications of pregnancy or childbirth than White mothers in the United States. Finally, White Americans are expected to live 3.8 years longer than African Americans.

It is hard to overstate the gravity of these inequalities in health. Dr. David Satcher, a former Surgeon General of the United States, and colleagues conducted a study of African American death rates and found 886,202 "excess" deaths could have been prevented between 1991 and 2000 had African Americans enjoyed the same health as Whites (Woolf, Johnson, Freyer, Rust, & Satcher, 2004). "That's the equivalent of a Boeing 767 shot out of the sky and killing everyone on board every day, 365 days a year," points out David Williams of Harvard's School of Public Health. And they are all black" (Smedley, Jeffries, Adelman, & Cheng, n.d., p. 2).

It is important to note that the health inequalities between African Americans and Whites are not static. In the period between 1990 and 2009, the inequality (or gap) in life expectancy between African Americans and Whites decreased by 2.7 years for men and 1.7 years for women. Some states moved closer to health equality than others; for example, New York State saw the biggest increase in African American life expectancy and greatest narrowing of the gap between Blacks and White, while the Black–White gap in life expectancy in Washington, DC, changed very little over the 20-year period studied (Harper, McLehose, & Kaufman, 2014).

- *What is the gap or inequality between life expectancy for African-Americans and White Americans in your city?*

- *What can CHWs do to narrow this gap and promote health equality?*

There are many examples of health inequalities changing over time. In 1950, African Americans were about 1.7 times more likely to die of influenza (flu) and pneumonia than Whites, but by the year 2000, that disparity was eliminated. Flu is an acute respiratory disease that presents obvious symptoms, can be treated with antiviral medications, and can be prevented through vaccination (quite different from chronic conditions like heart disease or cancer). The introduction of Medicare and Medicaid in the 1960s created more equal access to these medical interventions and contributed to greater health equality regarding flu. In the same time period, rates of heart disease became more unequal, even while the overall rates of heart disease decreased for both African Americans and Whites. Heart disease decreased much more in the White population than among African Americans between 1950 and 2000. Researchers suggest that multiple factors play a part in the higher rates of heart disease among African Americans, including education levels, income, health behaviors, stress, and racial segregation (Williams & Jackson, 2005).

The data regarding health inequalities for Latinos and Asian Americans in the United States are more mixed. For example, infant mortality for Puerto Rican mothers (7.10 per 1,000 live births) is significantly higher than for White mothers. However, the rates for other Latino groups are similar to or lower than the rate for White mothers (Mexican: 5.12; Cuban: 3.79; Central & South American: 4.43) (CDC, 2013a). Mothers classified as Asian and Pacific Islander (API) experienced an infant mortality rate of 4.27. Unfortunately, it is still rare to find health data that distinguishes among the many distinct API populations; when available, the data usually indicate wide variation in rates of disease or premature death among different API communities. For example, in Santa Clara County, California, residents of Vietnamese heritage were more than twice as likely than those of Chinese heritage to report poor health (Baath, Sujeer, Peddycord, Fenstersheib, & Luna, n.d.).

OTHER HEALTH INEQUALITIES

Other differences in social status and power are also associated with health inequalities. Many of these interact with race and ethnicity, yet also operate independently in shaping the population's health.

Immigration Status

Health inequalities also persist in the United States based on immigration status. While immigrants generally have a higher life expectancy than people born in the United States, they are much less likely to have health insurance or receive preventative health care services. Immigrant adults are twice as likely, and immigrant children more than four times as likely, to lack health insurance (Singh, Rodriguez-Lainz, & Kogan, 2013). Interestingly, new immigrants tend to have better health than do native citizens of the same sex, age, income, and educational level; this pattern is called the "Latino paradox" or the "immigrant paradox." However immigrants' health status declines the longer they live in the United States (Singh, Rodriguez-Lainz & Kogan, 2013; Smedley, Jeffries, Adelman, & Cheng, 2009). Changes in diet and activity levels can contribute to this decline, along with the loss of social ties with extended family, and increased exposure to discrimination (Life in America, 2014).

Gender

While women have a higher life expectancy than men in most nations, they experience disproportionately higher rates of domestic and sexual violence, with the resulting trauma, depression, and other chronic health conditions. They also face discrimination in the diagnosis and treatment of certain health conditions. Women tend to experience more days of illness per year, higher rates of disability and poorer health overall (Benoit & Shumka, 2009; National Center for Health Statistics, 2014b; Östlin, George, & Sen, 2003; Zack, 2013). While some inequalities in health can be directly tied to biological differences between the sexes (for example, higher rates of breast cancer in women than men), others are largely influenced by the status and treatment of women and girls (for example, higher rates of depression in women than men).

TG: Most of my clients have HIV, and most of them are people of color, gay men, and injection-drug users—people who face discrimination on a daily basis just because of who they are. They risk losing their families, get discriminated against when they look for work, or housing, or health care, and sometimes just when they are walking down the street. All of this takes a big toll on their health. It keeps them from getting basic things that they need, and after awhile, for some of them, it just sort of beats them down. They can lose confidence and faith in themselves. This is why I became a CHW—to work with other people like me who had experienced discrimination, to let them know that someone wants the best for them, and to advocate for them to be treated like they should be treated—with respect.

Sexual Orientation and Gender Identity

Health inequalities also exist based on sexual orientation and gender identity. Studies have documented higher rates of depression and attempted suicide among lesbian, gay, bisexual, and transgender (LGBT) youth compared to heterosexual youth. Interestingly, youth who experienced a positive school environment and were not subject to homophobic teasing had much lower rates of depression, suicide, substance use, and skipping school (CDC, 2014a). Transgender and gender-variant communities experience some of the highest rates of HIV infection in the United States, as well as high rates of violence, depression, unemployment, and attempted suicide (National Center for Transgender Equality, n.d.). Due to persistent discrimination and related stigma, comparably little research is available regarding the health status of transgender and gender-variant communities. Fortunately, this is beginning to change.

4.3 Awareness of Health Inequalities As a Catalyst for Change

Health inequalities are neither natural nor unchangeable. That inequality exists is not surprising; however, the large scale and enduring nature of many health inequalities—and the impact they have on human lives—still has the power to shock.

When new information about health inequalities is highlighted in a place where local public health or political leaders and residents are open to taking action, the result can be a campaign to address those inequalities. Berkeley, California, offers one such example. The catalyst, in this case, was the 1999 City of Berkeley Health Status Report, which pointed to a 20-year gap in life expectancy between men (mostly White) who resided in a wealthy district of the city and men (mostly African American) who lived in a low-income district. Even more surprising was the fact that the health inequalities in Berkeley (a famously liberal city) were higher than those in the surrounding regions (Ellis & Walton, 2012). The response was immediate.

> *Two prominent local policymakers used the occasion of the report's release to call a town hall meeting on the topic of health disparities in the city. Approximately 220 South and West Berkeley residents, policymakers, health care providers, and others participated in this lively meeting. Residents of many different racial and ethnic groups from the flatland neighborhoods and elsewhere voiced the strong conviction at this meeting that they themselves needed to do something about the disparities problem, including organizing, collecting their own data, and working to address racism. (Ellis & Walton, 2012)*

This initial meeting led to a variety of actions to address the root causes of inequality and improve health outcomes, as residents, community-based organizations and city agencies joined together in the South and West Berkeley Health Forum. A few of the actions undertaken to reduce health inequalities included:

- The creation of Community Action Teams (CATs), led by and composed of community residents, who took on CHW roles of community diagnosis, advocacy, and connecting residents to health services.
- The launch of the CHW-centered Black Infant Health Project in Berkeley, profiled in the section titled CHW Case Studies in Health Equality, in this chapter.
- Tackling hypertension in the community, including improving access to healthy food and physical activity, and opening a free weekly hypertension drop-in clinic.

Through these efforts, some health inequalities were reduced. For example, the likelihood of an African American woman having a baby with low birth weight was 4 times that of a White woman in 1991, and by 2011 this inequality was reduced to 2.5 times as likely. As low birth weight is associated with so many poor health outcomes later in life, this reduction is an important contribution toward closing the health gap between Whites and Blacks in Berkeley.

It is a sign of just how complex and entrenched patterns of social inequality are that other inequalities have not improved as much or at all. The 2013 Berkeley Health Status Report showed that the death rate (the percent of the population that dies in any given year) of African Americans in Berkeley was twice that of Whites, and the gap was actually increasing. Health equality and cultural humility are explicit priorities for the city's Health, Housing, and Community Services Department and their work to reduce inequalities is ongoing.

- *What has your city or county done to research and analyze local health inequalities?*

- *What are local communities doing to increase health equality?*

4.4 Social Determinants of Health

Health is shaped by the conditions we live in. In public health, these are called the social determinants of health: "the conditions in which people are born, grow, work, live, and age" (WHO, 2015, para.1). These conditions, in turn, are shaped by larger social, economic, and political forces that give some people more advantages or resources than others (see Chapter 3).

Our physical, social, economic, and political environment has a significant impact on human health. Our environment can pose physical hazards (such as pollution or radiation); it can influence behaviors around eating, exercising, driving, and so forth; it can present barriers to getting adequate health care services; and it can expose people to toxic levels of uncertainty and stress, with physiological effects on the cardiovascular system, the immune system, and other systems of the body (see Chapter 12 for more discussion of the effects of chronic stress). Below we provide a few examples of how social determinants can cause health inequalities. Keep in mind that each person is affected by multiple social factors—and that social determinants interact with one another.

INCOME AND WEALTH

In recent decades, economic inequality has grown dramatically in the United States and many other advanced economies. The United States had a Gini index (a measure of inequality in a society, where 0 means perfect equality, and 100 means perfect inequality) of 41.1 in 2010 (World Bank, 2015)—significantly higher than other wealthy countries, and similar to the levels of inequality found in the United States in the late 1920s, before the Great Depression. The Congressional Budget Office (2011) notes that incomes for the bottom 80 percent of households actually dropped between 1979 and 2007, and only the top 20 percent saw their income grow. While economic recessions tend to reduce inequality temporarily, the recovery from Great Recession (2008–2009) in the United States increased the concentration of wealth at the very top; the top 1 percent of households received 95 percent of the economic gains made in 2009–2012 (Saez, 2013).

It is well established that income (the money a person or household makes during a year) and wealth (the total value of a person's property, possessions, and money) are closely correlated to health, along a social gradient. The *Poverty and Inequality Report* from Stanford University points out that those with lower incomes are more likely to report being in poor health, to have children with asthma, and to report serious psychological distress (Stanford Center on Poverty and Inequality, 2014). Poverty can lead to fewer choices for good nutrition and physical activity. Yet even among those who share the same health behaviors, those with fewer resources tend to experience worse health outcomes. Sir Michael Marmot gave an example of this phenomenon found in his study of public employees in the United Kingdom: "If a poor person's smoking, he or she has a higher rate of disease than if a wealthy person is smoking" (Adelman, 2008, p. 3 of transcript, first episode). The many stresses that go along with poverty or limited resources help to explain this difference.

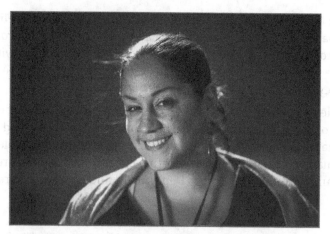

CHWs typically work with communities that experience the highest rates of illness, disability, and death.

While controversial, a growing body of research demonstrates that it is not just low income that leads to poor health; high levels of inequality itself can lead to worse health outcomes on a population level. The effect of inequality itself—separate from the effects of low income, for example—is likely to be small, yet still very important, because it affects so many people. It may be that inequality affects population health only after it reaches a certain point, like a Gini score of 30 or higher (Rowlingson, 2011). One possible explanation for why inequality would negatively affect health is "status anxiety" or stress caused by having low status in a hierarchical society (Wilkinson & Pickett, 2009). We discuss status in more detail further on.

SOCIAL STATUS

The stress of lower social status (e.g., being perceived or treated as "less than" on the basis of race, ethnicity, gender or gender identity, sexual orientation, educational level, immigration status, national origin, age or disability status) causes physiological reactions in the human body that contribute to chronic disease. Toxic stress can affect the immune system, the cardiovascular system, the body's use of insulin, and even brain development (Adelman, 2008). Toxic stress exposure over a lifetime helps explain why a person who changes social status—for example, someone who starts out living in poverty and later enters the middle class—may still have higher levels of chronic disease than those who experienced higher status all their lives—even when both groups have similar health habits as adults.

EMPLOYMENT AND WORK

Unemployment rates are higher among African Americans, youth, and less-educated workers. Jobs in the unionized manufacturing sector that used to provide good wages to blue-collar workers have declined sharply; the majority of jobs available in the 21st-century economy in the United States are lower-paid service jobs, many of them temporary or on-call positions, often without benefits. The instability of employment and low levels of control at work contribute to high levels of stress. With low pay, workers also have less opportunity to relieve their stress, or even take time off to care for a sick relative or see a doctor themselves.

EDUCATION

Education is still one of the most important routes to economic mobility. Those with a higher education earn more on average and tend to live longer (Robert Wood Johnson Foundation, 2011). However, great inequalities persist in regarding who has access to a high-quality education. Schools in the United States are highly segregated; most White children attend schools that are majority White, and most African American and Latino children attend schools that are majority non-White (Jordan, 2014). The amount of money invested in education per child varies a lot by state, and even more by locality—which has serious implications for racial inequalities. The Center for American Progress reports that ". . . schools with 90 percent or more students of color spend a full $733 less per student per year than schools with 90 percent or more white students" (Spatig-Amerikaner, 2012, p. 4). In addition, the cost of higher education has soared in recent decades, with an increasing share of the cost, even at public institutions, charged to students directly, leading to high levels of student loan debt.

Education is associated with better health overall. There are at least three ways that education can improve health (or that the lack of education can diminish health):

- People with higher levels of education have more health knowledge and health literacy, and can better use that information to improve health habits.

- More education often leads to better pay and more benefits at work. Jobs may also be less stressful or offer more choices than the work available without education. Stress is easier to manage with vacation time, and benefits such as sick leave and health insurance make it easier to take good care of one's own health or the health of family members.

- People with higher levels of education tend to have a larger and more diverse social network, along with higher social status and a greater sense of being able to control or influence what happens to them. These are associated with better stress management and healthy behaviors (RWJF, 2011).

- *Does the quality of education vary across different areas of the city or county where you live?*

- *What role does education play in promoting the health and well-being of the communities you serve?*

- *How accessible and affordable is a college education to low-income students in the city, county, or state where you live?*

NEIGHBORHOOD QUALITY

Access to nutritious and affordable food is essential for good health. Yet many low-income neighborhoods lack a single grocery store (See Chapter 17 for more discussion of how neighborhood quality affects eating and active living). Tobacco and alcohol are heavily marketed in low-income communities, as well. Inadequate transportation can also affect health; it affects the likelihood of getting a good job or education, or even reaching a health clinic, while also requiring a lot of time that could otherwise be used for health-promoting activities. Limited access to health care facilities in some neighborhoods affects preventative care, timely diagnosis of life-threatening illness, and management of chronic conditions. Violence in the community not only causes injury and death, it discourages people from engaging in outdoors activities. The combination of less physical activity and more psychosocial stress can lead to more cases of chronic illness. Recently, more public health efforts have taken a comprehensive look at the places people live, to try to improve their chances of a long, healthy life by improving neighborhoods. Examples of efforts to study and promote place-based health are documented by the Prevention Institute (http://preventioninstitute.org).

PUBLIC POLICY

Inequalities in the distribution of resources to support health and well-being that exist both within and among nations, do not occur randomly. To a large extent, they are created by public policy decisions. Policies use incentives or penalties to implement certain processes, procedures, or behaviors. Policy can be set by legislation (laws), by regulations (rules about how laws are implemented), by local ordinances (laws at the municipal or county level) or institutional policies (rules within a given institution like a school or a bank). Policies that are put in place by government entities are called public policies. You can read more about advocating to change public policies in Chapter 23.

The practice of **redlining**, a form of discrimination in financial services and home ownership, is another example of how policies have given an unfair advantage to one group over another. Redlining has had lasting effects on neighborhood quality and economic inequalities in the United States. Between the 1930s and the 1960s, the percent of Americans who owned homes skyrocketed—but people of color were largely locked out of this version of the American Dream. "The Federal Housing Administration and the Veterans Administration financed more than $120 billion worth of new housing between 1934 and 1962, but less than 2 percent of this real estate was available to non-White families—and most of that small amount was located in segregated areas" (Lipsitz, 2009, p. 6). Neighborhoods where African Americans or other people of color lived were "redlined" on city maps, and those areas were systematically denied loans or mortgages. Simply *because African Americans or other people of color lived there*, property values were expected to go down. This became a self-fulfilling prophesy: houses were difficult to sell without loans, and property values *did* go down. In a prac-tice called "block busting," speculators would use scare tactics to get White homeowners to sell at low prices, then turn around and sell those same properties to black families at higher prices. As most African Americans could not get bank loans, the speculators loaned money to African Americans at high rates, and often on a "contract" system that turned over full ownership of the house to the speculator if the family was even slightly late with a payment (Coates, 2014). As a result of federal housing and lending policies, fewer African Americans than Whites were and are homeowners.

Home ownership is a primary way that people in the United States gain wealth, as property values tend to rise over time. But most people of color were excluded from the government programs and subsidies that would have made home ownership possible. In the 1990s and 2000s when financing became available, African Americans and Latinos were often sold loans on less-favorable terms than Whites with the same credit history (Rothstein, 2012). The foreclosure crisis that began in 2008 hit African American and Latino communities par-ticularly hard, especially as many families of color had no reserves other than a house. Through racial inequali-ties in housing and banking, the inequalities in wealth were made greater, and neighborhood stability suffered. These factors influence neighborhood quality, access to healthy food, opportunities for employment or small business development, crime levels, and eventually, human health and life expectancy. Federal housing policies were not necessarily intended to add to health inequalities, but that was their effect.

In a similar vein, we could look at nearly any area where stark inequalities are present—such as employment, wealth accumulation, college completion, segregation, or the ease of obtaining citizenship upon immigration—and we would find that public policies have played a large role in creating and maintaining those inequalities.

Patricia Barahona, Senior Director of San Francisco Programs, Youth Leadership Institute

Patricia Barahona: Policy matters. This policy [an ordinance that limited the number of places selling tobacco, achieved through six years of advocacy] is sustainable in that we will start to see health dispari-ties lessen for the next 10 to 15 years. We are also already seeing some initial changes, in terms of changes in tobacco density improving health. We will see a decrease in health disparities—and we are excited to be able to say we were a part of it, the impact it has on the residents in those particular communities. We are working to get to the place where we can tell that story, how this one ordinance is making a difference in specific communities. The San Francisco Department of Public Health is tracking the decrease in tobacco permits over time—this ordinance put a cap on the number of permits to sell tobacco, to eventually make the concentration of tobacco outlets even throughout the city. Areas that are now over the cap can't get any new licenses until they drop below that cap of 45 tobacco outlets. [For more about this campaign, see Chapter 23.]

HOW DO DIFFERENT DETERMINANTS OF HEALTH INTERACT?

The focus in recent decades on the social determinants of health has helped CHWs and other public health pro-fessionals to better understand and address health inequalities. Traditionally, other causes of poor health have received more attention, yet these factors are also affected by social determinants. Let's take a closer look at a few of these other causes or contributors to poor health outcomes: genes, health behaviors or lifestyle, culture, access to health care, and quality of health care.

Genes

Genes certainly influence human health. Some illnesses tend to run in families, and some of those illnesses are influenced by genes that are passed down, biologically, from parent to child. Some illnesses are caused by a difference in a single gene; everyone with that gene mutation will have the same disease. Some genes, or combinations of genes, give people a certain weakness or predisposition toward an illness; in these cases, not everyone with the gene will have the disease, but people with the gene (or gene combination) are more likely to develop the disease than others. However, while genes do a great deal to explain health inequalities (or differences) between one family and another, they do very little to explain health inequalities among people of different races or classes. As noted above, race is a social category rather than a biological one, and there is at least as much genetic variation within any racial group as there is between racial groups (American Anthropological Association, 2011). This fact is surprising to many people, given our culture's focus on the superficial genetic traits that affect appearance. In fact, a recent review of genomic studies of heart disease, the main contributor to the gap between White and Black mortality, found no clue in human genes to explain the enormous racial health inequalities. As the authors of the review put it, "Despite the rapid increase in the number of genomic studies over the past decade that covered many outcomes, the accumulated evidence for a genetic contribution to CVD [cardiovascular disease] disparities in blacks versus whites has been essentially nil" (Kaufman, Dolman, Rashani, & Cooper, 2015).

Genes interact with the social and physical environment, and the new science of epigenetics helps to explain these interactions. **Epigenetics** studies how genes get turned on or off by exposures to chemicals, stress, and other environmental factors. These environmental exposures start at a very early age—in the womb, where a fetus's environment is affected by what happens to the mother. While a person's genes don't change, the *behavior* of those genes can change, showing how complex the relationship is between "nature" and "nurture," between our human biology and our physical and social environment.

Health Behaviors

Health behaviors are often presented as the leading cause of illness, especially illnesses that are sexually transmitted (such as HIV) or strongly affected by nutrition and physical activity (such as diabetes and hypertension). Yet health behaviors themselves are strongly influenced by social determinants. Low-income neighborhoods have less green space, fewer parks, less safe streets, more liquor stores, more stores that sell tobacco, fewer places to buy affordable healthy food, etc. Even among low-income neighborhoods, those with a higher density of fast food restaurants also have a higher rate of diabetes (California Center for Public Health Advocacy, PolicyLink & the UCLA Center for Health Policy Research, 2008). While personal behaviors do influence health—many CHWs work specifically on helping clients adopt healthier behaviors—efforts to improve health behaviors are generally more effective if they take into account the social environment. Likewise, changes in the community or in public policy can make personal behavior change easier to accomplish.

Access to Health Care

Access to health care is still not universal, and the lack of access contributes to health inequalities between populations. When health care is not available or affordable, many people will miss out on preventative care (vaccinations, screening tests, health advising). Chronic conditions are less likely to be well managed, and diseases like cancer may be diagnosed later in their development. The Commonwealth Fund, for example, reports that in 2012 (shortly before implementation of the main parts of the Affordable Care Act) that 47.3 million Americans were uninsured, and another 31.7 million were underinsured (Schoen, Hayes, Collins, Lippa, & Radley, 2014). Low-income communities and people of color are the most likely to experience barriers in accessing health care, especially high-quality health care (DHHS, 2011).

Differences in the Quality of Health Care

Differences in the quality of health care also contribute to inequalities. ". . . (R)acial and ethnic minorities often receive poorer quality of care and face more barriers in seeking care including preventive care, acute treatment, or chronic disease management, than do non-Hispanic White patients. Minority groups experience rates of preventable hospitalizations that are, in some cases, almost double that of non-Hispanic Whites" (DHHS, 2011). Several factors lead to uneven quality of health care. Many doctors and some hospitals do not serve the uninsured and may not accept Medicaid, reducing the choices or creating delays in treatment for low-income people. Attitudes and assumptions about ethnicity and race can also influence medical decisions (Smedley, Stith, & Nelson, 2003), through both conscious and unconscious preferences. For example, one experiment demonstrated that doctors who had no conscious racial bias still showed implicit bias (unconscious bias), which influenced their treatment decisions—White patients were more likely than African American patients to receive prescriptions for state-of-the-art treatment (Green et al., 2007).

While health care is important, it is not the most significant factor that drives health inequalities. It is difficult to state with certainty the exact proportion of illness or premature death that is due to each of the major determinants of health, as they interact with each other and some are difficult to measure. Nonetheless, several studies have at least estimated their relative importance to our health. Booske and her colleagues at the University of Wisconsin reviewed many studies and arrived at this conclusion about what most influences health (apart from genetics, which they left out of their report): 40 percent social and economic factors; 30 percent health behaviors; 20 percent clinical care; and 10 percent environmental factors (Booske, Athens, Kindig, Park, & Remington, 2010). Dr. David Satcher, former surgeon general of the United States, reached a similar conclusion in his research with Higginbotham: "Although critical to eliminating disparities, access to health care only accounts for 15–20 percent of the variation of morbidity and mortality that we see in different populations in this country" (Satcher & Higginbotham, 2008, p. 400). (Note: **morbidity** refers to the rate of illness or disability, while mortality refers to the rate of death.)

- *In the communities where you live and work, how do health care access, health care quality, health behaviors, and the social and physical environment influence health?*

- *Take a moment to read the case study of Keisha Mitchell at the start of Chapter 16. (The case study continues throughout the chapter—you can read more of it, if you like.) What social determinants of health do you think influenced Keisha's health, and the health of her family?*

4.5 Overcoming Health Inequalities

Understanding the root causes of a problem is the first step toward overcoming it. In our discussion of health inequalities, we have identified the social determinants of health as important root causes of preventable differences in population health. Because these root causes are strongly influenced by policies, advocating for policies that support health equality is crucial. Increasingly at the local, state and national levels, health advocates, community leaders, public health departments, and other health professionals are engaging in advocacy to improve the conditions for health.

Public Health and Social Justice Are Linked

Taking action on avoidable inequalities, inequities, is the right thing to do; it is a matter of social justice. We put at the center empowerment of individuals, of communities, and indeed of whole countries. We think of empowerment as material—if you do not have the money to feed your children, you cannot be empowered; as psychosocial, having control over your life; and as political, having your voice count. We must create the conditions for people to take control of their lives to lead flourishing lives. (Marmot, 2009, p. 1)

The Ecological Model—first introduced in Chapter 3—is useful in analyzing health inequalities. Changes can be made at all levels of the ecological model that promote social justice. Whether CHWs are working with individual clients, families, groups or communities, they are helping to promote greater health justice. Linking vulnerable clients to more effective services and supporting them to gain greater autonomy in managing their health and wellness helps to diminish persistent inequalities.

There is also important work to be done at the levels of the community and the society, through changing social environments and improving public policies. CHWs also play a vital role in this kind of work. When CHWs and the people they serve speak up at city council meetings or before state legislators, they are influencing public policy. When they mobilize community action to build more parks or close down a source of pollution, that mobilization contributes to health equality. When they partner with other organizations to confront racism or sexism or any other form of oppression, helping institutions recognize and address bias in any of their practices, CHWs are changing the social determinants of health for the better.

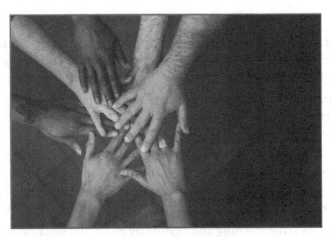

Promoting health equality requires building alliances among communities and organizations.

Advocating for social equality often means swimming against the tide of policies that produce greater inequalities in income, wealth, and health status. It requires confronting all forms of discrimination, not only on the interpersonal level but also on the institutional level. It calls us to find ways to ensure that everyone has access to sufficient resources and opportunities for health. Some are calling the medical personnel, public health workers, and CHWs who practice this approach to health "upstreamists" (Manchanda, 2013), building on the common public metaphor you saw in Chapter 3, of addressing the problems "upstream" where they start, instead of "downstream."

We can look to other nations for examples of how to reduce health inequalities. Sweden has promoted health and health equality through public policies that establish higher taxes and invest this money to provide universal access to basic resources. Education through college is free to all citizens. So are health care, child care, family leave, and other resources that promote public health. The child poverty rate in Sweden is around 7 percent, while in the United States it is about 23 percent (UNICEF Office of Research, 2013).

We can also look to our own history for inspiration. During the first part of the twentieth century, average life expectancy in the United States increased by approximately 30 years. These gains were not achieved, as many believe, by new advances in medicine, but rather by advocating for new social policies that improved working conditions and wages and increased access to education and civil rights.

Successful advocacy for policies that promote social justice requires the participation and leadership of representatives from communities that currently suffer the consequences of health inequalities, including low-income communities of color. It also requires building broad-based coalitions of diverse stakeholders who can work together. Fruitful partnerships can be formed among people and organizations working in public health and those working in other sectors, such as affordable housing, urban planning, rural development, food security (or uninterrupted access to affordable and nutritious food), economic security, workers' rights, and civil and human rights, including women's rights and LGBT rights.

Increasingly, public health professionals are pushing for an examination of "health in all policies." This approach develops methods and procedures for reviewing all new policies—whether it's a policy about transportation or one about shopping centers—in light of their potential impacts on health. California has been a leader in this movement; its Health in All Policies Task Force has developed guides for state and local governments to implement this kind of comprehensive health review. Because the social determinants of health are so diverse, this approach opens the door for public health professionals, communities and policymakers to predict consequences (ones that might have slipped by, intended or unintended, otherwise) and to modify both policies and governmental projects for the sake of the community's health (Public Health Institute, California Department of Public Health, and American Public Health Association, 2013).

POLICIES DESIGNED TO PROMOTE HEALTH EQUALITY

Public health professionals have identified a wide range of public policies to promote health equality. Here we summarize and adapt key examples from California Newsreel's *Policy Guide* and the *Unnatural Causes* documentaries produced for public television (Adelman, 2008).

Policies designed to promote health equality include the following examples:

1. *Promote understanding of the social determinants of health:* Such as educating decision makers and the general public about how patterns of inequality in the larger environment—where we live, work, and play—influence inequalities in health.

2. *Improve income and reduce wealth inequalities:* Such as raising the minimum wage to a livable level; increasing income supports, including unemployment insurance; ensuring secure retirement and pension plans and expanding access for nonstandard workers; supporting the right to organize; and repealing tax loopholes for the rich.

3. *Improve the physical and built environment:* Such as creating more low-cost housing; creating more safe and inviting parks and green spaces; providing appropriate clean-up and removal of toxic material; working to mitigate and adapt to climate change; and providing reliable and low-cost public transit.

4. *Promote racial justice:* Such as strengthening and rigorously enforcing existing antidiscrimination, voting rights, and equal opportunity laws; desegregating schools and neighborhoods; providing resources for jobs and educational access and retention; monitoring and eliminating environmental health threats; addressing arrest and sentencing discrimination and promoting rehabilitation in corrections facilities; increasing access, quality, and cultural competence of medical care and social services; and protecting the civil rights of undocumented workers.

   We would advocate broadening this proposal to include promoting justice and civil rights for all communities, including women, immigrants, lesbian, gay, bisexual, transgender, and intersex communities. Some groups have also advocated for a "truth and reconciliation process" as well, to acknowledge and address the impacts of our history of slavery, colonization of Native American lands, forced sterilization of Puerto Rican women and people with disabilities, and other major historical forms of oppression.

5. *Promote better working conditions:* Such as strengthening and reinforcing occupation health and safety laws; legislating paid sick leave (including parental and family leave) and vacations; and removing unfair barriers to unionization and strengthening collective bargaining.

6. *Improve conditions for children:* Such as guaranteeing universal quality preschool and day care; providing quality public schooling and safe places to play; and ensuring good nutrition and preventive (health) care.

7. *Improve social inclusion:* Such as strengthening democratic decision making, community organizations, and opportunities for civic engagement; strengthening laws against discrimination and segregation; and investing in jobs and public infrastructure in resource-poor communities.

8. *Improve education:* Such as reforming school financing to equalize school spending and access to quality Pre-K–12 education, and improving teacher compensation, training, and support.

9. *Improve food security and quality:* Such as providing affordable and nutritious food for all, especially the most vulnerable; limiting fast food and alcohol outlets; and supporting sustainable agriculture and local food production, especially organics.

10. *Improve public and sustainable transportation:* Such as giving precedence to cycling and walking; discouraging out-of-town malls and residential sprawl; and improving public transit.

11. *Use health impact assessments (HIAs):* Such as requiring the use of HIAs to evaluate the consequences of proposed development and policy initiatives on population health.

12. *Provide universal health care:* Such as supporting guaranteed and culturally competent, quality health care, access, and treatment for all.

- *Can you think of other policies that would promote health equality?*

- *Of the policy ideas listed here, which ones seem most urgent to you?*

What Do
YOU?
Think!

4.6 CHW Case Studies in Health Equality

There are many ways that CHWs work throughout the United States and throughout the world to promote health equity. We highlight two examples from the San Francisco Bay Area below.

Reducing Maternal and Child Health Inequalities: The Berkeley Black Infant Health Project

Babies who weigh less than 5.5 pounds at birth are considered low birth weight and face significantly increased risks of many health problems including asthma, cerebral palsy, hypertension, cardiovascular disease, and learning disabilities. When the City of Berkeley began issuing periodic "Health Status Reports" in the late 1990s, many were shocked to see how large the racial inequalities in health were in a city best known for its university and its progressive politics. *Black infants were four times more likely than White infants to be born with low birth weight* during the period from 1993 to 1995 (City of Berkeley, 2002).

The City of Berkeley evaluated the causes of this inequality and recognized that "being at risk for having a low birth weight baby is not a genetic predisposition but is due to many factors including stress that may be related to discrimination and racism" (City of Berkeley, 2002).

In response, the public health department developed the Berkeley Black Infant Health Program based on a community empowerment model. While other Black Infant Health Programs around the state were primarily focused on reducing infant mortality, Berkeley's was the first program explicitly focused on reducing the rate of low birth weight, and one of the few at that time to use community health workers. Two CHWs, Ramona Benson and Yvonne Lacey, were hired to conduct health outreach to invite pregnant and parenting women to participate in an ongoing support group. The group combined health education and stress reduction with empowerment, and linked their work to neighborhood community action teams.

Ramona Benson: In our group we talk about relationships, including relationships with mothers, with the baby's father, and a circle of friends. We talk about how to create support in our lives and to provide it to others. We talk about finances, education, racism, stress reduction, personal and community empowerment—and how to have a healthy baby. If our moms aren't stressed, if they have support in their life and are empowered to advocate for themselves, to navigate systems and ask for what they need, that will help their pregnancy and help them to raise a healthy baby.

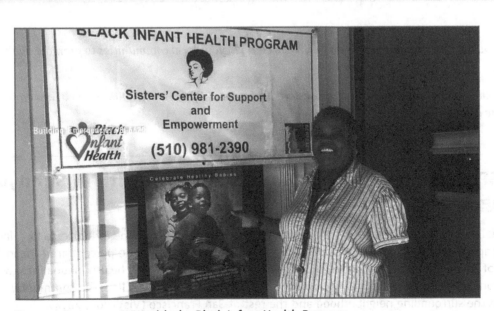

Ramona Benson, a CHW with the Black Infant Health Program.

The CHWs also helped women navigate the health system and overcome obstacles, so that Black women could get earlier and more consistent prenatal care.

> **Ramona Benson:** When we started in 2001, they told me I needed to reach 50 women in the first three months. Outreach was our first task. When I went out there, I reached 50 women in a week. It was easy. I was talking to women about what the program was about, what services we had to offer, and they were interested. But to bring them in [to use the services] was not always easy. We needed to identify other obstacles that got in the way of their coming in. . . . By helping them to navigate these obstacles, we developed a bond. I was able to identify with them, and helped them to eliminate the barriers.

By 2005, four years after the Black Infant Health Program was started, the inequality in rates of low birth weight between Black and White babies had been reduced from 4-to-1 to 2-to-1, and the inequality in access to early prenatal care (first trimester) had been virtually eliminated (City of Berkeley, 2007). The 2013 Health Status Report, following the greatest economic crisis in the United States since the Great Depression, showed that some inequalities had increased again. The gap between Black and White mothers accessing prenatal care in the first trimester reappeared (although much smaller than it had been in the 1990s), and the inequality in low birth weight increased slightly (due to a decrease in the rate of low birth weight among Whites, not an increase among Blacks). As of 2011, the ratio of Black babies with low birth weight to White was 2.5-to-1 (City of Berkeley, 2013). If anything, this increase demonstrated the importance of maintaining programs like the Black Infant Health Project. The number of CHWs and other health personnel focused on maternity had decreased sharply during the economic crisis. Despite setbacks, the achievements of the Black Infant Health Project and allied programs were substantial. While Black babies in Berkeley were still more than twice as likely as White babies to be born with low birth weight, huge progress had been made. The program continues to work to eliminate inequalities.

> **Ramona Benson:** I helped them identify what those challenges were [that got in the way of their health], and also where those challenges came from. We let them know it's a system thing, and in order for that system to change, you have to be present to give your voice. That's what CHW programs give to the community.

- *What are public health professionals and activists doing in your local communities to promote health equality?*

- *What policies and programs exist that are designed to reduce higher rates of illness and death among vulnerable communities?*

Hope SF: Altering the Basic Conditions of Health in Sunnydale Housing Project

The Sunnydale public housing project is the largest in San Francisco. It is home to a diverse low-income population; approximately half of the residents are immigrants and almost 40 percent are African Americans. Two thirds of the households have children. Sunnydale is greatly affected by health inequalities, with high rates of chronic disease, violence, and unemployment. Despite one good bus line, the community is largely cut off from the surrounding neighborhood and the rest of San Francisco (VisVision, 2014).

(continues)

Hope SF: Altering the Basic Conditions of Health in Sunnydale Housing Project

(continued)

Sunnydale is one of four public housing sites being redeveloped by a city-led initiative called Hope SF (www.hope-sf.org). The core strategy is focused on social cohesion, to assist residents as they transition into the new housing that will be built on the same site. The multiyear plan aims to redesign the housing development for better health and safety, while supporting the existing residents prior to, during and after the construction period, to prevent displacement. Residents have been involved in the planning process, alongside nonprofits and city agencies, to establish goals and programs in health, education, employment, safety, transportation, local amenities, and housing. The vision is to fundamentally alter the social determinants of health and well-being in Sunnydale (VisVision, 2014).

Residents have been hired as peer leaders, connectors, and community builders—in other words, community health workers—to work with residents on changing the conditions in Sunnydale. In the component focused on health equality, four peer leaders develop activities around physical activity and healthy eating. They also offer workshops and outreach around health in the home, including pest control, mold removal, and lead testing. Access to health care has been improved, as well, with a nurse available onsite twice a week.

"Helping people out, making a difference in people's lives, and helping them transition to a healthy lifestyle—that's basically what's going on around here," said Lafu Seumanu, a peer leader involved in organizing activities like a walking group, Zumba classes, and a cooking class using food that is available at the community food bank. "I see myself growing as a part of it, and I tend to share that story, as a kind of motivation."

Social cohesion and engagement with new programs is not something that happens overnight. High levels of mistrust and memories of broken promises from the city linger. For that reason, community health workers are central to the success of the program. Their knowledge and relationships in the community are what make the program relevant and inviting to the residents.

Reflecting on a leadership workshop about health inequality, program coordinator Emily Claassen observed, "People here know that things are not as they should be, they know that they've been neglected, they understand the systemic history of racism and disenfranchised communities, but it's hard to put your finger on exactly how it translates to health outcomes. Helping residents understand the link between their health and way it is impacted by their behavior, as well as how their behavior is affected by inequalities related to race and education, has proven to be a powerful tool among the Sunnydale Peer Leaders."

Lafu Seumanu shared her vision for Sunnydale as this redevelopment proceeds: "I would love to see residents moving to a unit where there's no pests, no mildew, a healthier unit, more standard and more modern. I'd like to see a lot of resources centered around the area, and more jobs for the youth. I wish that there was less of a stereotype about our community. Get the stereotype to die down, and it will help."

- *What links do you see between social conditions and health behaviors where you live?*

- *What parts of your city, town, or county have you never visited?*

- *Are some areas of your city or town more segregated or isolated than others?*

- *If you were designing an ideal housing development or neighborhood, from the ground up, what would it look like? What role would CHWs play in your project?*

What Do YOU Think?

4.7 The Role of CHWs

CHWs play an important role in promoting social justice and health equality, whether they are supporting individuals to manage chronic conditions, facilitating support groups, or engaging in community organizing campaigns. Part Five of this book provides greater detail about the work that CHWs do at the community level, and Chapter 23 illustrates how CHWs can facilitate grassroots community organizing and advocacy efforts.

CHWs have a responsibility to be knowledgeable about health inequalities and their causes, to acknowledge their impacts on clients and communities, and to address the social determinants that lead to health inequalities. Many CHWs work with others to advocate for policies that will promote greater social and health equality. CHWs encourage communities that face the highest rates of illness and premature death to fully participate in these efforts, and to advocate for new policies and programs that represent the vision of those communities.

CHWs also play a unique role within their places of employment (or volunteer service) to teach other professionals about the community, often calling for greater participation by clients and community members in the evaluation and development of programs and services. CHWs have, in a sense, one foot in the organization they work for, and another foot in the community. CHWs can help organizations to shift the way they provide services to better address the consequences of health inequalities, and to promote greater health equality. This is the focus of "upstream medicine," well described in a short book and videotaped TED talk by Dr. Rishi Manchanda (Manchanda, 2013). Manchanda provides an example of upstream medicine in which a doctor and a CHW (community coordinator) teamed up to survey patient needs, and to take medical personnel out of the clinic and into the neighborhood on "house calls" to see where and how their patients lived. They partnered with patients to identify strategies to address not only the patient's immediate medical needs ("downstream"), but also the social conditions like housing and neighborhood safety that affected their health ("upstream") (Manchanda, 2013). While efforts to be more accountable to the clients served may originate in the actions of a doctor, quite often it is the CHW who raises questions, shares information and persists to create changes in organizational practices, to better serve the community.

When we confront health inequalities and other forms of injustice, we may feel overwhelmed, depressed, or hopeless. Historian Howard Zinn (2004) reminds us of the key role that hope and faith play in keeping us moving forward to create a better and more just world:

> To be hopeful in bad times is not just foolishly romantic. It is based on the fact that human history is a history not only of cruelty but also of compassion, sacrifice, courage, kindness. What we choose to emphasize in this complex history will determine our lives. If we see only the worst, it destroys our capacity to do something. If we remember those times and places—and there are so many—where people have behaved magnificently, this gives us the energy to act, and at least the possibility of sending this spinning top of a world in a different direction. And if we do act, in however small a way, we don't have to wait for some grand utopian future. The future is an infinite succession of presents, and to live now as we think human beings should live, in defiance of all that is bad around us, is itself a marvelous victory. (para. 11)

Nancy Krieger and Anne-Emanuelle Birn (1998), public health researchers and advocates, write:

> To declare that social justice is the foundation of public health is to call upon and nurture that invincible human spirit that led so many of us to enter the field of public health in the first place: a spirit that has a compelling desire to make the world a better place, free of misery, inequity, and preventable suffering, a world in which we all can live, love, work, play, and die with our dignity intact and our humanity cherished. (p. 1603)

- *Who inspires you to work for social justice and health equality?*

- *How do you hope to promote greater health equality?*

- *What brings you hope and energy for your work as a CHW?*

Chapter Review

To assess your understanding of the key concepts presented in this chapter, reflect on how you would answer the following questions:

1. You are talking with a friend, family member, or client about your work as a CHW. How would you explain the following concepts, *in your own words*:
   - What are health inequalities?
   - What causes health inequalities?
   - Why are the consequences of health inequalities (how do they harm local communities and our society at large)?
   - What can we do to reduce or eliminate health inequalities?

2. Conduct research to answer the following questions about health inequalities in the city, county or state where you live:
   - Where can you find reliable information and data on health inequalities that impact your city, county, state, or nation?
   - Which communities in your city (or county or state) experience higher rates of illness, disability and premature death?
   - What organizations are working to eliminate these inequalities and to advocate for social justice?
     - What policy changes are these organizations advocating for?
     - What else needs to happen in your local area in order to promote health equality?
     - What role can you play in these efforts?

References

Adelman, L. (2008). *Unnatural causes: Is inequality making us sick?* 240 minutes. San Francisco, CA: California Newsreel with Vital Pictures.

American Anthropological Association. (2011). *Race: Are we so different?* Retrieved from *www.understandingrace. org/home.html*

Baath, M., Sujeer, A., Peddycord, D., Fenstersheib, M., & Luna, R. (n.d.) *Health disparities among the Asian Pacific Islander subgroups in Santa Clara County.* Retrieved from *www.sccgov.org/sites/sccphd/en-us/Partners/Data/ Documents/Asian%20subgroups%20poster%20combined%20final.pdf*

Benoit, C., & Shumka, L. (2009). *Gendering the health determinants framework: Why girls' and women's health matters.* Vancouver: Women's Health Research Network.

Booske, B. C., Athens, J. K., Kindig, D. A., Park, H., & Remington, P. L. (2010, February). *County health rankings working paper: Different perspectives for assigning weights to determinants of health.* Retrieved from *www. countyhealthrankings.org/sites/default/files/differentPerspectivesForAssigningWeightsToDeterminantsOfHealth.pdf*

California Center for Public Health Advocacy, PolicyLink, & the UCLA Center for Health Policy Research. (2008, April). *Designed for disease: The link between local food environments and obesity and diabetes.* Retrieved from *www.publichealthadvocacy.org/PDFs/RFEI%20Policy%20Brief_finalweb.pdf*

Centers for Disease Control and Prevention. (2014a, November 12). *Lesbian, gay, bisexual, and transgender health: LGBT youth.* Retrieved from *www.cdc.gov/lgbthealth/youth.htm*

Centers for Disease Control and Prevention. (2014b, December 23). *Reproductive health: Pregnancy mortality surveillance system.* Retrieved from *www.cdc.gov/reproductivehealth/maternalinfanthealth/pmss.html*

Centers for Disease Control and Prevention. (2013a, December 18). *Infant mortality statistics from the 2010 linked birth/infant death data set.* Retrieved from *www.cdc.gov/nchs/data/nvsr/nvsr62/nvsr62_08.pdf*

Centers for Disease Control and Prevention. (2013b, July 2). *Minority health: Asian American populations.* Retrieved from *www.cdc.gov/minorityhealth/populations/REMP/asian.html*

City of Berkeley, Public Health Division. (2002). *Health Status Report.* Retrieved from *www.ci.berkeley.ca.us/Health_Human_Services/Public_Health/Public_Health_Reports.aspx*

City of Berkeley, Public Health Division. (2007). *Health Status Report.* Retrieved from *www.ci.berkeley.ca.us/Health_Human_Services/Public_Health/Public_Health_Reports.aspx*

City of Berkeley, Public Health Division. (2013). *Health Status Report.* Retrieved from *www.ci.berkeley.ca.us/Health_Human_Services/Public_Health/Public_Health_Reports.aspx*

Coates, T. N. (2014, June). The case for reparations. *The Atlantic.* Retrieved from *www.theatlantic.com/features/archive/2014/05/the-case-for-reparations/361631/*

Commission on Social Determinants of Health. (2008). *Closing the gap in a generation: Health equity through action on the social determinants of health.* Final Report of the Commission on Social Determinants of Health. Geneva, Switzerland: World Health Organization.

Congressional Budget Office. (2011). *Trends in the distribution of household income between 1979 and 2007.* Retrieved from *www.cbo.gov/publication/42729*

Ellis, G. & Walton, S. (2012). Community building practice: An expanded conceptual framework. In Minkler, M. (Ed.), *Community organizing and community building for health and welfare,* (3rd ed.). New Brunswick, NJ: Rutgers University Press.

Evans, W. N., Wolfe, B., & Adler, N. (2012). The SES and health gradient: A brief review of the literature. In B. Wolfe, W. N. Evans & T. E. Seeman (Eds.), *The biological consequences of socioeconomic inequalities* (pp. 1–37). New York, NY: Russell Sage Foundation.

Green, A. R., Carney, D. R., Pallin, D. J., Ngo, L. H., Raymond, K. L., Iezzoni, L. I., & Banaji, M. R. (2007). Implicit bias among physicians and its prediction of thrombolysis decisions for black and white patients. *Journal of General Internal Medicine, 22,* 1231–1238. doi:10.1007/s11606-007-0258-5

Harper, S., MacLehose, R. F., and Kaufman, J. S. (2014). Trends in the black-white life expectancy gap among U.S. states, 1990–2009. *Health Affairs, 33,* 1375–1382. doi:10.1377/hlthaff.2013.1273

Hofrichter, R. (2007). *A brief lexicon for health equity and social justice.* Washington, DC: National Association of County and City Health Officials.

Jordan, R. (2014). *America's public schools remain highly segregated.* Retrieved from *www.urban.org/urban-wire/americas-public-schools-remain-highly-segregated*

Kaufman, J. S., Dolman, L., Rushani, D., & Cooper, R. S. (2015). The contribution of genomic research to explaining racial disparities in cardiovascular disease: A systematic review. *American Journal of Epidemiology, 181,* 464–472.

Kawachi, I., Daniels, N., & Robinson, D. E. (2005). Health disparities by race and class: Why both matter. *Health Affairs, 24,* 343–352.

Kawachi, I., Kennedy, B. P., Gupta, V., & Prothrow-Stith, D. (1999). Women's status and the health of women and men. In I. Kawachi, B. P. Kennedy, and R. G. Wilkinson (Eds.), *The society and population health reader: Income inequality and health* (pp. 474–491). New York, NY: New Press.

Krieger, N. (2006, June 7). *If "race" is the answer, what is the question?—on "race," racism, and health: A social epidemiologist's perspective.* Retrieved from *http://raceandgenomics.ssrc.org/Krieger/*

Krieger, N., & Birn, A. E. (1998). A vision of social justice as the foundation of public health: Commemorating 150 years of the Spirit of 1848. *American Journal of Public Health, 88,* 1603–1606.

LaVeist, T. A., Gaskin, D. J., & Richard, P. (2009). *The economic burden of health inequalities in the United States (summary of study produced for the Joint Center for Political and Economic Studies).* Retrieved from *http://jointcenter.org/sites/default/files/Economic%20Burden%20of%20Health%20Inequalities%20Fact%20Sheet.pdf*

Life in America: Hazardous to immigrants' health? (2014, Autumn). *UCLA Fielding School of Public Health Magazine.* Retrieved from *http://ph.ucla.edu/news/magazine/2014/autumn/article/ life-america-hazardous-immigrants-health*

Lipsitz, G. (2009). *The possessive investment in whiteness: How white people profit from identity politics.* Philadelphia, PA: Temple University Press.

Manchanda, R. (2013). *The upstream doctors: Medical innovators track sickness to its source* [E-Book]. New York, NY: TED Books.

Marmot, M. (2009). *Building a global movement for health equity.* Retrieved from www.gih.org/files/usrdoc/ Marmot_Speech_Report_July_2009.pdf

National Center for Health Statistics. (2014a). *Detailed tables for the National Vital Statistics Report (NVSR) "Deaths: Final data for 2013" Tables 7 & 21.* Retrieved from *www.cdc.gov/nchs/data/nvsr/nvsr64/nvsr64_02.pdf*

National Center for Health Statistics. (2014b). *Health, United States, 2013: With special feature on prescription drugs.* Retrieved from http://stacks.cdc.gov/view/cdc/23136/Print.

National Center for Transgender Equality. (n.d.) *Issues.* Retrieved from *http://transequality.org/issues*

Office of Minority Health and Health Disparities. (2007, June 6). *About minority health.* Retrieved from *www.cdc .gov/omhd/AMH/AMH.htm*

Östlin, P., George, A., & Sen, G. (2003). Gender, health, and equity: The intersections. In R. Hofrichter (Ed.), *Health and social justice: Politics, ideology, and inequity in the distribution of disease. A public health reader* (pp. 132–156). San Francisco, CA: Jossey-Bass.

Public Health Institute, California Department of Public Health, & American Public Health Association. (2013). *Health in all policies: A guide for state and local governments.* Washington, DC and Oakland, CA: American Public Health Association and Public Health Institute.

Robert Wood Johnson Foundation. (2011). *Education and health: Issue brief #5 exploring the social determinants of health.* Retrieved from *www.rwjf.org/content/dam/farm/reports/issue_briefs/2011/rwjf70447*

Rothstein, R. (2012, January 23). *A comment on Bank of America/Countrywide's discriminatory mortgage lending and its implications for racial segregation.* Economic Policy Institute Briefing Paper 335. Retrieved from *www.epi.org/ publication/bp335-boa-countrywide-discriminatory-lending/*

Rowlingson, K. (2011). *Does income inequality cause health and social problems?* Retrieved from www.jrf.org.uk/ report/does-income-inequality-cause-health-and-social-problems

Saez, E. (2013). *Striking it richer: The evolution of top income in the United States (updated with 2012 preliminary estimates).* Retrieved from *http://eml.berkeley.edu//~saez/saez-UStopincomes-2012.pdf*

Satcher, D., & Higginbotham, E. J. (2008). The public health approach to eliminating disparities in health. *American Journal of Public Health, 98,* 400–403.

Schoen, C., Hayes, S. L., Collins, S. R., Lippa, J. A., & Radley, D. C. (2014, March). *America's underinsured: A state-by-state look at health insurance affordability prior to the new coverage expansions.* Retrieved from *www.commonwealthfund.org/publications/fund-reports/2014/mar/americas-underinsured*

Singh, G. K., Rodriguez-Lainz, A., & Kogan, M. D. (2013). Immigrant health inequalities in the United States: Use of eight major national data sets. *Scientific World Journal, 2013,* 22 pages (unnumbered). Retrieved from www. hindawi.com/journals/tswj/2013/512313/

Smedley, B., Jeffries, M., Adelman, L., & Cheng, J. (2009). *Race, racial inequality, and health inequities: Separating myth from fact* [briefing paper]. Retrieved from *www.unnaturalcauses.org/assets/uploads/file/Race_Racial_ Inequality_Health.pdf*

Smedley, B. D., Stith, A. Y., & Nelson, A. R. (2003). *Unequal treatment: Confronting racial and ethnic disparities in health care.* Washington, DC: The National Academies Press.

Spatig-Amerikaner, A. (2012, August 22). *Unequal education: Federal loophole enables lower spending on students of color.* Retrieved from www.americanprogress.org/issues/education/report/2012/08/22/29002/unequal- education/

Stanford Center on Poverty and Inequality. (2014). *State of the union: The poverty and inequality report.* Retrieved from *http://web.stanford.edu/group/scspi/sotu/SOTU_2014_CPI.pdf*

United Nations Development Programme (UNDP). (n.d.) *Millennium Development Goals: Eight goals for 2015.* Retrieved from *www.undp.org/content/undp/en/home/mdgoverview/mdg_goals.html*

UNICEF Office of Research. (2013). *Child well-being in rich countries: A comparative overview, Innocenti Report Card 11.* Florence, Italy: UNICEF Office of Research. Retrieved from *www.unicef-irc.org/publications/pdf/rc11_eng.pdf*

United States Department of Health and Human Services (DHHS). (n.d.). *About Healthy People.* Retrieved from *www.healthypeople.gov/2020/About-Healthy-People*

United States Department of Health and Human Services. (2011). *HHS action plan to reduce racial and ethnic disparities: A nation free of disparities in health and health care.* Retrieved from http://minorityhealth.hhs.gov/npa/files/plans/hhs/hhs_plan_complete.pdf

U.S. Census Bureau. (2015). *Current Population Survey, 2014 Annual Social and Economic Supplement.* Retrieved from www.census.gov/hhes/www/poverty/publications/pubs-cps.html

VisVision: A transformation plan for San Francisco's Sunnydale and Visitacion Valley. (2014, October). Retrieved from *www.mercyhousing.org/file/VisVision-Transformation-Plan-Final-web.pdf*

Wilkinson, R., & Pickett, K. (2009). *The spirit level: Why greater equality makes societies stronger.* London, UK: Bloomsbury.

Williams, D. & Jackson, P. B. (2005). Social sources of racial disparities in health. *Health Affairs, 24,* 325–334.

Woolf, S. H., Johnson, R. E., Fryer, G. E., Rust, G., & Satcher, D. (2004). The health impact of resolving racial disparities: An analysis of US mortality data. *American Journal of Public Health, 94,* 2078–2081.

World Bank. (2015). *Data: Indicators.* Retrieved from *http://data.worldbank.org/indicator?display=graph*

World Health Organization (WHO). (n.d.) *Global health declarations.* Retrieved from *www.who.int/trade/glossary/story039/en/*

World Health Organization (WHO). (2015). *Social determinants of health.* Retrieved from *www.who.int/social_determinants/en/*

Zack, M. M. (2013, November 22). Health-related quality of life: United States, 2006 and 2010. *Morbidity and Mortality Weekly Supplements, 62,* 3, 105–111.

Zinn, H. (2004, September 20). The optimism of uncertainty. *The Nation.* Retrieved from *www.thenation.com/article/optimism-uncertainty*

Additional Resources

Bay Area Regional Health Inequalities Initiative. (n.d.). Retrieved from *www.barhii.org/*

Brennan Ramirez, L. K., Baker, E. A., & Metzler, M. (2008). *Promoting health equity: A resource to help communities address social determinants of health.* Atlanta, GA: U.S. Department of Health and Human Services, Centers for Disease Control and Prevention. Retrieved from *www.cdc.gov/nccdphp/dch/programs/healthycommunitiesprogram/tools/pdf/SDOH-workbook.pdf*

California Newsreel. (n.d.-a). *The raising of America.* [Video and website]. Retrieved from *www.raisingofamerica.org*

California Newsreel. (n.d.-b).Unnatural causes. [Video and website]. Retrieved from *www.unnaturalcauses.org*

Centers for Disease Control and Prevention. (2014, December 14). *A practitioner's guide for advancing health equity: Community strategies for preventing chronic disease.* Retrieved from *www.cdc.gov/nccdphp/dch/health-equity-guide/index.htm*

Economic Policy Institute. (n.d.). Retrieved from *www.epi.org*

The Equality Trust. https://www.equalitytrust.org.uk

Henry K. Kaiser Foundation. (2012, November 30). *Disparities in health and health care: Five key questions and answers.* Retrieved from *http://kff.org/disparities-policy/issue-brief/disparities-in-health-and-health-care-five-key-questions-and-answers/*

Hofrichter, R. (2006). *Tackling health inequities through public health practice: A handbook for action.* Washington, DC: National Association of County and City Health Officials.

Hope SF. (n.d.). Retrieved from *http://hope-sf.org/*

Institute of Medicine. (2002). *Unequal treatment: Confronting racial and ethnic disparities in health care.* Washington, DC: National Academies Press.

Institute of Medicine. (2014). *Supporting a movement for health and health equity: Lessons from social movements: Workshop summary.* Washington, DC: The National Academies Press. Retrieved from *www.nap.edu/catalog/ 18751/supporting-a-movement-for-health-and-health-equity-lessons-from*

LaVeist, T. A., & Isaac, L. A. (2012). *Race, ethnicity and health: A public health reader* (2nd ed.). San Francisco: Jossey-Bass.

National Association of City and County Health Officials (NACCHO). (2014). *Expanding the boundaries: Health equity and public health practice.* Washington, DC: NACCHO.

National Association of County and City Health Officials. (n.d.a). *Health equity and social justice program.* Retrieved from *www.naccho.org/topics/justice/*

National Association of County and City Health Officials. (n.d.b). *Roots of health inequity: A web-based course for the public health workforce.* Retrieved from *naccho.org/topics/justice/roots.cfm*

National Partnership for Action to End Health Disparities. (2011, April). *National stakeholder strategy for achieving health equity.* Rockville, MD: U.S. Department of Health & Human Services, Office of Minority Health.

Race Forward: The Center for Racial Justice Innovation. (n.d.). Retrieved from *www.raceforward.org/*

Robert Wood Johnson Foundation. (2014, August 21). Health policy brief: The relative contribution of multiple determinants to health outcomes. *Health Affairs.* Retrieved from *http://healthaffairs.org/healthpolicybriefs/ brief_pdfs/healthpolicybrief_123.pdf*

Robert Wood Johnson Foundation. (n.d.). *Social determinants of health topic area.* Retrieved from *www.rwjf.org/en/ our-topics/topics/social-determinants-of-health.html*

Unhealthy Work. (n.d.). *A project of the Center for Social Epidemiology.* Retrieved from *http://unhealthywork.org/*

University of Utah, Health Sciences. (n.d.). *Learn genetics: Epigenetics.* Retrieved from *http://learn.genetics.utah. edu/content/epigenetics/*

Vital Pictures. (2014). *American denial* [Film and website]. Retrieved from *www.pbs.org/independentlens/ american-denial/*

Wilkinson, R., & Marmot, M. (2003). *Social determinants of health: The solid facts* (2nd ed.). Retrieved from *www. euro.who.int/__data/assets/pdf_file/0005/98438/e81384.pdf*

World Health Organization. (n.d.). *Social determinants of health: Learning and tools.* Retrieved from *www.who.int/ social_determinants/tools/en/*

An Introduction to Health Care and Health Policy in the United States

5

Len Finocchio and Ellen Wu

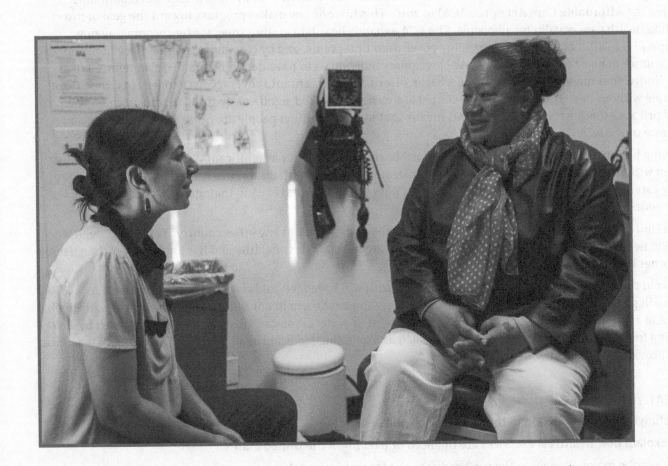

That's what the Affordable Care Act, or Obamacare, is all about—making sure that all of us, and all our fellow citizens, can count on the security of health care when we get sick; that the work and dignity of every person is acknowledged and affirmed.

—*President Barack Obama, April 2014*

Introduction

Our health care system is very complicated. As you will learn in this chapter, health services are paid for and provided to people differently depending on immigration status, age, race, or ethnicity, where they live, whether they are employed, and how much money they make. Receiving care in the United States generally requires having health insurance—through your job, a government program, or by purchasing it—or by having enough money to pay for care directly.

After nearly 100 years of efforts by some lawmakers to build a system that serves all people in the United States equally, President Obama and Congress passed the Patient Protection and Affordable Care Act (commonly called the **Affordable Care Act** or the ACA) in 2010. This historic law makes progress toward the goal of providing health care equally for all people. The ACA expands health insurance coverage by encouraging most employers to offer coverage, by expanding government programs, and by creating a "marketplace" to shop for comprehensive insurance. The ACA also requires individuals to have health insurance, also referred to as an **"individual mandate."** Since the ACA began offering enrollment into coverage in October 2013, the rate of people without health insurance in the United States has decreased significantly from 21 percent to 15.3 percent in April 2014 (Sommers et al., 2014). This means that nearly 11 million people are newly insured as a consequence of the ACA (Long et al., 2014).

Having health insurance coverage is now accessible and affordable for a significant proportion of U.S. residents. Even with insurance, some groups, such as immigrants or people with disabilities, experience challenges getting care. For example, the ACA rewards but does not require states to expand their government programs for the poor—called Medicaid—to include all adults.

The United States spends more money on health care per person than any other country. Yet even though we spend nearly $3 trillion each year on health care, we are generally less healthy and live shorter lives than people in other industrialized countries.

Most of the clients and communities you will work with will have Medicaid coverage or be uninsured. As a CHW, you will guide clients through our complicated system to assist them in enrolling into programs they are eligible for and also getting the right health care from the right providers. You can also play an important part by advocating for changes to our health care system, such as expanding Medicaid in all states and ensuring that services are provided to undocumented people.

WHAT YOU WILL LEARN

By studying the information in this chapter, you will be able to:

- Explain how health care services are financed or paid for in the United States
- Describe major changes to the system due to the federal Patient Protection and Affordable Care Act
- Describe who provides health care services in the United States
- Analyze why health status in the United States ranks so far behind that of other nations
- Identify health care programs, insurance coverage, and other resources that serve low-income clients
- Discuss how public policy is made, including policies about access to health care for low-income communities
- Describe the remaining gaps in the coverage and care delivery systems and who is left out
- Discuss and provide examples of how CHWs can participate in the public policy process

WORDS TO KNOW

Advance Premium Tax Credits

Affordable Care Act

Children's Health Insurance Program (CHIP)

Copayments

Deductible

Electronic Health Records

Federal Poverty Level

Grassroots Organizing

Health Insurance Marketplaces

Individual Mandate

Market Forces

Medicaid

Medicare

Premiums

Safety Net

Scope of Practice

Small Business Health Options Program (SHOP)

Stakeholder

Universal Health Care

5.1 What Health Care "System" Do We Have?

The purpose of any health care system is to organize and pay hospitals, health professionals, drug manufacturers, and others so that people can get preventive care to stay healthy and quality medical care when they are sick or injured. The definition of a *system* is "a regularly interacting or interdependent group of items forming a unified whole" (Merriam-Webster Dictionary, n.d.).

In most countries with large industrialized economies, the national or federal government ensures that the health system serves *all* people equally. They do this by passing laws to make access to health care a legal right for all persons; to collect taxes to pay for services; and to regulate providers and other parts of the system so that people receive affordable, quality health care services.

While the structure of these **universal health care** systems (systems that provide health care for everyone) vary, people living in a country with a universal health system, such as Canada, Sweden, Japan, or France, are guaranteed access to necessary medical care. Using tax dollars, the government budgets what it will spend on health care and negotiates prices for services. Care is coordinated among clinics, hospitals, doctors, and other providers through unified, or centralized, systems. The government also sets priorities about which services are most important to ensure the overall health and well-being of the population, with an emphasis on promoting the health of *all* people.

CREATING A HEALTH CARE "SYSTEM" IN THE UNITED STATES

The United States is the only country with a large, industrialized economy that does not have a universal, centrally run, and coherent health care system. While the ACA brings more organization and government control, health care in the United States is still very disorganized and piecemeal. While more people are insured, many still go without coverage. As a result, people in the United States are not served equally, and many, especially low-income working adults and the undocumented, do not get health care when they need it.

The ultimate goal is to have a health care system that serves everyone, with each of the different components working together to achieve a common goal. In 1946, the World Health Organization (WHO) declared that "The enjoyment of the highest attainable standard of health is one of the fundamental human rights of every human being without distinction for race, religion, political belief, economic or social condition" (World Health Organization, n.d.).

The ACA made fundamental changes to our existing system of insurance coverage and care delivery and makes a lot of progress toward a creating a "system." Yet there is still no constitutional right to health care for all persons in the United States. Rather, access to health services depends upon having health insurance from your job, qualifying for affordable government coverage, or buying insurance or services directly with your own money. For example, in 16 states that have not expanded their government Medicaid program, many poor adults without children do not have insurance coverage. Consequently, across the nation about half of all Americans get health insurance from their employers, and one in three from a government insurance program like Medicare or Medicaid (see Table 5.1). This leaves one in every six people, or about 42 million Americans, without any health insurance at all. Clearly the United States has a long way to go to creating a true health care system that serves everyone equally.

Since there is no strong and comprehensive central coordination of health care in the United States, influence and control comes from many places, mostly governments, employers, and insurance companies.

Table 5.1 Health Insurance in the United States (2013)

COVERAGE TYPE	PERCENT
Any private plan	64.2%
Employment-based	53.9%
Direct-purchase	11.0%
Any government plan	34.2%
Medicare	15.6%
Medicaid	17.3%
Military health care	4.5%
Uninsured	13.4%

Source: U.S. Census Bureau (2015).

The federal government is solely responsible for all aspects of health insurance for the elderly (Medicare). The federal government sets the rules for health insurance programs that cover low-income residents as well: Medicaid and the Children's Health Insurance Program (CHIP). And through the ACA, the federal government also sets the rules for both the federal and state health insurance "marketplaces," which offer tax subsidies to individuals and families to purchase standardized health insurance plans.

State governments follow federal rules for the Medicaid and CHIP programs and, if they have elected to establish one, the state insurance "marketplace" as well. The federal rules allow states some flexibility in how they develop and administer these insurance programs for poor and low-income children and adults. States also receive federal dollars to run these programs.

Local governments, like cities and counties, can be also responsible for health care for some people in need. In California, for example, counties are legally the "provider of last resort" and therefore responsible for some health services for the undocumented population who are uninsured and need care.

Employers wield a great deal of control and influence over the health care system as well. Currently, about half of all insured people in the United States get their coverage from their employers. Although the ACA does have new rules in place requiring large employers to pay for health insurance for full-time employees, employers still have a lot of control. Most large employers offer very good benefits, including health insurance, retirement plans, and so on. Small businesses are less likely to offer health insurance, because these benefits are very expensive and increasing in cost every year. The number of employers in the United States who offer health insurance to their employees has been steadily declining over the past decade due to increasing costs. At the same time, the cost to employees has been increasing through escalating premiums and rising copayments. These are the out-of-pocket expenses that we pay to cover part of the costs for insurance (premiums are usually paid monthly) or a share of costs for receiving services at a clinic or hospital or for medications (**copayments**).

Health insurance companies offer products to governments, employers, and individuals. Nationwide, there are dozens of insurance companies offering dozens of different insurance plans, so choosing among them can be difficult. Insurance companies also have influence over hospitals and physicians that participate in their care networks by how much they pay for services, how they link providers together, and what services they authorize for patients.

Other organizational influence and control of the health care system comes from the providers of health care, like physicians, hospitals, and manufacturers of drugs, technology, and medical devices. Physicians exert a lot of control because they make most of the decisions about what health care services people get. Hospitals control some of the system in the way they organize services and employ the health care workforce. Big drug companies produce new drugs and influence consumption and spending on those drugs through their marketing to doctors and consumers.

While federal and state governments do create laws governing many aspects of health care delivery, the U.S. system relies heavily on **"market forces"**—or competition between different products and services—to determine how health services are delivered and paid for, and who gets them, and how affordable they are. In fact, there is frequent tension between the role of the government and market forces in shaping the system, how it works, and whom it serves. Governments pass laws shaping the health care system since market forces don't always work well in meeting the goals of a health care system. The ACA includes many laws that control the insurance market because the forces of competition and profit were not serving all of these in need of insurance.

- *Can you think of other differences between health care and other products or services that are bought and sold in the United States?*

- *Should health care be a right or a product that people have to buy?*

HOW MUCH DO WE SPEND AND WHAT DO WE GET?

In 2013, about one of every six dollars in the U.S. economy (or about 17 percent) is spent on health care. This totals more than $2.9 trillion (yes, trillion!), or about $8,700 per person living in the United States (see Figure 5.1). By comparison, our northern neighbor Canada spends about half as much at $4,600 per person.

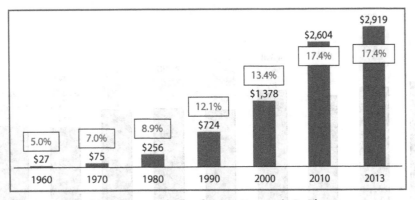

Figure 5.1 Health Care as a Share of Gross Domestic Product
Source: Centers for Medicare & Medicaid Services, Office of the Actuary, National Health Statistics Group; U.S. Department of Commerce, Bureau of Economic Analysis; and U.S. Bureau of the Census.

WHY IS HEALTH CARE SO EXPENSIVE IN THE UNITED STATES?

There are many factors that contribute to why health care is so expensive. As the size of our population increases, more people are using health care services. Life expectancy has also increased, resulting in the need for more services, prescription drugs, and technology later in life. And finally, our services cost more. For example, Canadians get more medical services but the country still spends less on health care than the United States.

People have different perspectives about why health care costs so much. Some say it's because health plans, pharmaceutical companies, and some hospitals are making a profit from our health care system. Others claim that our system encourages the creation and use of expensive medical technology. Doctors have said they that need to practice "defensive medicine" such as ordering more tests because of the cost of malpractice insurance.

For decades, one of the most serious consequences to the high cost of health care was an increasing number of uninsured people. Another result is that as the government spends more of its resources on health care, less funding is available to be invested in other areas such as education, housing, or social services that promote the public's health. In addition, the costs to businesses that provide employees with health insurance benefits have also increased, often putting them at a disadvantage in the global economy. These high and ever-increasing costs are motivating governments, employers, health care providers, and consumers to find ways to make services more affordable.

WHAT DO WE GET FOR ALL THE MONEY WE SPEND?

The United States spends more on health care than any other industrialized country (for example, Canada, France, Japan, and New Zealand). Figure 5.2 compares health spending per capita (per person) across several countries with industrialized economies. Figure 5.2 also show what portion of health care expenditures come from the private and public sectors, as well as out-of-pocket spending by consumers.

Despite this spending, the United States scores poorly on many important system and health outcomes indicators when compared to other countries (Davis, Stremikis, Squires, & Schoen, 2014). Compared to 11 other industrialized nations with universal health systems, the U.S. system has worse quality, poorer access to services, and less efficient care delivery. More troubling is that the U.S. system is less equitable for the poor and people of color. Finally, the United States ranks last in how healthy we are and how long we live compared to people in other industrialized countries with universal health systems.

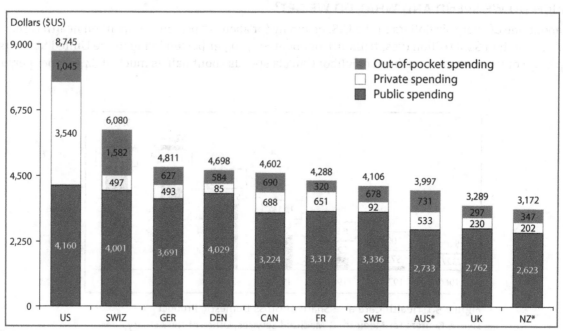

Figure 5.2 Health Care Spending per Capita by Source of Funding, 2012 (Adjusted for Differences in Cost of Living)

Source: OECD Health Data 2014 (Anderson, 2014, p. 5).

The overall health of the United States has improved over the past century and continues to do so each year, due in large part to public health programs, medical services, and health education. Our most basic measure for improved health is that we live much longer than we did 50 years ago. This progress, however, has come with several important consequences. Our longer lives mean we have more people with chronic diseases and disabilities living a long time. Our system is not well set up to take care of people with complicated long-term needs.

In addition, the successes of the public health and medical systems have not benefited all people in the country equally. In general, low-income people and people of color are more likely than Whites and middle-income people to experience barriers to getting services, and when they do get them, the services are often of poorer quality. As discussed in Chapter 4, low-income people and people of color are more likely to have chronic diseases and disabilities, and to live shorter lives. For example, African Americans are more likely than Whites to die from stroke and coronary artery disease and have twice the rate of infant mortality (CDC, 2013a).

These inequalities are the result of many factors, including health insurance coverage and access to routine preventive services. Furthermore, serious social and economic conditions contribute to poor health, such as lack of educational and employment opportunities, violence in neighborhoods, and inadequate public health protections. For example, nearly two in five Latinos in the United States were uninsured in 2010. The ACA has reduced this rate significantly but the disparity for Latinos remains. The differences in the health status and shorter lives between low-income people and people of color compared to Whites are one of the country's greatest failures.

5.2 How Do We Pay for Health Care?

- If you have health insurance, how much does it cost each year, including the costs of copayments, deductibles, and premiums?
- Has the cost increased in the past several years?

FINANCING

Where does the money come from to pay for insurance, hospital visits, lab tests, and physician care? Nearly half of all health care dollars come from the local, state, and federal taxes that support public programs such as Medicare, Medicaid, the Children's Health Insurance Program (CHIP), and local programs for the uninsured. The other half comes from the private sector, mostly from employers. During the past 20 years, the proportion (percentage) of public dollars paying for health services has increased, while the proportion of private dollars has decreased (see Figure 5.3). And the portion of health care costs paid for by the government will only continue to increase as the federal government subsidizes the expansion of Medicaid and health insurance marketplaces.

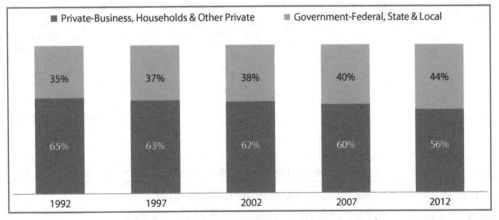

Figure 5.3 National Health Care Expenditures by Sector (1992–2012)
Source: Centers for Medicare & Medicaid Services, n.d.

HEALTH INSURANCE

Most health care dollars are not paid directly to health care providers, but to health insurance companies. The primary goal of insurance is to spread the financial risk for an unexpected, random event, such as an accident or serious illness, across a large group of people. A good example is car insurance. The consumer pays a set amount, usually monthly, to an insurance company for "coverage." This regular payment is called a **premium**. If that insured driver has an accident, that person will be required to pay an initial fixed amount (**deductible**), and the insurance company will pay the rest. The likelihood of an accident is small but may cost a lot when it occurs. The larger the group of contributors, the more effectively the insurance system works. In universal systems of care, everyone contributes, and everyone is insured.

In the United States, health insurance is very important in determining our access to health care services and the quality of those services. Most people can't afford to pay for health care on their own because the costs are so high. Numerous studies have shown that people with health insurance are more likely to have a doctor (primary care provider) whom they visit regularly, and are more likely to get preventive care services. The insured are also more likely to be treated earlier for health conditions and, as a result, have lower risks for mortality.

EMPLOYER-BASED HEALTH INSURANCE

More than half of all people with health insurance in the United States get it through their employers. Historically, businesses offered health insurance as a benefit to attract the best employees, and after many decades, "salary and benefits" became inseparable for most large employers and employees. Businesses receive a large tax deduction for providing such benefits to employees.

As health care costs increased over several recent decades, many businesses decided to pay less of these costs and to shift this economic burden to employees instead. Many businesses, especially small ones, could not afford the high cost of insurance for employees and dropped coverage altogether. As a result, employer-sponsored insurance for employees has been steadily declining for years (see Figure 5.4). The majority of the uninsured are employed but do not receive health insurance benefits from their employer, or they cannot afford to participate in their employer-sponsored health benefit.

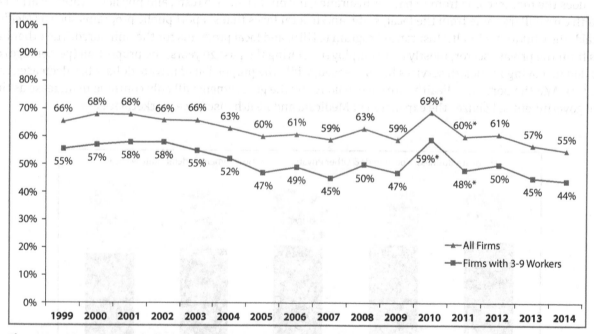

Figure 5.4 Percentage of All Firms Offering Health Benefits, 1999–2014

*Estimate is statistically different from estimate for previous year shown ($p < .05$).

Note: Estimates presented in this exhibit are based on the sample of both firms that completed the entire survey and those that answered just one question about whether they offer health benefits. The percentage of firms offering health benefits is largely driven by small firms. The large increase in 2010 was primarily driven by a 12-percentage-point increase in offering among firms with three to nine workers. In 2011, 48 percent of firms with three to nine employees offer health benefits, a level more consistent with levels from recent years other than 2010. The overall 2011 offer rate is consistent with the long-term trend, indicating that the high 2010 offer rate may be an aberration.

Source: Kaiser/HRET Survey of Employer-Sponsored Health Benefits, 1990–2014. (Kaiser Family Foundation and Health Research and Education Trust, 2014, p. 8)

This decline in employer coverage and the ever-increasing number of uninsured motivated many lawmakers and other stakeholders to push for fundamental changes to the health care system. Until the passage of the ACA, businesses were not legally required to provide insurance coverage to employees. The ACA now *encourages* employers with more than 50 employees to provide coverage to full-time workers and if they don't, are assessed a penalty fee of $2,000 per employee. Businesses with fewer than 50 workers are not required to provide insurance by the ACA but the law does provide these companies with incentives, in the form of tax credits, to help employees purchase coverage.

GOVERNMENT PROGRAMS

In a system where employers provide the majority of health insurance, this leaves those without jobs—the unemployed, children and the elderly—uncovered. In addition, too many people work for low-wages with employers who don't provide coverage. This leaves millions of people without coverage, or the money to pay for expensive health care.

The role of government is to pass laws and use taxes to promote and protect public health, and to provide for society's most vulnerable people—children, the poor, and the elderly. For decades, federal and state governments struggled to address the needs of these uninsured groups, but nothing comprehensive was done. In the 1960s, when these gaps in the employer-based coverage system were too large to ignore, Congress finally acted. In 1965, President Johnson and Congress created two major public health care programs in the existing Social Security Act: Medicare for those over 65 years old and Medicaid for specific groups of poor children, families, and disabled people. A third program, the federal Children's Health Insurance Program (CHIP), was created in 1997 to provide health coverage for low-income children in families whose income is higher than Medicaid limits. Since each of these programs was established, Congress and federal and state agencies have made many changes to the policies that determine who's eligible, what benefits are provided to them, and how many tax dollars are spent on the programs.

Most recently, in 2010 President Obama and Congress passed the Patient Protection and Affordable Care Act that makes significant improvements to our existing system. As this chapter describes, the ACA expands insurance coverage by encouraging most employers to offer coverage, by expanding the Medicaid program, and by creating a "marketplace" to shop for affordable and comprehensive insurance. The ACA also requires individuals to have health insurance, also referred to as an "individual mandate."

Medicare

Medicare is a federally funded and administered program that provides universal medical care for the elderly. Generally, someone is eligible for Medicare if they are 65 years old or older and are a citizen or permanent resident of the United States. In 1972, the government also included coverage for people who are disabled or have end-state renal (kidney) disease. Medicare has four different parts:

1. **Medicare Part A** covers hospital care, skilled nursing facilities, hospice care, and home health care related to hospital services. Part A is automatic, which means that people are enrolled once they turn 65 without filling out any paperwork or paying any money.

2. **Medicare Part B** covers physicians' services, outpatient care, and other medical services that Part A doesn't include, in addition to preventive care. Unlike Medicare Part A, which is automatic, you have to enroll in Medicare Part B. Once enrolled, it works like any other insurance, with premiums, deductibles, and copayments. Copayments are the amount that we pay for each health care service or medical prescription.

3. **Medicare Part C** is known as Medicare Advantage Plans. It is a program offered by private health plans approved by Medicare to provide Medicare services. Medicare Advantage Plans may also offer extra coverage but can charge different out-of-pocket costs and have different rules than standard Medicare for how you get the services, such as whether you need a referral to see a specialist.

4. **Medicare Part D** is insurance for prescription drug coverage that started in 2005. Up until that time, a major health care cost for the elderly—prescription drugs—was not covered. Each year you have to enroll in Medicare Part D and pay premiums, deductibles, and copayments.

Medicare does not cover long-term care, dental, or vision services, although some health plans offer these benefits as well as Medigap plans. Medigap are separate insurance plans that provide coverage for services not provided by Medicare. More information about Medicare can be found at the Center for Medicare and Medicaid Services website (www.medicare.gov/MedicareEligibility).

Medicaid

Medicaid is the single largest source of health coverage, providing care for more than 60 million Americans. It was initially designed to help some, but not all, low-income individuals and families get health care. Low-income children, parents of these children, pregnant women, seniors, and person with disabilities were eligible for Medicaid. However, low-income adults without children and undocumented immigrants were not covered by Medicaid.

Medicaid is funded by both the federal and state governments and administered by each state. The federal government provides specific rules and guidelines for the program, and each state develops policies to follow these.

The ACA made it possible for states to expand Medicaid programs to cover adults without children, and made the application process easier. The new requirements to Medicaid increase the program's consistency in eligibility and benefits across the states. For example, the income requirement for adults without children is set at 133 percent of the Federal Poverty Level or below (see further on for more information about the FPL) for all of the states. In 2015, this is about $32,000 a year for a family of four. Undocumented immigrants are still not eligible for the program.

As a result of a Supreme Court ruling in June 2012, the federal government cannot require the state to expand their Medicaid program. As a result, as of May 2015, 30 states (including the District of Columbia) were expanding their Medicaid programs, three states continued to debate whether or not to expand, and 18 states were not expanding their programs (Kaiser Family Foundation, 2015). This Supreme Court ruling undermined the ACA's intention to provide coverage to all low and moderate-income legal residents.

Medicaid provides benefits at little or no cost to enrollees. The mandatory benefits that all states program must provide include hospital and physician services, nursing home care, preventive care, family planning, labs, and x-rays. The ACA expanded the mandatory benefits to include behavioral health and substance use disorder benefits as well. States may also provide "optional benefits" that include prescription drugs, physical therapy, dental care for adults, and many others.

You can find general information about Medicaid at the Medicaid website (www.medicaid.gov/) and information about Medicaid for each state (www.statehealthfacts.org).

- *Who is eligible for Medicaid in your state?*

- *What are the income eligibility requirements?*

- *How often do people have to reapply for Medicaid?*

Children's Health Insurance Program

Children's Health Insurance Program (CHIP) is funded by both the federal and state government and administered by the states. Like Medicaid, the federal government provides general guidelines and each state develops its own program. Generally, children whose family income is below 200 percent FPL qualify for CHIP, although some states have expanded eligibility above 200 percent. CHIP programs must provide comprehensive benefits similar to Medicaid program benefits. The ACA continued CHIP eligibility standards until 2019 and in early 2015 Congress reauthorized funding for the program through September 2017. The federal government will have to reauthorize funding for the program for it to continue after that date.

For more information about the Children's Health Insurance Program, go to www.cms.hhs.gov/MedicaidGenInfo and www.statehealthfacts.org.

- *Who is eligible for SCHIP programs in your state?*

- *How much of the insurance premium do families have to pay?*

- *What do you think the income eligibility requirement should be—200 percent of FPL or higher, and why?*

Health Insurance Marketplaces

Health Insurance Marketplaces were established by the ACA to help individuals and small businesses buy more affordable health insurance. In the previous section about Health Insurance, we discussed how having more people participating in an insurance pool, helps to share risks and reduce costs. Before the marketplaces, individuals and small businesses who had to purchase insurance on their own had to pay much more than large employers. Health insurance marketplaces allow individuals and small businesses to more effectively share the risks and costs.

In June 2015 the Supreme Court will rule on another important case about the ACA (as of this writing, the court had not yet reach a decision). The case of King V. Burwell challenges subsidies to low-and moderate-income people in states that chose to use the federal health insurance marketplace instead of establishing their own state marketplace. If the court rules against the ACA, some 13 million Americans currently receiving health insurance through the federal exchange could lose coverage (Altman, 2014).

States had the option to set up their own health insurance marketplaces. For people living in a state that does not have a state marketplace, they can participate in the federal marketplace. A marketplace has different health insurance options (Qualified Health Plans) that consumers can choose from. These insurance options have to meet minimum requirements set by the state and federal governments. There is also a **Small Business Health Options Program** (SHOP) marketplace that helps small businesses provide health coverage to their employees.

Individuals who make less than 400 percent Federal Poverty Level (about $47,080 in 2015) can get help from the federal government in the form of tax credits used to subsidize, or offset, the cost of premiums for health plans purchased through marketplaces. **Advance premium tax credits** are calculated based on the reported income and can be used right away to lower the cost of the monthly premium. In addition, individuals who make less than 250 percent FPL (about $29,425) can also get their shared of cost reduced, such as lower deductible and co-pays. Individuals who qualify for Medicaid cannot participate in the marketplace. Undocumented immigrants are also not allowed to buy health insurance through the marketplace, even with their own money. You can find general information about health insurance marketplaces at the website www.healthcare.gov.

Other Government Programs

Other Government Programs such as the Veterans Administration and Indian Health Services provide health care. The federal government also finances, purchases, and organizes health services to military personnel. In addition to these federal programs, states, counties, and cities often have initiatives to provide coverage to the uninsured.

THE FEDERAL POVERTY LEVEL

When creating public programs to help vulnerable populations, lawmakers include specific criteria that individuals or families must meet in order to qualify. One of the most important criteria is income—to be eligible, a family or individual must demonstrate economic need or be living in poverty. Lawmakers established a dollar amount to determine what it means to live in, or at levels near, poverty.

Different levels, or multiples, of this **"federal poverty level"** (FPL) are used to determine eligibility and to provide help for state and federal health programs. For example, the ACA set a new Medicaid eligibility level at 133 percent of the FPL. The CHIP program minimum eligibility level is 200 percent FPL. And the maximum eligibility level to receive advance premium tax credits to buy insurance in "marketplaces" is 400 percent FPL. Medicare, however, does not have any income limits for eligibility.

Because so many policies use the FPL to determine eligibility, it is important to understand how this guideline affects the lives of individuals and families. It is especially relevant to the clients and communities with whom CHWs work. Many people consider the FPL to be an outdated measure that fails to take into account the reality of today's families. For example, the poverty level does not take into account the cost of child care in determining what makes up a family's basic needs. It also does not take into consideration the high cost of living in some regions and states. The federal poverty line is updated each year. The guidelines for 2015 are presented in Table 5.2.

Table 5.2 Federal Poverty Guidelines, 2015

HOUSE-HOLD SIZE	100%	133%	150%	200%	250%	300%	400%
1	$11,770	$15,654	$17,655	$23,540	$29,425	$35,310	$47,080
2	15,930	21,187	23,895	31,860	39,825	47,790	63,720
3	20,090	26,720	30,135	40,180	50,225	60,270	80,360
4	24,250	32,253	36,375	48,500	60,625	72,750	97,000
5	28,410	37,785	42,615	56,820	71,025	85,230	113,640
6	32,570	43,318	48,855	65,140	81,425	97,710	130,280
7	36,730	48,851	55,095	73,460	91,825	110,190	146,920
8	40,890	54,384	61,335	81,780	102,225	122,670	163,560

Source: Families USA, 2015.

- *In your city or county, can a family of four making $24,250 a year afford basic needs, including rent, food, clothes, transportation, and health care?*

- *What is the minimum wage in your city or state?*

- *What do you think about the level at which the federal government draws the poverty line? Where would you draw the line, and why?*

5.3 Who Provides Health Care Services?

As you have read in the previous sections of this chapter, money to pay for health services comes from the government, employers, and individuals. Insurance companies take these dollars and pay the providers of health services. Hospitals and physicians develop contracts with insurance companies to provide services for a negotiated price. We spend the majority of our health care dollars on hospitals and physicians. Figure 5.5 shows the distribution of all health care spending.

HOSPITALS

In 2012, there were nearly 5,000 hospitals nationwide. Of these, more than 3,000 were located in urban areas and approximately 2,000 were located in rural areas (American Hospital Association, 2014). Three out of five hospitals belong to a multihospital system. Hospitals provide a wide range of health care services from basic primary care to very high-tech and expensive specialty care. Most hospitals have both outpatient facilities, or clinics, and inpatient services. In clinics, people receive services for health care needs that can be addressed without being admitted into the hospital for inpatient care. Most hospitals and clinics accept all types of insurance and types of payments, including government-sponsored coverage. In a clinic, your visit may last a few minutes or up to a few hours. Inpatient care, where you stay overnight, is for more complicated needs that require specialists and high-tech interventions like surgery. Inpatient care is typically *very expensive*. A hospital stay usually costs around $2,157 per day, *plus* the cost of services provided by physicians (Kaiser Family Foundation, 2015).

General hospitals provide a wide range of services. Specialty hospitals focus on specific services, such as cardiology or pediatrics (for children). Many communities have at least one hospital, and it is commonly an

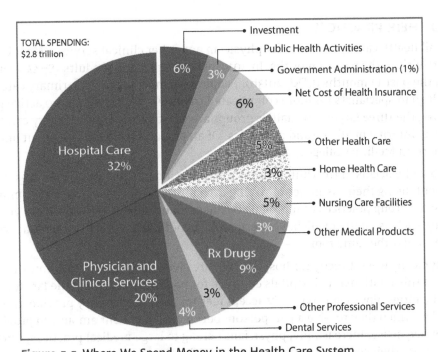

Figure 5.5 Where We Spend Money in the Health Care System

Note: Health spending refers to National Health Expenditures. For additional detail on spending categories, see the appendix. Further definitions are available at www.cms.gov. Segments may not total 100 percent due to rounding. See page 12 for trend data.

Source: Centers for Medicare & Medicaid Services (CMS), National Health Expenditures, 2014 release, *www.cms.org*

important source of employment. However, there are many communities, including Native American nations, without hospitals. Hospitals link with many other services and providers, such as physician groups, laboratories, imaging services, and long-term care facilities such as nursing homes. Hospitals may also serve as teaching sites for nurses, CHWs, allied health providers, and physicians.

Some hospitals have emergency departments (ED) to treat life-threatening conditions. In large urban areas, emergency departments are commonly used by the uninsured and some insured persons as their primary source of health care. Emergency departments make up one part of what is the health care **safety net** through which those without insurance seek care. *Safety net* is the term used to refer to those parts of the system that provide care to people without insurance, or who are having difficulty finding an accessible practitioner.

Public hospitals, supported largely through taxes, have an obligation to serve the poor, and they play an important safety net role for people who are uninsured. Public hospitals, also known as "essential community hospitals," take care of the vast majority of the nation's uninsured and low-income patients (America's Essential Hospitals, 2015). In addition to public hospitals, the safety net includes community health centers (discussed next) and nonprofit hospitals that have a legal obligation to provide a community benefit such as care to the uninsured. In return for providing free care to some patients, nonprofit hospitals typically receive additional tax benefits.

Of those hospitals that are privately owned, half are not-for-profits. For-profit hospitals are more likely to be specialty hospitals and serve a more narrow population, nearly all of which is insured.

- *Where do uninsured patients in your city or region go to receive health care?*

- *Does your city or region have a public hospital, a community health center, a free clinic?*

PHYSICIANS AND THEIR PRACTICES

Twenty percent of all health care spending is for physician and other clinical services. Most U.S. residents report having a health care visit in the past 12 months. In 2012, about 75 percent of adults 18–44 years of age reported a health care visit in the past 12 months (CDC, 2013b). People with insurance see a primary care doctor for most of their needs and will go to specialists for more complicated treatments. Of the 830,000 active physicians in the United States in 2013, the three largest specialties groups are those considered "primary care"—family medicine/general practice, internal medicine and pediatrics. Of all practicing physicians, about one third are women (Association of American Medical Colleges, 2014).

Until the 1980s, most physicians in the United States worked in individual private practices. Patients would make an appointment, using their insurance or paying cash for the visit. It is now more common for physicians to work in large private group practices that provide business management services. Most group practices focus on a single specialty, such as family medicine or dermatology, but there are also group practices that have many different specialties under the same roof.

Physicians do not typically work directly for hospitals but are given "privileges" to admit their patients into hospitals. Because of this relationship, hospitals compete for patients by offering the latest technology, best nurses, and nicest facilities. Physicians typically accept fees for each service they provide, though they also accept "capitation" in which they receive a per-person-per-month payment amount to provide all necessary services within their expertise. Increasingly, physicians belong to large medical practices, often with multiple specialties, that contract their services to hospitals and health plans.

Physicians have the broadest scope of practice of all health professionals and generally direct the medical care that each patient receives. **Scope of practice** refers to the skills and services that professionals are qualified and competent to provide. Other health professionals typically take direction from physicians who are often team leaders. You will learn about the scope of practice for CHWs in Chapter 7.

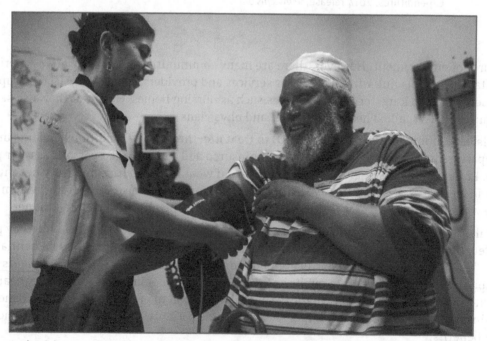

A physician monitors a patient's blood pressure and talks with him about his health.

COMMUNITY HEALTH CENTERS

More than 9,000 community health centers across the country form an important part of the health care delivery system. Community health centers often serve as the only affordable and accessible source of care in a community, and are also consider "essential" community providers. These not-for-profit outpatient clinics have a mission to serve the neediest in every community: 36 percent of their patients are uninsured, 39 percent have Medicaid, and nearly all are low income (National Association of Community Health Centers, 2013).

These centers receive most of their funding from Medicaid, a combination of state and federal dollars, and federal grants that support their services to the uninsured. Most of the clinics provide primary health care services, some specialty services, and some dental and mental health services. They are especially committed to and capable of providing culturally and linguistically competent health care services.

Like public hospitals, community health centers play a critical role in the health care safety net; they primarily serve low-income individuals, persons of color, the uninsured, immigrants, and those on Medicaid. These clinics are often the only source of health care for these populations, particularly in rural and other medically underserved areas. Increasingly, community health centers and clinics employ CHWs.

- *Where are the closest community health centers in your city or county?*

- *What types of services do they provide?*

- *What communities do they serve?*

- *Do they have special programs for clients who speak languages other than English?*

HOW HEALTH CARE PROVIDERS WORK TOGETHER

Some providers, such as large physician group practices, multihospital systems, and managed care plans, tend to work closely together. Some community health centers work closely with public hospitals, since both contribute to the health care safety net in a community.

But overall, the pieces of the U.S. health care system do not fit together very well, and health care is not well coordinated. Coordination is important for people with chronic diseases, including behavioral health needs, because the management of such conditions requires the services of many different providers. A person with diabetes, for example, may need to consult with their primary-care provider and specialists such as an endocrinologist, ophthalmologist, podiatrist, neurologist, cardiologist, urologist, a dentist, and the nutritionist. (Information about medical specialists can be found online. See the list of resources provided at the end of this chapter.)

Increasingly, practitioners, clinics, and hospitals make use of **electronic health records** (EHRs) to maintain all of a patient's medical information in one system. These EHRs offer the opportunity to help integrate and coordinate the different types of health services provided by different practitioners in different locations. The federal government has provided financial incentives for providers to adopt and use these EHRs. While they offer a great deal of promise, EHRs can be challenging to adopt, train providers to use, and keep up to date. Moreover, different EHRs in different health systems don't necessarily allow for sharing patient data.

HEALTH PLANS AND MANAGED CARE

Despite the overall poor coordination within the health care system, there have been some improvements over the past 25 years. In particular, managed care insurance plans have been established that aim to organize medical services and payment to offer better care at a lower cost. Managed care developed in response to many pressures, including spiraling health care costs, poor coordination of patient's health care, and the need to focus on health promotion and disease prevention. All managed care plans use similar mechanisms to coordinate care and manage costs, the most common being primary care providers as "gatekeepers" to services. In other words, you have to see your primary care provider before you can access other health services.

THE ROLE OF CHWs IN HEALTH CARE

CHWs are increasingly being recognized as a vital part of the health care system and are hired to work in clinics and hospitals as part of a health care team. Whether they work for a hospital, clinic, local health department, or community-based organizations, CHWs often work to ensure that clients understand their health and receive the best health care possible. The ACA has increased the opportunities for optimizing CHWs in the health system. For example, the spread of patient-centered medical homes and strategies to manage chronic diseases frequently relies on CHWs as a key member of the care team. Moreover, CHWs:

- Provide outreach to assist community members to understand and access health care services available in their communities

- Link people to health care services and follow up to ensure that clients understand their health issues and treatment

- Provide health education to assist individuals, families, and communities in learning about health and factors that affect their health and well-being

- Assist clients in enrolling in health insurance programs such as CHIP for the children of low-income families

- Act as navigators, assisting clients to figure out how to access the proper providers and services within a clinic, hospital, or health plan

- Advocate for clients within the health care organizations and systems to aid in ensuring that they are provided with culturally competent services, including, for example, interpretation services

- Provide client-centered health education and counseling services to assist clients to understand their health conditions and treatment regiments, how to follow treatment guidelines, and how to make changes that promote their health

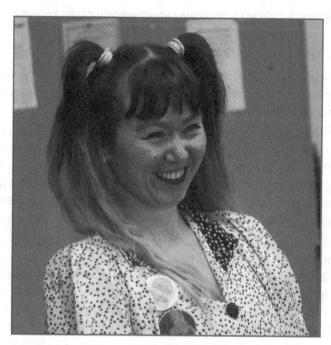

Increasingly, CHWs are key members of health care teams, supporting patients to access relevant services and to develop skills for self care.

- *Can you think of other ways that CHWs work within the health care "system" to promote health?*

What Do YOU? Think

5.4 More Work Needed to Get the System We Want

A lot of progress has been made in improving the U.S. health care system through the implementation of the Affordable Care Act. Millions more Americans now have access to affordable health insurance through the Health Insurance Marketplaces and the expansion of Medicaid. The law also makes changes to better regulate insurance companies, improve access to health care services, and improve quality of care. However, there is much more that needs to be done to get the kind of health care system that ensures everyone can get affordable and quality care.

COVERING THE REMAINING UNINSURED

Undocumented immigrants are still largely locked out of our health care system. Undocumented immigrants are not allowed to purchase insurance through the health insurance marketplace, even with their own money, and are not eligible for Medicaid. However, there are many efforts to expand health insurance options to undocumented immigrants. Many local jurisdictions, such as counties, are trying to cover undocumented immigrants in their area. Not only are they doing this because it's the right thing to do, it can also save them money. For counties that have public hospitals, it can cost them less to provide immigrants with services that keep them healthy, such as preventive care, than it does to pay for costly emergency care. In addition, states can cover undocumented immigrants in their Medicaid program using state funds. For example, California's state-funded Medicaid program includes services to immigrants who came to the United States before the age of 16 through the Deferred Action Childhood Arrivals (DACA) program.

Lastly, advocates for a single-payer approach to universal health care continue their fight statewide and nationally. Single-payer proposals insure *everyone*, in one common insurance risk pool, usually with the government paying providers directly for services. Single payer is the only model that provides universal coverage; it is used in Canada and throughout Europe. This model would save money overall, through the government's ability to negotiate lower rates and decrease administrative costs. The State of Vermont is considering a single-payer program.

In addition, many people who are eligible for health insurance do not enroll. They may not enroll because they don't know about the program, they don't think they are eligible, or the enrollment information is not in a language they understand. We hope that with funding and extensive outreach efforts through the ACA, more people will know about and enroll in available health insurance programs. However, there will still be people who are eligible but uninsured.

ACCESSING CARE

With millions more Americans insured through the ACA, there is a deep concern that there aren't enough medical providers available to see patients in a timely manner. Even before the ACA, patients often had problems with getting appointments when they wanted them. And if you had Medicaid, you often had trouble finding a doctor who would take you as a patient. There are many reasons why there aren't enough Medicaid providers, one of which is the low reimbursement rates they get paid.

The ACA included several provisions that addressed these issues. As a result of the law, Medicaid providers received an increase in payment for three years. Community health centers also received additional funding. There was also an investment in expanding the health care workforce, including the role of CHWs. These are only a few elements in the ACA that try to address access issues.

Whether these changes are enough to ensure that people who are covered through the ACA and Medicaid gain access to essential health care services is yet to be determined. We do know that some enrollees in the health insurance marketplaces have experienced trouble seeing their doctor. This may be the result of several factors, such as a "pent up" demand by patients who have not seen a doctor in a while, or the limited provider network available, which helps keep costs lower. Whatever the reason, we know that while having insurance helps you have access to more affordable health care, it does not guarantee that you will get the care you need, when you need it.

IMPROVING THE QUALITY OF CARE

While the quality of health care for some patients in the United States is excellent, the care delivered on average is inconsistent. Research has shown that patients get recommended care only 70 percent of the time, and 26 percent of patients experience difficulties with getting care. In addition, the quality of care people get differs across geographic regions (AHRQ, 2013a).

Each year since 2003, the Agency for Healthcare Research and Quality (AHRQ) has reported on progress and opportunities for improving health care quality and reducing health care disparities. The health care elements assessed are effectiveness, safety, timeliness, patient centeredness, care coordination, efficiency, and adequacy of health system infrastructure.

In AHQR's 2013 report, they state that "quality of health care in America is only fair." They found that the quality of care in hospitals is improving quickly, but the quality of care in ambulatory settings (where medical care is provided on an outpatient basis such as a clinic) is not. They also cite that for health care measures that are addressed in public reports from the Center for Medicare and Medicaid, there is more improvement. This is often the case with publicly reported measures, as there is more attention paid to them. Many advocates call for the public reporting of quality data for this reason.

There are many efforts to improve the quality of care in the United States. One framework that is being used, developed by the Institute for Healthcare Improvement, is the "Triple Aim":

- Improving the patient experience of care (including quality and satisfaction)
- Improving the health of populations
- Reducing the per capita cost of health care

Currently, there is a big difference between the best possible care and the care that is routinely delivered. We still have a lot of work to do.

ELIMINATING HEALTH INEQUALITIES

As mentioned above, the advances of our public health and medical systems do not benefit everyone equally. In general, low-income people, immigrants and people of color, receive less preventive care, have more chronic conditions, and die younger than Whites. As discussed in Chapter 4, there are many causes for these differences, including "root causes" such as poverty, racism, and lower quality education. These structural inequities already put low-income communities and communities of color at a health disadvantage. Without a good education you are less likely to get a job that pays a living wage, which impacts the neighborhood in which you live and the ability to get the services you need. In addition, even with similar income, education, and health insurance as Whites, communities of color still experience worse health status.

In conjunction with their annual quality reports, AHRQ also publishes a National Health Disparities report. More than 200 health care process, outcome, and access measures are tracked, covering a variety of health conditions and health care settings (AHRQ, 2013b). Some of the findings from the 2013 report included:

- African Americans and Latinos received worse care than Whites for about 40 percent of the quality measures.
- American Indians/Alaskan Natives received worse care than Whites for about 33 percent of the quality measures.
- Low-income patients received worse care than high-income people for about 60 percent of the quality measures.

There are probably many other disparities that we don't know about because we don't have the data to measure them. A major issue in being able to identify and then begin to eliminate health disparities is being able to collect and analyze demographic data such as race, ethnicity, income, sexual orientation, and gender identity. For example, because of sample size, many times Asians, Native Hawaiians, and Other Pacific Islanders are combined under a broad "Asian" category, although we know the experiences and health status of these populations are very different. Collecting and analyzing data is a critical component for our health care system to begin providing quality care, equally, to everyone.

REDUCING HEALTH CARE COSTS

The high cost of health care impacts everyone. Businesses that have paid for employees' health insurance are trying to reduce their costs by putting more of the responsibility on their employees or decreasing the benefits available. Local, state, and federal governments that pay for health care for vulnerable populations know that the increasingly high cost of health care is unsustainable for their budgets. Over the past few decades, the cost of health care has increased much faster than wages and inflation.

Health policy experts and policy makers are working on solutions to slow down or decrease our high cost of care. Some are focusing on creating more efficiencies, such as implementing health information technology (i.e., electronic health records) so that all of our medical providers can communicate with one another, preventing unnecessary or duplicative tests. Others are working on "payment reform," changing the way medical providers are paid. For example, there's movement away from getting paid for every service to getting a set amount for treating certain conditions or achieving quality health outcomes. There are also efforts to regulate how much health insurance plans can increase their rates every year.

It will take everyone working together and many solutions to address the increasing cost of health care in this country.

WHAT CAN WE DO TO IMPROVE OUR HEALTH CARE SYSTEM?

To change the health care system to provide better care for more people, we must get involved with how health policy is made. *Policies* are rules that guide how something works. Families often set household policies, including curfews and bedtimes for children. Many people and organizations develop and advocate for policies that impact our health care system. For example, the Center on Medicare and Medicaid Services writes regulations that govern how these two major public programs (Medicare and Medicaid) are run. States have ballot initiatives through which people can vote on policy. The local school board can pass a health and fitness plan for schools. In order to achieve a better health care system, we need to understand the process of how policies are made and seek opportunities to influence these policies.

THE POLITICS OF CHANGING HEALTH POLICY

There are many stakeholders with different interests and perspectives trying to influence the health care system, and this makes negotiations and compromise extremely challenging. A **stakeholder** is anyone who has an interest in the outcome of a decision (usually a policy change). Some stakeholders are well organized and have a lot of money to invest in their advocacy efforts; others do not. Stakeholders in our health care system include:

- Individuals, families, and communities
- Physicians
- Hospitals
- Health plans
- Pharmaceutical companies
- Businesses
- Unions
- Advocacy organizations representing patients and communities

IMPROVING ACCESS TO QUALITY HEALTH CARE FOR EVERYONE
REQUIRES CHANGING HEALTH CARE POLICIES

Each of these stakeholders has a unique view of the health care system and how it should be "fixed," and they lobby to influence changes to policy. Some, like insurance and pharmaceutical companies, have substantial resources to spend on advocating for their position, and others, like consumers, low-income communities, and the advocacy organizations that represent them, do not.

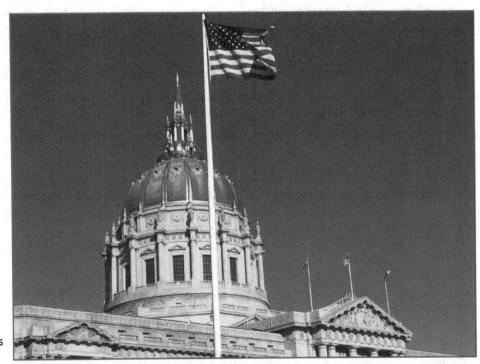

Improving access to quality health care for everyone requires changing health care policies.

- *How might the interests of consumers (or patients) be different from the interests of pharmaceutical companies or health plans?*

- *What is the primary concern of patients?*

- *What are the primary concerns of insurance companies and other stakeholders?*

THE ROLE OF CHWs IN CHANGING HEALTH POLICY

Part 5 of this textbook focuses on the role that CHWs play in facilitating community-level interventions and organizing efforts. Just as CHWs may serve as links between communities and health care systems, they may also link communities to the public policy process, assisting to mobilize grassroots participation and leadership. **Grassroots organizing** efforts are characterized by the participation of the communities that will be most affected by the proposed policies.

CHWs often play a vital role in supporting communities to organize and advocate for policy changes on the local, state, and national levels. While CHWs may themselves become visible leaders in these efforts, speaking to the media or testifying before policymakers, their primary role is to support community members to raise their own voices in support of social change. We will address these roles in greater detail in Chapter 23.

CHWs may contribute to changing public policies in the following ways:

- Conduct research on health inequalities and outstanding needs in the community
- Facilitate a community diagnosis in which community members identify their own resources and needs (see Chapter 22)
- Conduct outreach, education, and mobilization to inform community members and voters about important health issues
- Participate in media advocacy efforts by talking to reporters and writing opinion pieces or letters to the editor
- Testify to policymakers who are considering legislation on specific health issues important to your community
- Participate in public meetings and rallies on health issues
- Write letters to legislators, regulators, and providers about issues of concern in your community
- Collect stories about important health issues or encourage your clients to share their stories and speak out
- Partner with other advocacy organizations and collaborations working on issues of importance
- Train and support community members to engage in direct advocacy efforts, including protests, media advocacy, and testifying before policymakers
- Become a policymaker by serving on a local or state board, commission, advisory committee, or run for office!

- *Can you think of other ways that CHWs can participate in efforts to advocate for new public policies?*

- *Have you ever participated in such advocacy efforts?*

- *What was your role?*

- *What policies does your local community currently advocate to change?*

Chapter Review

1. You have been asked to make a presentation to a local community group about the health care system. How will you answer the following questions from the community:

   o Approximately how many people lack health insurance in the United States?

   o What is universal health care?

   o How does the U.S. health care system compare with those of other countries? Do we have the healthiest society?

   o Why is health care in the United States more expensive than in other countries?

   o What types of health insurance programs are available to low-income people?

   o What can we do to change the system and to get better health care for our community?

   o If you could make any changes you wanted to the U.S. health care system, what changes would you make and why?

2. Identify the following resources for low-income and uninsured clients in your community, city, or county:

   o Which hospitals provide care to uninsured patients? Do these hospitals publicize their policies and make it easy for uninsured patients to access free care?

   o Are there free clinics in the city or county?

   o Where and how can people with limited English proficiency access health care? Are there clinics or hospitals that provide services in languages other than English or that provide trained health care interpreters?

   o Where can clients go to enroll in Medicaid, Medicare, or SCHIP programs? What are the eligibility requirements for these programs in your state?

   o What local organizations are advocating for expanded access to quality health care for low-income and other vulnerable communities?

   o What policies are currently being debated in your city or county that will have an impact on access to health care services?

References

Agency for Healthcare Research and Quality. (2013a). *National healthcare quality report.* Retrieved from www.ahrq.gov/research/findings/nhqrdr/nhqr13/index.html

Agency for Healthcare Research and Quality. (2013b). *National healthcare disparities report.* Retrieved from www.ahrq.gov/research/findings/nhqrdr/nhdr13/index.html

Altman, D. (2014). *How 13 million Americans could lose insurance subsidies. Perspectives: November 19, 2014.* Kaiser Family Foundation. Retrieved from *http://kff.org/health-reform/perspective/how-13-million-americans-could-lose-insurance-subsidies/*

American Hospital Association. (2014). *Trend watch chartbook 2014.* Retrieved from *www.aha.org/research/reports/tw/chartbook/2014/14chartbook.pdf*

America's Essential Hospitals. (2015). *Essential hospitals vital data — results of America's essential hospitals' annual hospital characteristics survey, FY 2013.* Retrieved from *http://essentialhospitals.org/wp-content/uploads/2015/03/Essential-Hospitals-Vital-Data-2015.pdf*

Anderson, C. (2014). *Multinational comparisons of health systems data, 2014.* OECD Chartpack. The Commonwealth Fund. Retrieved from *www.commonwealthfund.org/~/media/files/publications/chartbook/2014/nov/pdf_1788_anderson_multinational_comparisons_2014_oecd_chartpack_v2.pdf*

Association of American Medical Colleges. (2014). *Physician specialty data book.* Center for Workforce Studies. Retrieved from *https://members.aamc.org/eweb/upload/Physician%20Specialty%20Databook%202014.pdf*

Center for Disease Control and Prevention. (2013a). *Health disparities and inequalities report—US 2013.* Retrieved from *www.cdc.gov/mmwr/pdf/other/su6203.pdf*

Centers for Disease Control and Prevention. (2013b). *Health, United States, 2013—At a glance.* Retrieved from *www.cdc.gov/nchs/hus/at_a_glance.htm*

Centers for Medicare and Medicaid Services, Office of the Actuary, National Health Statistics Group. (n.d.). *National health expenditure data.* Retrieved from *www.cms.gov/Research-Statistics-Data-and-Systems/Statistics-Trends-and-Reports/NationalHealthExpendData/NationalHealthAccountsHistorical.html*

Centers for Medicare and Medicaid Services. (2014). *National health expenditures 2014 release.* Retrieved from *www.cms.gov*

Davis, K., Stremikis, K., Squires, D., & Schoen, C. (2014). *Mirror, mirror on the wall: How the performance of the U.S. health care system compares internationally.* The Commonwealth Fund. Retrieved from *www.commonwealthfund.org/publications/fund-reports/2014/jun/mirror-mirror*

Families USA. (2015). *Federal poverty guidelines.* Retrieved from *http://familiesusa.org/product/federal-poverty-guidelines*

Kaiser Family Foundation. (2015). *Current status of state Medicaid expansion decisions.* Retrieved from *http://kff.org/health-reform/slide/current-status-of-the-medicaid-expansion-decision/*

Kaiser Family Foundation and Health Research and Education Trust. (2014). *Employer health benefits survey.* Retrieved from *http://files.kff.org/attachment/ehbs-2014-abstract-chartpack*

Long, S. K., Karpman, M., Shartzer, A., Wissoker, D., Kenney, G. M., Zuckerman, . . . Hempstead, K. (2014, December 3). *Taking stock: Health insurance coverage under the ACA as of September 2014.* Urban Institute, Health Policy Center. Retrieved from *http://hrms.urban.org/briefs/health-insurance-coverage-under-the-aca-as-of-september-2014.html*

Merriam-Webster Dictionary. (n.d.). Retrieved from *www.merriam-webster.com/dictionary/system*

National Association of Community Health Centers. (2013). *Community health centers at a glance.* [Infographic]. Retrieved from *www.nachc.com/client/documents/Infographic--CHCs.pdf*

Obama, B. (2014, April 1). *Remarks by the President on the Affordable Care Act.* Washington, DC: Office of the Press Secretary. Retrieved from *www.whitehouse.gov/the-press-office/2014/04/01/remarks-president-affordable-care-act*

Sommers, B. D., Musco, T., Finegold, K., Gunja, M. Z., Burke, A. & McDowell, A. M. (2014). Health reform and changes in health insurance coverage in 2014. *New England Journal of Medicine, 371,* 867–874. doi:10.1056/NEJMsr1406753

World Health Organization. (n.d.). *Preamble to the World Health Organization's Constitution.* Retrieved from *www.who.org*

Additional Resources

Centers for Medicare and Medicaid Services. (n.d.). Retrieved from *www.cms.gov/*

The Commonwealth Fund. (n.d.). Retrieved from *www.commonwealthfund.org*

Families USA. (n.d.). Retrieved from *http://familiesusa.org/*

HealthCare.gov. (n.d.). Retrieved from *www.healthcare.gov/*

Kaiser Family Foundation. (n.d.). Retrieved from *www.kff.org*

Medicaid general information. (n.d.). Retrieved from *www.medicaid.gov/*

Medical specialties. (n.d.). Retrieved from *www.medicare.gov/physiciancompare/staticpages/resources/specialtydefinitions.html*

Medicare eligibility. (n.d.). Retrieved from *www.medicare.gov/MedicareEligibility*

National Association of Community Health Centers. (n.d.). Retrieved from *www.nachc.org*

State Health Facts. (n.d.). *Medicaid information by state and children's health insurance programs by state.* Retrieved from http://kff.org/state-category/medicaid-chip/

CORE COMPETENCIES FOR PROVIDING DIRECT SERVICES

Practicing Cultural Humility

Abby Rincón

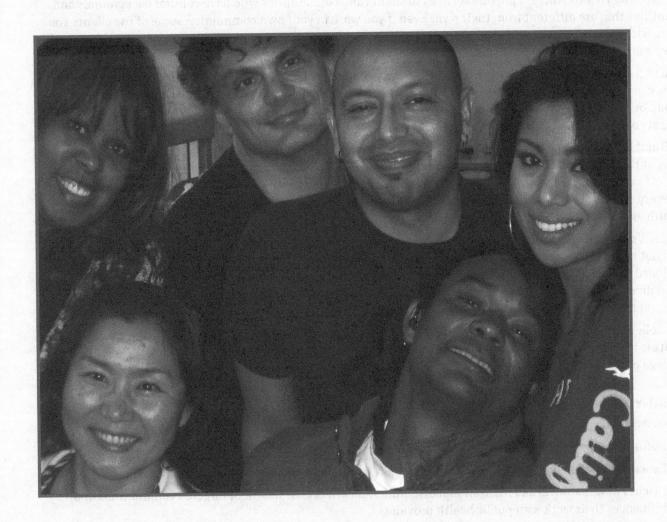

"More than a concept, Cultural Humility is a communal reflection to analyze the root causes of suffering and create a broader, more inclusive view of the world... Cultural Humility is now used in public health, social work, education, and non-profit management. It is a daily practice for people to deal with hierarchical relationships, changing organizational policy and building relationships based on trust."

Melanie Tervalon

Introduction

Community Health Workers provide services to clients and communities who have cultural backgrounds and identities that are different from their own. Even if you work in your own community, some of the clients you work with will come from a different generational, economic, ethnic, religious, or linguistic background or will have a different gender, gender identity, or sexual orientation than you.

The rich cultural diversity that surrounds us can pose challenges for CHWs and other helping professionals. How can we learn to work effectively with all clients? What if we don't know much about a particular cultural group or community? What if we grew up in households or communities that taught us to view people from different communities with bias or prejudice?

Cultural humility is an approach to providing services to clients and communities that emphasizes an awareness of the limitations of our cultural perspectives, and an acknowledgment of the risks of imposing our own beliefs on those we work with. It provides a framework for demonstrating respect for the cultural identities of every client and community you may work with as a CHW, and for interacting in ways that promotes their health and supports their autonomy.

As CHWs, we are committed to becoming compassionate providers to people of all backgrounds. One chapter will not make you an expert in how to do this, but by studying the concepts, questions, knowledge, and skills included in this chapter, you can enhance your understanding and ability to respond to the complexities of cultural diversity. This chapter invites you to make a commitment to become a lifelong learner and practitioner of cultural humility.

We believe that cultural humility is a foundational concept to guide the work of CHWs. We will continue to address it throughout this textbook, just as we do throughout the course of the CHW Certificate Program at City College of San Francisco.

WHAT YOU WILL LEARN

By studying the material in this chapter, you will be able to:

- Define the concept of cultural humility

- Describe the changing population in the United States and how this affects the work of CHWs

- Discuss how historical and institutional discrimination affects the health of targeted communities and influences their work with public health providers

- Analyze the importance of becoming lifelong learners and practitioners of cultural humility

- Discuss and analyze concepts of traditional health beliefs and practices and how they may influence the delivery of services to clients

- Identify, analyze, and apply models for practicing cultural humility and conducting client-centered interviews regarding health issues, including the Tool to Elicit Health Beliefs and the LEARN Model

- Create a personal learning plan in order to become a culturally effective CHW

WORDS TO KNOW

Gender Identity

Heterogeneity

Structural Racism

Structural Discrimination

6.1 Defining Cultural Humility

Cultural humility is essential for working effectively with diverse clients and communities. Cultural humility acknowledges histories of discrimination and current dynamics of power and privilege, and asks service providers to examine their own biases in order not to impose assumptions—about behaviors, beliefs, or values—onto the clients they work with. Cultural humility guides us in overturning traditional power dynamics between providers and clients that emphasizes the knowledge and skills of providers and assigns clients to a secondary position and role. When your work is guided by cultural humility, you will recognize that only the client is the expert in their own life (including their cultural identity, values and belief) and act in ways that enhance client autonomy and opportunities for empowerment.

A good place to start when studying the concept of cultural humility is with the meaning of the word "humility." Humility signifies not raising one's own significance or value too high, or above the value of others. It implies recognizing the limits of one's own wisdom and skills, and acknowledging and appreciating the wisdom, value, and skills of others.

When the word humility is used to create the term cultural humility, it emphasizes the limits of our ability to know or truly understand the culture of others. It also advances values of equity, and an understanding that no cultural identity or tradition has more or less value than any other. Cultural humility is designed to challenge and prevent the type of cultural arrogance that has led individuals, communities, organizations, and nations to impose their own beliefs and standards upon others.

Cultural Humility and Client-Centered Practice

Cultural humility is a foundational concept and skill for guiding the work of CHWs. We will refer to cultural humility throughout this textbook, drawing connections with other key concepts and skills. For example, cultural humility informs all of the work that CHWs do directly with clients and communities. It is also a key component of the client-centered approach (addressed in Chapters 8 through 11), which is designed to support a client's autonomy and self-determination.

Cultural humility goes beyond previously taught concepts—such as cultural competence or cross-cultural work—that emphasize the importance of learning about other cultures in order to provide services. What is the difference between cultural competence and cultural humility? According to Melanie Tervalon and Jane Murray-Garcia (1998)

> cultural humility incorporates a lifelong commitment to self-evaluation and critique, to redressing the power imbalances in the physician-patient dynamic, and to developing mutually beneficial and non-paternalistic partnerships with communities on behalf of individuals and defined populations. (Tervalon & Murray-Garcia, 1998, p. 123)

THE LIMITS OF OUR KNOWLEDGE ABOUT OTHER CULTURES: A WORD OF CAUTION

Some resources designed to promote an appreciation of cultural diversity and skills for working across cultural identities may do more harm than good. They teach seemingly definitive information about specific cultural groups. The assumption is that once people have learned about the culture and traditions of Mexican Americans (or another cultural group) related to health issues such as diet, death and dying, or sexuality, they will then *know* how to provide more sensitive or culturally competent services to members of that community. From our perspective, there are several key problems with this approach:

- It essentializes culture by assuming that there is such a thing as *the* Mexican American culture or *the* Mexican American diet. In reality, there is tremendous diversity within Mexican American or Chicano cultures or Vietnamese or Italian American cultures, or within any other culture.

- It fails to recognize, honor, and appreciate the tremendous richness and complexity of what we call culture (and the tremendous diversity *within* cultures).

- It promotes the idea that cultural communities and identities can be deeply and accurately understood by participating in trainings or another course of study.

- It may foster the very stereotypes that have proved so harmful in the past.

- It focuses on knowing specific information about the cultures, beliefs, and customs of others rather than the process and interaction between providers such as CHWs and the clients and communities they serve.

- It ignores power differences between people of different identities or cultural backgrounds (such as a CHW and a client).

- It fails to focus our attention on our own cultural traditions, values, and beliefs, and how these may cause us, unintentionally, to make assumptions about the beliefs, values, feelings, and behaviors of others.

While learning about different cultures can certainly strengthen your understanding of the communities you work with, *assuming that we understand or know something definitive about other cultures can result in harm.* When we assume that we understand where others are coming from, we may fail to ask for or to listen to the information that they provide, and may provide guidance that is based on faulty assumptions or misinformation.

To illustrate, let's consider the following scenario. Your agency sends you to a training that focuses on the *Cultural Health Beliefs and Practices of the Hmong Community.* The training is two days in length and exposes you to knowledgeable speakers, including leaders from the Hmong community, social workers, CHWs, and anthropologists. Detailed information is presented about Hmong history, culture, and customs, and the challenges Hmong immigrants face in the United States. You leave with a sense of understanding key aspects of Hmong culture, their history in the United States, and some of the most pressing health issues the community currently faces. There is a risk that the next time you encounter a Hmong client, you may assume to know a lot about her. You may not ask appropriate questions and fail to learn important information about the client and her health. As a result, the client may not receive an accurate assessment, relevant health education, case management services, or referrals from you.

While there is considerable value in learning as much as possible about the cultures of the communities that you will work with, *we encourage you to balance your desire for learning with a cultural humility framework.* Cultural humility reminds you of the limits of our own knowledge or understanding about the lives of others, and guides you in highlighting the expertise of the clients and communities you work with.

6.2 Practicing Cultural Humility

Many clients and communities face bias and discrimination when they attempt to access health and social services and, as a result, receive fewer services or services of poorer quality. As we addressed in Chapter 4, this is a significant reason for persistent health inequalities. In order to be successful in your ultimate goal of promoting health equality and social justice, you must develop your capacity to reach and provide quality services to people from many different backgrounds, cultures, and identities.

As CHWs, it's important to acknowledge what we don't know about cultural diversity. This is the first step toward improving our ability to work with people effectively, regardless of their identity and life experience. Learning how to work effectively across cultures is not just an intellectual endeavor: We must open our hearts as well as our minds in order to develop cultural humility.

This process requires a willingness to acknowledge the history, pain, and past hurts of our own communities as well as others. It also entails acknowledging our own biases and judgments about others. This may be uncomfortable and provoke strong emotion. In these moments, it can be helpful to stay humble and remember that we have all made mistakes and are capable of personal growth and change. Learning about cultural diversity can be a challenging, lifelong, and transformative journey.

Practicing cultural humility isn't easy. It requires:

- Studying histories of oppression and discrimination
- Examining our own assumptions and prejudices about people who come from communities different from our own

- Engaging respectfully with all clients and recognizing that they are our guides in determining their own cultural identity, values, knowledge, behaviors, and decisions

- Engaging in self-reflection and self-critique, including reflection about our own assumptions and biases and our interactions with clients

- Understanding that our own culture is no better than any other—all cultures deserve our respect

- Learning to be comfortable not knowing about the experience, culture, identity, values, or beliefs of others

- Recognizing that only the client is the expert about her own culture, values, and beliefs

- Placing our assumptions aside when working with others, and asking clients and communities to share their own experiences, knowledge, resources, needs, and priorities with us so that we may best support their health and well-being

By practicing cultural humility with our clients, we build a welcoming and respectful working partnership. In this partnership, we recognize that we need to learn about the client's experience, culture, values, beliefs, and behaviors, and we remember that the way to do that is *to ask* and *to listen* deeply to what they tell us.

> **Andrew Ciscel:** The first thing that comes to mind about working with clients is the piece about cultural humility. I really like to find out as much as possible about the client's life, their concerns and experience. Cultural humility guides me in doing this. It helps me so that I am making a conscious effort to check any assumptions I may have about any client. By asking questions and listening, I get to know who the client really is and, well, whatever they choose to share with me about what they might need and where they want to go. The frame of cultural humility has been so wonderful for guiding my work, and keeping it client-centered.

6.3 The Culturally Diverse Context for Community Health Work

Ismael Reed has said that, as a society, the United States is unique in the world because "the world is here." In America, "the cultures of the world crisscross" on a daily basis (Takaki, 1993, p. 16).

Think about where you fit in this multicultural mix.

What Do YOU? Think.

- *Were you born in the United States?*

- *What about your parents and grandparents?*

- *What about your neighbors, the people you encounter at the grocery store, the bank, or in your children's schools?*

- *What are the languages, cultures, and other identities of the students in your classes and the people in your community?*

- *What about the people who are your local politicians or in charge of large businesses and government institutions?*

The population of the United States is rapidly changing. Our nation looks quite different today from the way it did 50 or 100 years ago. Across the United States, our diversity is growing, including the number of languages spoken, the number of people who identity as biracial and multiracial, the types of food that are available, the range of cultural, religious, and community-based organizations and events. New legal protections have been passed (and are still being debated and advocated for) that benefit lesbian, gay, and transgender people.

The majority of children born in the United States today are people of color (U.S. Census Bureau, n.d.). Communities of color are in the majority of the population in in 49 of 366 metropolitan regions in the United States, and in four states: California, Hawaii, New Mexico, and Texas. Data and analysis from the U.S. Census Bureau predicts that by the early 2040s, whites will no longer be a majority and will constitute less than 50 percent of America's population. By 2050, people of color will comprise over 50 percent of the U.S. population (U.S. Census

Bureau, n.d.). Contrary to popular belief, the increase of communities of color in the United States is not the result of more immigration, but rather due to more births within the communities of color that are already here. This is especially true for Latino and Asian populations.

Each of the categories of the Census Bureau includes a wide array of ancestral countries of origin, cultural backgrounds, tribal affiliations, customs, religions, or life experiences. The United States has a rich linguistic diversity as well: it is estimated that there are between six and seven thousand languages spoken in the world, and many of these are also spoken within the U.S. Add to this rich diversity of cultures the differences emerging from life experiences and opportunities, such as poverty, political experience, and educational opportunity, and individual differences, such as gender identity, disability, family history, or sexual orientation.

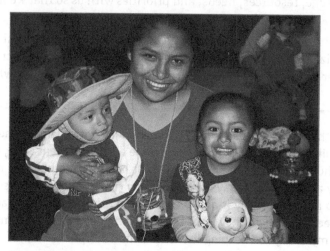

Family forms a key part of our identities and cultures.

The diversity of our nation's population is a tremendous strength, and it supports our economy. Richard Florida has noted, "the evidence is mounting that geographical openness and cultural diversity and tolerance are not by-products but key drivers of economic progress" (Florida, 2011).

IMMIGRANT COMMUNITIES

The population of the United States continues to be shaped by the histories of its many immigrants (Passel & Cohn, 2012):

- As of 2012, there were an estimated 40.8 million immigrants in the United States.

- The majority of immigrants come from four nations: Mexico, India, China, and the Philippines.

- There are an estimated 11 million undocumented immigrants in the United States. The majority of Latinos living in the United States were born here, and are not immigrants.

- The states with the highest number of immigrants are: California, Texas, Florida, and New York.

Most immigrant groups have faced prejudice and discrimination as they struggle to establish themselves in the United States. Unfortunately, there is still a strong backlash against immigrants today. Some people argue that immigrants are a drain on the U.S. economy, taking resources away from more established communities (most of whom were once immigrants themselves). Yet research evidence clearly shows that immigrants—both legal residents and undocumented—support our society through the payment of significant taxes which support our infrastructure and public services including schools, parks, and health care services: in 2010, immigrants paid $11.2 billion in state and local taxes alone (American Immigration Council, 2011).

6.4 Histories of Discrimination

Your ability to work effectively with diverse communities will also depend on your willingness to examine how larger societal policies and practices influence health status. As CHWs, we must be ready to understand the impact of discrimination based on ethnicity, nationality, immigration status, sex, gender identity, sexual orientation, and other identities on the lives and health status of the clients and communities you work with.

Racial discrimination is an integral part of U.S. history. African Americans/Blacks, Latinos, American Indians, Pacific Islanders, and some Asian populations are disproportionately represented in the lower socioeconomic ranks of our multicultural society. Racial discrimination across generations has also meant that a greater majority of children of color attend lower-quality schools; more adults of color work in lower-paying jobs; and disproportionate percentages of Black and Latino males end up in our prison systems. Ultimately, racial discrimination results in higher rates of illness and lower life expectancy (see Chapter 4). The government and institutional policies that created these inequalities in the past and that sustain them in the present are referred to as structural racism. **Structural racism** means that inequities are built into the key systems of a society, such as the educational, legal, employment, housing, and health care systems.

Other groups in the United States have also experienced individual and **structural discrimination**. For example, women still experience high levels of domestic violence. In the workforce, they receive less pay and fewer opportunities for promotion and experience higher rates of sexual harassment. Most recently we've seen many states address structural discrimination of lesbian and gay people by passing laws that allow same sex couples to marry legally.

- *Can you think of other examples of structural racism or structural discrimination?*

- *How might structural discrimination have affected a client you are working with?*

- *Have you experienced structural discrimination?*

DISCRIMINATION IN PUBLIC HEALTH

The field of public health itself harbors notorious instances of racism and other forms of discrimination that have led some people to have a deep mistrust of the public health system. One of the most notorious examples was a clinical study of the effects of untreated syphilis conducted on African Americans. In 1932, the Public Health Service, a branch of the U.S. government, carried out an infamous study known as the "Tuskegee Study of Untreated Syphilis in the Negro Male." This study focused on the effects of untreated syphilis among African American men in Macon County, Georgia. For more than 40 years, African American men who had the disease were given a placebo (a treatment that the patient does not know is ineffective) for what they were told by the U.S. government was "bad blood." They were each given $50 to participate in the study, offered a decent burial when they died, and were under the impression that the treatment for "bad blood" was helpful. Even though in 1942 it was well known that penicillin could cure syphilis, it was never offered to the men in the study. As a result, many of the men died, and others were disabled.

The Tuskegee study was officially ended in 1972 after it was exposed and publicized by the media. However, the memory of this unethical study, a blatant form of racism, remains strong in many African American communities. On May 16, 1997, President Bill Clinton issued a formal apology on behalf of the nation to the family members of the men who took part in this study.

Another example is the role of the U.S. government in the sterilization of women in Puerto Rico. When the United States assumed governance of Puerto Rico in 1898, the U.S. government worried that overpopulation of the island would lead to disastrous social and economic conditions. In 1937, a law was passed to implement a "population control program." Rather than providing Puerto Rican women with information and access to alternative forms of safe, legal, and reversible contraception, the U.S. government actively promoted the use of permanent sterilization through tubal ligation (tying off the fallopian tubes). Women were pushed toward having *la operacion* through door-to-door visits from health workers, with financial subsidies, and by favoritism toward sterilized women from industrial employers. Sterilization was not only provided by government clinics but also by factories where women provided cheap labor for overseas corporations. Rather than pay women maternity leave and benefits, factories did the calculations and found that by providing "operations" they would save millions of dollars.

Without informed consent, many women didn't understand that sterilization through tubal ligation was permanent. The phrase "tying the tubes" made women think the procedure was easily reversible. In 1936, 6.5 percent of Puerto Rican women had been sterilized. By 1953, 20 percent of women had had the operation, and by 1980, 30 percent had been sterilized. When word of this practice got out to the public, Puerto Rican community leaders and others were outraged.

Another example is the systematic discrimination that lesbian, gay, bisexual, transgender, and intersex (LGBTI) communities have experienced in health care, education, employment, marriage, and housing. Transgender communities lack civil rights protections at the federal level and in most states. When transgender and gender-variant people seek assistance from health professionals, their very identity may be pathologized and labeled as "gender identity disorder." Rather than providing transgender clients with the health care they seek, health professionals may diagnose their identity as an illness and, in some cases, have committed transgender clients against their will to mental wards or hospitals.

Actions such as these destroy public trust and create barriers between the communities who have experienced discrimination and our public health system. While you don't have the power to undo history, as a CHW you can work to ensure that gaps in your own knowledge, attitudes, and professional competencies do not cause further harm to your diverse clients.

- *What are your thoughts and feelings when you read about the government-sanctioned Tuskegee study or the sterilization of Puerto Rican women?*

- *How do you think these actions have affected Black and Puerto Rican communities?*

- *Are you aware of current structural or institutional injustices that harm people of color or other communities?*

- *How might these injustices influence your work as a CHW?*

- *How can you work to build trusting relationships with communities that have experienced such injustices?*

6.5 Defining and Understanding Culture

In essence, culture includes the beliefs, behaviors, attitudes, and practices that are learned, shared, and passed on by members of a particular group. Medical anthropologist C. G. Helman defines *culture* as:

> *a set of guidelines (both explicit and implicit) that individuals inherit as members of a particular society, and that tell them how to view the world, how to experience it emotionally, and how to behave in it in relation to other people, to supernatural forces and gods, and the natural environment. (Helman, 1994)*

According to Judith Carmen Nine Curt (1984):

- Culture cannot be shed.
- Every cultural detail is incredibly old.
- Culture functions in "out-of-awareness."
- In order to understand others, we must first understand our own culture.
- Culture is better understood by observing and studying the cultures of others.
- Cultures are neither better nor worse, simply different.
- Every human being is bound by his or her culture.
- In order to be free from the hidden constraints of culture, we must study it.
- This study is new in our society and our educational world.
- Behind the differences among people, there are basic similarities, such as love, family, loyalty, friendship, joy, and the belief in transcendence.

Culture is not static—it doesn't stand still. It is dynamic, constantly changing and evolving with us. Culture is also multifaceted. It incorporates and includes ethnic identity, immigration status and experience, sexual orientation, gender identity, religion or spirituality, social class, family background, language, physical ability, traditions, and much more.

Because culture is multifaceted and dynamic, there is a lot of diversity or **heterogeneity** *within* any culturally defined community. It is important to keep in mind that there may be as many differences within the community as there are similarities.

- *What are some of differences between people within the communities you belong to?*

- *As a CHW, why may it be important to understand that differences exist within communities who share a common culture?*

Keep in mind that it is not unusual for people to have more than one ethnic identity. For example, someone who has an African American father and a Chinese American mother may identify with both African American and Chinese American communities. But is this person's cultural identity based solely on ethnic roots and traditions? Probably not. This same individual may have other cultural affiliations that exert a strong influence on her identity, such as gender, class, disability or immigration status, sexual orientation, or religion. For example, an elderly, Buddhist, Latino male potentially shares experiences with many different cultural groups. For this reason, it's important as CHWs to allow our clients to define their cultural identities for themselves.

Gender identity is an important cultural consideration. Simply stated, **gender identity** is someone's own sense of being female or male, both or neither, and what that means to him or her (more information about gender identity is also provided in Chapter 10). Gender identity is an internal perception and may not be visibly apparent to others. Social definitions of what it means to be a man and what it means to be a woman vary across cultures. Like racial stereotypes, gender stereotypes and assumptions can be deeply harmful.

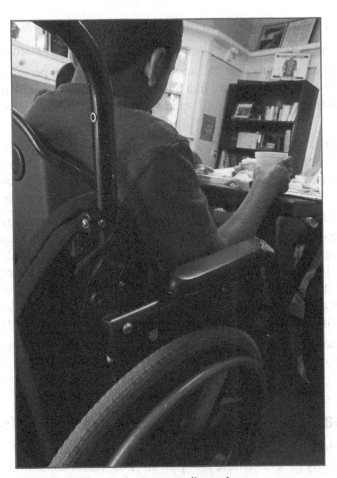

Culture and identity have many dimensions.

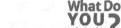

- *Have you ever had someone ask you, "Where are you from?" or "What are you?"*

- *Have you ever had someone mistakenly assume one of your cultural identities?*

- *How did this make you feel?*

- *How did you react?*

- *How do you define your cultural identities?*

- *Does this change depending upon the circumstances?*

6.6 Building Cultural Self-Awareness

Take a few minutes to answer the following questions.

1. What types of clients/communities do you think might have the greatest difficulties in accessing health or social services? Why?

2. What types of clients and communities do you lack experience with and knowledge about?

3. What types of clients or communities may you be less comfortable working with? Why?

4. How can you keep your personal attitudes and feelings from influencing the way you work with diverse clients?

5. What can you do to acknowledge your own stereotypes and prejudices? Why is this an important step to becoming an effective CHW?

6. Is it okay to be uncomfortable at times with clients of a particular cultural identity, or does this make you an unskilled CHW?

7. Is it okay to talk with your colleagues when you find that you are challenged in working with a client?

8. How can you learn to accept critical feedback about your work with diverse clients?

Now take a moment to reflect on your answers. Becoming aware of your own perceptions of others, your attitudes and behaviors, will aid you to work and live in a more culturally appropriate and sensitive manner. All of us have ideas and beliefs about people based on our upbringing and the prejudices that were passed on to us by our families.

Self-reflection is a powerful process for understanding our own cultural backgrounds and identities, as well as our own "hot-button issues"—the strong feelings, attitudes, and values that may arise during our work with others and that can have a negative influence on our ability to counsel a client effectively. Can you identify opportunities and areas for further learning? Are there communities that you are less comfortable working with?

Taking the additional step of acknowledging when the communities you belong to are the beneficiaries of unearned privilege in our society (for example, White people, males, heterosexuals and the physically able) may be more challenging, because we are socialized to assume that our experiences are shared by others around us—that everyone has access to the same level of benefits enjoyed by all. Consider where you have privilege in our society, and where you may lack it. These dynamics of power and privilege are not abstract or theoretical: they may be played out in your working relationships with clients, communities, and colleagues. Cultivating a high degree of self-awareness is the first major step in becoming a culturally effective CHW.

Please view the following video [▶] interview with Abby Rincón, the author of this chapter. Ms. Rincón talks about the challenge and the value of developing your skills for practicing cultural humility.

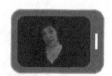

CULTURAL HUMILITY: FACULTY INTERVIEW

🔗 *http://youtu.be/ yV3DxgK5pn4*

6.7 Building Capacity as Culturally Effective CHWs

With time, study, training, and self-reflection, you will build your understanding of cultural humility and your ability to demonstrate it in your working relationships.

TRANSFERENCE OF POWER

An important component of cultural humility is the ability to promote the *transference of power*. While this concept has mostly been applied to the physician/clinician and patient scenario, it has important implications for CHWs as well. Traditionally, during a health care appointment, the health care provider asks most of the questions and leads the appointment with what they think is most important to talk about and/or ask about.

Reflect on your last appointment with your health care service provider:

- Who asked most of the questions?
- Were the questions the ones you wanted to answer in order to get to the problem and/or issue at hand?
- Were you able to fully express yourself, or did you find the appointment limiting?

Changing our approach can make it possible for the visit to be client-centered and to support the client to take the lead in identifying the concerns that are most important to them. This is what is known as a *transference of power*. While some questions need to be asked to begin the client intake or interviewing session, we want to create an atmosphere that invites and supports the client to tell her story and assert her needs. This transference of power allows the client to be the expert and the CHW or other caregiver to be the student. This produces a powerful change in the caregiver-client dynamic.

How can the CHW facilitate this transference of power? Client-centered interviewing and counseling are the best approaches for changing the power dynamic. This is a skill based on the concept of cultural humility. Chapters 8 through 11 provide detailed information about the client-centered approach, but let's start here by reviewing a particularly helpful model for interacting with clients.

Please note that several of the models introduced later in this chapter (the explanatory model, tools to elicit health beliefs, and the LEARN model) were developed to be used by physicians or other clinicians in health care settings. However, these tools and many of the questions may be adapted and used by CHWs to guide their work with clients.

THE EXPLANATORY MODEL

The explanatory model, developed by anthropologist Arthur Kleinman, is a client-focused health assessment that is respectful of the clients' views, perceptions, and definitions of *their* current concerns (Kleinman, 1980). Rather than imposing our own understanding of health conditions and related behavior, Kleinman recommends asking clients basic questions (what, why, how, and who) about their illness, to learn about their own experience and understanding.

Questions that may be used in the explanatory model include:

- *What* do you call the problem?
- *What* are the signs and symptoms of the illness that you are experiencing?
- *What* are your concerns or fears?
- *Why* do you think this illness or problem has occurred?
- *How* does the illness affect you and your family?
- *How* do you think the sickness should be treated?
- *How* do you want us to assist you?
- *Who* do you turn to for assistance?
- *Who* should be involved in decision making?

Interactive client interviewing techniques will enable clients to tell you about the primary issue at hand and assist you to understand how their cultural identities come into play.

Think about the following scenario with Luisa M.

Client Scenario: Luisa M.

Luisa M. comes to your agency and you are the first one to see her. Luisa is a recently arrived immigrant from Honduras and currently works as a domestic helper during the day and at night she washes dishes at a restaurant. She has three children, who are all living with her mother in Honduras. She has limited English language proficiency, wants to take ESL classes, and thinks she might be pregnant.

In the client interview, you learn of the many facets of Luisa's life. Because Luisa tells you about what is most pressing for her at this time, you learn that she has an undocumented immigrant status and she is very fearful of being deported; she is also very worried about being unable to support her family back home. As a result she has trouble sleeping at night and suffers from severe stomachaches. Finally, you learn that one of the reasons she left Honduras was to escape from a domestic violence situation and now has severe anxiety, which she refers to as *nervios*.

You started the interview most concerned with her pregnancy and wanting to assist her with prenatal care; however the new information that you learned means that you will need to learn more about her *nervios*, whether she may be experiencing post-traumatic stress (PTS), and how her severe stomachaches may affect her prenatal nutritional plan.

If you practice cultural humility and view learning about a client's reality as part of your core competencies, a client will tell you what her multiple cultural identities are. Only she is qualified to tell you what is most important to her. Listening in a nonjudgmental and compassionate manner, as well as validating her, will be critical to establishing trust, learning what is really going on for her, and creating a positive encounter so that she will return for a follow-up visit.

WHAT IF YOU MAKE A MISTAKE?

Cultural humility is an approach that acknowledges the limits of our understanding and our tendency to make mistakes when working with clients. Consider this scenario:

Reflecting on Your Practice of Cultural Humility

A CHW is working with a client in a health education session. The client has diabetes and her health has been getting worse. The client is from a cultural group that is different from that of the CHW. Throughout the session the CHW is compassionate; however, the client reacts negatively to the manner in which the CHW explains certain health information, particularly the information about healthy nutrition and eating. While the client doesn't say anything, the information the CHW presents is directly in conflict with the client's dietary traditions and family practices. The client feels that the CHW is trying to change her diet and doesn't understand or respect her traditions. Visibly offended and upset, the client leaves the session early.

Afterward, the CHW spends time thinking about what happened with the client, and talks with his supervisor. Through an examination of the session, the CHW and the supervisor determine that it is likely that the client was offended. The CHW realizes that he did not take time to ask the client about her own dietary beliefs and practices before presenting her with guidelines for a healthy diet, and is committed to doing so when working with future clients.

The CHW demonstrated cultural humility by acknowledging and desiring to learn about the problem, by acknowledging his mistake, and seeking to improve his skills. In this case, the CHW is "flexible and humble enough to then reassess anew the cultural dimensions of the experiences of each client" (Tervalon & Murray-Garcia, 1998).

What Do YOU? Think

- *Have you ever been offended by assumptions that a health care or social services provider made about you or a family member?*

- *What else could you do to demonstrate cultural humility in working with the clients described above?*

Please view the following short video, 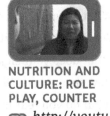 which shows a CHW working with a client who wants to change her diet and to control her diabetes. In the counter role play, the CHW does not do a good job of demonstrating cultural humility.

NUTRITION AND CULTURE: ROLE PLAY, COUNTER

🔗 *http://youtu. be/2Ck3V4johPM*

- What happened between the client and the CHW in this role play?
- What mistakes did the CHW make in terms of demonstrating cultural humility?
- What would you do differently to support this client?
- How would you demonstrate cultural humility?

6.8 Cultural Health Beliefs

Every cultural group has its own beliefs, values, and practices related to health issues, such as pregnancy and birth, death and dying, gender roles, familial responsibility, disease causation, religion and spirituality, traditional healing, and alternative healing practices. Your cultural group is no exception to this rule.

What Do YOU? Think

- *What are the health beliefs in your family or culture?*

- *Where did your family go to receive health care?*

- *What were the home remedies for illnesses?*

- *How were they used?*

- *What do you still practice today?*

- *Were there health topics or issues that were considered "taboo" or were forbidden to discuss?*

Earlier we discussed why CHWs must exercise caution and not generalize or stereotype about people from any cultural groups. Yet CHWs must still acknowledge and appreciate that individuals are indeed members of one or more cultural groups and may hold values rooted in those cultures. As CHWs, our goal should be to bring an open mind and to listen deeply to "where the client is coming from."

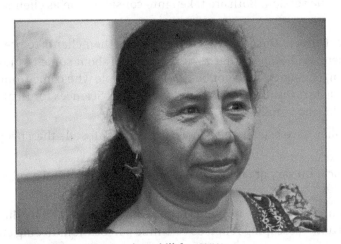

Cultural humility is a key skill for CHWs.

TOOL TO ELICIT HEALTH BELIEFS IN CLINICAL ENCOUNTERS

Arthur Kleinman's Tool to Elicit Health Beliefs in Clinical Encounters is an excellent resource for working with a client to define a health belief (Kleinman, 1980). Though it was developed to inform the work of nurses, physicians, and other clinicians, Kleinman's tool is also applicable to the work of CHWs.

- What do you call your problem? What name does it have?
- What do you think caused your problem?
- Why do you think it started when it did?
- What does your sickness do to you? How does it work?
- How severe is it? Will it have a short or long course?
- What do you fear most about your sickness?
- What are the chief problems that your sickness has caused for you?
- What kind of treatment do you think you should receive?
- What are the most important results you hope to receive from the treatment?

CHWs are not expected or required to be experts about the cultural health beliefs of their diverse clients. Rather, as a regular part of their practice, CHWs learn about these beliefs from their clients. Clients will answer these or any other questions based on their own belief systems, attitudes, and values.

THE LEARN MODEL

Another useful model when working with diverse clients is the LEARN model of Cross Cultural Encounter Guidelines for Health Practitioners (Berlin and Fowkes, 1983):

LEARN:

   L: listen with sympathy and understanding to the client's perception of the problem

   E: explain your perceptions of the problem

   A: acknowledge and discuss the differences and similarities between the perceptions of the client and the CHW

   R: recommend resources

   N: negotiate agreement

The LEARN model acknowledges cultural health beliefs held by the client and allows for CHWs to share what they know about a specific health condition. Neither perception is negated or devalued, and both are acknowledged and incorporated into the session. Both are taken into consideration as clients choose a course of action to promote their health.

As CHWs engage with their clients in this fashion, they are aiding their clients to preserve their own cultural health belief systems. Remember, however, that what may be true about some or most individuals from a particular cultural group, region, or country may not be true of all people who come from the same background. According to the *Provider's Guide to Quality and Culture* (Management Sciences for Health, n.d.), as you work with diverse clients, keep the following in mind:

- People from rural areas may have been living a more traditional lifestyle than people who have been living in urban areas.
- Economic status and education vary greatly among people within a cultural group or people who come from the same country.
- People from the same country may have migrated to the United States for very different reasons, including seeking economic opportunity, escaping religious or ethnic persecution, fleeing civil strife, or joining relatives in America.
- Generational differences may exist among people of different ages within the same cultural group and may include different belief systems.

TRADITIONAL HEALTH PRACTICES

Given that a significant percentage of the U.S. population are new immigrants or the children of immigrants, many people have recent experiences with traditional healing methods. Traditional health practices are different from the biomedical or Western medicine approaches used by nurses, physicians, and other health care providers in clinics and hospitals in the United States. Biomedical approaches are commonly said to focus more on treating disease than promoting health. Interestingly, many of today's biomedical treatments for disease are derived from traditional healing practices throughout the world, though this is not widely understood or acknowledged. Traditional health practices are often discounted or viewed as dangerous by Western medical providers. However, the recognition of traditional health practices is growing in the United States in two ways:

1. **Alternative medicine:** Traditional health practices are used instead of Western medicine (in the United States, the medical profession classifies any health practice that is different from its own biomedical model as "alternative"). Examples of alternative medicine are the use of acupuncture to treat asthma and the use of a special diet and herbs to treat cancer instead of being treated with radiation or chemotherapy.

2. **Complementary medicine:** In this approach, Western or biomedical practices are integrated and provided along with one or more other health traditions (such as Ayurvedic, chiropractic, acupuncture, or Chinese medicine). Some medical schools and hospitals in the United States are beginning to recognize and support complimentary medicine.

- *What traditional health practices are you familiar with?*

- *Do you know of clinics or hospitals in your area that practice complimentary medicine?*

- *What has your experience been with biomedical and alternative medical traditions?*

The following scenarios illustrate how traditional healing practices or cultural health beliefs may affect the care provided by health institutions.

The Influence of Cultural Beliefs

- A young Cambodian mother brings her eight-year-old daughter to a health center with a fever and bad cough. During the physical examination, the clinician discovers multiple red marks across the child's chest and back. The clinician could mistake this as a sign of parental child abuse. However, it is not. The mother practices "coining," a traditional, common practice in Southeast Asia. Coining entails rubbing heated oil on the skin and vigorously rubbing a coin over the area in a linear fashion until a red mark is seen. This is used to allow a path by which a "bad wind" can be released from the body. People use this method to treat a variety of minor ailments, including fever, chills, headache, colds, and cough.

- At a hospital, the nursing staff alerts a doctor about a patient who is agitated. The nurses want the doctor to order medication to calm the patient down, since he does not want to stay in bed. He is an elderly Japanese man who became upset and "uncooperative" because his bed was situated in the direction used to lay out the deceased in traditional Japan.

- A patient is seen at a health clinic for persistent, abdominal pain. The clinician suspects a stomach ulcer, prescribes medication, and sends the patient to speak with the CHW about following a new dietary regimen, eating several small meals throughout the day to minimize stomach acid buildup and pain. As the CHW explains the diet prescribed by the doctor, the patient remains quiet and appears uninterested. Finally, at the end of the session, the CHW asks if he has any questions. The man doesn't have any questions, but states that he is Muslim, this is Ramadan, and he cannot follow the prescribed diet. Ramadan is the ninth month of the Islamic lunar calendar, and every day during this

(continues)

The Influence of Cultural Beliefs
(continued)

month, Muslims around the world spend the daylight hours in a complete fast. Muslims abstain from food, drink, and other physical needs during the daylight hours as a time to purify the soul, refocus attention on God, and practice self-sacrifice.

Having the awareness and sensitivity to work effectively with diverse people is a critical skill for the twenty-first century. CHWs often play a vital role in aiding clients to access alternative or complimentary medicine and to advocate for these choices with Western or biomedical providers. As cultural brokers who build "bridges" between poor and underserved communities and health care providers, CHWs can play a role in assisting to foster a mutually respectful and cooperative partnership between biomedical providers and providers of other traditions.

6.9 Professional Roles of Culturally Effective CHWs

In Chapter 1, you read about the core roles of CHWs. Here, we look at those roles again and provide an example or idea for how to apply cultural humility. As you read, think of examples of your own.

1. **Cultural mediation between communities and health and social services systems:**
   - Help clients to better understand the nature of the services, treatments, and systems they access. Clients may also need support in expressing key concerns or posing questions.
   - Support other providers and colleagues to demonstrate cultural humility as they work with diverse clients. Encourage them to refrain from making assumptions about the lives and health-related behaviors of new clients, and to consult directly with clients to better understand their priorities, values, and goals.
   - If possible, encourage your colleagues or agency to participate in a training about cultural humility, and to examine how they can put key concepts and skills into practice.
   - *What else might you do, in your role as cultural mediator?*

2. **Providing direct services and referrals:**
   - As you provide services to clients, ask yourself if the questions you ask or the suggestions you provide are culturally biased. For example, when talking about diet and nutrition, are you referring to dietary guidelines that are inclusive of diverse cultural traditions? Are your questions sensitive to the client's experience, culture, and behaviors?
   - Be familiar with referral resources in the community that are culturally or linguistically appropriate. Assist your clients in navigating the system in the best way possible for them. Know which languages are spoken at various agencies for your clients who have limited English proficiency.
   - *What else might you do, in your role providing services and referrals?*

3. **Providing culturally appropriate health education and information:**
   - Participate in local cultural events and opportunities to increase your knowledge and cultural humility skills.
   - Support clients to understand their health and medical care by providing easy-to-understand health information and health education materials in the appropriate language and literacy level. Don't assume everyone can read.
   - Create a checklist to guide you in providing health education. For example, did you remember to ask the client how she understands her illness? Did you acknowledge his cultural traditions respectfully? Did you avoid professional jargon and technical words that the client may not understand?
   - *What else might you do while providing health education and information?*

4. **Advocating for individual and community needs:**

   o Consider how well the program and agency you work for demonstrates cultural humility. Are agency policies and practices inclusive and supportive of diverse cultural backgrounds and identities? Does the agency have a good reputation of respecting the cultures and identities of the clients or customers they serve? If necessary, advocate within the agency you work for and ask for additional professional development regarding cultural humility. Support your colleagues and your agency to improve the quality of services to diverse clients and communities.

   o Advocate for your agency to expand its capacity to provide services in multiple languages and to use qualified health care interpreters.

   o Advocate for agency forms and policies to be changed to be inclusive of lesbian, gay, bisexual, transgender, and intersex identities.

   o *What else might you do to advocate for your clients' and communities' cultural needs?*

5. **Assuring that people get the services they need:**

   o By welcoming all clients, putting your cultural assumptions aside, and inviting them to share their experiences, knowledge, concerns, and questions, you will form a positive connection intended to promote their health and link them with necessary services. Be patient. Learn to take the client's lead.

   o Learn to work with qualified interpreters.

   o *What else might you do to address culture issues that come between people and the care they really need?*

6. **Building individual and community capacity:**

   o Invite community members to provide input into the design of the services you provide. Facilitate a focus group to determine, for example, if community is comfortable with the idea of support groups, or would social groups or events be a better way to build mutual support? Adapt programs and services to what will work for *this* community.

   o Work with community members to learn new concepts and skills—such as how to conduct a community diagnosis—that will enhance their capacity to take action to promote their own health.

   o *What else might come up as you work to build individual and community capacity? How might you address those cultural differences effectively?*

Please view these short videos ▶ that show a CHW working with a client with depression. In the counter role play video, the CHW does not do a great job of working with the client; while in the demo role play video, the CHW demonstrates cultural humility.

DEPRESSION, RELIGION AND CULTURAL HUMILITY: ROLE PLAY, COUNTER

http://youtu.be/ y6d-GdXi8go

- What mistakes did the CHW make in the counter role play?

- How may the lack of cultural humility impact this client, or the relationship between the client and the CHW?

- What did the CHW do differently in the demo role play video?

- What else would you do to demonstrate cultural humility and support this client?

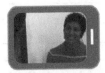

DEPRESSION, RELIGION, AND CULTURAL HUMILITY: ROLE PLAY, DEMO

http://youtu.be/ Bgr6TXWknQQ

CULTURAL DIVERSITY: IT'S PERSONAL, IT'S PROFESSIONAL, AND IT'S RIGHT

Cultural diversity is not something to tolerate, but to embrace and celebrate. Diversity brings richness to our society and keeps our work as CHWs fascinating, dynamic, and rewarding.

As you continue with your training and your career, remember to keep an open mind and an open heart. Respect and honor the differences of the clients and communities you have the opportunity to work with. Demonstrate compassion and a nonjudgmental perspective along the way.

We encourage you to take risks and expand your understanding of what cultural diversity means. Ask hard questions of yourself, examining your own cultural upbringing and values, including any bias that you may have toward others. Learn to acknowledge and accept your own limitations and mistakes. At times you may not be comfortable as you examine your own life and attitudes, and expand your horizons to study the history and perspectives of others. But the very moments when you are most uncomfortable may be your greatest opportunities for personal and professional growth.

Chapter Review

As in any other area of **professional development** (the process of learning new or enhancing existing professional knowledge and skills), building our capacity to practice cultural humility requires planning. The following questions and strategies for learning are based on a suggested approach from California Tomorrow's *Change Starts with the Self* (Chang, Femella, Louie, Murdock, & Pell, 2000). Spend some time answering the preliminary questions. Then identify specific steps or actions you will take to strengthen your knowledge and skills over the next three to six months.

1. What three strengths do I bring to this work on cultural humility? In what ways could I build on these strengths?

2. What three gaps (or challenges) do I want to work on?

3. Did any data, discussions, definitions, principles, or questions in this chapter provoke a strong emotional reaction for me? What are those feelings? What can I do to respond to my feelings in a way that honors my own experiences and perspectives and at the same time assists me to understand and honor the experiences or perspectives that are provoking those feelings?

4. Over the next six months to a year, what activities could I undertake to strengthen my capacity to work across differences of race, class, culture, and language?

   ○ Read the following books or articles: _____
   _____
   _____

   ○ View the following films or videos (in fictional movies, look especially for movies made *by* members of a culture, *about* their own culture): _____
   _____
   _____

   ○ Meet with and discuss these issues with: _____
   _____

   ○ Attend a lecture or presentation on: _____
   _____

   ○ Participate in the following training or workshops: _____
   _____

   ○ Participate in the following cross-cultural community events: _____
   _____

   ○ Join or organize a small discussion or study group focused on: _____
   _____

- ○ Volunteer with the following organization that promotes or organizes cross-cultural work in my community: _____

_____

- ○ Join or support the work of the following organization that advocates or organizes for the cultural diversity or equity concerns of a group that is marginalized or discriminated against in my community:

_____

_____

- ○ Other activities: _____

_____

5. What resources would I draw on to assist me in these activities? Who can I go to in my organization or agency to seek support and guidance in carrying out my learning plan? Which friends, family members, and colleagues do I feel most comfortable talking with about these issues, and why?

I will sit down again on the following date to evaluate my progress and development and to update my learning plan: _____

References

The American Immigration Council. (2011). Unauthorized immigrants pay taxes, too. Retrieved from *www.immigrationpolicy.org/just-facts/unauthorized-immigrants-pay-taxes-too*

Berlin, E. A., & Fowkes, W. C. Jr. (1983). A teaching frame-work for cross-cultural health care—application in family practice, in cross-cultural medicine. *Western Journal of Medicine, 139*, 934–938. Retrieved from *www.pubmedcentral.nih.gov/picrender.fcgi?artid=1011028&blobtype=pdf*

Chang, H. N.-L., Femella, T. S., Louie, N., Murdock, B., & Pell, E. (2000). *Walking the walk: Principles for building community capacity for equity and diversity: Accompanying tool change starts with the self.* Oakland, CA: California Tomorrow.

Florida, R. (2011). *How diversity leads to economic growth.* The Atlantic CityLab. Retrieved from *www.citylab.com/work/2011/12/diversity-leads-to-economic-growth/687/*

Helman, C. G. (1994). *Culture, health and illness.* Oxford, UK: Butterworth-Heinemann.

Kleinman, A. (1980). *Patients and healers in the context of culture: An exploration of the borderland between anthropology, medicine, and psychiatry.* Berkeley: University of California Press.

Management Sciences for Health. (n.d.). *Provider's guide to quality and culture.* Retrieved from *http://erc.msh.org.*

Nine Curt, C. J. (1984). *Non-verbal communication in Puerto Rico* (2nd ed.). Cambridge, MA: Assessment and Dissemination Center.

Passel, J., & Cohn, D. (2012). *Unauthorized immigrants: 11.1 million in 2011.* Washington, DC: Pew Research Center.

Takaki, R. (1993). *A different mirror.* New York, NY: Little, Brown.

Tervalon, M. (n.d.). *Cultural Humility: People, Principles and Practices.* Retrieved from *http://melanietervalon.com/wp-content/uploads/2013/08/Cultural-Humility-A-Video.pdf*

Tervalon, M., & Murray-Garcia, J. (1998). Cultural humility versus cultural competence: A critical distinction in defining physician training outcomes in multicultural education. *Journal of Health Care for the Poor and Underserved, 9*(2), 117–125.

U.S. Census Bureau. (n.d.). 2010 Census Data. Retrieved from *www.census.gov/2010census/data/*

Additional Resources

Cardenas, V., & Treuhaft, S. (Eds). (2013). *All-in-nation, an America that works for all.* Washington, DC: Center for American Progress and PolicyLink. Retrieved from *http://policylink.org/sites/default/files/AllInNation -book.pdf*

Chavez, V. (2012). *Cultural humility: people, principles, & practices.* [Video]. Retrieved from *www.youtube.com/ watch?v=SaSHLbS1V4w*

A 30-minute documentary that mixes poetry with music, interviews, archival footage, and images of community, nature and dance to explain what Cultural Humility is and why we need it.

Wah, L. M. (2013). *The color of fear* [Video excerpts]. Retrieved from *www.youtube.com/watch?v=2nmhAJYxFT4*

An insightful, groundbreaking film about the state of race relations in America as seen through the eyes of eight North American men of Asian, European, Latino, and African descent. Portions of this film are available on YouTube, such as this segment entitled "What it means to be American."

Guiding Principles

Tim Berthold and Edith Guillén-Núñez

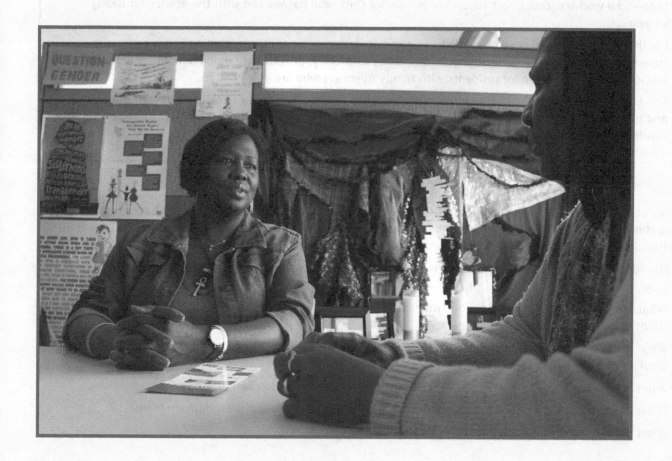

> ## CASE STUDY — Your First Job as a CHW
>
> *A month ago you started your first paid job as a CHW.* You work for a large nonprofit agency that provides a range of services in the low-income neighborhood where you grew up. The agency is known for its client-centered approach.
>
> You are the newest member of a team that includes five CHWs, a public health educator, and two part-time social workers. Your direct supervisor is a senior CHW who has worked with the agency for nearly 10 years.
>
> For the past month, you have been shadowing and observing other CHWs—including your new supervisor—as they conduct health outreach in the community, provide case management services, and facilitate a support-group for residents with family members who are incarcerated.
>
> You are impressed with the quality of services the CHWs provide. You really want to fit in with the team, and to make a good impression. You are also worried about making mistakes that could jeopardize your continued employment.

As you complete the first stage of your orientation and training at the new agency, you still have many questions about your role, the services you should or should not provide to clients, and how best to facilitate their health without doing harm to them or others. These questions include:

- How do I preserve the confidentiality of clients when I am working in the same community where I grew up?
- What are the limits of confidentiality? Under what circumstances may I break confidentiality and share client information with another agency?
- What is my scope of practice when I am conducting outreach and providing care management? What types of services can I provide to clients?
- What gets in the way of behavior change? How can I support clients to change behaviors?
- What do I need to know in order to be successful working as part of a multidisciplinary team?
- What are the key elements of client-centered practice?

Introduction

This chapter provides an introduction to seven topics and guiding principles that will inform your work as a CHW. These essential guiding principles include:

1. Ethics
2. Professional Boundaries
3. Self-Awareness
4. Scope of Practice
5. Working as part of a Multidisciplinary Team
6. Understanding Behavior Change
7. Client-Centered Practice

These principles will be referred to throughout the *Foundations* textbook, and provide a framework for the direct services that CHWs provide to clients and communities. For example, guiding principles such as Ethics, Scope of Practice, and Client-Centered Practice are critical concepts for CHWs who conduct initial client interviews or provide client-centered counseling or care management services.

WHAT YOU WILL LEARN

By studying the information in this chapter, you will be able to do the following:

Ethics

- Define ethics and explain how ethics are different from laws
- Discuss key articles from the CHW Code of Ethics
- Explain ethical guidelines relating to informed consent and confidentiality
- Apply the Framework for Ethical Decision Making to resolve ethical questions

Professional Boundaries

- Define and discuss professional boundaries and dual or multiple relationships
- Explain how CHWs may cross professional boundaries, and the potential risks of doing so
- Explain self-disclosure and analyze the potential risks and benefits for clients and CHWs

Self-Awareness

- Define self-awareness
- Explain the importance of self-awareness to the work of CHWs
- Identify practical strategies for enhancing self-awareness

Scope of Practice

- Define scope of practice
- Identify competencies that may lie within and outside the CHW scope of practice
- Analyze the potential consequences of working outside of the CHW scope of practice
- Explain how to respond when confronted with a challenge regarding your scope of practice as a CHW

Working as Part of a Multidisciplinary Team

- Explain the key elements for successful teams
- Identify common challenges to team work
- Discuss strategies for working successfully as part of a multidisciplinary team

Understanding Behavior Change

- Identify behaviors that clients may wish to change
- Apply the ecological model to analyze individual, family, community, and societal factors that influence behavior and behavior change
- Discuss and analyze four common mistakes that CHWs make when supporting clients to change behaviors

Client-Centered Practice

- Discuss the central concepts of client-centered practice
- Explain the value of a strength-based approach to working with clients
- Discuss implicit theory and how you will develop your own implicit theories of behavior change

WORDS TO KNOW

Boundary Crossing

Confidentiality

Dual or Multiple Relationships

Ethics

Informed Consent

Media Advocacy

Professional Boundaries

Self-Disclosure

Treatment Adherence or Compliance

7.1 Ethical Guidelines for CHWs

This section presents ethical guidelines for CHWs, drawing on a range of sources, including the Code of Ethics developed at the CHW Unity Conference in 2008 and widely used by state and national CHW organizations today. We will highlight several key ethical issues and present a framework for ethical decision making. As you read the ethical guidelines presented here, keep in mind that they are meant to be a guide to standards of conduct and practice in the profession. However, they do not provide an answer for every dilemma you will encounter. Consult your supervisor for additional information, including relevant laws, that will govern your conduct in the program, agency, and state where you are working.

- *Does the state where you live have a CHW Association?*

- *Does this association have a code of ethics?*

What Do **YOU?** Think

DEFINING ETHICS

Ethical standards provide guidance for professionals regarding "right conduct," and what to do when faced with a challenge or dilemma. Most professions—including those that provide direct services to clients or patients in the fields of health care and social services—establish a code of **ethics** in an attempt to standardize behavior and professional accountability.

COMMON ETHICAL CHALLENGES

CHWs are motivated by a deep and abiding commitment to promoting the health and welfare of the clients and communities with whom they work. No CHW wants to cause harm to their clients. Sometimes, however, CHWs face professional situations in which it isn't clear how to achieve these goals and what course of action to take. For example, what should you do if you are faced with the following ethical challenges?

- Your supervisor assigns you to provide a service that you haven't been adequately trained to provide.
- A homeless client with two children is late for an important medical appointment. They have no money to get to their appointment. Can you give them money for a bus ticket? Or take them to the appointment in your car?
- A client pressures you to sign a form that includes inaccurate information so that they will qualify for a key benefit
- A coworker asks you to look the other way and ignore their violation of an ethical code.
- A client reports that her 14-year-old niece is being sexually abused by an older male relative.
- A client with HIV disease informs you that she hasn't disclosed her HIV status to her partners, and she is continuing to have unprotected sex. One of these partners is also a client.
- A former client asks you out on a date. You are single, available, and interested.
- You observe a coworker using drugs on the job.
- A client reports that the agency you work for discriminates against the community they belong to.
- A client offers to loan you $3 so you can take the bus home. You forgot your wallet, and could definitely use a loan.

ETHICS AND VALUES

How you handle an ethical dilemma will be influenced by your values. Values are beliefs and attitudes about what matters in life. Personal values vary widely and are influenced by culture, community, family upbringing, personal experiences, and society. Values guide the decisions we make every day, including how we treat others.

Examples of values that guide the CHW field include honesty, respect, integrity, open-mindedness, self-determination, acceptance, trust, and tolerance.

At times, however, the personal values of CHWs may be in direct conflict with the values of clients, or the ethical guidelines of the profession. Knowing your own values is a tremendous resource for identifying and resolving these potential conflicts.

ETHICS AND THE LAW

Ethics and the law are integrally related, yet distinct.

Ethics is about doing what is morally right. Codes of ethics aim to standardize professional behavior and accountability. They are designed to inform clients and the public about the types of services they can expect to receive from professionals, and to ensure that clients are protected from inappropriate conduct or abuse from professionals. Typically, codes of ethics address issues such as informed consent, confidentiality, professional training, protections against discrimination, and maintaining clear professional boundaries with clients.

Laws are established by governments to prevent and punish behavior that is harmful or destructive to a society's well-being. Laws define the minimal standards that a society will tolerate that are enforced by government (Corey, Corey, & Callanan, 2011). Laws include statutes, regulations, agency policies and procedures, and court decisions and may be local (city laws), state, federal (national), or international. The consequences of breaking a law tend to be more severe than a violation of a professional code of ethics. For example, the penalty for breaking the law can include imprisonment, whereas the penalty for violation of a professional code of ethics may include being fired from your job or barred from future employment in your field. Keep in mind that violations of the law and of the professional code of ethics can impact your reputation and relationship with colleagues, clients, community members and, ultimately, yourself. Additionally, violations of ethical guidelines are sometimes also legal violations. For example, if you break the confidentiality of a client by disclosing her HIV positive status to another without written consent, you are violating both your ethical guidelines and laws that protect the privacy of people with HIV disease.

Chapters 1 and 2 of this book explained that the CHW profession in the United States is still in the process of seeking formal recognition, status, and financing mechanisms. As the CHW field continues to develop, the code of ethics presented here may be refined and revised.

The Community Health Worker Code of Ethics

Note: This Code of Ethics was developed during the 2008 Unity Conference (an annual conference of CHWs). It was later adopted by the short-lived American Association of CHWs. While the AACHW no longer exists, the CHW Code of Ethics continues to be referenced and used by regional, state, and national organizations (CHW Unity Conference, 2008).

A CHW is a frontline public health worker who is a trusted member of and/or has an unusually close understanding of the community she or he serves. This trusting relationship enables the CHW to serve as a liaison/link/intermediary between health/social services and the community to facilitate access to services and improve the quality and cultural competence of service delivery. A CHW also builds individual and community capacity by increasing health knowledge and self-sufficiency through a range of activities such as outreach, community education, informal counseling, social support, and advocacy.

(continues)

The Community Health Worker Code of Ethics

(continued)

Purpose of This Code

The Code of Ethics outlined in this document provides a framework for CHWs, supervisors, and employers of Community Health Workers to discuss ethical issues facing the profession. Employers are encouraged to consider this Code when creating CHW programs. The responsibility of all Community Health Workers is to strive for excellence by providing quality service and the most accurate information available to individuals, families, and communities.

The Code of Ethics is based upon commonly understood principles that apply to all professionals within the health and social service fields (e.g., promotion of social justice, positive health, and dignity). The Code, however, does not address all ethical issues facing Community Health Workers and the absence of a rule does not imply that there is no ethical obligation present. As professionals, Community Health Workers are encouraged to reflect on the ethical obligations that they have to the communities that they serve, and to share these reflections with others.

Article 1. Responsibilities in the Delivery of Care

Community Health Workers build trust and community capacity by improving the health and social welfare of the clients they serve. When a conflict arises among individuals, groups, agencies, or institutions, Community Health Workers should consider all issues and give priority to those that promote the wellness and quality of living for the individual/client. The following provisions promote the professional integrity of Community Health Workers.

1.1 Honesty

Community Health Workers are professionals that strive to ensure the best health outcomes for the communities they serve. They communicate the potential benefits and consequences of available services, including the programs they are employed under.

1.2 Confidentiality

Community Health Workers respect the confidentiality, privacy, and trust of individuals, families, and communities that they serve. They understand and abide by employer policies, as well as state and federal confidentiality laws that are relevant to their work.

1.3 Scope of Ability and Training

Community Health Workers are truthful about qualifications, competencies, and limitations on the services they may provide, and should not misrepresent qualifications or competencies to individuals, families, communities, or employers.

1.4 Quality of Care

Community Health Workers strive to provide high quality service to individuals, families, and communities. They do this through continued education, training, and an obligation to ensure the information they provide is up-to-date and accurate.

1.5 Referral to Appropriate Services

Community Health Workers acknowledge when client issues are outside of their scope of practice and refer clients to the appropriate health, wellness, or social support services when necessary.

(continues)

The Community Health Worker Code of Ethics
(continued)

1.6 Legal Obligations

Community Health Workers have an obligation to report actual or potential harm to individuals within the communities they serve to the appropriate authorities. Additionally, Community Health Workers have a responsibility to follow requirements set by states, the federal government, and/or their employing organizations. Responsibility to the larger society or specific legal obligations may supersede the loyalty owed to individual community members.

Article 2. Promotion of Equitable Relationships

Community Health Workers focus their efforts on the well-being of the whole community. They value and respect the expertise and knowledge that each community member possesses. In turn, Community Health Workers strive to create equitable partnerships with communities to address all issues of health and well-being.

2.1 Cultural Humility

Community Health Workers possess expertise in the communities in which they serve. They maintain a high degree of humility and respect for the cultural diversity within each community. As advocates for their communities, Community Health Workers have an obligation to inform employers and others when policies and procedures will offend or harm communities, or are ineffective within the communities where they work.

2.2 Maintaining the Trust of the Community

Community Health Workers are often members of their communities and their effectiveness in providing services derives from the trust placed in them by members of these communities. Community Health Workers do not act in ways that could jeopardize the trust placed in them by the communities they serve.

2.3 Respect for Human Rights

Community Health Workers respect the human rights of those they serve, advance principles of self-determination, and promote equitable relationships with all communities.

2.4 Anti-Discrimination

Community Health Workers do not discriminate against any person or group on the basis of race, ethnicity, gender, sexual orientation, age, religion, social status, disability, or immigration status.

2.5 Client Relationships

Community Health Workers maintain professional relationships with clients. They establish, respect, and actively maintain personal boundaries between them and their clients.

Article 3. Interactions with Other Service Providers

Community Health Workers maintain professional partnerships with other service providers in order to serve the community effectively.

3.1 Cooperation

Community Health Workers place the well-being of those they serve above personal disagreements and work cooperatively with any other person or organization dedicated to helping provide care to those in need.

(continues)

The Community Health Worker Code of Ethics

(continued)

3.2 Conduct

Community Health Workers promote integrity in the delivery of health and social services. They respect the rights, dignity, and worth of all people and have an ethical obligation to report any inappropriate behavior (e.g., sexual harassment, racial discrimination, etc.) to the proper authority.

3.3 Self-Presentation

Community Health Workers are truthful and forthright in presenting their background and training to other service providers.

Article 4. Professional Rights and Responsibilities

The Community Health Worker profession is dedicated to excellence in the practice of promoting well-being in communities. Guided by common values, Community Health Workers have the responsibility to uphold the principles and integrity of the profession as they assist families to make decisions impacting their well-being. Community Health Workers embrace individual, family, and community strengths and build upon them to increase community capacity.

4.1 Continuing Education

Community Health Workers should remain up-to-date on any developments that substantially affect their ability to competently render services. Community Health Workers strive to expand their professional knowledge base and competencies through education and participation in professional organizations.

4.2 Advocacy for Change in Law and Policy

Community Health Workers are advocates for change and work on impacting policies that promote social justice and hold systems accountable for being responsive to communities. Policies that advance public health and well-being enable Community Health Workers to provide better care for the communities they serve.

4.3 Enhancing Community Capacity

Community Health Workers help individuals and communities move toward self-sufficiency in order to promote the creation of opportunities and resources that support their autonomy.

4.4 Wellness and Safety

Community Health Workers are sensitive to their own personal well-being (physical, mental, and spiritual health) and strive to maintain a safe environment for themselves and the communities they serve.

4.5 Loyalty to the Profession

Community Health Workers are loyal to the profession and aim to advance the efforts of other Community Health Workers worldwide.

4.6 Advocacy for the Profession

Community Health Workers are advocates for the profession. They are members, leaders, and active participants in local, state, and national professional organizations.

4.7 Recognition of Others

Community Health Workers give recognition to others for their professional contributions and achievements.

DISCUSSION OF KEY ETHICAL CONCEPTS

There are certain ethical issues and concepts that CHWs frequently encounter in the course of their work. These include informed consent and confidentiality.

Informed Consent

Informed consent is related to Article 1.1 Honesty and Article 3.3 Self-Presentation in the CHW Code of Ethics. **Informed consent** is the obligation to provide clients with the information they need in order to make a sound decision about whether or not to participate in a program, service, or research study. This should include information about anything that could be potentially difficult for or harmful to the client, as well as information about any costs, insurance coverage, program requirements for participation, limitations of program services, and confidentiality.

One of the reasons we highlight informed consent as an ethical issue is because organizations sometimes fail to fully inform clients about the services they are receiving. There is also a history of coercing clients into services they may not be interested in. Notorious examples include the Tuskegee Syphilis Trials and programs that sterilized Puerto Rican women, discussed in Chapter 6.

Informed consent is an ongoing responsibility of CHWs. We recommend that you review the informed consent policies used by the programs you work for. Is all relevant information shared with clients in order to assist them in deciding whether or not to participate in services? Is the information presented in a way that your clients can understand? Is the same information provided to clients who speak languages other than English? If not, the ethical principle of informed consent has been devalued.

Confidentiality

Article 1.2 of the AACHW Code of Ethics addresses confidentiality. **Confidentiality** protects a client's communication with a CHW and forms an essential component for establishing a trusting and productive professional relationship. Unless clients are confident that the CHW will not disclose their information to others, they will be reluctant to share personal information.

The Health Insurance Portability and Accountability Act (HIPAA)

If you work in a health care setting, every new client or patient will be asked to read and sign a Health Insurance Portability and Accountability Act (HIPAA) form. HIPAA is a federal law that requires the protection and confidential handling of all health information.

Sergio Matos: Our access to communities is based on trust. We can't betray that trust. That trust defines us and it defines our role in these communities. And we're not at liberty to betray that trust for program goals or any other reason.

CHW

CHWs should address issues of confidentiality and its limits with new clients before services begin or before clients have an opportunity to disclose personal and intimate information. This should include an explicit discussion of the exceptions that would cause the CHW to "break" a client's confidentiality and report private information to others, including a supervisor and legal authorities such as the police or local child protection services. It is essential for CHWs to explain confidentiality and its limits using clear and accessible language, and to make sure that clients understand the concept and policy before addressing other topics in detail.

Ramona Benson: I had this big problem when I was starting out as a CHW, because some of my clients would say things to other providers, things that they thought were private, and then the provider would say: "I'm a mandated reporter. I have to report that to the authorities." That is the wrong way to handle things, especially with the ladies I work with. They have experienced so much racism and discrimination that it is already hard for them to trust people—and I know why! So when I start working with a client at the Black Infant Health Program, I always tell them up front what the rules are and what kind of information I will have to report to others. They have a right to know, and it's a matter of respect.

In general, CHWs do not share private information about their clients with others, including the client's identity (such as the client's name or Social Security number), unless the client provides written consent. For example, as described in Chapter 10, a client may be working with providers at more than one agency or program, and may ask these providers to consult with each other. In this case, the client could ask both providers and agencies to sign a Release of Information permitting them to share information about specific issues over a specified period of time.

However, there are several important exceptions that limit a CHW's ability to keep a client's information private. If clients disclose information about harm or the threat of harm to themselves or others, CHWs may have an ethical or legal obligation to report this to a third party, such as their supervisor, the local department of human services (such as a child protective services or elder abuse division), or the police. The types of harms that could require a breach of confidentiality include, for example, physical and sexual abuse and suicide. In such circumstances, CHWs have an ethical obligation not only to the client, but to anyone who may be harmed. This ethical obligation requires them to report the harm or threat of harm in order to protect the safety and health of the victim or potential victim.

When CHWs face a situation in which they must break the confidentiality of a client, we recommend that you consider if and how you may be able to involve the client in the reporting process. This can aid in preserving a positive working relationship between the client and the CHW. The decision about whether or not to participate, of course, must be left to the client. In cases of mandated reporting, it is important that the CHW fully and accurately understand the consequences of such reporting and be prepared to discuss these with the client. When necessary (or possible) the CHW may seek supervisory support in these situations.

Consider the case of a CHW working at a health clinic serving youth (see the featured example).

Client Scenario about the Limits of Confidentiality

A CHW works in a busy clinic that features specialized services for youth. Multiple signs are clearly posted throughout the clinic—including in the waiting room, at the front desk, and in meeting and exam rooms—explaining the limits of confidentiality. The CHW begins all client sessions by reviewing the limits of confidentiality and describing the types of information that cannot legally be kept private, including physical and sexual abuse and intended suicide.

After discussing the limits of confidentiality, a 15-year-old female client discloses that she is being sexually abused by her stepfather. Legally and ethically, the CHW has a clear duty to report this information to local law enforcement authorities. Despite having discussed the limits of confidentiality previously, the client begs the CHW not to make a report: the client is scared about what her stepfather and mother might do.

The CHW listens to the client's experience and concerns, and offers validation and support. The CHW then explains their legal duty to report the sexual abuse to the police. The CHW emphasizes concern for the client's safety and welfare. The CHW also explains why it would be wrong not to make a report: they have an

(continues)

Client Scenario about the Limits of Confidentiality

(continued)

obligation to do everything they can to protect clients from harm. Failing to report the abuse could send a message to the client that she shouldn't talk about what is happening to her or that the sexual abuse is acceptable or somehow doesn't matter.

The CHW calmly explains the need to call the police immediately, and asks the client if she would like to help make the call or to wait with the CHW and speak with authorities at the clinic. The client is also free to leave, although she and her parents will be contacted later by the police. The client decides to listen in on the call to the police. The CHW also asks the client if she would like to call the local rape crisis center and explains the type of services they offer. The client calls the local rape crisis center with the CHW, explains what is happening, and asks for a rape crisis counselor to come to the clinic to be her advocate when she speaks with the police. Throughout this process it is important to assess the client's safety and make an appropriate plan to prevent further harm to her or others.

As soon as the client leaves, the CHW documents the session and sends an email to their supervisor explaining that they called the police to provide a mandated report about the sexual assault of a minor. The next day, the CHW meets with their supervisor to review the case, complete documentation, and plan for how to check-in on the status of the client.

The client scenario described above presents a highly challenging situation. In the example provided, the CHW clearly explained the rules of confidentiality and its limits, and took time to listen to the client's questions, concerns, and feelings. The CHW also provided the client with several choices and supported her decisions. Ultimately, the CHW and the client acted together to report the sexual abuse to the authorities and to contact additional resources (the rape crisis center). While the situation was stressful for the client, providing her with choices also aided in giving back to her a measure of control. This is an important feature of working with victims of trauma (addressed in greater detail in Chapter 18). It is also a central feature of client-centered practice, discussed below.

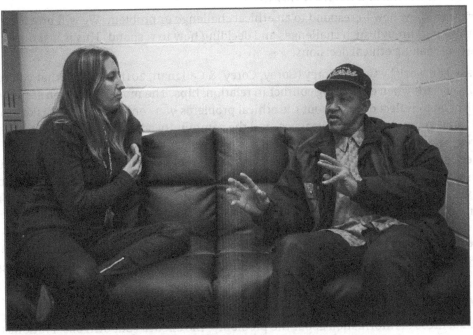

Listening with interest and respect encourages a client to talk about his life.

- *What do you think of the way in which the CHW handled this situation?*

- *Is there anything else you would want to do?*

- *Anything you would want to do differently?*

Please watch the following video 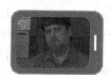 interview about explaining the limits of confidentiality policies, and responsibility for mandated reporting.

HOW ETHICAL CHALLENGES AFFECT CHWs

The types of situations that raise ethical issues are often stressful for CHWs and other helping professionals. It is difficult to witness clients in distress and at risk of harm, particularly when it isn't easy to figure out what the best course of action is. Ethical challenges may also place you in conflict with a client. For example, you may learn that your client is abusing her or his children, and have an ethical obligation to report this abuse to the authorities.

CONFIDENTIALITY AND REPORTING: FACULTY INTERVIEW
http://youtu. be/7oOGAAmQK6o

Don't forget to pay attention to your own feelings and concerns when you are in the midst of an ethical challenge. Try to develop an awareness of how these situations affect you, develop skills to manage your stress (Chapter 12), and consult with your supervisors.

> **Phuong An Doan Billings:** Some Asians don't set the boundaries like we do in the United States. One of our doctors was approached and asked to lend some money to a Vietnamese patient. He doesn't speak much Vietnamese, so he came and told me. I said, "Leave it for me. Let me handle it." I came to talk to the patient. I talked to her with real care, like a sister, so that I didn't upset her—if I talked like a professional, it would upset her. And I said, "I understand you have real difficulty, so we have a few agencies that can provide urgent relief. You let me know what you need, and I will look around for you. But don't approach a doctor like that. Here in America, we don't do it that way."

A FRAMEWORK FOR ETHICAL DECISION MAKING

It isn't always easy to know how to respond to an ethical challenge or problem. We will provide a seven-step framework for thinking through such challenges and deciding how to respond. This is just one of many ways to frame the process of making ethical decisions.

This model is based on work by Gerald Corey (Corey, Corey, & Callanan, 2011) and asks that you consider issues that are important when evaluating conflict in relationships. The model has seven steps with questions designed to assist you to reflect deeply about the ethical problems you confront. You are asked to consider yourself, your client, your supervisor, your colleagues, and the community when examining each of the steps in the model. As you review each step, consider its importance in the work that you do with clients and in your community. The questions that you choose to answer can vary depending on the ethical challenge you are facing, your experience with similar ethical challenges, time, and other limitations. Once you have sufficient practice and familiarity using the framework's seven steps, you will be able to develop your own process in thinking through such dilemmas.

Step 1: Describe the Problem or Dilemma

Write down as much as you know about the problem or dilemma. The following questions may assist you to gather relevant information:

- What has happened so far?

- What are your sources of information about the problem—the client? Your own observations (what you have seen or heard—not your judgment or opinions)? Reports of facts from others?

- When did you first become aware of the problem? Is this a new situation or an ongoing problem?
- Who is involved? Who else knows about the problem?
- What have you learned from the client about the client's experience, opinions, and concerns? What does the client want to see happen?
- Do cultural differences play a role in this problem? Are you making assumptions—based on your own cultural perspective—about others who are involved in this situation?
- What have you done so far in relation to the problem?

Try to consider the experiences and values of your client, your agency and supervisor, your community, and yourself. Pay attention to your intuition, which could be the reason that you are thinking through this ethical problem.

Step 2: Review Relevant Ethical Guidelines or Codes

Review the CHW Code of Ethics for guidance about the problem. Are there any Principles in the CHW Code of Ethics that address the problem? For example, does the situation raise concerns about confidentiality, scope of practice, or discrimination?

Step 3: Review Applicable Laws and Regulations

Are there any laws or regulations that speak to the issues in the problem? Are there any issues in the problem where you may be breaking the law if you don't address it, or vice versa? Does the situation involve any allegations of harm or violence? Don't forget to review your agency's policies and procedures.

Step 4: Seek Consultation

Consult supervisors, colleagues, and other professionals who may assist you in processing ethical problems. It is important to receive consultation because a third person, preferably someone removed from the problem and more experienced in the field, can offer feedback, support, and most important, assist you in thinking through the situation. When you seek consultation, remember to maintain client confidentiality. Explain the situation, but leave out the client's name and identifying details.

Step 5: Consider Possible Courses of Action

What possible courses of action can you take in response to the ethical challenge you face? Do you need to do anything at all? If it is appropriate and feasible, include your client as part of this discussion. If the challenge is one that you consider serious, however, and may result in harm to a client or other party, consult your agency's policies and your supervisor.

Step 6: Outline Possible Consequences of Decisions

Reflect on and write down the possible consequences of the various choices that you identified during Step 5. How might these courses of action and decisions impact the client, the agency, the community, and yourself? Might these decisions lead to further harm to any party? Again, consider inviting your client into this conversation about the consequences that may have an impact on the client's life and, as always, consult other CHWs and your supervisor if you are uncertain about your various options.

Step 7: Decide on What Appears to Be the Best Course of Action

When you think you've identified the best course of action, spend a little time reviewing and evaluating it first. Questions to consider may include: How does this choice fit with the ethical code? Will anyone be harmed by this course of action? How would I feel if my actions became public knowledge? Did I practice cultural humility? How were my client's cultural values and experiences taken into consideration? How were my own values affirmed or challenged? What did I learn from the struggle to resolve this ethical dilemma?

The goal of this seven-step framework is to assist in guiding you through the ethical decision-making process when you are faced with challenging dilemmas. It is important to engage in self-reflection throughout the steps so that you think about balancing all of the various needs involved in the problem. Implementing the framework takes practice.

7.2 Establishing and Maintaining Professional Boundaries

Establishing and maintaining appropriate professional boundaries protects CHWs as well as the clients and communities they serve, and the programs and agencies they represent. It is an ethical duty related to Article 2 of the Code of Ethics.

Professional boundaries are the limitations or ethical guidelines that define professional working relationships. Professional boundaries are established to protect both clients and providers from conduct that may violate ethical standards. Identifying what you can or cannot do for the client is an important part of building trust in your relationship. Your clients should know what to expect from your behavior at the outset of the relationship. The moment when a CHW deviates from a strictly professional role is known as a **boundary crossing**.

Examples of professional boundary issues include physical contact with a client, romantic or sexual involvement with a client, a CHW's self-disclosure of personal information to a client (see the section on self-disclosure below), and managing **dual or multiple relationships** with clients. **A dual or multiple relationship** exists when you have another type of relationship or connection with someone who is also a client. For example, a client may be a former coworker, a neighbor, a friend of a family member, or a member of your church, synagogue, or mosque.

CHWs confront potential boundary dilemmas frequently, including offers of gifts from clients, requests from clients to borrow money, or invitations to develop a romantic relationship. Whether it is lending a client money, being invited to become the godmother to the client's daughter, or seeing a client at your neighborhood grocery store or school, it is sometimes difficult to know what to do.

- *Can you think of other situations that fall within a boundary dilemma?*

What Do YOU Think?

Not every boundary crossing is unethical. Because CHWs often work in the same community where they live, it is difficult to avoid dual relationships with clients. In fact, those relationships may be part of what makes the CHW a trusted member of the community. CHWs must stay aware of their influential position with respect to clients, however, protect the confidentiality of the information they share, and avoid exploiting the trust of clients. Understand that some dual relationships can impair professional judgment or increase the risk of harm to clients. The guiding principle here should be: What is in the best interest of the client? If it could be harmful for a client to work with a CHW with whom the client has a dual relationship (member of the same social circle or religious community), then the CHW should refer that client to a colleague.

Please watch the following video 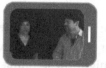 interview about the challenge of setting professional boundaries.

Taking time to review the CHW Code of Ethics can help to clarify the boundary issue you are facing. There are also questions that you can ask yourself as you reflect on the boundary dilemma:

SETTING PROFESSIONAL BOUNDARIES: FACULTY INTERVIEW

🔗 *http://youtu.be/ WXn-tvVILbY*

- Who benefits from the boundary crossing?
- Is the boundary crossing necessary, or are there alternative courses of action to take?
- Did the client receive informed consent about the potential risks involved in the boundary crossing?
- How will the boundary crossing affect the relationship?
- Is there a cultural context to consider in this situation?
- As always, if you have questions about when and where to draw healthy professional boundaries with clients, consult with your colleagues and, most importantly, your supervisor.

An Example of a Boundary Crossing

Anonymous: I made the mistake of giving a homeless client $10 to get some food. It was raining hard, and she and her son hadn't eaten that day. I just felt powerless to offer anything meaningful. They got a meal at Carl's Jr. and were able to sit there away from the rain. But from then on, every time I saw the client, she kept asking me for money. I had to explain that I couldn't give her money again, and why. She never understood this, however, because I gave her money before. We were never able to get past this situation, and eventually I had to stop working with her and referred her to a colleague. She was really angry with me, and I can understand why. I messed up.

In the situation described above, the CHW gave money to a client when motivated by concern for her and her child. While on the surface, offering money to a family in need may seem like a kind thing to do, it is an example of boundary crossing, and in the long run, it may be harmful to the client, the CHW, the community, and the agency that the CHW works for. When the CHW gave money to the client, their relationship changed. From then on, the client saw the CHW as a potential source of money. The CHW, of course, was not able to continue to give money to the client. The CHW also wasn't able to change the relationship back to the way it was before, or to continue providing effective client-centered services. If the employer found out that the CHW was giving money to clients, it would likely take disciplinary action that could include termination (firing the CHW). Once word gets out that a CHW is giving away cash, this is what other clients will come to expect and demand. It also undermines the reputation of the program and the agency that the CHW works for.

* *What do you think about this ethical challenge? What could the CHW have done differently?*

* *What are the guidelines in place at the agency where you work or volunteer regarding the exchange of gifts or loans?*

What Do YOU Think?

Please watch the following videos ▶ that show a CHW working to set a professional boundary with a client. In the counter role play, the CHW struggles to establish a clear boundary. In the role play demo, the CHW does a better job of establishing a clear boundary.

* What type of professional boundary was this CHW trying to establish?

* How well did the CHW establish a clear professional boundary in the Counter and Demo videos?

* What would you do differently to establish a boundary with this client?

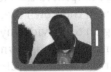

SETTING BOUNDARIES WITH CLIENTS: ROLE PLAY, COUNTER

🔗 *http://youtu.be/ kziHCHrwtzo*

SELF-DISCLOSURE

Self-disclosure is when a CHW—or another service provider—reveals personal or private information about themselves to a client they are working with. For example, a CHW might disclose that they have experienced homelessness, incarceration, or trauma, or that they are living with cancer, mental health challenges, or HIV disease.

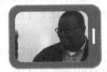

SETTING BOUNDARIES WITH CLIENTS: ROLE PLAY, DEMO

🔗 *http://youtu.be/ pX9x_w8ME9s*

Self-disclosure is a controversial issue that risks crossing professional boundaries. Some organizations and professionals feel strongly that providers should never disclose personal information to a client. Others argue that limited self-disclosure can help clients who face stigma and isolation to access supportive services. *The essential concern is whether self-disclosure may harm or benefit the client and the client-provider relationship.*

There are different types of self-disclosure (Zur, 2011). Personal information is sometimes disclosed to others in an accidental or unavoidable manner. Some disclosure of information is unavoidable, such as revealing to clients that you are pregnant or disabled and using a wheelchair. A CHW may also disclose personal information in an accidental way, such as through unplanned contact with a client outside of the office (for example, when a CHW sees a client at church or in another member organization). However, most self-disclosure is deliberate: the provider makes a decision to share personal information with the clients and communities they are working with.

Potential Risks of Self-Disclosure

The key reason why health and mental health providers do not disclose personal information to the clients they work with, is due to the potential risks or harms that may result. These risks may include:

- Self-disclosure may shift the focus from the client to the provider. It may interrupt or take time away from the client's story or concerns.

- A provider's self-disclosure may imply or unintentionally send a message that the client should think, feel, or make choices that are the same or similar (i.e., take the same path to recovery from substance use).

- It may leave the CHW/provider vulnerable to further inquiries about their personal life.

- It may change the nature of the relationship between the client and the provider. For example, some clients may want to develop a friendship with the CHW, and self-disclosure may lead them to believe that this is possible.

- *Can you think of other potential risks from self-disclosure?*

What Do YOU Think?

Potential Benefits of Self-Disclosure

Limited self-disclosure can be beneficial when clients face stigma, shame, or isolation, and related challenges in accessing services and support. For example, clients may be struggling with issues such as addiction, schizophrenia or depression, cancer, HIV disease, sexual orientation, or surviving trauma experiences. Sometimes, it can be helpful to the client for a service provider to briefly disclose that they have faced similar experiences and issues in their own life. For example, a CHW might say "I was in prison too," or "I have HIV disease." Without going on to provide any further details, this type of self-disclosure can help clients to feel more comfortable talking about their own lives and sharing their thoughts, concerns, and feelings. If the client continues to ask questions about the CHW/provider's experience, the CHW can always explain and shift the focus back to the client's experience: "This is a place to focus on your experience and concerns, not mine. Can you tell me more about what you have been going through?"

There is a strong tradition of limited self-disclosure among CHWs and other peer providers working in certain fields, such as programs and agencies that provide services to people living with mental health challenges, veterans, survivors of sexual assault and domestic violence, formerly incarcerated people, and people living with chronic health conditions including HIV disease.

Considerations for Self-Disclosure

We encourage you to consider the following questions as you determine if, when and how you may disclose personal information to the clients you work with.

1. **Benefit:** How may your client benefit from your self-disclosure? How may you benefit from the self-disclosure? Whose needs are being met?

2. **Alternatives:** Are there alternative ways that you can support the client other than disclosing personal information about yourself? Have you already tried using client-centered skills such as motivational interviewing skills?

3. **Burden on client:** Will your self-disclosure shift the focus of your work or conversation away from the client's experience and priorities? Will the nature of your self-disclosure place a burden upon the client?

4. **Nature of information being disclosed:** Is the information related to the topic that the client is discussing?

5. **Context:** What is happening at the moment when you are considering self-disclosure? What has been the primary focus of the meetings? Is your self-disclosure consistent with the client's priorities and goals?

6. **Condition of the client:** What is the client's emotional state? Are they highly distressed or vulnerable? Are they addressing issues in a comfortable manner?

7. **Timing:** When in the relationship with the client are you disclosing personal information? Is it in the beginning, after a couple of weeks, or at the end of our work together, that is, termination? Is the timing of your self-disclosure appropriate? Why are you self-disclosing this information now?

Be prepared that if you do decide to self-disclose, you may open yourself up to further questions from clients who want to know more about your life. You may need to explain your policy about self-disclosure and why you won't share more personal information. Be prepared to explain that your work is to support clients in making their own decisions, and you don't want to impose your own beliefs or values on others. In this sense, the issue of self-disclosure is related to the concept of cultural humility addressed in Chapter 6.

If you have questions or concerns about self-disclosure, please consult with your supervisor and review any guidelines or policies that your program or agency may have established.

Suggested Guidelines for Self-Disclosure

In general, we suggest that you err on the side of not disclosing personal information to the clients you work with. This is the best way to prevent the potential harms highlighted above.

If you are uncertain about why you are disclosing and how it may benefit the client, **please don't disclose!**

Don't disclose simply as a strategy for building a connection or trust with the client. Rather, let your client-centered practice speak for you. For example, use motivational interviewing skills (see Chapter 9) to ask open-ended questions and listen deeply to what the client has to share. Provide affirmations and support the client to make informed decisions about what they will do to enhance their health.

If you decide to disclose personal information with a client because you determine that it is likely to benefit them (and not you):

- Keep it brief (don't go on and on!). In general, the best self-disclosure is provided in just a few seconds by sharing just a few words (the equivalent of one or two sentences).

- Keep it limited. While you may disclose, for example, that you were incarcerated or are living with HIV disease, don't go on to discuss the details about your experiences and conditions. Remember that the focus of your work is not your own experiences, challenges, values, or beliefs, but to support clients to reflect and better understand their own experiences.

- Quickly refocus the discussion on the life, questions and concerns of the client.

Please watch the following videos, ▶️ including role plays and an interview, on the topic of self-disclosure.

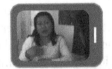

SELF-DISCLOSURE: ROLE PLAY, COUNTER

🔗 *http://youtu. be/7CpFvjXO-rs*

- What personal information did the CHW disclose to the client, and why?

- What did the CHW do well—and not-so-well—in terms of self-disclosure?

- What would you have done differently if you were the CHW working with this client?

- What are your guidelines for providing a self-disclosure to the clients or communities you work with?

7.3 The Duty of Self-Awareness

In Chapter 1 we introduced self-awareness as an essential quality and skill for CHWs. A lack of self-knowledge can significantly undermine your ability to provide client-centered and culturally relevant services. When CHWs and other helping professionals are unaware of their own experiences, values, and beliefs, they are at risk of imposing them on others. This may result in harm to the very clients and communities you intend to support.

SELF-DISCLOSURE: ROLE PLAY, DEMO

🔗 *http://youtu. be/12s4zgUUJFs*

THE VALUE OF SELF-AWARENESS

When our own issues or challenges are present, powerful, and unresolved, we may not be fully aware that they are influencing our ability to listen to, work with, and support others. We may unconsciously guide, direct, or pressure clients to talk about or avoid certain topics, to consider or make certain choices that are more about our own needs than the interests of the client.

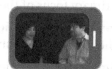

SELF-DISCLOSURE: FACULTY INTERVIEW

http://youtu.be/ ihcr6GvBAAg

For example, a CHW who is uncomfortable with aspects of human sexuality may communicate this discomfort to clients. A CHW with strong values and beliefs about reproduction, including pregnancy, abortion, and adoption, may impose these beliefs on a client who is pregnant. CHWs with a history of substance use may have difficulty separating their own experiences and beliefs from those of clients who are currently using drugs. CHWs who have been exposed to trauma, such as child abuse or sexual assault, may become restimulated and overwhelmed by their own memories and responses when working with clients who have also survived trauma. CHWs who are unaware of what triggers their anger and defensiveness are less prepared to handle these emotions when they are triggered during interactions with clients.

- *Can you think of other examples of how a CHW's own issues may interfere with their ability to work effectively with clients and communities?*

- *Have you ever worked with a helping professional who seemed uncomfortable or judgmental about your identity or behaviors?*

- *Can you identify past experiences or personal issues that could be restimulated through your work as a CHW?*

What Do YOU? Think?

Developing self-awareness is a lifelong task. It involves an ongoing process of identifying and working to better understand yourself, including your:

- *Life experiences:* Such as experiences of divorce, incarceration, immigration, chronic illness, discrimination, homelessness, trauma, and the deaths of family and friends

- *Values and beliefs:* Topics such as reproduction, religion, sexual orientation, gender identity, substance use, the criminal justice system, and death and dying

- *Prejudices:* Most of us have grown up in a community or a society that values certain groups of people more than others based on factors such as ethnicity, nationality, religion, age, immigration status, sex, gender identity, sexual orientation, and disability status. While many of us don't want to acknowledge it, growing up surrounded by prejudice influences our own thoughts, feelings, and behavior, often in subtle ways. We may be more comfortable working with certain groups of people than others, and we may provide more attention and better services to some types of clients than others. Examining our assumptions and prejudices is an essential first step in developing the ability to provide equal treatment and quality services to all clients and communities without discrimination.

SELF-EVALUATION

No matter how much you already know about yourself and others, you can always learn more. Please reflect on the following questions:

- What types of situations may provoke strong emotion or judgments for you? What provokes your anger or defensiveness?

- When do you find it most difficult to listen to others?

- When are you most tempted to tell others what to do?

- What health and health-related topics are you least prepared to address with clients? For example: How prepared are you to deal with experiences of trauma such as exposure to war, domestic violence, child abuse, and sexual assault?

- What health behaviors are you less familiar or comfortable with? For example: Which aspects of human sexuality are you least prepared to address effectively with clients?
- What populations are you less familiar with and least prepared to work with? For example, are you equally capable of working effectively with men and women? With people of all sexual orientations? With people of all gender identities? People of all ages including children, teenagers, and seniors? People who do not speak the same language as you? Are you comfortable working with interpreters?

ENHANCING SELF-AWARENESS

We encourage you to take an active approach to increasing your self-awareness. There are many ways to do this, including the following options:

- **Self-reflection:** Make time to think about your own life experiences, beliefs, and values. How might these influence the way you work with clients and communities?
- **Learning to identify issues that come up in the course of your work:** With time and practice you will begin to notice when your own issues arise in the course of your work with colleagues or clients. Successful CHWs learn how to note this and put the issue or issues aside in the moment. They continue to focus on the client or group they are working with, and after their work is done, they take time to reflect on what happened and how they can best move forward to learn more about these issues.
- **Writing/journaling:** All CHWs document their work with clients and communities. Many CHWs also keep a separate journal to write about their own work experiences, including their accomplishments, challenges, insights that assist them to better understand themselves, and questions that emerge through practice.
- **Counseling, supervision:** All CHWs should receive regular supervision. This is an opportunity to talk further about your own issues in order to better understand them and to enhance your ability to ensure that they don't interfere with your work. You may also seek to participate in counseling or therapy outside of the work environment to enhance self-awareness and to address particularly challenging issues.
- **Support from classmates, colleagues, family, and friends:** Talk with someone you trust and who can support your effort to better understand the issues that may get in the way of client- and community-centered practice.
- **Training and other professional development opportunities:** Seek out opportunities to learn more about the communities you work with, the topics and issues that arise in your work, and how to enhance cultural humility and other client-centered skills.
- **Formal education:** You may wish to continue your formal education by taking courses at a local college or university on issues that will assist you to better understand yourself, your own community and history, and how to work effectively with communities that are different from your own. This may include vocational or academic courses in psychology, ethnic studies, art, or history.

7.4 Scope of Practice

Scope of practice is a concept commonly used in most professions—including the health care and mental health fields—to determine which skills and services workers are competent and authorized to perform on the job, and which lie outside their expertise. For example, doctors are trained to diagnose illness and to prescribe treatment, including medications. These functions lie within their scope of practice. But doctors are not trained to provide legal advice (within the scope of practice of attorneys-at-law) or to install an electrical circuit in your home (within the scope of practice of electricians); these competencies lie outside their scope of practice.

Scope of practice is also an ethical issue, and relates to several of the ethical principles introduced above, including Article 1.3: Scope of Ability and Training.

More established professions, such as medicine and social work, have well-developed scope-of-practice guidelines. Because the CHW field is still developing, however, it lacks well-defined guidelines. *For CHWs, the lack of formal guidelines significantly complicates the challenge of determining which skills or competencies you can and cannot practice.* Unfortunately, questions and concerns related to scope of practice may not be raised until someone— usually a supervisor or colleague from another profession, such as nursing or social work—tells the CHW that they shouldn't have done something on the job. We hope this chapter will assist you to understand and to clarify your scope of practice, and to prevent conflict with colleagues and supervisors.

As we discussed in Chapters 1 and 2, the CHW field is not always recognized or adequately respected by other professions. Other occupations often try to limit the scope of work of CHWs, questioning the ability of CHWs to provide certain types of services. As their numbers grow, however, CHWs are negotiating a clearer and more expanded scope of practice.

FACTORS THAT INFLUENCE THE CHW SCOPE OF PRACTICE

The role and the work of CHWs can appear to be so large and all-encompassing that it feels overwhelming. Understanding where your role begins and ends, and when to make a referral to another professional, can provide clarity and comfort to CHWs and assist you to prevent mistakes that may harm your clients, your agency, and your own career. The scope of practice for CHWs varies considerably from one place to another, and may depend on a variety of factors, such as:

- State and local laws (including employment, mandatory reporting, and Medicaid reimbursement statutes)
- The agency, program, and supervisor you work for. For example, some employers may train CHWs to cofacilitate support groups, while others do not. Some employers or unions negotiate employment contracts that specify or limit scope of practice
- The type of health issue you focus on. For example, CHWs who work in the chronic conditions management field may be trained to support patients with medications management
- Your background, training, and skills
- Your own level of comfort and competency
- Overlapping scopes of practice of other colleagues such as nurses, medical assistants or medical evaluation assistants, senior health educators, and social workers
- Politics and competition among professions and professional associations for status, recognition, control, and pay
- The context of the work, including issues raised by clients

One way to think about scope of practice is to brainstorm a list of tasks and services that CHWs commonly provide, and those that are generally considered to lie outside the scope of practice of CHWs. These are not definitive lists and may vary in your state, agency, or health program.

TASKS AND SERVICES WITHIN OR OUTSIDE OF THE CHW SCOPE OF PRACTICE

Within the CHW Scope of Practice

The following tasks and services generally lie *within* the CHW scope of practice:

- Recruitment of clients or research study participants, including the provision of informed consent
- Conducting initial interviews with new clients
- Supporting clients to access new services
- Supporting clients in better understanding their own questions, resources, knowledge, and options for action and services
- Supporting clients in communicating their questions or concerns
- Providing culturally and linguistically appropriate health education and information
- Supporting clients to develop and implement a plan to reduce risks and to enhance their health
- Supporting clients in changing behaviors
- Providing informal counseling or coaching services (also referred to as peer counseling)
- Providing case management services (although some have challenged the use of this term and would reserve case management for nurses, social workers, and other licensed professionals) and referrals

- *What other competencies do you think generally lie within the CHW scope of practice?*

Outside the CHW Scope of Practice

The following competencies are considered to lie *outside* the CHW scope of practice:

- Diagnosing illness and other health conditions
- Prescribing treatment or medication
- Counseling severely mentally ill clients (although CHWs will often provide outreach, peer support, health education, and case management services to clients living with severe mental illness)
- Providing therapy (rather than more limited peer counseling)
- Providing advice on legal or medical issues

- *What other competencies do you think generally lie outside the CHW scope of practice?*

What Do YOU Think?

Services That May Be within or outside of the CHW Scope of Practice

It is generally easiest to determine competencies that lie within or outside of the CHW's scope of practice. However, there are a number of competencies that are sometimes considered to lie within, and sometimes considered to lie outside of the CHW scope of practice, depending on the factors identified above (state law, policies of the employer, professional politics, and training). In order to avoid confusion, conflict with colleagues, and harm to your clients, seek clear guidance from your supervisors regarding what you are and are not permitted to do on the job.

The following competencies may require specialized training and supervision and *sometimes lie within* and *sometimes outside* the scope of practice of CHWs.

Counseling

While some professionals argue that CHWs shouldn't perform "counseling" and object to the use of this term, there is a strong tradition of CHWs and others providing peer-based and client-centered counseling. For example, both the Centers for Disease Control and Prevention and the World Health Organization advocated for CHWs working in the field of HIV prevention to be trained to provide client-centered counseling services to support clients to reduce risks for transmitting HIV and other sexually transmitted infections, and to prevent the progression of HIV disease. In many agencies, CHWs are trained to use motivational interviewing and other client-centered counseling skills with clients. The topic of client-centered counseling is addressed in Chapter 9.

Interpretation and Translation Services

Bilingual CHWs are frequently asked to interpret oral conversations between clients and providers, or to translate written documents from one language to another. Some CHWs and their employers have advocated for CHWs to provide these services. Others have advocated for interpretation and translation services to be provided only by those with specialized training or certification because the potential consequences of mistakes made during interpretation or translation can be harmful for clients.

Home Visiting

Many CHWs visit with clients outside of the office including in their homes, in homeless shelters, on the streets, and in jail, hospitals, or residential program settings (see Chapter 11). While many organizations train and support CHWs to conduct home visiting, others do not and may assign other professionals to provide these services.

Medications Management or Treatment Adherence Counseling

Increasingly, CHWs work in partnership with clinicians to support clients in understanding and following medications and other treatment guidelines—sometimes referred to as medication management or **treatment adherence or compliance**. For example, CHWs at San Francisco General Hospital work with families to aid them to better understand their children's asthma medications and know how to use them properly to prevent symptoms. The CHWs work under the close supervision of a nurse practitioner. To read more about medications management, please see Chapter 16.

Accompanying Clients

CHWs may accompany clients during visits to other agencies, appointments with physicians or other professionals, or even court appearances in order to lend support or provide advocacy.

Media Advocacy

Some organizations train and support CHWs to take a lead role in **media advocacy**—working with print, radio, TV, or social media to promote programs, policies, or health information—while others do not.

Community Diagnosis and Community Organizing Efforts

In some settings CHWs take an active role in facilitating a community diagnosis or community organizing campaigns or movements. In other settings, these efforts are lead by other professionals. For more information, please see Chapters 22 and 23.

Facilitating Training or Community Education Sessions

Many CHWs are trained and supported to develop and/or facilitate educational trainings or health education sessions for groups in a variety of settings, addressing a variety of health topics. See Chapter 20 for more information about facilitating health education trainings.

Facilitating Social or Support Groups

There are different points of view regarding the level of education or training required to facilitate groups. Some groups may be facilitated by licensed professionals, others by CHWs. For more information about group facilitation, please see Chapter 21.

Crisis Intervention and Working with Survivors of Trauma

CHWs may provide crisis intervention or work with a client in crisis, such as a client recently exposed to sexual assault or domestic violence or other trauma, or someone who is thinking of suicide.

On the one hand, some professionals argue that CHWs do not have sufficient training to provide these services, and the risk of inadvertently causing harm to clients is too great. These advocates believe that clients in crisis should be referred as soon as possible to licensed professionals.

On the other hand, some CHWs and professionals argue that CHWs can be trained to provide crisis intervention services. They argue that it is not possible for many clients in crisis to be seen by a licensed clinical provider. These advocates also point to the rape crisis and domestic violence movements as models for the provision of culturally competent crisis intervention services by unlicensed staff. To read further about the scope of practice concerns, please see Chapter 18.

Research Projects

CHWs may provide assistance with research projects such as by recruiting or enrolling participants, as interviewers or focus group facilitators.

Determining Eligibility Status

CHWs may assist in determining the client's eligibility for state and federal Medicaid, Medicare, SCHIP, and other programs, as discussed in Chapter 5.

- *What other competencies do you think may sometimes lie within or outside of the CHW scope of practice?*

TG: There have been lots of times when other professionals have tried to tell me that I'm not qualified to provide some kind of service just because I don't have a graduate degree. A social worker at the hospital told me that I shouldn't call myself a case manager. I told her that was my title—Prevention Case Manager. And I told her that my work was funded by the State AIDS Office, and that they could look on the CDC (Centers for Disease Control and Prevention) website to learn more about how CHWs do case management. It made me angry, but I also had to stay professional, because I know that I will continue to refer clients to that social worker.

WHEN CHWs WORK OUTSIDE THEIR SCOPE OF PRACTICE

CHWs may be influenced to work outside of their scope of practice by the desire to help and support clients and communities. CHWs may do this when they perceive that their clients are at risk and lack access to important resources and services, such as health care or legal assistance. CHWs sometimes get caught up in the dangerous notion that it is their responsibility to rescue their clients or solve their clients' problems.

- *Can you think of situations where you might be tempted to exceed your scope of practice?*

Consequences of Working outside of Your Scope of Practice

Imagine that a CHW:

- Advises a client about cancer treatment
- Provides a client in a domestic violence situation with legal advice about whether or not to file a report or to seek an order of protection
- Provides ongoing counseling to a highly distressed and suicidal client

- *How might this impact the client?*

- *How might it impact the CHW?*

- *How might it affect the agency that the CHW works for?*

When CHWs step outside of their scope of practice, they risk doing harm to their clients and to themselves. CHWs do not have the required training or licensure to diagnose or treat medical conditions, to provide legal guidance, or to provide therapy to a suicidal or severely mentally ill client. For example, giving advice (rather than information) about cancer treatments could result in a client seeking inappropriate, ineffective, or harmful treatments. Under such circumstances, CHWs should refer the client to a medical provider.

Stepping outside of your scope of practice may negatively affect your professional reputation and could result in disciplinary action and the loss of your job. When you step outside of your scope of practice, you are likely to be usurping (taking over) the role of other professionals, such as nurses or social workers, and this may damage your relationship with these colleagues.

Providing services that you are not competent or licensed to provide may also seriously damage the reputation of your program or agency. News that a CHW has done something unethical or has harmed a client will travel quickly in the community and could result in diminished support for an important agency or program.

Exceeding your scope of practice also breaks trust with the communities that CHWs pledge to support. Most of the communities that CHWs serve have already experienced a long history of harmful treatment by health, medical, education, law enforcement, or other government agencies or representatives. Each betrayal takes a toll on the community and makes it harder for them to establish trusting relationships with service providers.

What to Do When You Are Uncertain about Your Scope of Practice

If your scope of practice has not been clearly defined by the agency that employs you, or you are uncertain about the type or level of service that you should provide in a certain situation, consider the following suggestions:

- Review your job description and your agency's policies regarding your scope of practice.
- If you are not certain that a certain duty lies within your scope of practice, *don't do it,* and consult with your supervisor.
- Examine the potential for causing harm to clients or communities.
- Be aware of your own risk factors for exceeding your scope of practice. For each of us, there may be particular types of situations or clients that may motivate our desire to go above and beyond the call of duty and may tempt us to step outside of our professional boundaries. *What are your risk factors?*

- Clearly explain to your client what services you can and cannot provide, and stay within these professional boundaries.
- Don't let the client be your guide regarding scope of practice. Some clients, out of an understandable desire to meet their needs, may try to pressure you to step outside of your scope of practice. Hold firm to your scope of practice and your ethical guidelines.
- When questions arise, ask for support and guidance from colleagues and your supervisor, as appropriate.

What to Do When You Disagree with How Your Scope of Practice Is Defined

As we noted above, professionals sometimes disagree about which competencies are within or outside of a CHW's scope of practice. As a result there may be times when you disagree with how your scope of practice is defined by your agency, your supervisor, or your colleagues.

Sometimes, a supervisor or colleague might ask you to perform tasks that you have not been trained to do. At other times, you may find that your agency has defined a scope of practice that is too restrictive and that keeps you from providing services that you are truly competent to provide.

Handle these challenges in a way that promotes the welfare of clients as well as your own professional reputation, and that of the program and agency you work for. Take this as an opportunity to advocate *within* your agency and with your supervisor for changes to your scope of practice. This might involve educating your colleagues and your supervisor about CHWs and their role and about your training, experience, and skills. It might involve finding out from your supervisor what additional training he or she would like you to have in order to provide certain services. It is likely to involve advocating for increased opportunities for professional development.

As CHWs organize on a local, state, and national level, they will be better able to advocate for recognition of their competencies and contributions, an expanded scope of practice, and increased pay.

7.5 Working as Part of a Multidisciplinary Team

CHWs often work as part of a multidisciplinary team that may include other CHWs as well as colleagues with a wide range of professional backgrounds, such as health educators, public health professionals, social workers, psychologists, nurses, and physicians. Sometimes, a majority of the team will be comprised of CHWs. In other settings, you may be the only CHW on your team.

Increasingly, as discussed in Chapters 1, 2, 5 and 16, CHWs are hired to work as part of a clinical team in health care settings, such as in primary health care clinics that focus on serving low-income clients with one or more chronic health conditions.

Learning how to work effectively as part of a team is a key skill for your long-term success as a CHW. In this section we will present information about working in teams, including common challenges and strategies for success. *While the emphasis of some of the information presented is on working with interdisciplinary teams in health care settings, the concepts and skills are relevant to any team work setting.*

THE USE OF CLINICAL TEAMS IN HEALTH CARE SETTINGS

Clinical teams are increasingly used to provide primary health care, especially in busy clinics that serve a high volume of patients who are living with chronic health conditions. While in the past, physicians worked more independently (and some still do), today they are more likely to work in close collaboration with other providers. The restructuring of primary health care toward the use of health care teams has also been promoted by recent health care reforms and the Patient Protection and Affordable Care Act. The use of health care teams is defined as:

> *Team-based health care is the provision of health services to individuals, families, and/or their communities by at least two health providers who work collaboratively with patients and their caregivers—to the extent preferred by each patients—to accomplish shared goals within and across settings to achieve coordinated, high-quality care.*
> *(Naylor et al., 2010)*

Providing primary care services through a team-based model is a way to address changes in health care delivery systems, including:

- A large ratio of patients to licensed primary care physicians
- The lack of sufficient time for physicians and other licensed providers to spend with all patients, and especially patients diagnosed with more than one chronic condition
- Research evidence that physicians interrupt patients during the initial discussion of their health issues within 23 seconds, and, that in 25 percent of visits, patients do not have any opportunity to voice their concerns (Bodenheimer & Liang, 2007)
- Research showing that 50 percent of patients leave medical visits without understanding the recommendations of physicians (ibid.)
- The increasing complexity of modern medicine and insufficient collaboration and communication among providers
- Increasing rates of chronic conditions
- The needs of patients living with chronic diseases for more intensive care in order to manage symptoms, change behaviors, and take any prescribed medications properly
- Risks for adverse health events (such as strokes or heart attacks) and medical errors
- Rising health care costs

There are many different ways to organize primary health care teams. Some teams are quite small, and others are quite large, depending upon the needs of the health care practice and the patients they serve. In general, primary health care teams include:

- The patient (the most important member of the team!)
- The patient's family
- One or more physicians
- A medical assistant

Some teams also include:

- Nurses or nurse practitioners
- Licensed mental health providers such as a social worker or psychologist
- Community health workers
- Front-desk receptionists
- Panel managers
- Health educators
- Pharmacists
- Other providers _____

THE BENEFITS OF TEAM-BASED CARE

There are many benefits to a team-based approach for the delivery of primary health care. Teams can improve the coordination of health care services for patients, their families, and providers, and often provide more timely access to health care (it is easier for patients to get an appointment with one of the team members). Team-based practices promote greater collaboration and consultation among health care providers, and have been shown to result in improved health outcomes for patients and their families (Bodenheimer, 2007; Stellesfon, Dipnarine, & Stopka, 2013). While improved patient health is the most important benefit, team-based practice has also been shown to reduce health care costs, a critical advantage at a time when our society is struggling to provide access to health care for all (or most) residents.

KEY CHARACTERISTICS OF EFFECTIVE PRIMARY HEALTH CARE TEAMS

As the use of health care teams has increased, a new literature has emerged that is striving to research, identify, and promote the key characteristics of successful teams. Pamela Mitchell and her colleagues (Mitchell et al., 2012) interviewed members of high-performing primary health care teams and identified the importance of shared values for successful team work including:

- **Honesty,** including open and transparent communication about goals, decisions, questions, and mistakes. Honesty is seen as an essential ingredient for fostering trust among team members.

- **Discipline,** including hard work and following the guidelines, policies, and protocols established by the team and the health care organization.

- **Creativity,** or the ability to adapt and develop new strategies for addressing common problems. Mistakes are viewed as an opportunity for problem solving and improving services.

- **Humility,** which includes respect for the training and skills of *all* members of the team and the different perspectives that each bring to their common work. Humility is also about recognizing that all members of the team will make mistakes from time to time.

- **Curiosity,** or the constant striving to understand mistakes and successes, with the goal of continuous improvement of the services provided to patients.

Researchers have also identified common principles for successful team-based health care (Mitchell et al., 2012). These include:

- **Shared goals:** All members of the team, including the patient, establish shared goals that reflect the priorities of the patient and their family. These goals should be clearly communicated, understood, and accepted by all team members.

- **Clear roles:** The roles and responsibilities of each team member are clearly communicated and understood by the team. This permits an efficient division of labor among the team.

- **Mutual trust:** Team members take time and make an effort to build trust with one another, creating a strong sense of team spirit and pride in team accomplishments.

- **Effective communication:** Clear and consistent channels for ongoing and honest communication among team members. This fosters team spirit and permits timely identification and resolution of questions and challenges, resulting in improved quality care for patients.

- **Measurable processes and outcomes:** Data is gathered and analyzed on an ongoing basis to identify patient or client needs, risks, and outcomes. Data provides opportunity for the comparison of performance indicators and patient outcomes over time, and drives continuous improvement of team systems and services.

To read more about these common principles, please go to the Institute of Medicine website at *www.iom.edu*. Another resource for further study of the principles of effective health care teams is the Interprofessional Education Collaborative (IPEC) (*https://ipecollaborative.org/*).

If You Are Working As Part of a Clinical Team

Take a moment to reflect on your experience working as part of a clinical team.

- How well do you think that your health care team performs?
- Does the team have clearly identified common values?
- Does the team do a good job of including patients and their families in key decisions?
- Are the roles and responsibilities of all team members clearly identified?
- How does the team work to develop and maintain trust?
- How often, and how well, does the team communicate with one another (including the patient)?
- What sort of data does the team use to measure processes (policies and protocols) and health outcomes? Is this data used to improve team systems and the delivery of patient-centered health care?

THE ROLE OF THE CHW WITHIN HEALTH CARE TEAMS

The role of the CHW as a member of a primary health care team will vary depending upon the size and make-up of the team. It will also depend upon the training and skills of the CHW. For example, some CHWs are also trained to serve as Medical Assistants, and some may also serve as Panel Managers. In general, however, CHWs serve on the front lines and provide the following types of services:

- **Outreach** to recruit new patients and maintain contact with existing patients
- **Home visits** (when patients are too ill to come to the clinic, or are out of communication with the clinic)
- **Patient education** (such as providing and reinforcing information about how to manage chronic conditions)
- **Client-centered counseling and case management services**, including the development and monitoring of Action Plans
- **Medication management**
- **Communication** with patients (via phone, text, email, and regular mail) and reminders about appointments, medications, behavior change, and so forth.
- Other _____
- **What other services may CHWs provide?**

CHWs often spend more time with patients than other members of the health care team. This is particularly true if the CHW conducts patient education, counseling, and case management services. This, in turn, frees up physicians and other licensed providers to see more patients, and to focus on issues of diagnosis and treatment. Because the CHW may spend more time with patients, and may visit them at home or in other community settings and engage in more frequent email, text, and/or phone communications, the CHW often has a better understanding of the patient's current health risks and concerns, and can play a vital role in sharing this information with the rest of the team.

THE CHALLENGES OF TEAM WORK

Team work is often challenging. However, CHWs are likely to face unique challenges due to their professional roles. These challenges may include:

- A lack of information and understanding about the CHW scope of practice, and qualifications. As a result, CHWs may have to spend extra time explaining their role and job duties to new members of the team (and members who do not have previous experience working with CHWs).
- A lack of understanding and respect for the services that CHWs provide outside of the agency office or clinic (such as outreach and home visits).
- Being treated, at times, with less respect than other members of the team, particularly those who are licensed providers.
- A perception that CHWs are more closely allied with clients than with the agency, program, or other providers (of course such a divide—client versus provider/agency—is detrimental to the very concept of effective client-centered team work).
- Less job security arising from the way that services and provider positions are financed and paid for. For example, many organizations still rely upon temporary grant funds to pay for CHW positions.

- *Can you think of other types of challenges that CHWs may face?*

- *Have you faced other challenges as a member of a health care team?*

What Do YOU Think?

SURVIVAL STRATEGIES FOR EFFECTIVE TEAM WORK

As a CHW, you will always be working with some type of team. Learning how to be a valued team-member is critical for the long-term success of your career. Strive to become the type of professional that others can rely on and are excited to work with day to day. Consider the following suggestions for successful team work:

- Know your job description, scope of practice, and what is expected of you in the workplace day-to-day
- If you don't understand some aspect of your job or of the clinic or program where you work, speak up and ask for clarification

- Bring a positive attitude and your "best self" to work every day
- Participate actively in team meetings and case conferences
- Provide culturally sensitive client-centered services
- Keep up to date with your documentation
- Learn how to switch codes and adapt to the codes of the professional workplace including, for example, codes for dress, language, mode of communication, time management, and so forth
- Maintain close communication with your direct supervisor
- Reach out and ask for the support and guidance that you want and need
- Focus on solutions more than "problems." While it is important to be able to name challenges or difficulties, dwelling on them is rarely appreciated in a professional environment
- Take responsibility for the mistakes that you make without drama
- Learn how to receive and provide critical feedback professionally
- Don't avoid big or persistent problems in the workplace; find a professional and respectful way to raise them with your colleagues, in the appropriate forum (a meeting with your supervisor, a team meeting, a case conference, etc.)

- *What else might be helpful guidance for working effectively with a multidisciplinary health care team?*

7.6 Understanding Behavior Change

One of the most common roles for CHWs is supporting clients to change behaviors that influence their health. While supporting people to change behaviors may sound relatively straightforward, the process of changing behavior, and the art of supporting others in doing so, is a complex and challenging task. For these reasons, we will review some basic information and guiding principles about the behavior change process. Chapter 9 will build on this information and present skills for conducting behavior change counseling.

WHICH BEHAVIORS DO PEOPLE TYPICALLY ATTEMPT TO CHANGE?

Behaviors selected for change may include:

- Patterns of eating (including disordered eating) and nutrition
- Physical activity or exercise
- Stress management
- Building greater social support and connection to family, friends, or community
- Adherence or compliance to treatment guidelines (such as remembering to take medications at the proper times and in the proper doses)
- Sexual behaviors (such as regular and effective contraceptive use and safer sex practices)
- Smoking, alcohol, and drug use (reducing or eliminating use)
- Anger management
- Parenting practices (such as effective discipline)
- Screening for cancer (including regular self-exams for breast and testicular cancer)
- Driving (such as driving within the speed limit and not under the influence of alcohol or other substances)

- *Can you think of other behaviors to add to this list?*

Your Experience with Behavior Change

Before you begin to think about how to support others in changing their behaviors, we would like you to reflect on your own experiences. If possible, take time to discuss your responses with a friend or colleague.

- Which behaviors have you tried to change?
- What motivated you to change your behavior?
- Was it easy to make changes?
- Did change happen all at once?
- What factors supported you in making change?
- What got in the way of successful behavior change?
- Were you able to maintain change over time?
- Did you ever relapse or return to the old behavior you had hoped to change? If so, what influenced this? How did you feel when you relapsed?
- After a relapse, were you able to try again to change your behavior? How? What helped?

Most of us have struggled over the course of our lives to change certain behaviors: to stop smoking, to exercise regularly, to eat healthier foods, to turn in homework assignments on time, or to change the way we talk with loved ones when we are angry. We know from our own experience how challenging and frustrating it can be to make and sustain behavior change. If it were easy to change behavior, our society wouldn't experience such high rates of violence, addiction, cancer, heart disease, diabetes, HIV disease, or automobile accidents.

FACTORS THAT INFLUENCE BEHAVIOR: DEVELOPING AN ECOLOGICAL APPROACH

Imagine that you are working with a client who has expressed the desire to:

- Change their diet in order to manage diabetes and prevent heart disease
- Use condoms regularly to reduce the risks of sexually transmitted infections
- Leave an abusive relationship

Despite good intentions, clients may fail to meet their own expectations and may relapse for various periods of time to the very behaviors or situations they were attempting to change. *Why is changing behavior so difficult? What gets in the way?*

Table 7.1 identifies some of the factors that may get in the way of successful behavior change. These factors correspond to the ecological model presented in Chapter 3 and include individual, family and friends, neighborhood or community, and societal factors.

The table illustrates how a wide range of factors may influence the health and behavior of your client and complicate their efforts to change. We have categorized these factors at the level of the individual, family and friends, neighborhood or community, and the broader society or state. These factors will always depend on your client's identity (including life experiences, gender, age, ethnicity, nationality, immigration status, primary language, sexual orientation, disability status, and so on), and social context. Social context refers to the reality in which people live, and includes their families, friends, workplaces, homes, and the economic, cultural, and political dynamics affecting their neighborhood, city, state, or nation.

Table 7.1 Factors That Get in the Way of Behavior Change: An Ecological Model

CLIENT EXAMPLE	INDIVIDUAL FACTORS	FACTORS RELATED TO FAMILY AND FRIENDS	NEIGHBORHOOD AND COMMUNITY FACTORS	SOCIETAL FACTORS: MEDIA, ECONOMICS, AND POLITICS
The client wants to leave a relationship characterized by violence and threats of violence.	A long history of abuse—beginning as a child Lack of self-esteem Loneliness and fear of being on one's own Lack of formal education and job skills Age Love for the partner who hurts them Perceived need to preserve the family Shame about having stayed in the relationship so long; worried about what others will think *Other possibilities?*	Pressure from family and friends not to be single Concern for keeping the family intact, especially when there are children involved Judgment from friends about being with an abusive partner Cultural norms and attitudes A history of incarceration related to drug use *Other possibilities?*	Isolation from the spiritual community that used to be a source of faith and comfort Domestic violence is accepted as normal by many members of the local community Lack of job training and employment opportunities that could help with independence Lack of social services, including services for victims of domestic violence *Other possibilities?*	Discrimination based on ethnicity, nationality, immigration status, gender, sexual orientation, or other identity Poverty Lack of government support for educational and social service programs for low-income communities Lack of funding for victims of domestic violence, including counseling, legal assistance, and affordable transitional housing *Other possibilities?*

The list of factors provided in Table 7.1 is not meant to be exhaustive: it doesn't include every possibility. When students at the City College of San Francisco brainstorm a list of factors that influence behavior, the list typically fills up six to eight large pieces of flip chart paper and includes over a hundred distinct items. Additional factors that influence the ability of our clients to successfully change behaviors may include the following:

Individual Factors

- Emotions, such as embarrassment, shame, guilt, fear, love, or loneliness
- Desire for love, intimacy, and a sense of belonging
- Dependency—economic or emotional—on others
- Pleasure (the desire for pleasure, including pleasure from sex or drug use)
- Lack of confidence in the ability to succeed
- Thoughts, including self-defeating thoughts (such as "I always mess up," "I won't be able to," "I don't care what happens . . .")
- Self-esteem (how we think and feel about ourselves)
- Spiritual, religious, or metaphysical "faith," meaning, or purpose
- Knowledge relevant to behavior change (such as information about nutrition)
- History—what has happened before—including history of successful behavior change and history of trauma such as domestic violence and sexual assault
- Long-established patterns of behavior, including risk behaviors such as drinking or using drugs when under stress

- Choices, including choices regarding education, relationships, drug use, sexual behavior, nutrition, and so on
- Lack of formal education and employment skills

Family and Friends
- Level of family support and conflict
- Isolation
- Peer pressure—from friends and sexual partners
- Sense of belonging
- Healthy romantic and sexual relationships
- Exposure to violence in relationships with family or others

Neighborhood and Community Factors
- Social identity and sense of belonging to a defined community
- Availability of community-based resources such as health and social services agencies, good schools, faith-based institutions including churches and mosques, recreational and cultural programs including parks and after-school programs for youth, affordable and healthy food, public transportation, affordable housing
- Working conditions, including exposure to hazardous chemicals, low pay and lack of benefits, conflict with management, and other sources of stress
- Relative presence of potentially harmful dynamics and resources, such as a large number of bars and liquor stores; drug sales; or crime, including property theft, assault, gang-related activity, and violence
- Support from helping professionals, such as CHWs (or harmful interactions with helping professionals)
- Cultural or religious support or rejection
- Community norms and expectations
- Stigma and prejudice against one's identity or behaviors

Societal Factors
- Prejudice and discrimination based on ethnicity, nationality, immigration status, language, gender, gender-identity, sexual orientation, level of education, disability, age, history of incarceration, and so forth
- Government policies, including those determining access to necessary services such as safe housing, healthy nutrition, effective schools, after-school programs, health insurance, employment, drug treatment programs, residency or citizenship, health education programs, and civil rights
- Criminal justice approach to drug use, rather than a harm-reduction approach (people locked up for using drugs rather than provided with treatment and services to reduce harm)
- Economic policies and forces influencing wages, working conditions, employment benefits, and access to resources
- Corporate promotion of products such as fast food, low-mileage cars, or handguns
- Media promotion of harmful attitudes and behaviors
- Political events, including global economic practices and war
- Natural influences (often influenced by human actions), including natural disasters such as Hurricane Katrina

- *What do you think of these lists?*

- *Is there anything you would like to add?*

- *Is there anything listed here that you question or would like to see changed or omitted?*

What Do YOU Think?

As discussed in Chapter 3, research in the field of public health has demonstrated that social context and ecological factors influence human health far more significantly than the genetics, knowledge, or behavior of individuals. In order to become effective agents of change, CHWs must learn to view individual clients within the broad social context in which they live. An ecological approach to understanding and facilitating behavior change examines both the factors that an individual may be able to control, and the broader social, economic, cultural, and political factors that influence her choices, behavior, and health.

COMMON MISTAKES IN ATTEMPTING TO FACILITATE BEHAVIOR CHANGE

Before introducing resources designed to facilitate effective behavior change, we want to address several common mistakes that CHWs and other helping professionals often make when working with clients. We encourage you to understand what these mistakes are, and why we suggest that they may undermine your effective work with clients. The four common mistakes are:

1. Relying on information alone

2. Giving advice

3. Blaming the client

4. Failing to address issues of accountability

As we address each of these common mistakes in turn, we will apply them to the case of working with a client named L. described below.

The Client "L."

L. was recently diagnosed with gonorrhea and is worried about getting infected with HIV. L. is shy around people she or he is attracted to, and feels embarrassed in sexual situations when not drinking or using drugs. L. doesn't regularly use condoms and isn't comfortable negotiating safer sex. L. wants to change these behaviors, but doesn't feel confident that she or he can.

Common Mistake #1: Relying on Health Information Alone

Often, CHWs and other helping professionals (including nurses and physicians), work from the assumption that if they provide a client with clear and accurate information about a health condition, and what they can do to prevent the condition or improve their health, the client will apply that information to change the behavior.

For example, a CHW working with L. may focus on providing information about STIs and how to prevent them:

> **CHW:** Gonorrhea is one of the most common sexually transmitted infections or STIs. You can contract it from unprotected vaginal, anal, or oral sex. Fortunately, gonorrhea is a bacterial STI and can be effectively treated with antibiotics. If you don't get treated with antibiotics, and complete that treatment, a gonorrheal infection can result in a range of complications including sterility: the inability to have children. To prevent infection with gonorrhea or other STIs in the future, practice safer sex. This may include no penetrative oral, vaginal, or anal sex; monogamy with a committed and trusted partner who has been tested and proven to be free of STIs; and the use of condoms every time you have sex . . . . (*And the CHW goes on—and on!—providing information about safer sex, testing, and treatment of STIs.*)

While the information provided is accurate, in most cases it is unlikely to motivate the client to make immediate, significant, and lasting behavior change. It is common for people who fully understand the health risks of certain behavior, such as unprotected sex or smoking, to continue these behaviors. L. may already know a lot about STIs and how to use condoms. L. doesn't necessarily lack information: other factors are influencing L.'s behavior and getting in the way of successful behavior change.

- *Have you ever encountered a health care or other helping professional who focused exclusively on providing you with health information?*

- *How does this type of approach work for you?*

- *Do you think that this type of approach will be effective with most clients?*

- *Why or why not?*

We don't recommend this approach because:
- It is unlikely to result in effective and lasting behavior changes.
- This approach assumes that the client doesn't have complete or accurate knowledge about the health issue.
- The CHW dominates the session in providing information and does not make space for the client to share knowledge, questions, concerns, and ideas.
- It minimizes the difficulty of making changes in behaviors and doesn't provide meaningful support to assist in that process.
- The client may feel condescended or "talked-down" to, particularly if the CHW doesn't take time to acknowledge what the client already knows the information and wishes to talk about the challenges of behavior change in a more realistic way.
- The client may feel frustrated by the encounter and less likely to return to this or other similar providers in the future.

Please note: We want to underscore that the critique we offer here is not about the value of providing health information. Indeed, a vital role of CHWs is to educate clients about health conditions, under the guidance of other health professionals and within their scope of practice. CHWs provide health information to clients and assist them to better understand health conditions, their risks, and the options for reducing these risks. The problem arises when CHWs don't first assess what the client already knows, and when they assume that accurate health information alone is sufficient to support their clients in making healthy and lasting behavior changes.

Mistake #2: Giving Advice

Many helping professionals provide advice to clients about what they should and shouldn't do, and sometimes what they should think and feel.

For example, a CHW working with L. may make the following types of statements:
- "If you haven't been treated yet, you should go to a clinic immediately to get a prescription for the right antibiotic. Let's call up City Clinic right now to make an appointment."
- "You shouldn't feel embarrassed about sex, it's just a natural part of life."
- "You need to start using condoms every time you have sex, regardless of the circumstances." All you need to say is, "I don't have unprotected sex. My health is too important to me to take a risk."
- "I think you should go to a drug and alcohol recovery group. I facilitate a support group on Thursday nights for women/men like you. It starts at 4 PM."

In this example, the CHW not only wants to tell the client what to do ("Go to City Clinic" or "Attend a recovery support group"), they even want to tell L. what to feel ("You shouldn't feel embarrassed") and what to say ("All you need to say is . . .").

- *Have you ever encountered a health care or other helping professional who liked to give you advice?*

- *How does this type of approach work for you?*

- *Do you think that this type of approach will be effective with most clients?*

- *Why or why not?*

We don't recommend this approach because:

- It is unlikely to result in effective and lasting behavior changes.

- It assumes that clients cannot make informed decisions for themselves about what to do to promote their health. It assumes that clients require an "expert" to guide their behavior.

- It may undermine the client's autonomy and sense of competency. It fosters dependence on others.

- Many clients do not like to be told what to do. Such an approach may cause them to lose trust in and respect for health care and other helping professionals and could result in them avoiding services in the future.

Sometimes, we fall into a pattern of giving advice without even noticing it, generally out of a desire to be supportive. While providing advice may be an appropriate thing to do in your family or with your friends, it isn't something that we recommend you do with clients. Be aware of the words you use and be cautious about the times when you find yourself using phrases such as:

- *You should . . .*

- *You need to . . .*

Please note: There are many occasions when we encourage CHWs to share suggestions with clients about choices that they may make. Rather than telling a client what to do, however, we encourage you to present the choices as options for the client to consider. Instead of saying "You should," try saying something like:

- Have you thought about?

- Have you considered?

- What do you think about . . . ?

- I'd like to share a suggestion for something to consider as you decide what you want to do . . .

Please watch the following videos ▶ that show a CHW working with a client. In the counter role play, the CHW provides the client with advice in a way that we don't recommend. In the demo role play, the CHW shares information with the client in a different, more effective way.

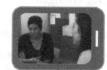

GIVING ADVICE: ROLE PLAY, COUNTER

🔗 *https://youtu. be/Our62-cDogk*

- What classic mistake does the CHW make in the counter role play?

  ○ How may this impact or affect the client?

- What does the CHW do differently in the demo role play?

- What would you do differently if you were working with this client, and why?

Mistake #3: Blaming the Client

Sometimes CHWs or other helping professionals focus primarily on what clients do that increases their health risks. This focus is sometimes accompanied by a tendency to blame clients for their illnesses or disabilities. This approach is deeply influenced by political and media messages that tend to blame people for unfortunate circumstances, including poverty and poor health outcomes. For example, when people engage in risky behaviors, others blame them. When people try but don't succeed in changing

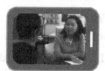

GIVING ADVICE: ROLE PLAY, DEMO

🔗 *https://youtu. be/J8Jn_okskAM*

behaviors, they may be blamed again. Sometimes, when people are diagnosed with cancer, diabetes, HIV disease, or other health conditions, they are blamed yet again. This perspective may unduly influence the approach and tone that CHWs take when working with individual clients.

Blaming the client is manifested both in the tone with which a CHW communicates with a client, and the content of what is said. For example, a CHW who is influenced by a "blaming the client" approach may ask or make the following types of questions and statements when working with L.:

- Why are you having sex with so many partners?
- You don't seem very concerned about your risks for sexually transmitted infections.
- Don't you know what gonorrhea can do to your body?
- If you don't stop having anal sex, you are going to end up with a disease that is a lot worse than gonorrhea.
- If you can't talk with your partners about using condoms, you shouldn't be having sex: "No glove, no love!"
- You seem embarrassed to talk about sex. It is just a natural part of life.

- *Have you ever encountered a health care or other helping professional who seemed to blame you in some way?*

- *How does this type of approach work for you?*

- *Do you think that this type of approach will be effective with most clients?*

- *Why or why not?*

We don't recommend this approach because:

- It is unlikely to result in effective and lasting behavior changes.
- It assumes that the client's health and behavior are determined 100 percent by the client.
- It fails to recognize social, political, economic, and cultural relationships and dynamics that influence our knowledge, attitudes, choices, and behaviors.
- It fails to recognize how difficult it can be to change behaviors such as alcohol and drug use, diet, and sexual behaviors.
- It isn't the proper role of CHWs to pass judgment on clients.
- It is likely to provoke feelings of embarrassment, shame, or anger in the client, especially if they have often been judged by others in the past.
- It is likely to prevent the formation of a trusting, supportive, and lasting relationship with the CHW.
- It may discourage a client from returning to the same agency for services or from accessing services elsewhere.
- It may be harmful to your client. Blaming people for poor health or for the inability to change behaviors is generally counterproductive; it contributes to a lack of confidence and may diminish their hope in the possibility of change. One of the key roles of CHWs is to carry hope for positive change for the clients and communities you work with, especially during difficult times when they are discouraged.

Ramona Benson: I don't put the blame on the client when she doesn't do something. She's probably blaming herself already. I look at the whole picture. I look at the system, too. Did the health care system treat her right? Give her an appointment on time? Cancel that appointment? Get her a prescription that she needed for her baby? Charge her too much? Mix up her health insurance?

Mistake #4: Failing to Address Issues of Accountability

Like most of us, clients sometimes engage in behaviors that may be harmful to their health or the health of others. When a client reveals that she or he is engaging in harmful behavior, you will be faced with the question of how to respond. Unfortunately, many CHWs and other helping professionals fail to take advantage of this opportunity and don't engage clients in talking further about these potential harms. This common mistake is the flip side of "blaming the client." In order not to make judgments about clients, the CHW may stay silent about potential harm, may focus the discussion on what clients are doing well to promote their health, or may otherwise avoid the conversation.

Some of reasons for making this common mistake may include:

- A mistaken notion that the role of the CHW is to accept and support everything their client *does* (rather than always accepting and supporting *the client*, but not necessarily the behavior or choices)
- Being uncomfortable with confrontation or conflict
- Fear of insulting, angering, shaming, or otherwise harming the relationship with the client

- *Have you ever encountered a health care or other helping professional who failed to talk with you about things that you were doing that could be harmful to yourself or others?*
- *How does this type of approach work for you?*
- *Do you think that this type of approach will be effective with most clients?*
- *Why or why not?*

We don't recommend this approach because:

- It is unlikely to result in effective and lasting behavior changes.
- It deprives the client of an opportunity to reflect in a deep way about behaviors that may be harmful to themselves or others.
- It does not respect your client's ability to address challenging issues.
- It sends and reinforces a message that the client should not discuss these issues.
- It may result in increased shame and guilt regarding the behaviors.
- It increases the likelihood that clients will continue to engage in the behavior and will indeed cause harm to themselves or others (imagine, for example, that your client has untreated gonorrhea and is continuing to have unprotected sex with others).
- It violates your code of ethics to do no harm to the client or others.
- It may discourage a client from returning to the same agency for services or even from accessing services elsewhere.

An alternative:

Rather than avoiding the situation, we encourage you to address these concerns directly and respectfully with the client. For example, when working with L., a CHW may say something along the lines of:

CHW: L., you told me that you want to prevent getting another STI in the future and that you are continuing to have sex without using condoms. How do you feel about this? (CHW pauses and listens). What are some of the factors that get in the way of using condoms? (the CHW pauses and listens). What do you want to do differently to prevent getting an STI in the future?

7.7 Client-Centered Practice

In the section above, we have presented four common mistakes that we hope you will avoid when working with clients. In this section, we will introduce concepts *that we do recommend* to guide your work with clients and communities.

The principal framework that we use to train CHWs at City College of San Francisco is client-centered practice (also referred to as person-centered practice). Client-centered practice is not a unified theory or concept, but draws upon a wide variety of theories, models, concepts, and skills. These include the work of Carl Rogers, the field of humanistic psychology, models of client-centered counseling promoted by leading public health organizations such as the Centers for Disease Control and Prevention and the World Health Organization, harm reduction, cultural humility, motivational interviewing, and self-determination. We will introduce and discuss these concepts and skills in more detail in Parts 2 (Chapters 6–11) and 4 Part 4 (Chapters 15–18) of this book.

Client-centered concepts and skills can be used to guide most of the services that you will provide, including health outreach and home visiting, care management, client-centered counseling, and chronic conditions management. It can be used when working with formerly incarcerated clients and when addressing mental health challenges or trauma. The concepts are even applicable when doing work at the group or community level (addressed in Part 5 of this book).

The essential value and guiding principle of client-centered practice is an emphasis on the experience, ideas, beliefs, and feelings of the client, and working in a way that enhances the client's autonomy. In this sense, client-centered practice may be contrasted with more traditional or provider-centered models that emphasize the knowledge, skills, and beliefs of the professional (such as a physician or social worker). In these models, the role of service providers is to advise clients or patients about what they should do (or know and believe), and the role of the client was to follow this expert advice.

The client-centered approach views CHWs as facilitators who support clients to make changes that promote their health. This approach recognizes that in order for these changes to be most valuable, effective, and long-lasting, they must come from the client, not from providers or outside "experts." In other words, it is not the role of the CHW to tell clients or communities what to believe or what to do in order to promote their health. Rather, your role is to support clients and communities in carefully analyzing the factors that both harm and promote their health, in identifying possible choices or courses of action and their consequences, and in developing and implementing a plan for individual or community-level change.

Please watch the following video interview [▶] about the problem of giving advice to clients.

- Why do some service providers rely on giving advice?
- Do you like it when service providers give *you* advice?
- How may giving advice impact clients?

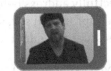

GIVING ADVICE: FACULTY INTERVIEW
🔗 *http://youtu.be/ ffFXsvPAKkA*

A CHW MODEL FEATURING BIG EYES, BIG EARS, AND A SMALL MOUTH

HIV prevention groups in Zimbabwe (International Training and Education Center on HIV [I-TECH], 2005) developed the following image (Figure 7.1) to depict client-centered practice.

This diagram represents a CHW who is working with a client. The big ears show a CHW who is listening carefully and deeply to the client. The big eyes indicate that the CHW is carefully observing the client and the surrounding world (social context). The small mouth indicates that the CHW is careful not to talk too much during the session. Rather than dominating the discussion, the CHW uses techniques such as asking open-ended questions to provide clients with an opportunity to reflect on their life and their health, to talk about their experiences, and to identity actions that will reduce harm and promote their health and well-being.

BIG EYES, BIG EARS, SMALL MOUTH: FACULTY INTERVIEW
🔗 *http://youtu.be/ jE9uNHRhLA4*

Please watch the following video [▶] interview about the concept of a CHW with Big Eyes, Big Ears and a small mouth.

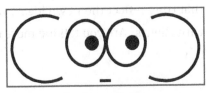

Figure 7.1 Big Eyes, Big Ears

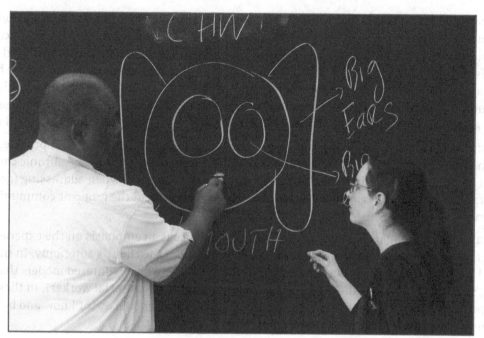

Students discuss the picture of a CHW with Big Eyes, Big Ears and a small mouth.

THE STRENGTH-BASED APPROACH

Client-centered practice is also strength-based. While traditional approaches often focused primarily or exclusively on the client's risk behaviors and lack of resources, a client-centered approach seeks greater balance. It emphasizes the internal and external resources that a client already has. External resources are often easier to identify. They are the resources that lie outside of the client and may include family and friends, stable housing, a trusted primary health care provider, spiritual faith or religious tradition, or a secure job at a living wage. Internal resources reside within the client, and may include knowledge, skills, talents, experiences, wisdom, courage, compassion, humor, and past accomplishments. The client-centered practitioner always looks for and acknowledges a client's internal and external resources and supports clients to draw upon these resources to promote their health (see Chapter 12 for more information about internal and external resources).

Client-centered practice does not mean that CHWs should always agree with or support everything that a client says or does. While CHWs should provide unconditional positive regard for clients, CHWs do not provide unconditional approval of their behaviors. Some of your clients will engage in behaviors or make decisions that may be harmful to themselves or others. These are opportunities for CHWs to ask questions, express concern, and offer other options for the client to consider. As we addressed earlier, occasionally CHWs will have an ethical and legal obligation to report behaviors that could harm the client or others. You also have a responsibility to directly and respectfully address behaviors or decisions that carry health risks such as skipping medical treatments, engaging in unprotected sex, smoking, or sharing needles to inject drugs. Knowledge and skills for how to address these issues in a client-centered way will be addressed in the chapters that follow.

ARE YOU DOING CLIENT-CENTERED WORK?

To assess whether or not you are doing client-centered work, reflect on the following questions:

- Are you providing clients with the space and the opportunity to voice their true feelings and opinions?
- Are clients making health decisions that truly reflect their own ideas, values, and reality?
- Are you dominating the discussions with clients? Are you talking more than the clients are?

- Are you bringing your own agenda into the clients' sessions?
- What is getting in the way of your ability to truly listen to clients?

Please watch the following video, which shows a CHW working with a client and making the common mistake of talking too much.

- In this video, what information is the CHW trying to share with the client?
- Why might this CHW—or other helping professionals—make the mistake of talking too much when working with a client?
- How might talking too much impact or affect a client?

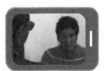

TALKING TOO MUCH: ROLE PLAY, COUNTER

🔗 *http://youtu.be/ VhDFNaFow6c*

Alvaro Morales: I started out doing a lot of HIV-antibody test counseling that really trained me in the client-centered approach. My job was to work with a client to assess their own risks for HIV infection—and what they could realistically do to reduce those risks. I would ask pretty straight-forward questions that just gave them a chance to talk, to identify their own resources, and any-thing else that they might want to learn or to get access to . . . like drug treatment or syringe exchange or parenting classes, anything. I still use this approach anytime I am working with clients and even when I am working with communities, because the same skills that you use to listen to clients and to support them to figure out what they can do to improve their health, it's the same thing you do to support communities to figure out what they want to do to improve things on a bigger level.

AN APPLICATION OF CLIENT-CENTERED PRACTICE

Above, we discussed four classic mistakes that CHWs might make when working with a client named L. Here, we wish to show how a client-centered approach could be used to work with the same client.

Using a client-centered approach, a CHW may ask a range of questions over the course of one or more sessions. These questions should not be asked all at once, but as appropriate and in response to what the client says. They may include:

Assessing Knowledge

- L., can you tell me what you know about STIs and how to prevent them?

Questions about Specific Behaviors

- Are there particular times or situations when you notice that you are more likely not to use condoms?
- What is it about these situations that makes it more difficult for you to use condoms?
- Can you tell me about a time when you did negotiate condom use or another type of safer sex?
- What made this possible? What was this like for you?
- It seems that when you are sexually attracted to someone, it is harder for you to talk with them about using condoms—is that right?
- Why do you think this is so?

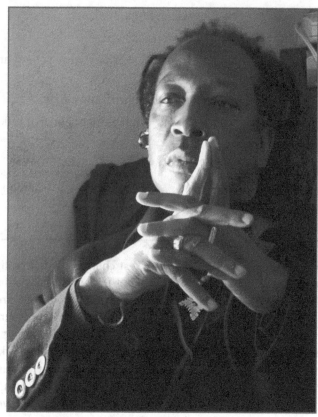

A CHW's ability to listen deeply is key to providing effective client-centered counseling.

Assessing Resources

- What kind of support do you have to make these changes in your life?
- Is there a particular family member or friend you feel comfortable confiding in?
- Do you have a good source of health care?
- Where do you usually go? Do you know about the free health clinic? What has your experience been with these medical providers?
- Can you tell me about a time when you were successful at making a change in your life?

Assessing Readiness

- What is it like for you to talk about these issues?
- How important is it to you to start using condoms more frequently when you have sex?
- It sounds like you are ready to try talking about condom use with your sexual partners—is that right?
- Would you like to schedule another time to meet and talk together?

Identifying Actions to Promote Health

- What can you start to do now to reduce your risk for STIs?
- What will you try to do differently in your next relationship?
- What will assist you to reduce risks for sexual transmission of HIV?

The CHW may make the following types of statements, as appropriate:

- I'm really glad that you talked with me tonight, and that you went to a clinic to get tested for STIs.

- It is up to you to decide what issues we talk about. I will ask you some pretty personal questions, including questions about your sex life, but it is completely up to you whether or not you want to answer or talk about these issues. I will respect whatever you decide about this.

- I talk with a lot of people who find it difficult to negotiate safer sex and condom use. Most people don't grow up being taught how to talk about sex. I think most people find it embarrassing at first.

- I'd really like to talk with you again. You can always find me here on Saturday nights. You can also call me at (gives business card and number).

This CHW asks open-ended questions designed to assist clients to reflect on their knowledge, behaviors, and feelings; their risks for HIV infection; and what they are ready to do to reduce these risks. The CHW doesn't judge clients' behavior or tell clients what to do, say, or feel. The CHW assesses and affirms the positive steps that clients have taken and aids in identifying their resources. While the CHW does affirm the efforts that clients are making to understand and change their behavior, the clients do most of the talking.

- *What else would you do or say to demonstrate a client-centered approach when working with L.?*

What Do YOU Think ?

IMPLICIT THEORY

When most people think of theory, they think of formal theories that have been researched and published in books and articles. Implicit theory refers to the concepts that each of us develop—in this instance related to behavior change—based on our own life and work experience. Over time, CHWs develop implicit theories about behavior change through the course of their work with hundreds of diverse clients. Typically, we don't have the opportunity to conduct research on these theories or to publish them, and they are not formally recognized by others working in the public-health field.

The Implicit Theories Project investigated beliefs about behavior change among CHWs doing HIV prevention work in the San Francisco Bay Area. Researchers from the University of California, San Francisco (UCSF), reported that CHWs develop their own theories about risk behaviors and the factors that influence behavior change based on their work with clients and communities (Freedman et al., 2006). The theories developed by CHWs often shared common ideas, including an emphasis on the influence of social context (or environmental factors) and the importance for clients of having a sense of community. Researchers also highlighted the importance of implicit theories to the development of effective community-based programs and services.

We strongly encourage you to continue to develop your own implicit theories as you build your career in the community health field. We encourage you to reflect deeply about the question of why people behave the way they do, and what supports people to change behaviors that are harming their health or the health of others. Consider the following resources for developing your own implicit theories:

- Examine your own biases and reflect on how your own identity, experience, and culture may influence your ideas about behavior and behavior change (you may wish to refer to Chapter 6).

- Research and read about theories of behavior change.

- Attend local workshops and classes that address issues related to behavior change.

- Ask your colleagues what they have found works in supporting the behavior change of clients.

- Share your implicit theories with colleagues, engaging in dialogue and refining your beliefs over time.

- Most importantly, don't forget to ask, and to listen carefully to, what your clients believe motivates their behavior and supports their ability to create lasting changes.

You will learn more about client-centered practice and how to apply it in your work with clients in Parts 2 and 4 of the *Foundations* textbook.

Please watch the following video interview about the process of developing your own approach to client-centered practice.

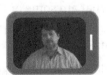

YOUR APPROACH TO CLIENT-CENTERED COUNSELING: FACULTY INTERVIEW

http://youtu.be/ yHIfoqqkxJI

Chapter Review

To review your understanding of the concepts and skills addressed in Chapter 7, please review the questions provided below and consider how you would answer them.

ETHICAL GUIDELINES

How would you respond to the following situations:

- A client asks to borrow $10 to get something to eat. What should you do? How will you explain your decision to the client?

- A client with HIV disease informs you that she hasn't disclosed her HIV status to her partners, and she is continuing to have unprotected sex. One of these partners is also a client. What should you do?

- Which articles in the AACHW Code of Ethics apply to these situations?

- Apply the Framework for Ethical Decision Making to one or more of these situations:

    Step 1. Identify and describe the problem or dilemma.

    Step 2. Review the relevant ethical guidelines or codes.

    Step 3. Know the applicable laws and regulations.

    Step 4. Obtain consultation.

    Step 5. Consider possible and probable courses of action.

    Step 6. Outline possible consequences of decisions.

    Step 7. Decide on what appears to be the best course of action.

SELF-AWARENESS

Review the questions posed earlier in the chapter for self-evaluation, such as: What populations are you less familiar with and least prepared to work with?

SCOPE OF PRACTICE

- What is scope of practice (SOP), and why is it important for CHWs to understand?

- Identify at least three tasks or services that are clearly within the CHW SOP.

- Identify at least three tasks or services that are outside of the CHW SOP.

    o What factors may determine whether or not this task is within the CHW's SOP?

    o What could the CHW do to determine whether the task was within their SOP?

    o What may happen when CHWs exceed their scope of practice?

SUCCESSFUL TEAM WORK

- What are some of the key characteristics of successful teams?

- What are some of the common challenges that you may face when working as a member of a multidisciplinary team?

- Identify at least 3 key strategies for successful team work.

PROMOTING BEHAVIOR CHANGE

Apply the ecological model to the issue of binge drinking. A client gets drunk on the weekend, blacks out, and can't remember what happened or what they did. Identify factors that influence behavior and may get in the way of successful behavior change at the following levels:

- Individual factors
- Family and friends
- Neighborhood and community factors
- Societal factors
- How might the "blaming the client" approach be used when working with the client who is binge drinking?
- Why would you discourage a new CHW from using the "blaming the client" approach?

CLIENT-CENTERED PRACTICE

- How would you briefly explain the central concept of client-centered practice to a new CHW?
- What does it mean to apply a strength-based approach to your work with clients, and how is this different from traditional approaches?

References

Bodenheimer, T. (2007). *Building teams in primary care: Lessons learned.* Prepared for the California HealthCare Foundation. Retrieved from *www.chcf.org/~/media/MEDIA%20LIBRARY%20Files/PDF/PDF%20B/PDF%20BuildingTeamsInPrimaryCareLessons.pdf*

Bodenheimer, T., & Liang, B. Y. (2007). The teamlet model of primary care. *Annals of Family Medicine, 5*(5), 457–461. Retrieved from *www.annfammed.org/content/5/5/457.full*

CHW Unity Conference. (2008). *Code of ethics for Community Health Workers.* Retrieved from *www.in.gov/isdh/files/CHW_CodeofEthics_approvedfinalJune2008.pdf*

Corey, G., Corey, M. S., & Callanan, P. (2011). *Issues and ethics in the helping professions* (8th ed.). Belmont, CA: Brooks/Cole.

Freedman, B., Binson, D., Ekstrand, M., Galvez, S., Woods, W. J., & Grinstead, O. (2006). Uncovering implicit theories of HIV prevention providers: It takes a community. *AIDS Education and Prevention 18*(3), 216–226.

International Training and Education Center on HIV (I-TECH) and the Ministry of Health and Child Welfare, Zimbabwe. (2005). *Integrated counseling for HIV and AIDS prevention and care: Training for HIV primary care counselors.* Unpublished training manual.

Mitchell, P., Wynia, M., Golden, R., McNellis, B., Okun, S., Webb, C. E., . . . Von Kohorn, I. (2012). *Core principles & values of effective team-based health care.* [Discussion Paper]. Institute of Medicine. Retrieved from *http://nam.edu/wp-content/uploads/2015/06/VSRT-Team-Based-Care-Principles-Values.pdf*

Naylor, M. D., Coburn, K. D., Kurtzman, E. T, Prvu Bettger, J. A., Buck, H., Van Cleave, J., & Cott, C. (2010). *Inter-professional team-based primary care for chronically ill adults: State of the science.* Unpublished white paper. Presented at the ABIM Foundation meeting to Advance Team-Based Care for the Chronically Ill in Ambulatory Settings, Philadelphia, PA.

Stellesfon, M., Dipnarine, K. & Stopka, C. (2013). The chronic care model and diabetes management in us primary care settings: A systematic review. Centers for Disease Control and Prevention. *Preventing Chronic Disease: Public Health Research, Practice and Policy, 10*, 120180. doi:10.5888/pcd10.120180

Zur, O. (2011). *Self-disclosure & transparency in psychotherapy and counseling: To disclose or not to disclose, this is the question.* Retrieved from *www.zurinstitute.com/selfdisclosure1.html*

Additional Resources

Bodenheimer, T. (2008). The future of primary care: Transforming practice. *New England Journal of Medicine, 359,* 2086–2089. doi:10.1056/NEJMp0805631

The California HealthCare Foundation. (n.d.). Retrieved from *www.chcf.org/*

Findley, S. E., Matos S., Hicks, A. L., Campbell, A., Moore, A., & Diaz, D. (2012). Building a consensus on community health workers' scope of practice: Lessons from New York. *American Journal of Public Health, 102,* 1981–1987. PMCID: PMC3490670

The Interprofessional Education Collaborative. (n.d.). Retrieved from *https://ipecollaborative.org/*

Temaner Brodley, B. (1991). *Instructions for beginning to practice client-centered therapy.* Retrieved from *http://world.std.com/~mbr2/cct.beginning.practise.html*

Willard, R., & Bodenheimer, T. (2012). *The building blocks of high-performing primary care: Lessons from the field.* The California HealthCare Foundation. Retrieved from *www.chcf.org/~/media/MEDIA%20LIBRARY%20Files/PDF/PDF%20B/PDF%20BuildingBlocksPrimaryCare.pdf*

Conducting Initial Client Interviews

Tim Berthold and Mickey Ellinger

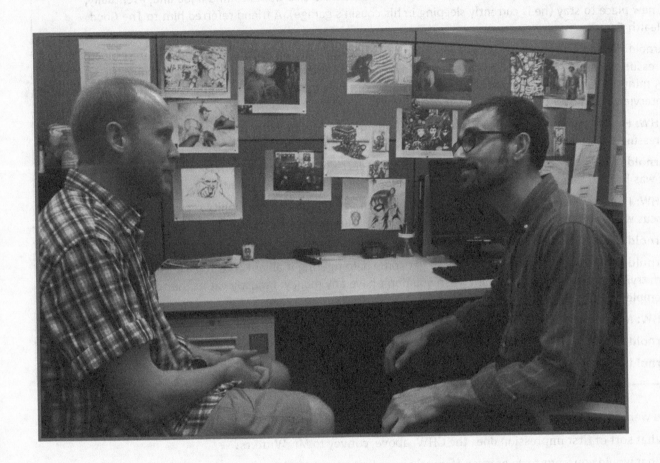

CASE STUDY Arnold

Arnold Winters is 52 years old and was recently released from prison after completing an eight-year sentence related to drug use. During his stay in prison, Arnold developed hypertension (high blood pressure), and it still isn't under control. He didn't receive good health care in prison, and the food and lack of exercise didn't support his health. Arnold wants to make changes in his life: to stay in recovery and to reunite with his family, particularly his children and grandchildren. He also wants to find a job and, eventually, a new place to stay (he is currently sleeping in his cousin's garage). A friend referred him to The Good Health Center.

Arnold fills out a form at The Good Health Center, providing a reason for the visit, and his latest blood pressure readings. The receptionist tells Arnold to take a seat and wait for his name to be called. He is 15 minutes early for his appointment. An hour later, Arnold's name is called, and he is escorted to an interview room by a CHW.

CHW: Hi, I'll be doing your intake today to see if you qualify for our services. I see here that your blood pressure has been really high. How did you let it get so out of control?

Arnold: Well … . (Arnold pauses). I guess the biggest factor was being in prison for the past eight years. It was hard to take care of myself there, and the health care wasn't so good either.

CHW: I understand, but our philosophy is that we each need to take responsibility for our own health. Our focus will be on what *you* can do to get your blood pressure under control.

Arnold (*thinks*): The only way you can *understand* is if you've been in prison. Have you been in prison?

Arnold: Well, I guess that's why I came, to get some help figuring it all out. I've started exercising, and I'm trying to eat good, but it's hard when you don't have any money. I mostly eat at the soup kitchen at Temple Church.

CHW: Maybe I could put you in Keith's group. He's another one of our clients and he's also an "ex-con."

Arnold (*thinks*): Here we go again with the "ex-convict" label. That isn't who I am!

Arnold: Okay.

If you were the CHW who is working with Arnold Winters, how would you answer the following questions?

- What sort of first impression does the CHW, above, convey to Mr. Winters?
- What would you want to do or say differently in order to greet Mr. Winters and to conduct the initial client interview?
- How will you explain your organization's confidentiality policies?
- How will you gather and document key information from Mr. Winters?
- How will you acknowledge the resources and strengths that Mr. Winters already has?
- How will end the initial interview?

Introduction

Think about a time when you have been a new client or patient at a clinic, hospital, or social-services agency. What was your initial interview like? How did you feel during the interview, and how did you feel about the clinic or agency afterward? What did the person who was interviewing you say or do to make the interview more (or less) comfortable and effective for you?

This chapter addresses how to conduct an initial interview with a new client who may be interested in participating in a particular program, service, or research study. These interviews are often the first contact that a client has with an agency, and the CHW's first opportunity to develop a positive connection or rapport with that individual or family. *These initial client interviews may also be referred to as an intake or assessment.* For the purposes of this chapter, we will focus on conducting initial interviews to determine eligibility and participation in a particular health-focused program or service. Guidelines for conducting research interviews tend to be much more extensive and strict, and the format, questions, and policies for research interviews vary widely. If you are hired to conduct research interviews, you will be trained to follow detailed procedures.

Our approach to client interviewing is informed by the guiding principles covered in Chapter 7. Our goal is to prepare you to conduct an ethical, client-centered interview that stays within the scope of practice for CHWs.

WHAT YOU WILL LEARN

By studying the information in this chapter, you will be able to:

- Describe the types of initial client interviews that CHWs are likely to conduct
- Explain confidentiality policies to a client
- Demonstrate how to obtain informed consent for an interview
- Discuss and demonstrate how to build rapport with a new client
- Conduct a client-centered interview, including the use of open and closed-ended questions
- Explain the value of the strength-based approach, and demonstrate how to conduct a strength-based assessment
- Explain the importance of documentation and specific strategies for taking notes during an interview
- Close an initial interview effectively

WORDS TO KNOW

Body Language

Closed-Ended Question

Open-Ended Question

8.1 An Overview of Initial Client Interviews

In general, CHWs conduct initial interviews with new clients in order to:

- Assess and determine whether the client is eligible for and interested in participating in the services provided by a particular agency or program
- Complete an initial assessment of the client's resources, risks, and priority concerns
- Obtain informed consent for participation in a research study, and in some cases, to initiate the research interview

The questions that you will ask, the length of the interview, and the forms used to document information about the client will vary depending on the purpose of the interview and the type of program or service that the client is interested in. Initial interviews may be fairly simple or very complex, and may consist of 10 to 50 or more questions. Some interviews are conducted in one session lasting 15 to 45 minutes or longer, and others take place during more than one session. The longest interview forms and most complicated procedures are used by research studies that may be conducted over multiple sessions.

During an initial interview, you will gather a range of information from the client. You will probably ask for basic demographic data such as date of birth, gender, gender identity, ethnicity, primary languages, address, income, and family status. This demographic information is sometimes sensitive in nature, and we will offer suggestions about how and when to gather it. You may also ask questions about the client's health status, including questions about their knowledge, attitudes, and behaviors in relation to a specific health condition or concern such as diabetes, hepatitis C, or a type of cancer. Interviews may also include questions about the client's support system; prior experience with similar programs and agencies; the client's current condition and concerns; and the client's expectations regarding the program or service your organization offers.

The type of questions you ask during initial interviews will vary depending on the program you are working for and the specific health issues you are addressing. The questions asked by CHWs working with a domestic violence agency will be different from those working for a perinatal health, drug counseling, diabetes management, or mental health program. Some questions may be highly personal in nature. For example, interviews regarding clients' risks for HIV disease typically include questions regarding their history of drug use and sexual behaviors.

You will use a form or forms, provided by your employer, to document the information that you learn from the client. Suggestions for how to document the interview are provided toward the end of this chapter.

Initial interviews or assessments may be stressful for a client. They may be worried that they or their family members won't qualify for services. They may have been mistreated or disrespected by health or social services providers in the past, and be worried about being judged by the interviewer. Clients may have engaged in activities that are illegal, such as drug use or prostitution, and be worried about whether telling you about such activities will be held against them. Undocumented immigrants may be worried about their security and the possibility that they will be reported to immigration authorities.

Can you think of other concerns or sources of anxiety for new clients?

CASE STUDY   **Arnold** (*continued*)

- For example, what might contribute to Arnold's stress as he prepares for his interview at The Good Health Center?
- What might he be hoping for?
- What might Arnold be worried about?
- What experiences might he have had before, at other agencies or clinics, including in prison?

Primary goals for conducting an initial client interview include:

- Welcome the client to the agency, and make the person as comfortable as possible during the interview process
- Build a positive initial connection
- Describe and explain the interview process and related services that the client may be eligible for
- Explain confidentiality and its limits
- Obtain informed consent from the client in order to conduct the interview, and in order to decide whether to participate in a particular program
- Assess not only the client's risk factors, but also the internal and external resources that promote their health
- Listen and respond to the client's questions and concerns
- Provide guidance and support to the client in making decisions about their next steps including whether to enroll in specific programs or research studies

What other goals might you have when you conduct an initial client interview?

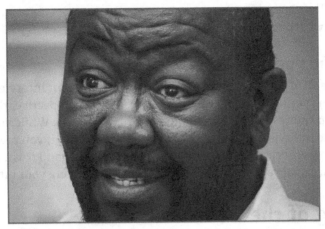

CHWs are often the first member of a team to welcome a client to a new program or agency.

A REMINDER ABOUT SCOPE OF PRACTICE

Your scope of practice (see Chapter 7) may limit the type of questions you ask and the type of information you gather during an interview. For example, when CHWs conduct a client interview at a hospital or health center, medical providers will assess medical conditions, such as hypertension or diabetes. In this context, the role of the CHW is to work in partnership with medical providers who will be responsible for diagnosing medical conditions and prescribing treatment. When working as part of a team, be sure to clarify your role and scope of practice with your supervisor and your teammates.

THE STRUCTURE OF A CLIENT INTERVIEW

A client interview, like a good story, has a distinct beginning, middle, and end.

The **beginning** of the client interview is likely to include:

- Welcoming the client and assisting the person to feel as comfortable as possible
- Introducing yourself, your agency and program, and the purpose of the interview
- Explaining the interview process and the types of information that you hope to learn
- Explaining confidentiality and its limits
- Obtaining informed consent to conduct the interview and initiate services
- Building rapport

The **middle phase** of the interview generally includes:

- Gathering detailed information from the client required in order to determine eligibility for the health program, service, or research study
- Answering the client's questions and concerns
- Assessing the client's risk factors, as well as the internal and external resources they bring to the task of improving their health
- Building rapport

The **ending phase** of the interview generally includes:

- Determining enrollment or participation in the program or service in question
- Providing other referrals, as appropriate
- Identifying the next steps for the client (such as scheduling a follow-up appointment)

- Asking if the client still has any outstanding questions or concerns
- Continuing to build rapport
- Closing the interview in a way that affirms and respects the client

JUGGLING ALL THE ELEMENTS OF THE INTERVIEW

It can be challenging to juggle all of the essential elements of an initial client interview. You have a lot to accomplish in a relatively short period of time. From a client-centered perspective, the most important thing about the interview is to listen and respond to the client's priority concerns. While you may feel pressure from your employer to complete the interview and all of the required paperwork, if you pressure the client to answer your questions and respond to your priorities, you may undermine rapport and trust. Be patient with the client and yourself. If necessary, you can always schedule another time to complete your intake questions and forms.

8.2 The Beginning of the Interview

In most, but not all cases, the interview will serve as your first interaction with a prospective client. It may also be the client's first interaction with anyone from the agency you work for. Making a positive first impression is important to conducting a productive interview. It is the first step toward establishing an ongoing working relationship, and it increases the chances that the client will return to the agency to participate in the services you provide.

- *What makes you feel comfortable and welcomed when you go to a new agency for services?*

What Do YOU Think?

CASE STUDY   **Arnold** (*continued*)

Do you think Arnold felt comfortable with the CHW who interviewed him?

Do you think Arnold would trust the CHW to support him to reach his health goals?

Is Arnold likely to recommend The Good Health Center to others?

Please view the following video [▶] interview about the importance of providing a new client with a warm welcome.

What else do you want to do or say to welcome a new client to the program or agency you work for?

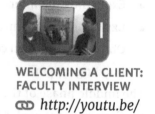
WELCOMING A CLIENT: FACULTY INTERVIEW
⚭ *http://youtu.be/ iQrImzhjAIs*

BUILDING A POSITIVE CONNECTION OR RAPPORT

Your success as a CHW will be influenced by your ability to create and maintain a positive, trusting relationship with clients. While trust will largely be based on the quality of services that you and your organization provide, it will also depend on how clients feel treated by you and by others who deliver services. Your own style or approach also contributes to building a trusting professional relationship. This personal style may include, for example, your tone of voice, your smile and sense of humor, and how you listen to clients and acknowledge their accomplishments and their challenges. Never fake your approach or style of working with clients: be true to your own experience, values, and personality.

Some of the clients you work with will have personal histories that include abuse, violence, discrimination, homelessness, addiction, and incarceration. Many clients have also had bad experiences with helping professionals that may influence their interactions with you. Some clients will observe you closely to see if you are going to be yet another person who in some way disappoints or disrespects them. While you can't do anything to change the past, you can treat all clients with respect and dignity and work to build a professional alliance that supports their health. We cannot emphasize enough the vital importance of building a warm and respectful relationship with your clients: It is the foundation for all the work that you will do together.

THE INTERVIEW SPACE

Not all client interviews take place in a quiet, comfortable, and private room. Often, the interviews will take place in the middle of waiting rooms, in homes, in shelters—or even outside, on the street or in a park. No matter where the interview takes place, you can find ways to make the best of a less-than-private situation to assist the client to feel safe and comfortable.

If you are working in a setting that is not ideal for conducting an interview, acknowledge this and ask the client to aid you in determining the best location for your conversation. For example, if you meet a client in a public space, such as a park, you might say:

> "How about sitting down together on that bench over there in the corner: It seems a little less noisy and more private. Would that work for you? Do you have another suggestion for where we can talk?"

If you have access to an office for conducting interviews, think about what you can do with the materials and budget at hand to make it as inviting as possible. Does the office have a comfortable chair for clients? Can you decorate the space? Is there a place for a client's children to sit and play while you conduct an interview? Can you purchase or seek donations of children's books or toys? Can you offer clients a glass of water, a cup of tea, or a snack? This attention to detail can be meaningful in conveying your commitment and concern for clients and your work. Seating arrangements are also important to consider. For example, asking a client to sit on the other side of your imposing desk may create a feeling of formality and distance that could get in the way of building rapport or connection. Sitting next to a client during an interview may create a more relaxed atmosphere and allow the information you write down to be shared. Think about the options available to you, and talk with colleagues about how they set up their interview space.

- *What kind of office makes you feel most comfortable?*

- *How would you decorate an office—with very little money—where you conduct client interviews?*

- *How would you handle the interview space when doing street outreach?*

INTRODUCING YOURSELF

You may have noticed that Arnold was never properly introduced to the CHW he met with. Please remember to introduce yourself to your clients: tell them your name, job title (if this is the first meeting), what you will cover during your meeting, and how you would like to be addressed. For example:

> "Hi, it's a pleasure to meet you. My name is Lucy Chang, and I'm a community health worker here at the clinic. I'll be talking with you today about our asthma management program. Please call me Lucy."

Sometimes people try to use a "professional" tone of voice that may seem impersonal, cold, or robotic to a client. We encourage you to be yourself, and to welcome a new client like you would a visitor to your home. Smile. Reach out to shake hands if appropriate. Use a warm and friendly tone of voice.

Greet the client, and if you know it, call them by name—it may be written down in an appointment book. In clinic or agency settings, it generally conveys respect to address clients by their last names—Mr. Dorman, Ms. Lee, Mrs. Ramaya—until or unless they ask you to address them differently. If the client is using a different name from the one you have written on the appointment form, clarify which name they would like to use in the documents you prepare and what name they would like to be called by. If you are ever unclear as to how to address new clients, ask them how they would like to be addressed.

> "Good morning, Mrs. Sanchez, how are you today? Should I call you Mrs. Sanchez, or do you prefer to be called by a different name?"

By asking the clients to tell you the name they would like to be called, you are demonstrating respect and flexibility, and your willingness to take their guidance. This sets a positive tone for a client-centered interview.

DETERMINE THE LANGUAGE OF SERVICE

You may be conducting an interview in English, American Sign Language, Farsi, Cantonese, or another language. Be sure to ask clients what their primary language is. You may need to provide them with an interpreter, if available, or find someone who speaks their language to conduct the interview. Don't proceed with the interview if you are not truly fluent in the language of service. This is essential so that no mistakes are made that could be harmful to the client's health or welfare.

ASK CLIENTS WHAT THEY WANT TO ACHIEVE

A good way to begin an interview is to ask some version of: "What brings you here today?" This gives clients an opportunity to share what they hope to get out of the meeting. It also conveys your interest in the client's priority concerns.

EXPLAIN THE INTERVIEW

Let the client know what to expect from the initial interview, by clearly explaining:

- The purpose of the interview
- How long the interview may take
- The type of information you will ask them for
- How this information will be used

You will speak more at the beginning of the interview, and should take time to explain the interview process. You will also explain confidentiality and obtain informed consent. For example, you might say something like:

> *"I understand that your daughter Christa has asthma. I'm here to talk with you about her asthma and to see how we might work together to improve her health. This first meeting will take about half an hour. Do you have that much time today?"*

(Assuming the client is prepared to spend half an hour with the CHW, continue . . .)

> *"I have a number of questions to ask about Christa and your family. The questions are about her symptoms, any medication she may be using, problems that she and you may be facing that influence her health—things like that. If I ask you a question that you would prefer not to talk about, please let me know, and I promise to respect your wishes."*

(Client responds.)

> *"You will see me writing down the information that you tell me on this client intake form. (Show the client the form, even if they are unable to read.) At the end of the interview, we can decide together whether our Pediatric Asthma Program would be a good fit for Christa and your family.*
>
> *If you do decide to participate in the program, the information I document will be placed in a file to be shared with your service provider. Do you have any questions about the interview before we begin?"*

EXPLAIN THE CONFIDENTIALITY POLICY

Confidentiality was introduced in Chapter 7, as one of the most important ethical obligations for CHWs. Part of this obligation is learning how to clearly explain confidentiality and its limits to your clients. You must do this at the beginning of your first session or interview with new clients, before they have an opportunity to tell you something that you may have to report to others. Check with your supervisor to be sure that you understand the confidentiality policy and protocols at your agency.

The Health Insurance Portability and Accountability Act (HIPAA)

If you work in a health care setting, every new client or patient will be asked to read and sign a Health Insurance Portability and Accountability Act (HIPAA) form. HIPAA is a federal law that requires the protection and confidential handling of health information. To learn more about HIPAA, please search online or see the resource from the U.S. Department of Health and Human Services provided at the end of this chapter.

Telling a family that an interview is confidential is not sufficient. Clearly explain what confidentiality means. Tell the client who will have access to the information you document.

While in general you are able to promise that the client's information will be kept private, there are important exceptions to this rule. For example, if you learn that any of your clients have harmed or are intending to do harm to themselves or others, or have been harmed by others, you have a duty to report this information. The harms that we refer to include suicide, child abuse, sexual abuse, physical assault, or threats.

Earlier, we suggested that when you welcome a new client, you ask: "What brings you to the clinic today?" However, if clients start to talk about a subject that you may need to report to legal authorities, we suggest that you interrupt them and take time to clearly explain the limits of confidentiality. If you don't explain this up front, and a client discloses a situation that you have a legal and ethical obligation to report, it is likely that the client may feel set up or betrayed. This is likely to destroy all hope of establishing trust.

The CHW might say something such as:

> *"I want to hear more about your daughter's asthma. But before we start to talk about that in greater detail, I need to explain our policy on confidentiality."*

> *"Everything that you tell me will be kept private. It will go into your client file here at the clinic. Only your service providers here, including the nurse practitioner, respiratory therapist, and community health worker will have access to the information in your file. They will not share this information with other service providers unless they talk with you first, and you sign a form giving them permission to share this information with others."*

Take your time. Don't rush this. Maintain eye contact and a friendly tone of voice. Pay attention to your client's body language and signs that the person may not understand you.

> *"However, there are a couple of exceptions to this policy that I need to discuss with every new client. If a client ever tells me that they are harming themselves or others or are being hurt by someone else, then by law I have to tell my supervisor, and they may have to tell law enforcement authorities. By hurting themselves or others we mean things like sexual or physical abuse or suicide. As a health worker, if I learn that someone is in danger, I can't keep silent. Do you understand these guidelines? Do you have any questions about the privacy of what we talk about today?"*

If you doubt that clients fully understand you, ask them to tell you what they understand about the privacy or confidentiality policy. This is the best way to be certain that you have been clear. For more information about confidentiality and ethics, please refer to Chapter 7 and, most important, remember to share any questions or concerns you may have with your supervisor.

How would you explain the concept of confidentiality to a client?

Please view the following video ▶ that shows a CHW talking with a new client about confidentiality.

CONFIDENTIALITY: ROLE PLAY, DEMO

⌘ *http://youtu.be/odhxp7ILWfc*

- What did the CHW do well in terms of explaining confidentiality to the client?
- What else would you want to say when explaining confidentiality to a new client?

OBTAIN INFORMED CONSENT

Before you conduct an interview or provide services to a client, you need to obtain the client's informed consent. Informed consent means that the client understands what the interview or service will consist of, and gives permission to participate in the interview or program in question. Generally, the client is asked to give informed consent in writing.

The biggest mistake a CHW can make is to rush this process. Sometimes clients are told to: *"Sign your name here so that we can do the interview [or before you start the program]."* This is *not* informed consent! In order to be certain that clients understand what the interview will consist of, explain it to them in simple language, then ask them to tell you what they have learned. *"Mrs. Sanchez, I want to be sure that you understand what this interview is all about before I start. Can you tell me what we will talk about and how the information will be used?"*

If the client does not fully understand what the interview will consist of (the types of questions you will ask, how the information will be used, and the limits of confidentiality), review the information again. Check to see if they have any questions or concerns: *"I don't want to rush you. Before we begin the interview, do you have any questions for me?"*

Note: Review your agency's policies about informed consent. Depending on the program you work for, there may be an age of consent for minors and guidelines for working with people who are developmentally disabled or mentally ill. In some instances, a parent or legal guardian must be consulted. People who are noticeably drunk or high on drugs cannot provide consent for services.

BE AWARE OF BODY LANGUAGE AND TONE OF VOICE

We communicate not only with words, but also through body language and tone of voice. Our facial expressions, how close we sit to others, how we hold our body and our arms, and the degree of eye contact we maintain often convey important messages about what we are thinking or feeling. The tone of our voice also tends to change with emotion and may invite connection or create distance. Try to build an awareness of the tone of voice and body language that you and your clients use.

Be cautious, however, about assuming that you understand what is meant by a particular physical expression such as avoiding eye contact, crossing arms over the chest, frowning, or rolling the eyes. Body language is influenced by cultural as well as individual differences. With experience, you will become more skilled in noticing the body language of others, and as appropriate, talking with your clients about them. For example: *"I notice that whenever you talk about residential treatment, your expression seems to change. I wonder what you are feeling when we talk about this. Is there anything else you would like to say about residential treatment programs?"* Remember that many people are unaware of their body language. Don't push clients to talk further about this, or anything else, if they don't want to.

- *How might your tone of voice and body language work to build a connection with clients?*

- *How might it get in the way of building a connection?*

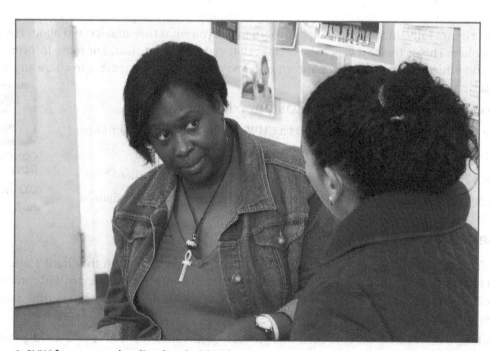

A CHW focuses on the client's priorities.

Please view the following videos, 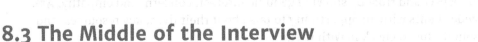 which show a CHW talking with a client. In the first counter role play video, the CHW does not do a good job of communicating with body language. In the second video, the CHW does a much better job.

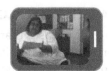

COMMUNICATING WITH BODY LANGUAGE: ROLE PLAY, COUNTER

🔗 *http://youtu.be/ DbsgG-LObPE*

- What mistakes did the CHW make in the first video in terms of communicating with body language? How may the CHWs behavior have impacted the client?

- What did the CHW do differently in the demo role play video?

- What would you do differently if you were the CHW working with this client? How do you use body language to communicate with the clients you work with?

COMMUNICATING WITH BODY LANGUAGE: ROLE PLAY, DEMO

🔗 *http://youtu.be/ WDV2OPRzfYo*

8.3 The Middle of the Interview

The middle of the interview is when you gather and provide information that will assist you and clients in determining whether they should participate in a particular health program or service.

> **Phuong An Doan Billings:** I try to understand people who come to us with a lot of problems. Sometimes they don't say all that's going on for them. When the doctors ask them, "How you feel today? How are you?" they'll say, "I'm good," but there's a lot inside that they cannot say. But because we CHWs are one of them, we are community people, and we use our client-centered skills. They can confide in us. They can tell us how they really feel.

LISTEN TO AND FOCUS ON THE CLIENT

Gathering the right information is an important part of providing quality services to clients. However, you don't have to be rigid in the way you gather information. Your focus should be on the client or family in front of you rather than on the form waiting to be filled out. Ask the questions on the form and document what you learn as the conversation flows. Maintain eye contact periodically even while taking notes, and be sure to explain why you are taking notes. For example, *"I want to make sure I accurately record the information you share with me."*

> **TG:** The forms are not the most important part of the interview. I want to make sure my families are doing okay. I check in with them first, and we talk. Most of the time, I get all the information I need by just talking with them. No one wants to be grilled with question after question.

Before you begin an initial interview, carefully review the forms your organization uses for assumptions that could make someone uncomfortable, such as assumptions about gender, gender identity, or who makes a family. If the forms you have been asked to use are biased, talk with your supervisor. When you are working with your clients, practice cultural humility. Frame your questions in ways that respect all kinds of individuals, and all kinds of families. Asking a client to tell you about their family, for example, is preferable to asking: "Are you married or single?"

USE LANGUAGE THAT IS ACCESSIBLE TO THE CLIENT

If you use words or phrases that a client doesn't understand, you will undermine your ability to conduct an effective interview. Similarly, if you present detailed information that a client already understands, you may also undermine rapport. A good way to start is to ask clients what they already know about a topic. For example: *"Can you tell me what you already know about mammograms?"* or *"Can you tell me what you remember about the HIV antibody test?"* If you use medical terms, such as mammogram, sputum, or antibody test, be sure to explain them using everyday language. Try to avoid using acronyms (initials or words made out of initials, like SSI or WIC), at least until you have first spelled them out and explained them (Social Security Income; Women, Infants, and Children). As you talk with clients, periodically check in to see whether they understand, by asking them to explain the information to you.

DEMONSTRATE YOUR CONCERN FOR THE CLIENT

Create an atmosphere of mutual respect and trust by showing genuine interest, concern, and empathy. Ask open-ended questions that provide clients with an opportunity to talk about their lives, key resources, and priority concerns. If the client sounds upset, check in with them:

> *"It sounds like you are upset. Do you want to take a break before we move on?"*

or

> *"It sounds like you had a really bad experience at the emergency room. It can be difficult to see your child so sick and not be able to do anything about it. Let's try to figure out what happened, and what can be done to prevent this from happening in the future."*

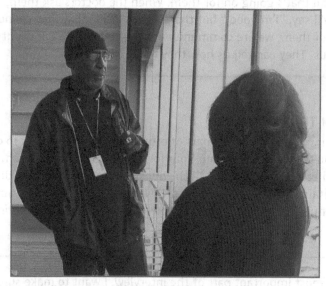

A CHW listens as a client shares her concerns.

GATHER DEMOGRAPHIC INFORMATION

The demographic information that you will document (information such as date of birth, nationality, ethnicity, sex, gender identity, family status, address, income, health insurance, and so on) can be highly sensitive. It can be awkward to ask for this type of information: It isn't something that you would ordinarily ask someone. For these reasons, we suggest that you don't start an interview by asking for demographic information. Even though these questions tend to be placed at the very beginning of the forms you use, you may want to leave them until later in the interview, after you have established a connection with the client. You could also ask clients to fill out the information themselves and then review it together (although keep in mind that not all of your clients will be able to read or write). As always, be respectful of the client's right not to answer any of the questions that you ask.

Francis Julian Montgomery: I know I am asking for a lot of personal information during an intake or assessment, so I try to make it more of a dialogue instead of an interrogation. I don't just read questions off of an intake list. I want to create a natural conversation, and I make sure to listen because clients will often tell me things in response to one question that fills in answers to other questions as well.

TIME MANAGEMENT

Part of your job is to juggle providing client-centered services with the need to complete the interview questions, all within the time frame that you and the client have allotted for your meeting. With practice, you will learn to listen to your client and to be aware of the time that remains in your session. If you scheduled 40 minutes, are you on track to finish the interview on time? Would it be possible to finish on time without unduly interrupting the client's agenda or damaging your rapport? If so, call this to the client's attention and make this decision together: *"Arnold, I don't mean to interrupt, but we have about 15 minutes left, and I think we can complete the intake form in that time. Should we move on to the next set of questions?"*

Sometimes, however, priority issues may emerge for the client during the course of the interview, and these are the most important issues for you to address in the moment. If and when this occurs, acknowledge this to the client. *"Arnold, we have about 15 minutes left, and I'd like to keep talking with you about your family. Is it okay if we schedule another meeting time to complete the interview form?"*

RESPECT YOUR CLIENT'S RIGHT TO PRIVACY

While it is your job to ask questions, clients have a right to decide what information they will and won't share with you. This is especially true with questions about immigration, welfare, substance use, sexuality, traumatic experiences, and any issue that may have legal consequences that may range from loss of housing to deportation. Even if you maintain confidentiality about such issues, the fears of your clients need to be respected. If you ask a sensitive question and you sense that the client is uncomfortable, move on—don't try to push or force an answer.

> *"These questions can be difficult to talk about. I don't want to push you to talk about anything that you may not want to discuss with me. Would you like to move on to the next question?"*

ASSESSING CLIENT RESOURCES: A STRENGTH-BASED APPROACH

You will be asked to assess clients' health risks and current needs including, for example, their needs for housing, legal assistance, mental health counseling, and health education. The forms will guide you in asking these questions.

However, helping professionals often focus primarily or exclusively on a client's problems, including what they have or haven't done that may increase their risks for disease or disability. In contrast, a client-centered approach also emphasizes the positive accomplishments, resources, and attributes of clients and communities. Every client has done something positive to promote their own health and wellness or that of their family.

When working with clients, guide them in assessing both external and internal resources that promote their health and wellness. External resources are sometimes easier for CHWs and clients to talk about. These are resources that lie outside of the individual and may include, for example, family and friends, spiritual or religious community, cultural traditions, employment, a safe home, health insurance coverage, or a skilled medical provider. Internal resources are unique to each individual and include, for example, life accomplishments, knowledge and skills, a sense of humor, spiritual or religious faith, intelligence, creativity, integrity, the ability to be a good friend, commitment to family, vocational skills, or the ability to survive difficult life challenges. For more information about external and internal resources, please refer to Chapter 12.

These strengths are often the most important resources that a client has for making changes in their life to promote their health. Every client you will work with has both external and internal resources, though, at times, it may be difficult for the client or the CHW to see these resources.

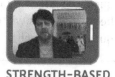

STRENGTH-BASED PRACTICE: FACULTY INTERVIEW

🔗 *http://youtu.be/ Cq4PX89tlZE*

Please view the following video ▶ interview about the advantages of working with clients from a strength-based perspective.

- Why else is a strength-based approach important for working with clients?
- What else do you want to do or say as a CHW to identify and build upon a client's resources and strengths?

Acknowledging a Client's Strengths

During a class at City College of San Francisco, a CHW student raised her hand to say: "All this stuff about resources sounds good in theory, but I'm working with homeless heroin addicts. I'm working with one man who has been out on the streets for almost 10 years. I don't think he has any of these resources!" In response, the other students in class validated her experience ("sometimes it is really hard to see the positive things"), and offered suggestions for how to move forward with the client. For example, classmates asked:

- "He must have been doing something right just to be able to survive the streets for so long. What has kept your client alive on the streets for almost 10 years?"
- "What do you like about this client?"
- "If he isn't in touch with any of his family, does he have any friends out on the streets?"
- "What else—other than heroin—is important to this client? What else does he really care about?"

As a consequence of this classroom discussion, the student began to view her client in a different way and to understand that he did, indeed, have both internal and external resources. For example, the client had developed strong survival skills from living on the streets for so long. He had a tremendous capacity to be kind to others: no matter how bad he was doing, he always asked how she (the student) was doing. He also had a best friend and they watched out for each other on the street, sharing places to sleep, drugs, and food.

At appropriate points in the interview, ask questions and create opportunities to focus on the client's strengths. There are many ways to do this. For example, ask clients about their past accomplishments, key relationships, their knowledge and skills, and what they most care about and who or what keeps them going. Listen closely to the information they share with you and build upon it in your future work. Remember to inquire about and to document a client's external and internal resources, even if this is not part of your agency's interview form.

Affirm the resources and strengths that you observe in your client (you will read more about this in Chapter 9). For example, you might say something like: *"You mentioned that you quit smoking. That seems like a really big accomplishment to me. What did you learn that you might be able to apply to your current health goals?"* or *"I respect how you have managed to survive. It can take a lot of strength and creativity to keep going after losing so much . . ."* A few kind words can mean a lot to a client who is struggling, and acknowledging a client's strengths often makes it more possible for that person to do so as well. These words have to be authentic, though, and true to the strengths you observe in a client.

Andrew Ciscel: Being client-centered is about forming a collaborative relationship with the person I'm working with. It means that I learn more from them than they learn from me. I use client-centered skills to learn about their life, their challenges and resources. I invite them to bring their whole person to the conversation, and to share what they want to about their life and work, school and family, their health and their living situations. I really want to show my appreciation when clients do this, and to help them to highlight their own strengths. With some clients, so much is happening in their life and it is easy for them to get lost in the difficulties and the problems, and I can help them to also see and really appreciate their strengths. And this makes it easier for them to reflect on the skills that they already have, and to focus on how to use them to move their life forward in the direction they want to go.

One of the key roles for CHWs is to hold onto hope for your clients, even in times when they can't hold it for themselves. Recognizing your clients' strengths and assisting them to draw upon those strengths as you work together should underlie all of your interactions with your clients.

CASE STUDY Arnold (*continued*)

- Think about Arnold, the client introduced at the beginning of the chapter. Based on the information provided, what strengths do you see?
- How would you work with him to identify other strengths?
- What are some of your own internal and external resources?

ASK FOR CLARIFICATION

If you don't fully understand what a client is saying, and are unable to record the information accurately, ask! Sometimes CHWs feel shy about interrupting a client or admitting that they did not understand what a client said. However, it is much worse to pretend to understand when you don't, to miss the opportunity to document important information, or to record misinformation. You might say something like: *"I'm not sure that I fully understood what you told me about Christa's symptoms. Could you tell me again?"* or *"I want to make sure I fully understand what you are saying about the mold in your apartment. Did you say that it was there when you moved in?"*

SUMMARIZE WHAT YOU HAVE HEARD

Depending on the nature of the interview, you may want to review some of what you learned in order to be certain that you are accurately documenting what the client shared with you. For example, you might say something like: *"I just want to make sure that I have documented everything correctly. Your daughter Molly is doing better with her new inhaler, but continues to have difficulty breathing at night. You are going to remove the carpet in her room to see if that makes a difference. Did I get that right?"*

DOES THE CLIENT HAVE QUESTIONS OR CONCERNS?

Check in regularly to see if your clients have questions or concerns, particularly if you sense that they may be confused or upset. Taking the time to address their questions as you go along aids in building trust. Talking about their questions or concerns may also provide you with important information about their lives, health issues, and situations so you can assist them to access relevant programs and services.

ASKING QUESTIONS: SOME EFFECTIVE TECHNIQUES

The key to a good client interview depends not only on the type of question you ask, but also on the ease of the conversation between you and the family member. You want to create a smooth conversation rather than an interrogation. Using a combination of open-ended and closed-ended questions can assist you to accomplish this goal.

Closed-Ended Questions

Closed-ended questions can be answered with a few words, like *yes* or *no*. They are used when you want to focus the conversation and get specific information. Closed-ended questions often start with *is* or *do*.

> *"Do you have your asthma medication?"*

> *"Is your Medicaid enrollment up to date?"*

Open-Ended Questions

Open-ended questions invites the client to respond with more than a *yes* or *no* answer. It encourages people to talk and may facilitate dialogue. Typically, open-ended questions use words such as *what, how, when,* or *would*.

> *"What brings you here today?"*

> *"What medications are you currently using?"*

> *"How did you feel when . . .?"*

> *"What are some the challenges that you are facing in terms of eating a healthier diet?"*

> *"Would you tell me more about that?"*

Questions at the Beginning of the Interview

Asking a broad open-ended question, such as "What brings you into the clinic today?" or "How have things been since we last talked?" or "What would you like to talk about today?" opens up discussion and leaves plenty of room for dialogue. If you start the interview with a closed-ended question, you are setting the direction of the interview and may miss important information that is critical to understanding the situation of the person or family you are interviewing.

The following are two examples of an interview: (1) starting the interview with a closed-ended question, and (2) starting the interview with an open-ended question. The interview is with the Sanchez family and their five-year-old daughter, Christa, who has asthma. Christa's asthma has been under control, and they are here at the clinic for a checkup.

Starting an Interview with a Closed-Ended Question

> *CHW: Hi, are you here for a checkup?*

> *Mrs. Sanchez: Yes.*

> *CHW: Great. Has Christa had any problems with her asthma?*

> *Mrs. Sanchez: No. She's been taking her medicines every day, and there hasn't been a flare-up.*

> *CHW: So is Christa's asthma under control?*

> *Mrs. Sanchez: Yes, it is.*

> *CHW: Good. So I'll see you in four months for a follow-up.*

Starting an Interview with an Open-Ended Question

> *CHW: Hi, how is everyone today?*

> *Mrs. Sanchez: We're okay, I guess. We're here for a checkup.*

CHW: *Great. How have you and Christa been doing since we last talked?*

Mrs. Sanchez: *It's been busy. Christa is starting kindergarten next month, so we're here for her school exam.*

CHW: *Wow. Starting kindergarten, that's exciting. We should probably get an extra spacer for Christa to bring to school and a copy of the asthma action plan for the school nurse.*

Mrs. Sanchez: *Oh, I didn't think of that.*

CHW: *After we talk, I'll get you another spacer and action plan. How have Christa's symptoms been?*

Can you see how starting the interview with an open-ended question enabled the family to disclose information important for Christa's asthma care?

Questions for Gathering Additional Information

There are times when clients will share information that is vague, such as: "Things could be better," or "I wasn't feeling well." To get a more accurate assessment of the issue or problem, you will need to ask an open-ended question.

"*Can you tell me more about . . . ?*"

"*How do you feel when that happens . . . ?*"

"*What else is on your mind . . . ?*"

"*Could you give me an example of . . . ?*"

If clients are being vague, there might be other reasons for this. If you press for more information and they are still resistant, check in and make sure you're not making them uncomfortable. For example: "Would you prefer to move on with the rest of the interview and we can come back to the subject later?"

Questions for a More Accurate Assessment

During initial interviews, you will gather information and assess what will motivate clients to better manage their health. The *who, what, when, where, how,* and *why* series of questions can serve as a guide to aid you in asking questions for a more accurate assessment.

WHO: *Who works with Christa to manage her medications?*

WHAT: *What happened next? What can assist Christa to manage her asthma? What is it that you are most worried about? What else do you think the family can do to aid in preventing Christa's asthma attacks?*

WHEN: *When did the asthma episode occur? When did it begin?*

WHERE: *Where does Christa tend to have the greatest difficulty breathing? Where does Christa seem to do best in terms of her breathing?*

HOW: *How did Christa learn to use her inhaler? (If the child is older than four years or so, ask him or her directly how he/she felt.) How does Christa's asthma impact the rest of the family?*

WHY: *Why do you think that it happened?*

Don't Interrogate!

Avoid the interrogation style of interviewing or asking a series of blunt questions at a relatively fast pace.

"*What's your name?*"

"*Your address?*"

"*Your nationality?*"

"*Your date of birth?*"

"*Why are you here?*"

Asking too many questions too quickly like this can make clients feel uneasy and defensive.

Don't Ask More Than One Question at a Time

Asking several questions at once can be confusing. "When did your daughter first show signs of asthma? Was it before or after the episode on the playground at school? Did your family physician ever notice symptoms or speak to you about asthma?" Ask one question at a time.

Pace Yourself

Building a positive relationship with the client is more important than finishing your intake interview or assessment form. You don't need to ask every question during one interview. When we asked experienced CHWs what is important for new CHWs to understand about client interviewing, they said: "Relax. Make sure the families know that you are there for them, not the forms." They also mentioned to pace the speed of the interview. Slow things down so that families can think about questions before answering. You might say something like: *"Take your time answering these questions."* Or, as appropriate: *"Let's put this interview form aside for a few minutes. Would you like to talk further about (whatever the issue is that seems to be a priority for the client)?"*

An Interview with the Pan Family That Didn't Go Very Well

In the following interview, Greg is a CHW at a neighborhood health center. He is interviewing the Pan family. Their child has chronic asthma.

Greg: Come in and take a seat. [points to two chairs on the other side of desk]

Pan family: [sits down]

Greg: Let's start with the forms, shall we?

Pan family: Okay. [phone rings]

Greg: [interrupts] Hold on a second. Let me get my phone. [turns away, speaking quietly into phone] Hello . . . [has a short conversation with another colleague] I have someone in my office. I'll get back to you later. [turning back to the Pan family] Okay, now where were we? Yes, the forms. We need to fill out these forms before you see the doctor.

Pan family: [silence]

Greg: Okay. Parents' first and last name?

Pan family (mother): Luanne and Charlie Pan.

Greg: Your child's name and age?

Pan family (mother): Mark—he's seven years old.

Greg: So Mark had a bad asthma attack last week?

Pan family: It wasn't that bad, but it scared us.

Greg: [writing in chart] According to parents, asthma attack was not severe.

Pan family: How long do you think this appointment will take? We need to get Mark back to school, and we need to get back to work.

Greg: We can give you a work and school slip, but I need to complete this form for my job.

There are several problems with the interview that Greg conducts with the Pan family. For example:

- Greg never welcomes the Pans or introduces himself.

- Greg doesn't clearly explain the purpose of the interview, or ask the Pan family how much time they can take for the interview.

- Greg takes a phone call during the interview.

  Don't take calls during a session with a client unless it is truly an emergency. Remember that their time is just as valuable as yours.

- Greg documents in Mark's chart that, "According to his parents, Mark's asthma attack wasn't severe."

  Greg didn't ask appropriate open-ended questions to learn detailed information about Mark's attack. He doesn't know what type of asthma attack the Pan family considers to be severe. This is important information to document accurately.

- Finally, Greg dismisses the Pan family's concern about school and work, and tells them that they have to stay and complete the paperwork. He tells them that he needs to complete the forms as part of his job.

  Greg's work duties are not as important as the needs of the clients. This is the Pan family's interview, and their needs should come first.

- *How would you conduct this interview differently?*

8.4 The End of the Interview Process

Don't rush the end of the interview process: this is a time to review questions, concerns, or decisions that the client has made. You don't want to undermine a good interview by rushing the client out the door or leaving the person confused about where to go next.

TIME MANAGEMENT

Toward the end of the interview, check the time remaining to see if it will be possible to complete the interview. You may need to allow time to schedule a follow-up appointment. If you need more time, you may be able to continue the interview for an extra 10 or 15 minutes. Ask the client if this will be possible: *"Arnold, I want to be respectful of your time, and I'd like to finish the interview form. Would you able to stay for an extra 15 minutes today, or would it be better to schedule a follow-up appointment?"*

If you routinely find that you need extra time to complete initial client interviews, in spite of effective time management, you may wish to talk with your agency to see if it is possible to schedule longer appointments.

REVIEW DECISIONS MADE AND NEXT STEPS

The interview may or may not have clarified the client's eligibility and interest in participating in a particular program or service. If decisions have been made, be sure to review them together. If the client has decided to participate in follow-up meetings or services, be sure to provide a written copy of this plan, including when and where to access services, who their contact person or service provider will be, and how best to contact that person.

> *"Okay, Arnold, you clearly qualify for our hypertension management program, and I'm glad that you have decided to enroll. You have an appointment with Samuel tomorrow at 3 P.M. in this same building, and he'll hook you up with all of the services."*

PROVIDE REFERRALS

In some cases, you will offer referrals to clients who have expressed an interest in additional services, such as transitional housing or legal assistance. Review what the referral is for, and provide them with clear information about where to go and who to contact.

> *"Arnold, you said you might be interested in the organization I mentioned, Joining Together. It is a group run by and for formerly incarcerated people. Here is their card. They do advocacy on behalf of formerly incarcerated communities, and they help connect people to educational opportunities, job training programs, and employment. They are located right on Market near 6th Street. I wrote down the name of Sally B. here. I really respect her and the work that she does. Do you have any questions about the referral? Do you think you might check them out?"*

For more information regarding how to make an effective referral, please see Chapter 10.

ASK CLIENTS IF THEY HAVE ANY REMAINING QUESTIONS OR CONCERNS

Check in one last time to see whether clients have any outstanding questions or concerns that they would like to talk about. Even if the answer is no, asking the question communicates your concern for their welfare.

THANK THE CLIENT

Regardless of how the interview went, and whether or not the client ultimately decided to enroll in a particular program or service, the person invested significant time and effort talking with you. Thank them and leave them with an encouraging word. For example:

"Arnold, I am really impressed with your motivation to . . ."

"Arnold, I really appreciate all that you shared with me today. I will be keeping you mind, and I hope that you are able to reconnect with your family in the ways that you talked about."

"I hope you will enjoy the support group we talked about. I know the other participants will benefit a lot from what you have to share. If you can, please let me know how it goes."

PROVIDE YOUR CONTACT INFORMATION

If it is appropriate for clients to contact you in the future, give them your business card and contact information.

"Arnold, here is my card. You can always reach me at this number. Don't hesitate to call me if you think I can be helpful. I won't always be able to get back to you right away, but I promise I'll always call back."

8.5 Documenting Client Interviews

Many CHWs dread the task of documenting their work. They may feel that they spend too much time filling out paperwork, that the forms take their attention and time away from clients. We want you to appreciate why documentation is such an important part of your work.

The primary purpose is to provide information that will be used to guide the delivery of care and services for clients. The information you document may also be used to evaluate services and programs, again with the purpose of improving the quality of services that clients receive. If you can't provide timely, clear, and accurate documentation of the services you provide, including initial client interviews, this could be harmful to the client and to your career.

BECOME FAMILIAR WITH THE FORMS YOU USE

The forms that you use to document client information will vary depending on the nature of the interviews you conduct and the program and agency you work for. A good starting point is to carefully review all the forms that your program uses, not just the ones you are responsible for completing. Next, take all the forms you are responsible for completing and review each question. You should understand all of the terms used, why each question is being asked, how to document a variety of common responses, how the information you document will be used, and how it may impact the health of the client. Talk with a colleague or supervisor to clarify anything that you don't fully understand and couldn't explain to a client. The more familiar you are with the forms, the better you will be able to focus on talking with and listening to clients during an interview without constantly referring to the paperwork.

EXPLAIN THE FORMS TO CLIENTS

Tell your clients that you will be writing down the information they share with you on forms provided by your agency. Depending on the nature of the interview and the literacy level of your clients, you may ask them to fill out part of the form on their own and review it with them later. You might also provide clients with a copy of the form as you conduct the interview.

Take time to clearly explain why you are using forms to document the interview, and how the information will be used in the future. Be prepared for clients to stop you during an interview to ask something like: "Why do you need to know that?" For example, clients may be concerned about why you need to know their Social Security number, or what may happen if they tell you that they are experiencing domestic violence at home. Learn to view these moments as opportunities for deeper engagement with a client. Affirm their right not to answer a particular question. It may or may not be essential for determining their eligibility and participation in services, and you may be able to return to these issues in the future, once trust has been established. Most important, be prepared to honestly and accurately respond to their questions. If you aren't sure, say so, and if possible, find someone who can answer their questions.

Please watch the following video that shows a CHW talking with a client about how and why she will be taking notes during their meeting.

TAKING NOTES: ROLE PLAY, DEMO

http://youtu.be/ yZ6FiTr3O4o

- What did the CHW do well in explaining note taking to the client?
- What else might you want to do and say to a client to help them understand the notes you take during a session?

HOW AND WHEN TO FILL OUT THE FORMS

Sometimes, CHWs think they can interview a client and document the interview later on. We strongly encourage you to fill out the documentation as you talk with clients. This is the best way to ensure that the information you record is accurate. If you wait to fill out the forms until after the interview, you may not remember all that they shared with you, and you may misrepresent important information. You may end up unintentionally harming your clients.

As you document the interview, explain to the client what you are doing. For example: *"Arnold, I'm going to take some notes as we talk. I want to make sure that I keep an accurate record of the information you share with me. Is that all right?"* Documentation doesn't need to get in the way of conducting an effective interview. The more familiar you are with the forms, and the more experience you have, the easier it will become.

> **TG:** I made mistakes in the past by delaying writing up client notes, thinking that I would remember it all. Now I always document client information while we talk. I explain what I'm doing and why I'm doing it. It has never been a problem with a client.

CHW

Most forms ask for specific information: name, address, phone number, medical history, and so on. Some forms, especially those used during home visits, will ask for more descriptive information, such as about conditions in the home. This is where your observation skills will be essential. Some agencies use SOAP notes. SOAP stands for: Subjective, Objective, Assessment, and Plan. Whether or not your agency or clinic uses SOAP notes, it is a good format to use while taking notes. You will learn how to take SOAP notes in Chapter 10, "Care Management."

IF THE FORMS ARE A PROBLEM

We hope you will work with programs that have already developed culturally relevant and inclusive forms that guide you in conducting client-centered interviews and reporting accurate client information. However, some of you will be working with forms that are problematic in different ways. They may not have places to document your client's identity (if they are Arabic, multiracial, lesbian and in a committed relationship, transgender, and so on), or they may have places to document your clients' health-related risks, but not their resources or strengths. Sometimes, forms can be changed, and your input as a CHW will aid in improving them. This isn't always possible, however, particularly when working with standard forms used by city, county, state, or federal government programs. You may, however, be able to write down additional information in the margins of the forms, or create an addendum (additional piece of paper) that can become part of the client's file. If the forms you use pose problems, speak to your colleagues and supervisor to see if you can develop some practical solutions.

Chapter Review

Imagine that you are a CHW at The Good Health Center and are scheduled to meet with Arnold—the 52-year-old client described at the beginning of this chapter—to conduct an initial client interview. You have reviewed the form he filled out, and understand that he is interested in participating in programs and services (such as primary health care, health education, support groups) that will assist him to better control his hypertension (high blood pressure). Based on what you have learned, *and in your own words:*

- How will you welcome Arnold?
- How will you explain the purpose of the interview to him?
- How will you explain confidentiality?
- How will you obtain informed consent from Arnold?
- How will you document the information that Arnold tells you, and how will you explain this process to him?
- What will you do and say to keep the interview client-centered?
- How will you assess Arnold's external and internal resources?
- What open-ended questions might you ask Arnold?
- What will you say when he tells you that he just got out of prison?
- What will you say when he tells you that, more than anything, he wants to rebuild a relationship with his family?
- What types of referrals might you provide to Arnold?
- What will you say to end your interview session with Arnold?

Additional Resources

Community Health Works. (2005). *Managing children's asthma: A community-focused, team approach.* Volume 3: Community Health Worker Manual. Retrieved from *www.communityhealthworks.org*

U.S. Department of Health & Human Services. (n.d.). *Health information privacy.* Retrieved from *www.hhs.gov/ocr/privacy/*

Client-Centered Counseling for Behavior Change

Tim Berthold and Darouny Somsanith

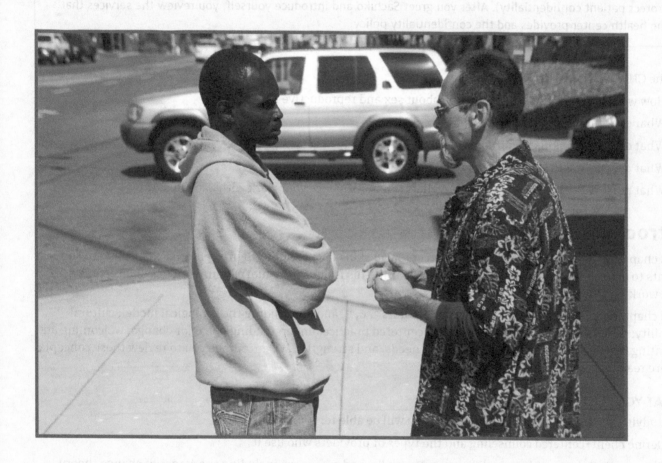

CASE STUDY	Sachiko

You are a CHW who works for a Community Health Center. Your focus is on working with youth and young adults.

Today, you meet a new client named Sachiko. She is 16 years old, and recently started her first sexual relationship with Keith, who is 17. Sachiko is really happy to be with Keith, but is also worried about getting pregnant. Sachiko comes to the clinic to talk about contraception. She is a bit nervous at first, because she has never had to talk about issues like sex or contraception during a health care visit. Sachiko worries that the staff might judge her for having sex.

Sachiko fills out a new patient information form at the front desk and signs a HIPAA form (a policy to protect patient confidentiality). After you greet Sachiko and introduce yourself, you review the services that the health center provides and the confidentiality policy.

As the CHW working with Sachiko:

- How would you support Sachiko to talk about sex and reproductive health?
- What concepts would guide your work?
- What counseling skills would you use?
- What questions will you ask Sachiko?
- What personal experiences, values, or beliefs might influence your work with Sachiko?

Introduction

This chapter provides an introduction to concepts and skills for providing client-centered counseling to support clients to change behaviors and enhance their health. This is one of the most common types of direct services that working CHWs provide.

This chapter builds upon information from Chapters 3, 6, 7, and 8, including the ecological model; cultural humility; ethics and scope of practice; client-centered practice; understanding behavior change; welcoming and orienting clients; and assessing clients' risks, needs, and strengths. We encourage you to review these concepts before reading this chapter.

WHAT YOU WILL LEARN

By studying the information in this chapter, you will be able to:

- Define client-centered counseling and the types of providers who use it
- Discuss client-centered counseling concepts, skills, and resources, including the stages of change theory, action planning, and harm reduction
- Explain key concepts and techniques for motivational interviewing
- Identify common challenges to providing client-centered counseling
- Evaluate your own performance in providing client-centered counseling
- Develop your own professional development plan to enhance your counseling knowledge and skills

WORDS TO KNOW

Ambivalence

Harm Reduction

Relapse and Relapse Prevention

Risk-Reduction Counseling

9.1 An Overview of Client-Centered Counseling

Client-centered counseling is not a unified theory or concept. It draws upon and incorporates a wide variety of theories, models, concepts, and skills including, for example, the work of Carl Rogers, the field of humanistic psychology, and models of client-centered counseling promoted by leading public health organizations such as the Centers for Disease Control and Prevention and the World Health Organization. It includes concepts and models of harm reduction, cultural humility, motivational interviewing, and self-determination theory.

The essential value of client-centered counseling is to honor and enhance the client's autonomy. It emphasizes the experience, ideas, beliefs, and feelings of the client. The role of the client-centered counselor is as a facilitator who supports clients to make changes that promote their health. This approach recognizes that in order for these changes to be most valuable, effective, and long lasting, they must come from the client, not from providers or outside "experts."

Precious Beddell: With client-centered counseling, the client is in the driver's seat. Providers are like the signs along the road that offer compassionate support to help the driver reach their destination. If the driver veers off course, they can consult a CHW or other provider who will always ask if they require support or resources to get back on track to continue their journey.

WHO PROVIDES CLIENT-CENTERED COUNSELING?

Client-centered counseling is provided throughout the world by people with a wide range of training. Some are also mental health clinicians with extensive education, clinical training, and licensure such as psychologists and licensed clinical social workers (LCSW) and marriage and family therapists (MFT). Unlicensed providers also use client-centered counseling to support clients with behavior change and other goals. These unlicensed and front-line providers include CHWs, HIV prevention workers, mental health peer specialists, drug and alcohol counselors, and sexual assault and domestic violence counselors. In some work settings, these unlicensed providers are referred to as "peer counselors" or "informal counselors."

CHWs provide client-centered behavior change counseling in a wide variety of settings including community-based organizations, hospitals, clinics, drug and alcohol counseling programs, and local health departments. CHWs apply client-centered counseling to support clients to change behaviors related to issues such as nutrition and physical activity; HIV disease; mental health challenges; tobacco, alcohol, and drug use; reproductive health; and the management of chronic health conditions such as diabetes, cancer, or hypertension.

SCOPE OF PRACTICE CONCERNS

It is important to distinguish client-centered counseling from therapy. Client-centered counseling is provided by public health and health care professionals of all levels. It is applied to support clients in changing behaviors related to a specific health topic. The emphasis of the work is on *what the client can do now* to achieve a health outcome in the near future (such as within 3–12 months). It does not focus on past issues. In contrast, therapy is provided by licensed mental health professionals with extensive training and the required skills to address more challenging issues, including trauma and crisis. Therapists are qualified and licensed to diagnose mental health conditions and to offer and provide recommendations for treatment.

As we address in Chapters 7, 18 and 21, CHWs who provide client-centered counseling should receive ongoing supervision and regularly consult with colleagues to monitor scope of practice concerns.

When clients face issues that are beyond the CHW's training level, skill, and scope of practice, they should be referred to a colleague with more advanced training and skills such as a physician or licensed mental health professional.

ONGOING PROFESSIONAL DEVELOPMENT

Professional development is a commitment to enhance your knowledge and skills, and your effectiveness in supporting the health of the clients and communities you serve. We strongly encourage you to seek out opportunities to continue to build your client-centered counseling skills over the course of your career. There are many ways to do this. For example, you may ask to shadow or sit in and observe a more experienced colleague as he or she provides client-centered counseling services. Supervision meetings and case conferences are also wonderful opportunities to pose questions, discuss challenges, and to learn from your colleagues. Free training opportunities (generally in exchange for a volunteer commitment from you) may exist in the city or county where you live in areas such as reproductive health counseling and HIV antibody test counseling. Suicide prevention/crisis intervention, domestic violence, and rape crisis centers are also outstanding resources. You will not only receive training in vital areas, and in some cases certification, but will have a chance to practice your skills as a volunteer and receive supervision. Other community-based organizations and community colleges also provide affordable workshops and classes that will enhance your counseling knowledge and skills.

- *What training have you already received in counseling skills?*

- *What educational and training opportunities exist in the area where you live?*

CHARACTERISTICS OF SUCCESSFUL CLIENT-CENTERED COUNSELORS

Your work with clients will be guided by concepts and skills of client-centered counseling. It will also be influenced by the personal qualities that you bring to your work. The following list of qualities and characteristics of successful counselors is adapted from a curriculum designed to train CHWs working to respond to the HIV epidemic in Zimbabwe (International Training and Education Center on HIV [I-TECH], 2004):

- Belief in the wisdom of their clients
- The desire to learn something new from each client and counseling session
- The ability to set aside personal issues, concerns, and beliefs when working with clients
- Cultural humility
- The ability to honor the life experience, feelings, opinions, and values of the client
- Acceptance of their own limitations and mistakes
- A deep commitment not to discriminate against clients on the basis of their identity, beliefs, behavior, or any other reason
- Acceptance of a client's ambivalence to change
- Understanding that resistance to change is natural and common
- The expression of empathy in a visible and authentic manner

- *What qualities or characteristics would you add to this list?*

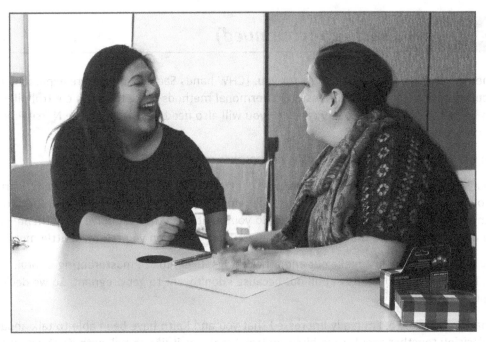

A client connects with a CHW.

9.2 Developing an Action Plan

Client-centered counseling often supports clients to develop an individualized action plan or behavior change plan. The plan clearly identifies the client's health goals, and outlines a set of specific and realistic actions or behaviors to reduce risks and promote health (the format of the action plan is also used when providing care management as discussed in Chapter 10). The first step to developing a plan is to support the client in identifying their current challenges, risks, and needs (see Chapter 8). Next, the client will prioritize these concerns to identity a goal or goals that they can work towards in the next three to six months or so. You will also support the client in identifying their internal and external resources (See Chapter 12), and to discuss how they can build upon resources as they implement their action plan.

Sometimes, you will conduct client-centered counseling with a client who has been referred to your program to address a specific health risk or issue such as prostate cancer, smoking, or pregnancy. At other times, the issues that the client is most concerned about will emerge during the assessment. In the case study, for example, Sachiko comes to the clinic with the goal of preventing pregnancy. As she talks with the CHW, a second goal of preventing sexually transmitted infections (STI) also emerges. The priorities and goals of a behavior change plan are revisited often, and they can always be revised according to the wishes and needs of the client.

CASE STUDY **Sachiko** (*continued*)

CHW: So Sachiko, your main priority is to get some birth control to help prevent pregnancy, is that right?

Sachiko: Yeah, that's the main thing. Do you think I could get something today?

CHW: Well, it may depend on what type of contraceptive method you end up selecting. My role is to tell you about the available methods, their effectiveness and risks, and to help you make an informed choice about

CASE STUDY	Sachiko (*continued*)

which method or methods will work best for you. [CHW hands Sachiko a brochure explaining different contraceptive options] If you are interested in hormonal methods—like the birth control pill—or barrier methods—like the diaphragm or cervical cap—you will also need to meet with the Nurse Practitioner today, and I can refer you.

Sachiko: Okay, I think I'm interested in the pill because some of my friends are on it . . .

CHW: Okay. Before we talk more about the birth control pill and other options, I'd like to learn a little bit more about your current sexual activity. This will help us to provide you with better information about how to prevent pregnancy and protect your health. So you mentioned that you have a boyfriend—is it Keith? [Sachiko nods] And you said that you've been "messin around." Can you tell me a little more about that?

Sachiko: Well, we mostly just make out and other things, like, um . . . masturbating or oral. We started to have sex before but I made him . . . pull out because I don't want to get pregnant. So we decided not to do it until I get on the pill.

CHW: Thanks Sachiko. So, I'm really impressed that you and Keith have been able to talk about this and made a decision together about using birth control. What was it like to talk with Keith about this?

Sachiko: Well, it was a little weird I guess. . . . I mean I've never had sex before so I never really had to talk about it. . . . But, I mean, I really didn't want to get pregnant so that kind of made me say something.

CHW: So you felt good about the conversation with Keith? You were both able to listen and express your concerns?

Sachiko: Yes, I mean, he doesn't want me to get pregnant either. That would. . . . We both knew this girl who got pregnant and she dropped out of school . . .

CHW: I am wondering, have you and Keith talked about using condoms? They are an effective method for reducing the risks for pregnancy and sexually transmitted infections like chlamydia or genital warts. . . .

Sachiko: I asked Keith. I mean, I said that we could have sex with a condom, but he said that he doesn't like them because they don't feel good for the guy. He said that if I got on the pill then we could do it natural and there wouldn't be anything in between us. . . .

CHW: Well the reason that I bring this up is that sexually transmitted infections are really common among young people and hormonal contraception, like the birth control pill, doesn't offer any protection at all for preventing STIs. Can you tell me what you know about STIs?

Sachiko: Well, we had a lecture about them at school, and I've heard of like, herpes, I guess and that chlamydia one, but I guess I didn't think that those infections were a big thing for girls like me?

CHW: Young women are particularly at risk [CHW provides Sachiko with a brochure about STIs]. And some of these sexually transmitted infections can lead to really serious health issues, like HIV disease, and genital warts that can increase risks for cervical cancer. I think it is important for anyone who is sexually active these days to know what the health risks are so that you can decide what you are willing to do to protect your health. Are you open to learn a little more about STIs?

Sachiko: Yeah, I guess that it is just a little . . . overwhelming.

CHW: There is a lot to know and to think about.

CASE STUDY   Sachiko (*continued*)

Sachiko: Yes, a lot more than I guess I wanted to really think about! But, but I'm glad I came. . . .

CHW: I'm really glad that you came too. Is this a good time to talk more about STIs, or would you like to take a break and schedule another time to talk?

Sachiko: [Looks at her watch] No, I mean, I did come here to find out about all this stuff, so let's go ahead and talk about it now. If I want to can I make another time to come back, too?

CHW: Of course. And if you'd like to meet with me again we can make an appointment. And sometimes I meet with couples too. So, if there is ever a time when you and Keith would like to come in and talk together, I'd be happy to do that too, but no pressure okay? [Sachiko smiles] Whatever you decide will be fine with me.

Sachiko: Thanks, I need to think about that. But I'm ready to talk more about the STIs. Can you tell me more about the warts thing that you mentioned, I think I remember my cousin saying something about it. . . .

Each agency you work for is likely to have a slightly different form and structure for developing an action plan (this may be called by different names such as a risk-reduction plan, treatment plan, action plan, health plan, and so forth). Ideally, the form will have a place to clearly document:

- Basic client information (including name, address, date of birth, sex/gender identity, primary language, and so on)
- Primary health risks
- Resource needs, such as mental health counseling, housing, or child care
- Strengths or internal and external resources
- Goals, such as to prevent pregnancy, reduce asthma symptoms, or prevent the further progression of HIV disease
- Actions or steps to reach the goal, such as consistent use of contraception, taking medications as prescribed and directed, eating a healthier diet, or reducing asthma triggers—such as dust, tobacco smoke, or animal dander—in the home.
- Notes or comments about the counseling session (see Chapters 10 and 16)
- Follow-up appointments and referrals

The behavior change plan form may be completed at the beginning of a session, but typically, the client's needs, strengths, and goals are identified over the course of one or more sessions.

TG: You might think you are going to sit down and do this all at once in some logical order—assess risks and resources, come up with goals and a plan. But that isn't how it usually goes, at least for me. Especially when I first meet with clients, I want to follow their lead about what is most important to talk about. I know that if the client decides that they want to keep working with me—that we will develop this plan together, and I will write it down. Like everything, it's a process, and the plan keeps developing. That's a good thing, because new goals or priorities come up, or the client realizes that some of their action steps are just too unrealistic.

CASE STUDY   Sachiko *(continued)*

Sachiko comes to the health center with a clear goal: to prevent pregnancy. She already has elements of a plan worked out as well: she wants to start using birth control pills and to stop having vaginal sex until the pill takes effect.

In talking with the CHW, another goal also emerges: to prevent STIs. Using the client-centered counseling skills presented later on in this chapter, the CHW supports Sachiko to explore her relationship with Keith, her concerns about STIs, and what she is ready to do to prevent infection. The CHW also talks with Sachiko about strengths and needs, including her relationship with her parents and friends, and her other life goals.

The following is a sample behavior change plan that could be developed with Sachiko:

The Community Health Center Action Plan

Client's Name ___(Sachiko Takahashi)_____

Client's Case Number _____

Demographic information (such as date of birth, address, gender identity, ethnicity, primary language)

_____

_____

_____

Health Goals

- To prevent pregnancy and STIs

Health Risks

- Having unprotected vaginal sex and oral sex
- Never used condoms before
- Hesitant to negotiate condom use with partner
- Partner says he doesn't like condoms
- Cannot talk with parents about sexual activity
- Other: _____

Internal Resources

- Wants to prevent pregnancy
- Came to clinic, is willing to talk openly about her health issues and concerns
- Is doing well in high school—wants to go to college
- Other: _____

External Resources

- Has friends she can talk with, including Esther
- Is enrolled in high school
- Has a loving family
- Other: _____

CASE STUDY   Sachiko (*continued*)

Action Plan

- Start using the birth control pill as of today (06/12)
- Stop having vaginal sex until pill is effective
- Get tested for STIs
- Will carry condoms and lubricant with her
- Will try to talk with Keith about condoms and getting tested for STI
- Will consider asking Keith to come to the health center to talk with the counselor together.
- Other: _____

Comments _____

Follow-up meeting scheduled

_____ Yes _____ No When? June 17, 3:30 pm

Referrals Provided _____

Comments: 16-year old girl in first sexual relationship. Nervous at first, but talked openly about her sexual behaviors, relationship, and concerns. Primary concern is pregnancy. Not thinking about STIs when she came to the clinic. Now states she wants to prevent STIs, but is worried that her boyfriend (Keith) doesn't want to use condoms. She is also worried that the relationship will be over if she insists on using condoms. She will talk with her best friend (Esther), and try to talk with Keith about condoms. Have scheduled an appointment for next week. She may invite Keith to come with her.

Follow-up meeting scheduled

_____ Yes _____ No When? _____

Referrals Provided: Sachiko met Nurse Practitioner at the Center for an exam, STI testing, and to get a prescription for birth control pills.

The client and the counselor will revisit the behavior change plan many times over the course of their work together. Goals and actions may be revised according to the progress and needs of the client.

USING A BUBBLE CHART

Bubble charts are a resource to assist a client in identifying options for reducing risks and promoting health. The bubbles may be left completely blank for the client to identify, or may be presented with some options already filled in. The tasks are to identify a wide range of actions that the client can take, and for the client to decide which of these options are best to begin with (Bodenheimer, MacGregor, & Sharifi, 2005).

In the example provided below, the CHW is counseling a client with diabetes (see Figures 9.1 and 9.2). The CHW fills in some of the bubbles and leaves others blank for the client to fill in:

CHW: *Let's talk about what you feel ready to do to better control your diabetes. I have a chart here* [shows chart in Figure 9.1 to client] *that shows some of the actions you might want to take to promote your health, such as checking your blood glucose levels regularly, physical activity or exercising, and eating a healthier diet. Can you think of other things that you could do to mange your diabetes?*

Client: *Well, I guess one thing is to keep coming here and working with you. Another thing is, if I am really going to change my diet I have to talk with my family about it and get some support. We all eat together, and if they can make at least some changes it would really help me to be more successful this time. I've tried before to eat better, but after I while I tend to slip back to old habits.*

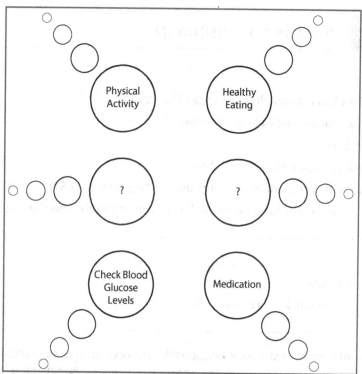

Figure 9.1 Bubble Chart from CHW
Source: Adapted from Bodenheimer & Laing, 2007.

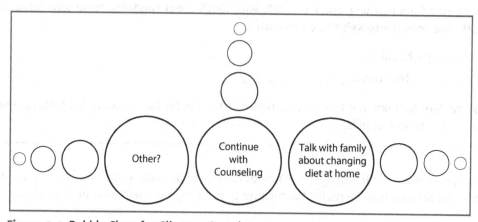

Figure 9.2 Bubble Chart for Client to Complete

CHW: Okay, let's add those to the chart. I think that talking with your family and asking them for support sounds like a really great idea. [writes them in the blank bubbles in Figure 9.2.]

CHW: Which of these options do you want to start talking about? Which seems like the most realistic action for you to start with?

Client: Well, diet is going to be the hardest thing to change. I mean, they're all going to be hard, but . . . can we start with the exercise? But I want to totally honest—I don't really do any exercise now.

CHW: I really appreciate your honesty. That is what this is all about—starting where you are today, and seeing what feels manageable for you to try to do to make a change. So you say that you don't do any physical activity now—but what about walking? How much do you walk in a day or a week?

- *What do you think of the bubble chart?*

- *Would you use it when you are doing client-centered counseling?*

- *How could the CHW use the bubble chart in working with Sachiko?*

9.3 Knowledge and Skills for Client-Centered Counseling

There are a wide range of skills and resources that can be used to conduct client-centerd counseling. The skills you use will depend upon the issues you are addressing, the agency or program you work for, your own level of knowledge and experience, and your scope of practice. With time, you may refine and adapt these skills and develop your own *implicit theories* of behavior change (see Chapter 7). Please refer to the resources provided at the end of this chapter for further study.

HARM-REDUCTION AND RISK-REDUCTION COUNSELING

Harm-reduction and risk-reduction counseling offer useful strategies for client-centered work and are commonly used by CHWs. Harm reduction is a philosophy about life and health, as well as an approach to behavior change that was started by a community of people who inject drugs. This community objected to the "abstinence-only" philosophy that usually guides health and social service providers in working with people who use drugs. The goal of abstinence-based programs and counseling is to support clients to stop using drugs as quickly as possible. Because abstinence-only programs focus only on supporting people to stop using drugs entirely, they offer little or nothing to clients who may not (or may not yet) want to quit using.

Harm Reduction

Harm reduction essentially views any action that will reduce harm to ourselves and to others as valuable and worthy of support. Not everyone will quit smoking, stop drinking sugary soda or eating "fast" food, or stop drinking alcohol completely. However, if they change or reduce their use in some way, they can significantly reduce their health risks. For example, if someone who eats fast food six to eight times a week reduces this to two to three times a week, they can reduce risks for heart disease, diabetes, and other chronic conditions. Injection drug users may reduce their use, start to use in other ways, or limit or stop sharing syringes and works (depending on the drug, this may include cottons and cookers, for example) with others. All of these actions can significantly reduce their risks for HIV, Hepatitis C, and other disease-causing agents that may be carried in human blood.

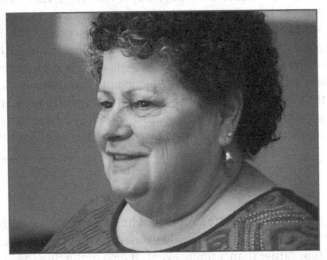

CHWs use client-centered counseling skills to support people in changing behaviors and making changes designed to improve their health and the quality of their lives.

Harm reduction is a highly practical approach to preventing risks and promoting health. Harm reduction recognizes how difficult it can be to stop using drugs and alcohol, and acknowledges that not everyone who uses wants to or is going to stop using immediately or at all. It recognizes people's autonomy, and understands that people will make these sometimes difficult and highly personal decisions for themselves.

Harm reduction remains a controversial philosophy and practice in the United States, particularly in relation to drug use. In countries such as Canada and the United Kingdom, however, governments have developed drug treatment policies guided by harm reduction. Local governments provide injection drug users with clean syringes and, in some cases, with uncontaminated drugs, such as heroin, along with counseling, employment assistance, and other social services. These policies and programs have been shown to dramatically reduce the harms associated with injection drug use, including rates of HIV infection, unemployment, and loss of family and home.

The harm-reduction philosophy and approach can be applied to any number of health-related issues, not just to issues of substance use. For example, it can be used to support clients to reduce health risks for conditions such as diabetes, pneumonia, sexually transmitted diseases, bicycle and driving injuries, depression, or cancer.

- *What do you think about the philosophy and practice of harm reduction?*

- *How does harm reduction apply in your life: what actions do you take that assist you in reducing health risks?*

Risk-Reduction Counseling

Risk-reduction counseling is a form of behavior change counseling based on harm reduction. Clients identify behaviors that place their health at risk, such as unprotected sex. The CHW then assists a client to identity options for reducing these risks by changing behaviors, such as having less sex or different types of sex, using condoms or other safer sex strategies. This is the predominant client-centered approach to HIV prevention throughout the world and promoted by leading public health organizations (Centers for Disease Control and Prevention, 2001; I-TECH, 2004; World Health Organization, 2006).

Increasingly, harm-reduction and risk-reduction counseling are used along with the Stages of Change theory and motivational interviewing (introduced later on in this chapter).

CASE STUDY **Sachiko (*continued*)**

Sachiko could use harm-reduction or risk-reduction strategies in several ways. For example, the most effective way to prevent pregnancy is to not have vaginal sex. However, if Sachiko decides to continue to have vaginal sex, a range of options will help to reduce this ongoing risk. These options include contraception, such as barrier methods (such as a condom, diaphragm, or cervical cap), hormonal methods (birth control pills, patches, or vaginal ring, etc.) and intrauterine methods (IUDs). Sachiko's task is to determine the level of risk that she is comfortable living with and to choose the risk-reduction method that best fits her goals, life style, and comfort level. The task of the counselor is to help her explore these options, understand her level of risk or safety with each method, and make an informed decision. Sachiko will also have to meet with a medical provider before being prescribed a hormonal method, being fitted for a diaphragm, or getting an IUD.

STAGES OF CHANGE THEORY

The Stages of Change theory provides a framework for understanding how people may change behavior (Prochaska, Norcross, & DiClemente, 1999). The model is widely used and describes behavior change as a process that usually involves many steps rather than a single event. It also highlights the fact that behavior change may be marked by both progress and setbacks, including relapse or returning to prior patterns of behavior. The model has been used to understand behavior change related to different health concerns including substance use, HIV/AIDS, nutrition, diabetes, mental health challenges, and other chronic conditions.

The Stages of Change theory (Table 9.1) is often used with motivational interviewing and other counseling skills and techniques. It can guide clients and CHWs in identifying where the client is in terms of their own process of behavior change.

Table 9.1 The Stages of Change

STAGE OF CHANGE	DEFINITION	BEHAVIORAL DESCRIPTION	ROLE OF THE CHW
Precontemplation	The individual is not thinking about the health risks of their current behaviors (such as the risks of unprotected vaginal sex).	The individual is not planning to change within the next six months.	To encourage the client to begin thinking about their risks and possible behavior change.
Contemplation	The individual is thinking about change in the near future (such as trying condoms).	The individual is planning to change within the next six months.	To support the client to begin actively planning steps for changing their behavior.
Preparation	The individual is ready and making a plan to change (for example, has purchased condoms and lube and has planned for how to use them).	The individual is actively preparing to make changes within the next month.	To support the client to develop an individualized and realistic plan for behavior change.
Action	The individual has started making changes (for example, is talking with partners and using condoms and lube for vaginal sex).	The individual has made the change for more than one day and less than six months.	To encourage and support the client to take actions and change behaviors in accordance with their plan.
Maintenance	The individual has committed to the change long term (is practicing safer sex regularly, including use of condoms and lube for vaginal sex).	The individual has maintained this change for more than six months.	To acknowledge and congratulate the client for their success, to support them in maintaining new behaviors, and to prevent relapse to the previous risk behaviors.
Relapse	Individual has "relapsed" to previous patterns and risk behaviors (has had vaginal sex again without using a condom).	Individual found it hard to maintain new behaviors or faced challenges that made it hard to be consistent with the new behavior. May have relapsed due to relationships, trauma, loss, doubt, or any number of factors.	Not to judge the client and to assist them in accepting that relapse is often a normal and anticipated part of the behavior change process. To assist the client in identifying what influenced their relapse, what they have learned, and what they want to do now. To revisit and revise the client's behavior change plan.
Return to precontemplation or action	Behavior change is a complicated process, and people frequently have to keep trying before they are able to maintain new behaviors (uses condoms during next sexual encounter).	As above.	As above, CHWs support clients to continue to think about and take actions to reduce health risks.

TG: Stages of Change—yeah, the stages of change is useful because the whole belief of harm-reduction and client-centered counseling is that you have to meet the client where they are. The Stages of Change method helps me to understand where the client is so that we can build from there.

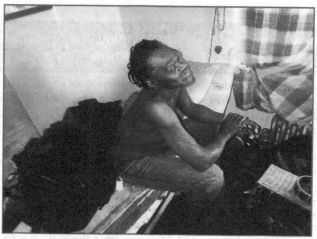

When they first met, the client was very sick with HIV disease. He had lost a lot of weight, and didn't have much hope for the future.

CASE STUDY   Sachiko *(continued)*

Sachiko is at the Preparation stage in terms of preventing an unplanned pregnancy. She is concerned about getting pregnant, thinking about it, and comes to the health center to ask about using the birth control pill.

However, when she first came to the health center Sachiko wasn't thinking about STIs: she said: *"I guess I didn't think that those infections were a big thing for girls like me?"* In terms of STI prevention, Sachiko was in the Precontemplation stage.

Once the CHW began to talk with her about STIs, Sachiko moved to the Contemplation stage. She began to think about and to talk about her risks for STIs. She agreed to talk more about STIs and stated: *"I'm ready to talk more about the STIs. Can you tell me more about the warts thing that you mentioned, I think I remember my cousin saying something about it."*

- *What do you think about the Stages of Change model?*

- *Does it seem like an accurate description of your own experiences with behavior change?*

- *Is there a behavior you are currently trying to change? If so, where are you on the Stages of Change?*

What Do YOU Think?

RELAPSE PREVENTION

As discussed above and in Chapter 7, relapse is a common and natural part of the behavior change process. **Relapse** means returning to the prior behavior that the client has been trying to change. For example, a client may relapse and start to drink alcohol again, stop exercising, skip their medications, have sex without a condom, or return to eating a less healthful diet.

Relapse prevention is working with clients to help them anticipate and prevent relapse, as well as to plan for how they may recover from a relapse. We recommend talking with clients about relapse as a common part of the behavior change process. This helps to "normalize" relapse and may support clients to feel more comfortable talking about it if they do relapse. For example a CHW might ask: "What may be your risk factors for relapse? What could make you more vulnerable to returning to _____ (the behavior they are trying change)?"

As a CHW, you can also help clients to anticipate the possibility of relapse and to come up with plan for what to do next. For example, you could ask the client: "What would like to do if you do relapse? How would you like to handle this?" This provides the client with an opportunity to come up with a plan that may help them to recover from a relapse more quickly and to either resume or revise their behavior change plan.

Please watch the following video, which shows a CHW talking with a client about Relapse Prevention.

In this video role play, how did the CHW support the client with relapse prevention?

- What else would you do—or do differently—if you were working with this client?

Please also watch the following video interview about Relapse Prevention:

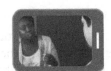

RELAPSE PREVENTION: ROLE PLAY, DEMO

http://youtu.be/ g7UiLRJ-QkE

9.4 Motivational Interviewing

Motivational interviewing (MI) is a form of client-centered counseling that is widely used throughout the world to support clients and patients to change behaviors and enhance their health. All types and levels of health and social services providers use MI, including CHWs, social workers, and physicians.

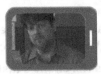

RELAPSE PREVENTION: ROLE PLAY, DEBRIEF, FACULTY INTERVIEW

http://youtu.be/ EaXhsT6B8y8

We recommend MI as one of the most important resources for CHWs to use in their daily work with individual clients, families, groups, and communities. We often return to the topic of motivational interviewing throughout this book to address how it may guide your work in providing services such as care management and chronic conditions management.

Motivational interviewing is defined as "a directive, client-centered counseling style for eliciting behavior change by helping clients to explore and resolve ambivalence. Compared with nondirective counseling, it is more focused and goal-directed. The examination and resolution of ambivalence is its central purpose, and the counselor is intentionally directive in pursuing this goal" (Rollnick & Miller, 1995).

Please note that we can only provide a very brief introduction to motivational interviewing in the *Foundations* textbook. The literature about motivational interviewing is large, complex, and growing. With further study and ongoing practice you will gradually be able to increase your understanding and skills for practicing MI. For further study, please see the additional resources provided at the end of this chapter.

KEY CONCEPTS FOR MOTIVATIONAL INTERVIEWING

Like all forms of client-centered counseling, motivational interviewing aims to support the autonomy of clients to make informed decisions about their health, and their lives more broadly. Before introducing MI techniques, we will review several key concepts.

Responding to Ambivalence

Behavior change implies giving up something that we have become used to and that may provide pleasure, comfort, or a sense of meaning or identity. It is natural that people feel **ambivalence**—or have contradictory thoughts and emotions—about changing familiar patterns of behavior such as eating, exercising, having sex, parenting, expressing anger, or using alcohol, tobacco, and drugs. Motivational interviewing not only accepts ambivalence to change as natural, it encourages clients to explore their ambivalence as a key part of the behavior change process. The techniques described later in this chapter—including the use of OARS and Rolling with Resistance—support the client in addressing and, if possible, resolving their conflicts related to behavior change.

> **TG:** I worked for a long time in the gay community, and I think we made some mistakes early on in the AIDS epidemic. We kind of pushed safer sex and condom use, and we didn't stop to acknowledge what a big change this was. I mean, sexual freedom and sexual pleasure are really important to most of the community. Motivational interviewing is a great resource for me to use when I counsel gay men, because it is a way to focus on what makes it so hard to change, how they feel about it, what they really want in their lives.

- *What behaviors have you tried to change over the course of your life?*

- *What did you have to give up in order to make these changes?*

- *Did you ever feel ambivalent or have doubts about changing these behaviors?*

What Do YOU Think ?

The Spirit of Motivational Interviewing

Practitioners of MI caution against focusing too much on its techniques alone. They argue that for the techniques to have value, they must always be guided by what they call the *spirit* of motivational interviewing. The spirit of MI highlights values related to the relationship between counselor and client, the importance of addressing ambivalence and supporting the client's autonomy. Rollnick and Miller highlight the following seven key points about MI spirit (Rollnick & Miller, 1995).

1. **Motivation to change is elicited from the client, and not imposed from without.** Other motivational approaches have emphasized coercion, persuasion, constructive confrontation, and the use of external contingencies (e.g., the threatened loss of job or family). Such strategies may have their place in evoking change, but they are quite different in spirit from motivational interviewing, which relies upon identifying and mobilizing the client's intrinsic values and goals to stimulate behavior change.

2. **It is the client's task, not the counselor's, to articulate and resolve his or her ambivalence.** Ambivalence takes the form of a conflict between two courses of action (e.g., indulgence versus restraint), each of which has perceived benefits and costs associated with it. Many clients have never had the opportunity of expressing the often confusing, contradictory, and uniquely personal elements of this conflict, for example, "If I stop smoking I will feel better about myself, but I may also put on weight, which will make me feel unhappy and unattractive." The counselor's task is to facilitate expression of both sides of the ambivalence impasse, and guide the client toward an acceptable resolution that triggers change.

3. **Direct persuasion is not an effective method for resolving ambivalence.** It is tempting to try to be "helpful" by persuading the client of the urgency of the problem about the benefits of change. It is fairly clear, however, that these tactics generally increase client resistance and diminish the probability of change (Miller, Benefield, & Tonigan, 1993; Miller and Rollnick, 1991).

4. **The counseling style is generally a quiet and eliciting one.** Direct persuasion, aggressive confrontation, and argumentation are the conceptual opposite of motivational interviewing and are explicitly proscribed in this approach. To a counselor accustomed to confronting and giving advice, motivational interviewing can appear to be a hopelessly slow and passive process. The proof is in the outcome. More aggressive strategies, sometimes guided by a desire to "confront client denial," easily slip into pushing clients to make changes for which they are not ready.

5. **The counselor is directive in helping the client to examine and resolve ambivalence.** Motivational interviewing involves no training of clients in behavioral coping skills, although the two approaches are not incompatible. The operational assumption in motivational interviewing is that ambivalence or lack of resolve is the principal obstacle to be overcome in triggering change. Once that has been accomplished, there may or may not be a need for further intervention such as skill training. The specific strategies of motivational interviewing are designed to elicit, clarify, and resolve ambivalence in a client-centered and respectful counseling atmosphere.

6. **Readiness to change is not a client trait, but a fluctuating product of interpersonal interaction.** The therapist is therefore highly attentive and responsive to the client's motivational signs. Resistance and "denial" are seen not as client traits, but as feedback regarding therapist behavior. Client resistance is often a signal that the counselor is assuming greater readiness to change than is the case, and it is a cue that the therapist needs to modify motivational strategies.

7. **The therapeutic relationship is more like a partnership or companionship than expert/recipient roles.** The therapist respects the client's autonomy and freedom of choice (and consequences) regarding his or her own behavior.

- *What do you think of the spirit of MI?*

- *How well does it fit with your own values and ideas about the work of CHWs?*

- *How does the spirit of MI fit with other concepts for client-centered practice, including cultural humility?*

> **TG:** Motivational interviewing is a lot different from the kind of counseling I got when I was going through recovery [from drug use]. In those days, they used a much more aggressive strategy to kind of break you down—to make you see and admit that you needed to change. But motivational interviewing doesn't force anything on the client, and I like that. I still have to challenge the client about what is keeping them from making the changes that they want to make. But they can choose to talk about it with me or not. And motivational interviewing gives me the tools to do this in a much better way.

ENHANCING MOTIVATION

Motivation is an important factor in determining successful behavior change. Our level of motivation for change often varies over time and in response to different events or circumstances. Motivation comes from within (sometimes referred to as intrinsic motivation), and is also influenced by external events and relationships with others including family and friends.

Motivational interviewing highlights the way that a client's motivation for change is shaped and influenced by the character of the relationship and interactions between a client and a service provider or counselor. The practice of MI was developed out of an understanding that the approach that counselors take—the skills they use, and the choices they make—can enhance or undermine a client's motivation for change. In other words, what you say and do when working with clients can make a *big difference* in whether they make progress in understanding and changing health-related behaviors. Some of these factors are represented in Figure 9.3 below.

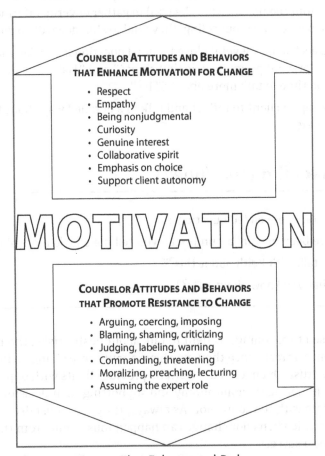

Figure 9.3 Factors That Enhance and Reduce Motivation for Change
Source: "YES WE CAN Toolkit: Community Health Worker Manual" by Community Health Works (2003).

- *What else might CHWs do to diminish or reduce a client's motivation?*

- *What else can CHWs do to enhance a client's motivation to change?*

- *Has your motivation for change ever been influenced by a counselor or other type of helping professional? In what ways?*

MOTIVATIONAL INTERVIEWING TECHNIQUES

Motivational interviewing features a variety of client-centered counseling techniques and resources. We will highlight three techniques and resources in this chapter.

The Use of OARS

OARS are skills that CHWs can use to guide conversations with clients. OARS stands for:

Open-ended questions

Affirmations

Reflective listening

Summarizing

Open-Ended Questions

Open- and closed-ended questions were discussed in detail in Chapter 8. Closed-ended questions generally prompt yes, no, or one-word answers from clients. They may be used to gather or verify information, but when they are used too often in the context of behavior change counseling, they tend to shut down dialogue rather than to open it up.

In the case study, the CHW asks Sachiko several closed-ended questions: "So Sachiko, your main priority is to get some birth control to help prevent pregnancy, is that right?" and "Have you and Keith talked about using condoms?" and "Is this a good time to talk more about STIs?"

Open-ended questions encourage a client to reflect and talk in a detailed way about their life experiences and their values, feelings, and beliefs.

CASE STUDY   **Sachiko** (*continued*)

The CHW asks Sachiko several open-ended questions:

- "You said that you've been messin' around—can you tell me a little more about that?"

- "What was it like to talk with Keith about this?"

- "Can you tell me what you know about STIs?"

Open-ended questions are used to encourage a client to talk about health risks, their readiness to change behaviors, and any ambivalence or resistance they may have about these changes. Providing space for dialogue without judgment also builds trust. Open-ended questions provide clients with opportunities to talk about sensitive health topics while honoring their autonomy and supporting their decision about what kind of information they are willing to share with the counselor. As always, the client must drive the behavior change process, and the solutions by which behavior change can happen must come from them. Without a client's buy-in, the process will not be a success.

Examples of other open-ended questions include:

- What do you think about that?

- What motivates you to think about changing this?

- What do you feel now—what is it like for you talk about these issues?

- What would you like to do about that?
- What else? Such as? How so? What happened then? What did you do then?
- What happened the last time that you _____?
- What would it be like for you to try _____? How might you begin? What might you say?
- What is it that most gets in the way of making these changes?
- What allowed you to accomplish this? What skills and resources did you bring to this situation?
- What have you learned from prior challenges and experiences that are similar to what you are facing now?
- What is different now?

- *Can you think of other examples of open-ended questions that you might ask when you are doing client-centered counseling?*

- *What are some of your favorite open-ended questions to ask clients?*

- *What is it about these questions that may be helpful to clients?*

> **TG:** My favorite questions are simple ones like: "What's going on?" or "What are your thoughts about this?" or " What was that like?"

Affirmations

As discussed in Chapters 7 and 8, many of the clients that you will work with rarely receive an acknowledgement of their strengths, internal resources, and accomplishments. Sometimes, when clients work with service providers, the focus is on what isn't working in their lives (rising blood pressure, a cancer diagnosis, a domestic violence situation), the "mistakes" they may have made, the risks they are facing, and their outstanding needs. Motivational interviewing places an emphasis on recognizing and affirming people's positive qualities, intentions, and accomplishments. These strengths are often the most important resources to support a client in making changes that will promote their health.

Affirming statements provide clients with direct and immediate positive feedback for their efforts and accomplishments, and encourage them to continue along the Stages of Change in reflecting about, planning for, and taking steps to change behavior. Providing affirmations should be done at the appropriate time—when clients have done or said something that is a positive contribution to their health—and in an authentic manner, using your own language and style.

CASE STUDY Sachiko *(continued)*

> The CHW makes the following affirming statement to Sachiko: "I'm really impressed that you and Keith have been able to talk about this and made a decision together about using birth control" and [further on in this chapter] "I thought it was *really* good. You were so clear and direct."

Other examples of affirming statements include:

- I respect how open you are to thinking about what you might want to change.
- It sounds like it took a lot of _____ (courage, strength, will power, and so on) to _____ (do that, talk with him, go to the meeting, and so forth).

- It seems like you learned a lot from that experience.

- Great job. I know that talking to your partner about condoms was a hard thing for you to do.

- I know things didn't turn out like you expected, but you took a big chance and did your best in a difficult situation.

- You've survived some really difficult things in the past, and I trust that you can figure this out too.

- I really appreciate how strong your sense of humor is, even in the midst of the challenges you have been facing.

- You have been very generous in supporting _____ (your friend or family member).

What Do **YOU?** *Think*

- *Can you think of other examples of affirming statements?*

- *Can you think of an affirming statement that you received in the last week?*

- *Are affirmative statements important to you and for your own attempts to change behaviors?*

Please watch the following video ▶ of a CHW working with a client and providing an affirmation.

- How well did this CHW provide an affirmation to the client?

- How may this affirmation have benefited the client?

- What value have affirmations had in your own life?

- When do you provide an affirmation to others?

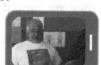

PROVIDING AN AFFIRMATION: ROLE PLAY, DEMO

http://youtu. be/FrggzUE 7Z_I

Reflective Listening

Reflective listening is the art and the skill of reflecting back to clients what they have shared with you about their experiences, beliefs, feelings, behavior, and intentions. By reflecting back what clients say, the CHW can:

- Clarify what clients have said, preventing miscommunication and wrong assumptions

- Let clients know that they are being heard and understood

- Provide clients with an opportunity to hear and reflect on their own statements

- Build and deepen the conversation

Reflective listening isn't easy to do: it requires commitment, concentration, patience, and cultural humility. There are different types of reflections that a CHW may share with a client, including those that attempt to echo back precisely or similarly what the client has said, and reflections that may add an interpretation or emphasis that permit the client to reflect and respond.

Reflective statements may include:

a. **Repeating:** Repeating back as precisely as possible words or phrases that the client has said.

  For example, later on in the Case Study, Sachiko says: "He [Keith] said that he tried them [condoms] before, but they just don't feel so good for the guy. He said he wants to 'go natural'." The CHW might repeat this statement: "Keith says that condoms don't feel so good for the guy and he wants to go natural."

  However, we caution you against repeating what a client tells you too often. If the CHW repeats back exactly what the client says too many times, it can be irritating and may begin to undermine the connection or rapport you are building with the client.

b. **Rephrasing:** Using different words to try to express the same meaning that the client has expressed.

  Such as: "So Keith doesn't want to use condoms when you have sex because he thinks that sex will feel better without them."

c. **Paraphrasing:** This is a step beyond rephrasing in which the client-centered counselor attempts to interpret and summarize what the speaker means. The purpose is to assist the client to better understand their own experience, feelings, and meaning.

Such as: "So even though you told Keith that you were scared of getting pregnant, he didn't want to use a condom because it might not feel as having sex without one."

d. **Reflection of emotions:** The CHW or client-centered counselor will attempt to assess what the client may be feeling and to ask the client about it. The emphasis on emotions comes from an understanding that they are powerful resources for guiding our behavior.

Such as: "You are worried about not using condoms," or "Are you shy about talking about this stuff with Keith?" or "I'm wondering if you are scared about what might happen if you don't use condoms."

You don't have to get the emotion "right." Right or wrong, you present clients with an opportunity to clarify for themselves what they are feeling. You may intentionally amplify an emotion to assist clients to clarify what they are feeling. For example, a client might say: "I guess I feel a bit nervous about talking with my partner about condoms. I don't want to mess up the relationship." The CHW might reflect back: "Are you scared that just talking about condoms could make your partner start to question your relationship?"

TG: Sometimes when I use the OARS and I reflect back something that a client said, it helps them to really hear their own words, the feeling and meaning of what they said. Even when I get it wrong it can help because if the client says, "No, that's not what I said!"—then I have an opportunity to show that I want to listen, I want to understand.

e. **Reframing:** Reframing means to take information given by the client and reflect it back with a different emphasis or interpretation. The goal is to suggest a different way of viewing or thinking about an experience or an issue—one that may be more affirming or supportive to their behavior change efforts. Reframing can be particularly useful in terms of changing patterns of negative thinking that undermine a client's efforts. As always, the client is free to accept, to reject, or to change any suggestion you offer for how to reframe an experience (see Table 9.2).

- *What benefit do you see to sharing reflective statements with clients?*

- *In what situations might you share reflective statements?*

Table 9.2 Examples of the Use of Reframing in Behavior Change Counseling

CLIENT SAYS:	CHW REFLECTS AND REFRAMES AS:
I just don't know what to do anymore . . .	You feel like you don't know what to do. But I see that you *are* doing something—you came here to talk with me and to ask for support.
I know I should start exercising, but I just can't fit it in. After work, taking care of kids, making dinner, I'm just too exhausted. I just don't have the motivation.	You feel like you don't have any motivation. But you must have a lot of motivation to work and raise a family. What motivates you to do these things so well?
I don't want to put myself at risk anymore, but I don't want to lose Keith either.	You care about Keith and want to keep your relationship, but you don't want to be vulnerable for STIs either. Maybe you feel like you will have to sacrifice one or the other. What would it be like to have them both?
I keep dieting and I lose weight, but then I gain back even more, and I think I'm making it even worse. I just can't control what I eat.	*How might you reframe this statement?*
Your example here: _____	Your example here: _____

Summarizing

Summarizing is a way to reflect back the main concerns, feelings, or decisions that a client shares with you. It is another way to demonstrate that you are listening deeply and that you have understood the most important information the client shared with you. It can be used to transition from one main idea or stage of change to another, to reflect the client's natural ambivalence about and resistance to change, and to clarify key decisions that the client has made. For example, the CHW might say to Sachiko:

- "I understand that you want to be able to have sex with Keith and, at the same time, to protect yourself from pregnancy and STIs, is that right?"
- "You and Keith are worried about pregnancy, but you haven't talked about STIs, right?"

Other examples of summaries may include:

- "To summarize, you are not ready to stop using meth, but you do think that you can stop sharing syringes with friends. Is that right? What will assist you in putting this plan into action?"
- "So you want to change your diet, but you are worried about giving up your favorite foods, is that right?"
- "Okay, let me see if I have heard you correctly: you really want to bring your blood pressure down, and you'd like to be able to manage it without using medications. But you aren't sure what changes you can realistically make in order to control your blood pressure."
- "So you are going to reach out to your friend _____ to share some of what you have been going through, and you are going to think more about the idea of going to a support group."

Use of a Motivation Scale

A resource that is sometimes used to support motivational interviewing and other forms of client-centered counseling is a simple scale from 0–10 (Figure 9.4). The scale can be used to assess how important it is to clients to change their behavior, how ready they are to make a change, and how confident they are that they will succeed in making changes.

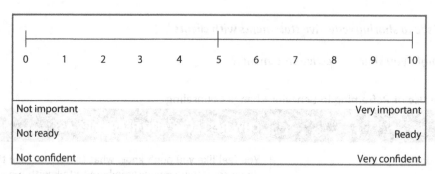

Figure 9.4 A Simple Scale

CASE STUDY **Sachiko** *(continued)*

CHW: Sachiko, on this scale from 0 to 10, how important is it for you to prevent pregnancy?

Sachiko: Like a 50! [Sachiko laughs] I *really* don't want to get pregnant right now, not for a long time, not until I know I'm ready.

CASE STUDY   Sachiko (*continued*)

CHW: Okay, so you are really clear about preventing pregnancy. Before we move on, I'm wondering how you're feeling about preventing STIs. Using this same scale from 0 to 10, how important is it to you to prevent getting an STI like chlamydia or genital warts?

Sachiko: I don't know . . . maybe like a 6 or 7?

CHW: So you aren't as concerned about getting an STI.

Sachiko: Well . . . I mean, not compared to getting pregnant. I guess that is just a much bigger worry for me, you know?

CHW: Let's just take these as separate health issues, okay. So you don't have to compare one risk against the other. [Sachiko nods] Now, just thinking about sexually transmitted infections, how important is preventing them.

Sachiko: Well, maybe 7 or an 8. I mean, I wouldn't want to have to come back to the clinic—no offense!— and get treated or anything. And I guess I would have to talk about it with Keith. . . .

CHW: So what would you say is the difference between a 7 and 10 in terms of how important it is for you to prevent getting an STI? Is there anything that might move your concern closer to a 9 or a 10?

Sachiko: Well, I guess that I just haven't been thinking about STIs, so maybe if I understood more about them—like what the risk is for somebody like me, and what the infections could do—then maybe I would be more worried about them.

CHW: Are you open to talking more about STIs now?

Sachiko: Yeah, I think I need to understand it better.

[The CHW provides more information about the health consequences of STIs.]

The following guidelines come from Thomas Bodenheimer, a physician, researcher, and advocate of new primary health care models that feature a central role for CHWs. He has promoted the use of the 0–10 scale in working with clients or patients with diabetes and other chronic conditions (Bodenheimer, MacGregor, & Sharifi, 2005).

The 0–10 scale may be used to assess how important a particular issue is to the client. If the level of importance to the client is relatively high (a 7 or higher), the CHW can move on to explore risk-reduction steps and the client's confidence in putting them into action. But if the level of importance is low, the CHW may take time to talk about the issue further, providing the client with information about the risks that the issue may pose to the client's health.

When clients develop behavior change plans, the scale may be used to assess how confident they are in putting the plan into action. If the client's confidence level is relatively low, such as a 4, the CHW might ask the client why they rate their confidence at a 4 rather than a 1. This can aid in identifying what the client *is* confident about changing. The CHW might also ask the client what would make it possible for the person to move up the scale in confidence from a lower score, such as a 4, to a higher score, such as a 7 or 8. This may assist the client to reflect further about behavior change, what is getting in the way, and what the client may need to keep moving forward.

If there is a high enough level of importance and confidence to make the behavior change, the CHW should suggest discussing an action plan. The action plan should be tailored to the importance and confidence level of the client.

CASE STUDY   Sachiko *(continued)*

The CHW working with Sachiko might ask her:

CHW: Okay, based on what you know now, and using the same scale of 0 to 10, how confident are you now of using condoms when you have sex?

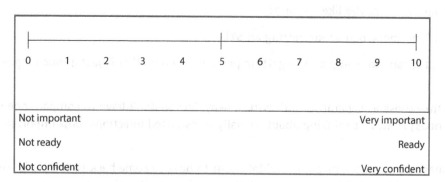

Not important	Very important
Not ready	Ready
Not confident	Very confident

Sachiko: I think condoms are a good idea and everything, but . . . I'd have to say like a 5 or 6.

CHW: Okay. Can you tell me more about why your confidence is at a 5 or a 6?

Sachiko: Well, because I still have to talk with Keith about them. I mean, he has to agree to use them, too, and he already told me that he doesn't like them.

Please watch the following video 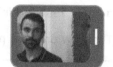 that shows a CHW using a motivation scale as they work with client.

- How did the CHW use a motivation scale in her work with this client?
- How might the use of a motivation scale be beneficial to this client?
- How and when do you like to use a motivation scale in your work with clients?

SAFER SEX & USING A
MOTIVATION SCALE:
ROLE PLAY, DEMO.
🔗 *http://youtu.be/
h9MP3W4vFFE*

Rolling with Resistance

As you work with clients, keep in mind that it is common and natural for them to express ambivalence and resistance to change. When clients express ambivalence about changing their behavior, motivational interviewing encourages counselors to "roll with resistance."

For example, if a client says: "I tried to stop partying, but if I totally stop using meth (methamphetamine) that would mean giving up all my friends, and I'm not ready to do that." In this moment, instead of trying to convince, persuade, or pressure the client to stop using meth, try reflecting this statement back and providing the client with an opportunity to reflect further. For example, you might say: "You aren't sure you want to give up meth if it means giving up friendships, too."

The technique of rolling with resistance honors the client's right to self-determination and offers a safer place to explore difficult emotions, relationships, and choices. If CHWs push back in the moment when clients are expressing resistance to change, they may push clients away altogether, and diminishing their ability to trust you or other service providers in the future.

TG: Sometimes, when a client is resistant to change—and haven't we all been resistant to change?—a counselor kind of digs in there, or the client and counselor can become kind of stuck. The counselor might think their job is to help to convince a client to change anyway, but with some clients—most of my clients—that will only make them even more resistant. So the rolling with resistance thing is just acknowledging that the client is having a hard time making these changes, or is having second thoughts, and just kind of normalizing that. I feel that talking about it in this way kind of takes some of the power or the energy away and makes it easier to talk about whatever the client is facing.

CASE STUDY   Sachiko (continued)

Sachiko and the CHW have been talking about using a condom to prevent STIs. Sachiko expressed ambivalence about making this change. The CHW continues to rely on her OARS and to roll with resistance to address these issues.

CHW: So, not having condoms and the objection of your boyfriend are the two things that are preventing you from using condoms. Is that right?

Sachiko: Yeah, but really, it is Keith . . .

CHW: Can you tell me a little more about why you think Keith doesn't want to use condoms?

Sachiko: I don't know . . . He just said that he tried them before, but they just don't feel so good for the guy. He said he wants to "go natural," with me on the pill but no condoms.

CHW: Sachiko, if Keith was all right with using condoms, would you want to use them?

Sachiko: Yes, that would be . . . I think I'd feel relieved. I wouldn't have to worry so much about everything that can go wrong. I think I'd feel more able to just . . . enjoy being with him.

CHW: You would feel a lot better if Keith agreed to use condoms.

Sachiko: Yes—that would make me feel much better about being with Keith, and about having sex.

CHW: Sachiko, I understand that Keith doesn't like to use condoms. They do reduce some of the pleasure. But it's also true that lots of guys use condoms all the time. They can still have satisfying sex and lower the risk for STIs. What would it be like for you to talk a little more with Keith about this?

Sachiko: I guess I'm worried about bringing it up because he already told me that he doesn't like them and . . . I just don't want to do anything that is going to mess it up.

CHW: You don't want to mess up your relationship . . .

Sachiko: Yeah, I mean being with Keith is like the best thing in my life right now. We hang out all the time, and I just feel like I can talk with him about anything. . . .

CHW: But talking about sex and condoms is different . . .

Sachiko: Well, I mean . . . I guess it is just a lot harder to talk about sex than I thought. Sometimes I . . . I guess I just feel embarrassed.

CASE STUDY   **Sachiko** (*continued*)

CHW: It is really common for people of all ages to have difficulty talking about sex. But I've also seen that, with practice, it gets easier for people to talk about.

Sachiko: [pauses, thinking]

CHW: Sachiko, I hope you know that I am not trying to tell you what to do about your relationship with Keith. My job, like I said before, is to help you think about options that can protect your health. But only you can decide what you want to do . . .

Sachiko: Yeah, I know. I'm just realizing that. . . . That when we talked about this before, we were both only thinking about pregnancy so. . . . So maybe I haven't even given Keith a chance to talk about the STI thing. . . .

CHW: So there may be more to say to Keith.

Sachiko: Yeah. It's just something that I need to think about more, you know? [Sachiko looks at her watch]

CHW: Okay. Shall we wrap up for today?

[Sachiko nods]

CHW: If you want to talk about it more, you can always send me another text and we can schedule a meeting time, okay?

Sachiko: I will. And thank you for listening to me. I just need to think this over before I can talk about it more.

CHW: I get it. And thank you for talking with me, Sachiko, I've really enjoyed it.

Please watch the following videos, which show a CHW working with a client who is experiencing ambivalence about how to move forward and promote his own health.

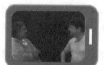

ROLLING WITH RESISTANCE: ROLE PLAY, COUNTER

🔗 *http://youtu.be/ x_hyIMRMy7A*

- In the counter role play, how did the CHW respond to the client's ambivalence? How did the CHW's response impact the client?

- In the demo role play, what did the CHW do differently to roll with resistance? What was the impact of the CHW's approach on the client?

- How would you demonstrate rolling with resistance in working with this client?

ROLLING WITH RESISTANCE: ROLE PLAY, DEMO

🔗 *http://youtu.be/ rgqrusY2MJI*

Now please watch the following interview about rolling with resistance.

- What are your thoughts about the technique of rolling with resistance? Is this a technique that you plan to use when working with clients?

9.5 Additional Resources for Client-Centered Counseling

There a number of other resources and techniques that CHWs may use to support clients to change behaviors and promote wellness. The following examples are adapted from a curriculum for training CHWs in Zimbabwe (I-TECH, 2004).

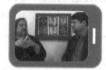

ROLLING WITH RESISTANCE: FACULTY INTERVIEW

🔗 *http://youtu.be/ 9vNeWuNUflo*

THE USE OF SILENCE

Silence can provide an opportunity for clients to reflect upon a question or decision, to identify their thoughts and feelings, and to find the words to express them. Some counselors become unsettled by silence and rush to fill it with their own words. In these moments, learn to pause, breathe, observe, and if necessary, count to 10 (or 20!) before you say something. Give the client space and time to think and feel. If the silence continues, you might comment on the process (see below) and seek clarification about how the client would like to proceed. For example, you might say something like: "You're very quiet. Do you want more time to think about the question I asked, or would you like to move on to another topic?"

Please watch the following videos on the use of silence that show a CHW working with a client.

- How well did the CHW use silence in working with this client?
- How would you have used silence in working with this client?

Please watch the following video interview about the use of silence.

- What are your thoughts about the use of silence? When and how may you use silence in working with clients?

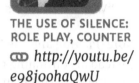

THE USE OF SILENCE:
ROLE PLAY, COUNTER

*http://youtu.be/
e98joohaQwU*

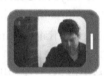

THE USE OF SILENCE:
ROLE PLAY, DEMO

*http://youtu.be/
N5NyZ7OLcMA*

THE USE OF SILENCE:
FACULTY INTERVIEW

*http://youtu.be/
DZNOeVxZfIs*

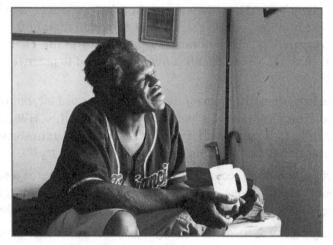

After working with a CHW for nearly a year, the client was taking HIV medications regularly, had gained weight, and was making new plans for his future.

Commenting on the Process

Commenting on the process draws the client's attention to what is happening in the moment, and often highlights dynamics between the client and the service provider. It can help to identify or resolve difficulties that the client may be experiencing in their work with you, and to shift the conversation or working dynamic between clients and counselor in a more productive direction. Learning to be aware of their thoughts and emotions in the moment and to express them to the service provider can help clients to enhance their ability to do this in other situations.

For example, if you sense a client's change of mood when a particular topic is raised, or feel there is a discrepancy between the client's verbal and nonverbal communication, you may wish to comment on the process. For example: "I notice that each time we talk about your husband, your voice drops to a whisper." Or, "You say that everything is fine at home, but when you talk about it your eyes fill with tears."

Commenting on the process can also be done as a way of acknowledging what the client has been through, while at the same time highlighting her strengths: "I am really impressed that you have been able to cope on your own for so long. How have you managed to do it?"

Finally, commenting can also highlight aspects of your interaction with the client: "I notice that you are trying to shift our conversation and to ask me questions about my life." Or "How you are feeling about the work that we are doing together?" Or "Would you like to talk about a different topic?"

Widening the System

When people are facing challenges, they often forget that others may be able to assist. "Widening the system" refers to reminding clients about their external resources, including friends, family, and others who may be able to provide meaningful support. For example:

- "Have you shared this with anyone else?"
- "Who do you usually turn to for support or to talk about issues like this?"
- "What would it be like to talk with a family member or friend about what you are going through?"
- "What additional support would be helpful to you right now?"

Role-Playing and the Empty Chair Technique

Instead of continuing to talk about a situation or challenge, consider asking the client to role-play or act it out in some way. This technique can assist clients to think through and prepare for challenging situations and to practice skills that will support their behavior change.

The Empty Chair technique is a form of role-playing. Sometimes a counselor might use an empty chair to represent another person in the client's life. The counselor might ask the client to imagine that this other person (a parent, partner, child, service provider, or other significant person in their life) is sitting in the chair and ask them what they would like to say to them: "If your husband was sitting in this chair, what would you like to say to him?" This may assist a client to rehearse difficult conversations and to practice effective communication skills in a safer environment.

Not only might the client practice addressing someone else in the empty chair, but they may also try sitting in the chair to role-play the responses of the other person. For example, the CHW might say: "I wonder if you would consider sitting in the chair for a moment and playing the role of your husband. I'm curious what you think he might say about the situation. Is this something you would like to try?"

Role-playing is not for everyone, and these techniques must always be offered as a suggestion to the client. If you want to learn more about this technique, we suggest that you talk with colleagues and your supervisor about how to use it. Try practicing with colleagues before you introduce the technique to clients.

When done correctly, role-playing can assist a client to "get in touch" with certain experiences, thoughts, and emotions that may otherwise be hard for them to identify or talk about. It can provoke insights that give clients an avenue to clarify complex issues and decide what they are ready to do to change their behaviors.

CASE STUDY   **Sachiko** (*continued*)

Sachiko and the CHW continue to talk about the issue of condom use.

CHW: I hear that you don't want to mess up your relationship with Keith, and you are also worried about the risks of not using condoms.

Sachiko: Yes . . . and I'm just not sure what to do about it. . . . It's a lot harder being in this situation than I thought.

CHW: Sachiko, why do these two things have to be in conflict? What if you could use condoms and stay with Keith?

Sachiko: That would be great, but . . . I still don't know what I can say.

CHW: I have an idea—but let me know what you think about it. Imagine that Keith is here right now. What would you say to him about using condoms?

Sachiko: You mean like *right now*?

[*CHW nods.*]

CASE STUDY   **Sachiko** (*continued*)

I don't know. I guess, I'd say, "I really want to talk to you about condoms. I know you don't like them and everything, but I'm really worried about us getting one of those diseases that are out there and I feel like protecting each other is the right thing to do. So I'm wondering—will you try using a condom with me?"

CHW: How did that feel?

Sachiko: It actually felt pretty good . . . I'm surprised I could even figure out what to say . . . That wasn't so bad, was it?

CHW: I thought it was *really* good. You were so clear and direct. [Sachiko smiles] What would it be like to actually say this to Keith?

Sachiko: I don't know. I have to pick the right time. I will try, but—I just don't know if I'll be able to do it.

CHW: If you do decide to say something, at least now you have an idea of what you might say.

Sachiko: That's true. At least I can feel a little bit more prepared.

- *Which of the techniques described above have you used before?*

- *How do you feel about role-playing or the empty chair technique?*

- *What other counseling, communication, or active listening skills might you use when conducting behavior change counseling?*

9.6 Common Challenges to Client-Centered Counseling

Because the behavior change counseling invites clients to address highly personal issues, challenges inevitably arise. The longer you work as a CHW, the more likely you will be to face the following types of challenges as you provide client-centered counseling.

MAKING MISTAKES

Students who are training to become a CHW often say, "I just don't want to make a mistake!" They don't want to do or say something that may be hurtful, disrespectful, or harmful to a client's health. However, despite your knowledge, skill, ethics, and best intentions, you *will* make mistakes: all of us do.

Anticipate that you will make mistakes, and consider how you want to respond when you do. Listen and observe clients carefully for signs that you may have made a mistake. Hopefully the client will tell you by saying something like: "That is *not* what I meant: don't put words in my mouth!" In this moment, please don't become defensive. Place your own issues and reactions aside and focus on your client's experience. Learn the art of offering an authentic apology. Saying you are sorry or apologizing can restore your connection with the client and in many cases it can even deepen it. A sincere apology can create a foundation for deeper work (see Chapter 13).

NOT UNDERSTANDING THE CLIENT

Sometimes CHWs feel embarrassed to admit that they haven't understood something that a client says. But if you don't stop to clarify what was said, you risk misunderstanding something important and continuing to work with a false assumption. When you don't understand something that the client has told you, *ask them about it.* For example, if a client talks with you about sexual or drug-use behaviors that you are unfamiliar with, ask for an explanation: "I'm not familiar with _____. Could you tell me more about it?" When you ask in this way, you are also expressing your interest in your client and your desire to learn about their life.

NOT KNOWING WHAT TO DO

As a CHW, you will face moments in your work when you are not sure what to say or do. With time and experience, this will happen much less frequently. In these moments, we recommend relying upon the client-centered skills that you do have—such as motivational interviewing or commenting on the process. For example, you might invite the client to talk with you about the challenge that you are facing in the moment, or ask them an open-ended question that provides them with an opportunity to reflect on a particular aspect of the issue you have been addressing together. You could ask a client "How can I best support you?" or "What would you like to talk about right now?"

After the session, reflect on your work and try to understand what you may have done (or not done) that contributed to the challenge or difficulty you faced. Use the Self-Assessment Form (provided later in this chapter) to review how well you applied client-centered concepts and skills. Consult with colleagues or a supervisor to talk about the experience, how you handled it, and to identify other options that you could use in the future. The goal here is to understand the type of challenge that you faced so that you can better respond next time in a way that benefits the client.

SCOPE OF PRACTICE

Keep your scope of practice in mind as you support clients to change behaviors. Identify any situations in which you may be at risk of working beyond your scope of practice due, for example, to factors such as the health risks that the client is facing or their level of distress. This may include issues such as mental health challenges, trauma, suicidal thoughts, or any issue that you have not been properly trained to provide. Consult immediately with a supervisor. Together you may determine that it would be best for the client to be referred to work with a colleague who has more training and skills, such as a licensed mental health professional. More information about scope of practice is provided in both Chapters 7 and 18.

ANGER, AGGRESSION, AND CONFLICT

As we have discussed in other chapters, there are many reasons why clients may feel frustrated or angry. They may sometimes express anger or other emotions in ways that seem disrespectful or even threatening. Being angry is natural, and learning to express it can be a powerful and positive resource for self-knowledge and behavior change. Yelling at or threatening a counselor, however, is not. When this happens, the challenge for the CHW is to de-escalate the conflict and to support the client to express themselves in a different way. If you are unable to de-escalate a situation, end the session as quickly as possible. Your work should never be done at the expense of your own safety needs. To read more about handling anger and conflict, please read Chapter 13.

CRISIS

Sometimes you will work with clients who are in crisis. They may relapse to drug use, stop using the medications they need, become homeless or incarcerated, or face domestic violence. These are the moments to remember your scope of practice, turn to supervisors for consultation, or make an immediate referral. Over the course of your career, seek out opportunities for additional training on working with clients in crisis.

Mandatory Reporting

As discussed in Chapter 7, there are limits to client confidentiality, and you have a legal and ethical duty to report certain kinds of behaviors and events. If you learn that a client is harming or threatening harm to themselves or others, you must immediately report this to your supervisor and to appropriate law-enforcement authorities. These events and behaviors include physical or sexual abuse of a minor, assault or threats of assault on others, and plans or attempts to kill oneself. Again, if you face these circumstances, *immediately contact your supervisor* for assistance in reporting these risks to a third party such as the police or child protection agencies. Your supervisor will also guide you in determining your next steps with the client, such as making an appropriate referral. Assessing a client's risks for suicide are addressed in Chapter 18.

- *Have you experienced these types of challenges with clients?*

- *Can you think of other types of challenges that you may face as a counselor?*

- *Which of these challenges do you feel least prepared to handle?*

- *Where can you go to access additional information and to enhance your skills for handling these challenges?*

9.7 Documenting Your Work

Other chapters in this book address the importance of documentation (see Chapters 8, 10 and 16). Please refer to the guidelines presented there, and *document each session as it happens or immediately afterwards.* If you wait too long before writing up case notes, you are likely to forget some of the essential details.

9.8 Team Work and Supervision

As we discussed in Chapter 7, most CHWs work in team settings, and many work as a member of a multidisciplinary team. Team work implies both benefits and challenges for all members of the team, including clients and CHWs. Do your best to develop and maintain positive relationships with all members of your team, and to consult them regularly as you face questions or challenges in your work. Your teammates can help to determine how best to support a client, can serve as the basis for a referral, and can help you to enhance your skills over time.

Working with supervisors is addressed throughout this textbook, including in Chapters 7, 14, and 21. If you provide client-centered counseling, your employer should arrange for you to receive ongoing supervision. Ideally, supervision will be provided by an experienced counselor or mental health provider. Supervision is an opportunity to support you to provide quality client-centered counseling by addressing issues such as:

- Ethics
- Scope of practice
- Safety and mandatory reporting
- Referrals
- Practicing cultural humility
- Challenges with documentation
- Personal issues that arise during or after counseling
- Understanding and resolving counseling challenges
- Counseling goals and developing risk-reduction or behavior change plans
- Counseling skills and techniques such as the use of motivational interviewing

You have an ethical duty to accurately reflect your counseling work to your supervisor. Don't waste this valuable time by avoiding difficult issues. If you are confused, uncertain, or struggling in your work with a particular client or bothered by personal issues, memories, or emotions, talk about these topics. The purpose of supervision is to protect the welfare of clients. It also supports your continued professional development and your well-being, so that you can continue to provide client-centered services.

9.9 Self-Awareness

Providing direct services to others will naturally touch upon your own life experiences, values, feelings, and beliefs. You have an obligation to ensure that your own issues do not get in the way of your work with clients. If your own cultural assumptions and beliefs, values, or emotional needs start to guide your work, you risk doing harm to your clients. If you become aware that this is happening, seek consultation immediately.

Signs that your own issues may be getting in the way of your work may include:

- Finding it difficult to listen to the client
- A strong need to talk about your own ideas or experiences
- Asking questions that are more related to your own needs and interests than those of the client
- Inability to demonstrate interest, curiosity, and interpersonal warmth to the clients you work with
- Becoming overwhelmed or distracted by difficult memories and emotions
- The desire to tell the client what to do
- Providing less counseling, or poorer-quality counseling, to certain clients (discriminatory treatment)
- Difficulty listening to particular types of issues (such as sexual issues)
- Difficulty providing affirmations to a client
- Becoming defensive with a client
- Treating a client with anger, disrespect, or contempt

- *Can you think of other ways that our own issues may get in the way of our ability to provide effective client-centered counseling?*

Many service providers are challenged to keep their own issues from interfering with their work with clients. Good supervision, as discussed above, should focus not only on the challenges and needs that your client faces, but also on your own issues that arise during counseling. If, for example, you are working with a client who is the victim of domestic violence, and you grew up in a home characterized by domestic violence, talk about this with your supervisor, another colleague, a therapist, or a friend. Don't talk about it with your client. For further discussion of these issues and guidelines for self-disclosure (if or when to share personal information with a client), please see Chapters 7 and 21.

- *What issues may be particularly difficult for you to discuss with a client?*

- *Are you comfortable talking about sexual behaviors?*

- *Are there particular client behaviors or choices that it may be difficult for you to accept?*

- *Are there communities that you know less about and that may be challenging for you to work with successfully?*

9.10 Self-Assessment

In addition to the supervision that you receive, and the evaluation of your counseling work by others (including clients and colleagues), we recommend that you regularly evaluate your own work as a client-centered counselor. Every once in a while, after you end a meeting with a client, or at the end of day, use the following Self-Assessment resource (see Table 9.3) to evaluate your performance.

- *When and how might you use this self-assessment?*

- *What else would you add to the checklist?*

Table 9.3 Self-Assessment for Client-Centered Counseling

COUNSELING SKILL	YES	NO	COMMENTS AND SKILLS TO IMPROVE:
1. Did the client identify his or her own health goals and risks?	_____	_____	_____
2. Did I identity client strengths or internal and external resources?	_____	_____	_____
3. Did the client determine a behavior change plan?	_____	_____	_____
4. Did I apply a harm-reduction approach?	_____	_____	_____
5. Did I ask open-ended questions?	_____	_____	_____
6. Did I provide the client with affirmations?	_____	_____	_____
7. Did I practice reflective listening?	_____	_____	_____
8. Did I summarize appropriately?	_____	_____	_____
9. Did I roll with resistance?	_____	_____	_____
10. Did the client speak as much or more than I did?	_____	_____	_____
11. Did my own agenda, values, or beliefs get in the way of client-centered practice?	_____	_____	_____
12. Did I identify personal issues that I should address in supervision?	_____	_____	_____
13. Did I share appropriate referrals?	_____	_____	_____
14. Did I document this counseling session for the client and the program?	_____	_____	_____
15. Were any ethical or scope of practice concerns identified that require follow-up?	_____	_____	_____
16. Other?	_____	_____	_____

9.11 Creating a Professional Development Plan

Throughout your career as a CHW, you will continue to learn and to enhance your skills. Figure 9.5 shows a sample Professional Development Plan that you can use to establish goals for building your client-centered counseling skills. There are many ways to engage in professional development activities, such as:

- Research and read about behavior change counseling and related issues including books, articles, and online resources
- Attend conferences and trainings, including free trainings
- Participate in case conferences (see Chapter 10 for more information)

- Shadow another counselor
  - ○ Ask to sit in and observe an experienced counselor at work. The client must give permission for you to observe before you join the session.
- Self-reflect
  - ○ Reflect on your own work. Keep a journal if that is helpful. Talk with family and friends about your work, your accomplishments, and the challenges you face. Use the self-assessment provided in Table 9.3.
- Debrief with colleagues
  - ○ Talk with a trusted colleague about your work, particularly the challenges you face and the personal issues that may get in the way of client-centered practice.

Professional Development Plan

Name: _____

Identify one or more health topics that you would like to learn more about:	
Identity one or more communities that you would like to learn more about:	
What I will do to enhance my counselling skills:	When I will do it:

Figure 9.5 Professional Development Plan

- Participate in supervision
  - Participate in ongoing supervision with an experienced behavior change counselor or therapist.
- Learn from clients
  - This may be the most valuable way to continue to enhance your skills. Listen to the feedback that your clients provide about your approach, style, and skills. Pay particular attention to any critical feedback that you receive. Try not to be defensive, but to reflect on what you may want to change about the way you work.

- *Have you participated in any of these professional development activities before?*

- *Can you think of other strategies and opportunities for professional development?*

- *Which type of professional development activities are you most interested in?*

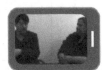

Please watch the following video ▶ interview:

- What types of concepts and resources guide your approach to providing client-centered counseling?
- What questions and concerns do you have about client-centered counseling?
- What is your strategy for continuing to enhance your skills for doing client-centered work?

DEVELOPING YOUR CLIENT-CENTERED PRACTICE: FACULTY INTERVIEW
http://youtu.be/ A71MPjMuYh8

Chapter Review

Jerome is 48 years old. He has been smoking cigarettes since he was 16. He smokes approximately half a pack of cigarettes a day. Jerome's wife and children have been trying to persuade him to stop smoking for many years. Recently, his good friend and neighbor died of lung cancer, and Jerome is newly motivated to stop. He has tried several times over the years to stop smoking on his own, but never lasted longer than a month or two. He says: "Smoking has been a part of my life for so long, I don't know what I'd do without it. It helps me to relax. It's what I do."

You are a CHW working with Jerome. He shares the following information with you:

- "I just don't want to let my family down, particularly my wife. I know she's scared that I could get it (cancer)."
- "You think I'm bad now. I tell you, when I was younger I used to smoke a pack a day or more. Cigarettes were a lot cheaper then, though."
- "You know, I wasn't gonna tell you, but I used to drink too much too. Almost ruined my marriage. My wife, she kicked me out at one point. Said she wouldn't take me back if I kept it up. And I did it. I quit, and I haven't had alcohol in 22 years!"
- "Is it gonna make any difference now—quitting? I've probably done enough damage already. Sometimes I lie awake at night and I worry that cancer is already there."
- "I don't know if I can quit. I used to think I'd give it up by the time I was 30 or 40 . . . but I just never did. It embarrasses me, but I don't know if I've got what it takes to do this. When I stopped, all I thought about was smoking."

Please practice answering the following questions about how you would work to support Jerome:

1. Where is Jerome on the Stages of Change in relation to stopping smoking?
2. What is an example of a harm-reduction strategy or approach that Jerome might take?

3. Use your OARS. Based on the information provided above, provide at least two examples of each of the following that you would ask or share with Jerome:

   - Open-ended questions
   - Affirming statements
   - Reflective statements
   - Summaries

4. Explain two different ways that you could use a 0–10 scale when working with Jerome:

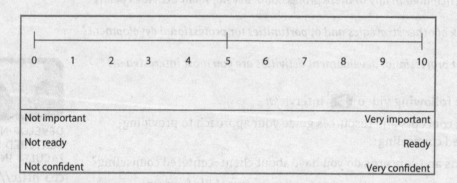

5. Jerome says to you: "I know my wife wants me to quit, but I don't think I can. I've smoked for too many years, and what good is quitting now gonna do me, anyway?" How would you respond in a way that demonstrates *rolling with resistance?*

6. What personal emotions, thoughts, and behaviors will you pay attention to as you counsel Jerome? What will you do if you become aware that your own issues are interfering with your ability to provide client-centered counseling?

7. Identify at least three things that you will do to continue to enhance your skills as a behavior change counselor, and when you will do them.

References

Bodenheimer, T., MacGregor, K., & Sharifi, C. (2005). Helping patients manage their chronic conditions. California Healthcare Foundation. Retrieved from *www.chcf.org/~/media/MEDIA%20LIBRARY%20Files/PDF/PDF%20H/PDF%20HelpingPatientsManageTheirChronicConditions.pdf*

Centers for Disease Control and Prevention. (2001). Revised guidelines for HIV counseling, testing, and referral. *Morbidity and Mortality Weekly, 50* (RR19), 1–58. Retrieved from *www.cdc.gov/mmwr/preview/mmwrhtml/rr5019a1.htm*

Community Health Works. (2003). YES WE CAN Toolkit: Community Health Worker Manual. Community Health Works, San Francisco State University. *www.communityhealthworks.org.*

International Training and Education Center on HIV (I-TECH) and the Ministry of Health and Child Welfare, Zimbabwe. (2004). *Integrated counseling for HIV and AIDS prevention and care: Training for HIV primary care counselors.* Unpublished manual.

Miller, W. R., Benefield, R. G., & Tonigan, J. S. (1993, June). Enhancing motivation for change in problem drinking: a controlled comparison of two therapist styles. *Journal of Consulting & Clinical Psychology, 61*(3), 455–61.

Miller, W. R., & Rollnick, S. (1991). *Motivational interviewing: Preparing people to change addictive behavior.* New York, NY: Guilford Press.

Prochaska, J., Norcross, J., & DiClemente, C. (1999). *Changing for good: A revolutionary six-stage program for overcoming bad habits and moving your life positively forward.* New York, NY: Avon Books.

Rollnick, S., & Miller, W. R. (1995). What is motivational interviewing? *Behavioral and Cognitive Psychotherapy, 23*, 325–334.

World Health Organization. (2006). *Prevention and control of sexually transmitted infection: Draft global strategy.* Report by the Secretariat. Retrieved from *www.raiseinitiative.org/library/pdf/A59_11-en.pdf*

Additional Resources

Center for Evidence-Based Practices (n.d.). *Motivational interviewing reminder card.* Retrieved from *www .centerforebp.case.edu/client-files/pdf/miremindercard.pdf*

The International Society of Behavioral Nutrition and Physical Activity. (2009). 9th Annual Meeting. Retrieved from *www.ijbnpa.org/series/Self_deter*

Karen, G., Rimer, B. K., & Lewis, F. M. (Eds.). (2002). *Health behavior and health education theory, research, and practice.* San Francisco, CA: Jossey-Bass.

Miller, W. R., & Rollnick, S. (2002). *Motivational interviewing: Helping people change.* New York, NY: Guilford Press.

Miller, W. R., & Rollnick, S. (n.d.). *The spirit of motivational interviewing.* Retrieved from *www.motivational interview.net/clinical/whatismi.html*

Motivational Interviewing. (n.d.). Retrieved from *http://motivationalinterviewing.org*

Oregon Reproductive Health Program, Oregon Health Authority. (2013). *The OARS model: Essential communication skills.* Retrieved from *http://public.health.oregon.gov/HealthyPeopleFamilies/ReproductiveSexualHealth/Documents/ edmat/Client-CenterCounselingModelsandResources.pdf*

Runkle, C., Osterholm, A., Hoban, R., McAdam, E., & Tull, R. (2000). Brief negotiation program for promoting behavior change: The Kaiser permanente approach to continuing professional development. *Education for Health, 13* (3), 377–386.

Ryan, R. M., Patrick, H., Deci, E. L., & Williams, G. C. (2008). Facilitating health behavior change and its maintenance: Interventions based on Self-Determination Theory. *The European Health Psychologist, 10.* Retrieved from *www.selfdeterminationtheory.org/SDT/documents/2008_RyanPatrickDeciWilliams_EHP.pdf*

Self-Determination.org. (n.d.). Retrieved from *www.selfdeterminationtheory.org/*

Sheldon K. M., Williams G., & Joiner, T. (2003). *Self-Determination Theory in the clinic: Motivating physical and mental health.* New Haven, CT: Yale University Press.

Sobell, L. C., & Sobell, M. B. (2008). *Motivational interviewing strategies and techniques: Rationales and examples.* Retrieved from *www.nova.edu/gsc/forms/mi_rationale_techniques.pdf*

World Health Organization. (n.d.). *HIV/AIDS Training.* Retrieved from *www.who.int/hiv/topics/vct/toolkit/ components/training/en/index4.html*

Care Management

Tim Berthold, Craig Wenzl, and Emily Marinelli

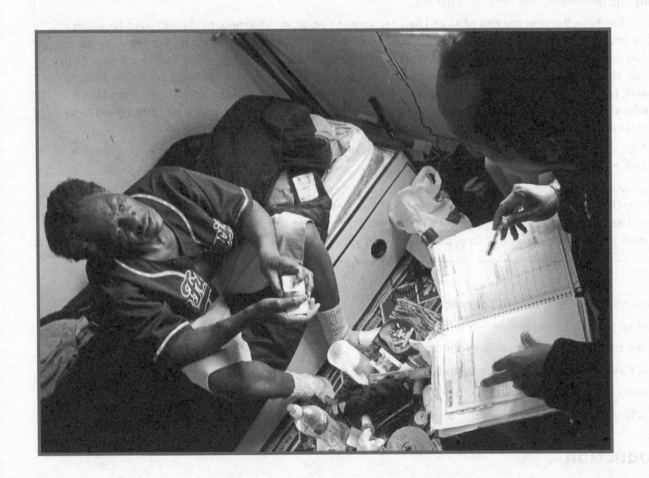

| CASE STUDY | Simone |

Simone is a 34-year-old transgender woman who was recently kicked out of a residential drug recovery program for getting into arguments with other clients. She grew up in a small town, earned a bachelor's degree in business from a local university, and had a good job at a local bank. When Simone told people that she was going to start living as a woman and was changing her name (from James), she was rejected by her family and her church, and fired from her job.

Simone has been living in the city of Saint Louis for almost two years. She thought things might be easier for her in a big city, but she faces constant harassment from people who stare at her and call her names. She has worked on and off in a variety of service sector jobs, but has quit or been fired from each one. At her last job, she started yelling at a customer who kept calling her "Mr." and "Sir." She has a hard time looking for work because she is worried that people will discriminate against her, and she doesn't tell them about her educational qualifications or past work experience because it is connected to her past identity and legal name James. She has lived on the street and in shelters.

She feels deep pain about the loss of her family, especially her younger brother, whom she helped to raise, and being estranged from her faith community.

You provide care management services to homeless adults. You meet Simone on the street outside a soup kitchen. One of your clients introduces you to her. The three of you spend some time talking. You make an immediate connection and are impressed with her charm and great sense of humor. When you tell her about the work that you do, she makes an appointment with you.

If you were the CHW working with Simone, how would you answer the following questions:

- What services can you provide to Simone in your role as a care manager?
- What strengths and resources does she possess?
- What risks and challenges is she facing?
- What resources might promote her health and well-being?
- What types of referrals might you share with her?

Introduction

This chapter provides an introduction to knowledge and skills for providing care management services (sometimes referred to as case management or care coordination as discussed below). As a care manager, you will support clients in creating a realistic plan to promote their own health and well-being and to take action to implement that plan. You will link clients to resources, programs, and services that will enhance their health and safety. You may also help them with navigating systems (such as health care and health insurance), advocacy and self-empowerment, peer counseling, and short- and long-term goal planning.

WHAT YOU WILL LEARN

By studying the information in this chapter, you will be able to:

- Define care management
- Explain your scope of practice as a care manager
- Understand the differences and similarities between working with an individual versus working with families as your client
- Analyze and examine concepts of gender identity and working with transgender and gender nonconforming communities

- Work with clients from a strength-based perspective to identify both strengths and needs
- Support clients to develop a detailed care management plan designed to promote their health and well-being
- Identify and provide meaningful referrals to community resources
- Organize your work and manage your files
- Clearly document the care management services you provide

WORDS TO KNOW

Care Management

Gender Identity

Homeostasis

Transphobia

Gender Identity

We chose a case study about a transgender women as the focus for this chapter in order to highlight the unique challenges that gender variant people face in our society, and to provide an opportunity for CHWs to enhance their knowledge and skills for working effectively and respectfully with gender variant clients and communities. We provide additional information about gender identity in textboxes throughout this chapter.

There is growing recognition in the fields of medicine and public health of a diverse range of gender identities. Some of these are considered under the umbrella of "transgender" and many fall outside of a binary or dualistic concept of gender (male/female). As a CHW you will most likely work with transgender communities and/or people with a variety of gender identities and expressions.

People may identify as female, male, transgender, male-to-female, female-to-male, gender queer, none-of-the-above, or a growing number of other identities. What is most important for CHWs is to practice cultural humility: Don't make assumptions or judgments about the gender identity of the clients you work with. Take time to learn from your clients about their identities, challenges, and strengths, and seek out educational resources to learn more about the communities you will be working with. Resources for learning more about gender identity are included at the end of this chapter.

The concepts and definitions related to gender identity have changed over time and will continue to evolve. Here are some terms that will be helpful to know (Sausa, 2008).

Gender identity: An individual's internal sense of being male, female, both, neither, or something else. Since gender identity is internal, one's gender identity is not necessarily visible to others.

Transgender: An umbrella term for people whose gender identity, expression, or behavior is different from those typically associated with their assigned sex at birth.

Gender variant: A term for individuals whose gender expression is different from societal expectations based on the sex at birth.

Cisgender: A term used for individuals who are not transgender. These individuals have an assigned sex at birth (usually male or female) that matches their gender identity. "Cis" comes from the Latin word that means "the same."

Sexual orientation: A self-identity that describes a sense of how individuals are attracted to other individuals, or not. This may change over time. Some examples might be queer, lesbian, gay, heterosexual, bisexual, asexual, pansexual, panromantic, and others.

(continues)

Gender Identity
(continued)

Transphobia: Fear based on a person's perceived and/or known gender variation; occurs on a localized and a global scale.

Transgender ally: Someone outside of a group or identity who advocates and takes positive action on behalf of that group. Consider the ways you can be an "Ally" to transgender and gender variant communities—these were mentioned in the digital story "Transgender 101" (adapted from Gender Diversity Project: Resources for Education). You can practice being an ally in your work as a CHW, as an advocate, even in your agency.

- Get educated and examine your own biases about gender roles, identities, and expressions. Don't rely on transgender people to educate you.

- Use appropriate pronouns and names. It is important to view people as their chosen gender and call them by their chosen name. If you're not sure which pronoun they prefer, ask.

- Create a safe and open environment. Support your friends or family members' gender explorations. Challenge homophobic and transphobic remarks or jokes.

- Do not "out" a transgender person (reveal someone's transgender/gender variant status). This is a safety issue: Many people are prejudiced against gender variant people. Finally, understand that gender identity is only one aspect of a whole person. Every person has many social identities, experiences, and personal history that make them unique.

10.1 Defining Care Management

Because we live in a world characterized by unequal access to basic resources, rights, and opportunities, many of our clients face significant barriers to health. Care managers work with clients to identify the resources they already have, as well as those that they would like to gain access to. Based on this assessment, clients develop a plan (we will refer to this as an Action Plan) to improve their health, and take realistic actions to implement this plan. As a care manager, you will develop an in-depth knowledge of local health, educational, and social service programs and work to link your clients to these essential resources. Occasionally, care managers also take a more active role in advocating with local agencies to provide services to clients in need. The challenge for CHWs is to provide care management services in a way that is client-centered and that supports the autonomy and empowerment of the client.

According to the Center for Health Care Strategies, Inc., **care management** can be defined by assisting

> *consumers and their support system to become engaged in a collaborative process designed to manage medical/ social/mental health conditions more effectively. The goal of care management is to achieve an optimal level of wellness and improve coordination of care while providing cost effective non-duplicative services. (Center for Health Care Strategies, n.d.)*

Please note that several different terms are used to describe these services including case management, care management, care coordination, and systems navigation. As a working CHW, the agency that employs you will orient you to the language, policies and protocols that they use to provide these services. For the purposes of this chapter, we will use the term care management.

Some people object to the term *case management* because it may be interpreted to suggest that clients are the "cases" who need to be "managed." That view of people would clearly undermine the client-centered practice of CHWs, who work to support the autonomy and self-determination of clients. We view the "case" that requires management as the social context that creates health inequalities and deprives low-income and other vulnerable clients and communities from access to the basic resources that will promote their health.

CHW care managers work for a wide variety of public and private sector agencies, including local health departments, community-based nonprofit health and social services agencies, hospitals, and clinics. They work for programs addressing a wide range of health issues such as homelessness, mental health, domestic violence, maternal and child health, infectious diseases such as tuberculosis or HIV/AIDS, and chronic conditions such as diabetes or asthma.

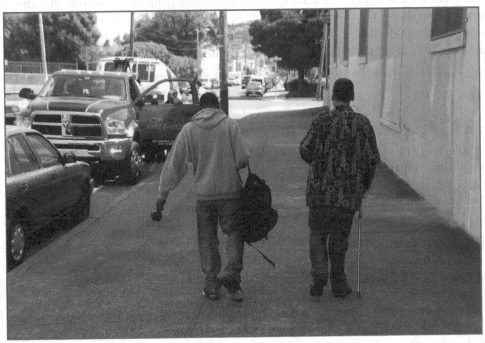

Care management services are provided in a variety of settings. A CHW provides case management services while taking a walk with a client.

Care management services are generally provided on an ongoing basis. It takes time to develop and implement a health plan and to successfully link clients to new services. Care managers may work with clients from two to three months to a year or more.

The number of clients you work with at one time (sometimes referred to as a "caseload"), can range widely from a dozen or so to 50 or more, depending on the nature of the program you work for, relevant policies, and how frequently you have contact with clients.

Care management services are provided in a wide range of locations, including your office, a client's home, in the hospital, in jails or prison, in a homeless shelter, soup kitchen, residential drug recovery program, on the streets, or through the Internet and mobile web.

> **TG:** At my agency, we are supposed to work with clients for about six months, but some of my clients need more time, and sometimes I don't see them for a while and then I start working with them again. One of my clients, we've been working together for 18 months. He just got out of jail and then went into the hospital, and he called me from there. I'm just glad that he keeps calling and reaching out to me, and even if he doesn't always succeed, I know that he wants a better life.

One of the challenges with the concept of care management is that it seems to imply that the services that clients need to access actually exist in all local communities. *The reality, however, is that many communities lack important resources* such as transitional or affordable housing options, food assistance programs, mental health services, legal services, and educational or employment opportunities.

Alvaro Morales: I was working for a program serving people who were homeless. I tried to link clients to the resources they needed, like housing or jobs or family therapy. Sometimes, no matter how hard I tried, those services just didn't exist, or there weren't any spaces right then, or my client didn't fit the eligibility rules. Often, the best I could do was to offer a guaranteed place in a shelter, but a lot of our clients don't like shelters. I usually opened the drop-in center early in the morning, and some clients had slept outside in the doorway. When I went home at night to my family, I knew that most of our clients were sleeping on the streets. I often felt angry and frustrated because the situation is just so overwhelming and unfair and totally preventable.

RESEARCH ON THE ROLE OF CHWs IN CONDUCTING CARE MANAGEMENT

Research on the roles of CHWs in conducting care management is still emerging as the field expands. Some key study findings demonstrate the effectiveness of CHWs working in team settings and coordinating care. For example, a study of patients with chronic obstructive pulmonary disease (COPD) showed that using individualized action plans, care managers supported patients by ultimately decreasing ". . . impact of exacerbations on health status," and thus accelerated recovery (Trappenburg et al., 2011).

For the Patient Centered Medical Home (PCMH) study, CHWs were hired as part of teams providing in-home patient care in South Bronx, New York. Findings from this study show that CHWs "developed a trusting relationship between the patients, serving as a two-way liaison between the community and health care system," and as a result, traditionally marginalized communities had greater access to medical and mental health care. In this integrated team approach, CHWs worked as are managers and supported the team of health providers to "understand the patient's backgrounds, constraints and preferences . . . [and] helped everyone genuinely focus on the patient" (Findley, Matos, Hicks, Chang, & Reich, 2014).

The Centers for Disease Control and Prevention released a report in 2015 on the role of CHWs in addressing chronic health conditions (Brownstein & Allen, 2015). This report highlights the unique role of CHWs as "culturally competent mediators, . . . between providers of health services and the members of diverse communities." The CDC findings support the integration of CHWs in the role of care managers in health care teams, including in the prevention and control of various chronic health conditions such as; hypertension, cardiovascular disease, breast, cervical, colorectal and prostate cancers, diabetes, and asthma. The effectiveness of CHW care management was measured in high-risk or priority populations that often do not receive or benefit from services they need. CHWs engage communities in care and provide coordination and management of care in teams that further support retention and wellness.

10.2 Basic Care Management Concepts

The approach to care management provided in this chapter draws on the concepts of client-centered practice discussed elsewhere in Part 2 of the *Foundations* textbook. Basic elements of care management include:

- Work from a strength-based perspective that emphasizes a client's internal and external resources
- Support the autonomy and decisions of clients
- Support clients in developing their own action plans that include clear goals, priorities, and realistic actions to achieve these goals
- Practice cultural humility: don't make assumptions about the knowledge, behaviors, or values of your clients or impose your own cultural norms. Work to transfer power to the client.
- Provide client-centered education and counseling, as necessary, about the health issues or conditions relevant to the client
- Understand the three phases of care management and when to end services
- Develop an in-depth understanding of available basic resources and services and maintain ongoing professional relationships with these service providers

- Provide clients with referrals to resources, including clear guidance about why and how to access these resources
- Set boundaries and stay within your scope of practice
- Consult regularly with a supervisor and or members of your program or clinic team
- Manage client files and stay organized
- Document your work accurately
- Present and discuss your work with individual clients to the health care team or your program coordinator or supervisor
- Accept feedback and be open to examining your own assumptions or bias

A note about strength-based care management: Some care managers focus exclusively or to a large extent on the problems or challenges that clients face and the resources they lack. Clearly, assessing a client's needs and challenges is essential to identifying basic resources that will promote their health. However, focusing primarily on what is lacking in a person's life can reinforce low self-esteem and the sense that they themselves are somehow lacking. Many clients, especially those who have been homeless, incarcerated, subjected to violence, or addicted to drugs or alcohol, have received these messages too many times already. This approach also overlooks the client's strengths, talents, and achievements. For all of these reasons, and with all clients, we ask you to use a strength-based approach in your work.

THE CARE MANAGEMENT PLAN

The focus of care management is to develop a client-centered plan documenting the strengths, needs, clear goals, and actions that will be taken to promote the client's health and well-being. Depending on where you are working, this document may be called an action plan, care plan, treatment plan, care coordination plan, service plan, care management plan, self care plan, or any number of other terms. The agency you work for will determine what the plan is called and what forms are used to document and monitor progress. For the purposes of this chapter, we will refer to it as a care management plan.

SCOPE OF PRACTICE AND WORKING AS PART OF A TEAM

As a care manager, you will always be working as part of a team. It may be a team of three, consisting of the client, yourself and your supervisor, or it may be a larger team and include other professionals such as social workers, nurses, or physicians. If you are working as part of a larger team, take time to clarify and understand the roles and scope of practice of each team member (review Chapter 7 for more on scope of practice and working with teams). Ideally, you will have a chance to meet together regularly to discuss your work, the client's progress, and how best to work together to assist the client to implement the plan. The agency and program you work for should provide you with clearly written policies and protocols to guide your work as a member of a team. These generally include participating in team meetings to discuss the welfare of specific clients (sometimes called "case conferences"), described at the end of this chapter.

One way to define your scope of practice is to look at how the responsibilities are often shared among the members of the care management team:

Client Responsibilities

Clients may take responsibility to:

- Decide to participate in care management
- Decide whom to work with, and provide informed consent to work together
- Provide accurate information in a confidential setting
- Identify strengths and needs
- Identify goals and develop a realistic plan of actions to meet those goals
- Communicate regularly with other members of the care management team, and attend appointments or call in advance to cancel if necessary

- Decide which other providers, if any, the care management team can share confidential information with (with a signed release)
- Ask questions and raise concerns related to care management services
- Strive to learn new information and skills to enhance their health and well-being
- Identify additional services they are interested in accessing, and speak up if they are reluctant to access a particular service
- Follow prescribed treatments and use of medications and communicate with the team if challenges or concerns arise
- Actively participate in deciding when and how to end care management

- *Have we left out any important responsibilities?*

- *What else might a client do to contribute to the success of care management?*

CHW Care Manager Responsibilities

CHW care managers may take responsibility to:

- Conduct an initial assessment with clients; orient individuals or families to the program, services, and policies, including confidentiality
- Obtain informed consent to provide services
- Honor principles of client-centered practice, including the client's right to self-determination
- Work with the client to assess their strengths or internal and external resources, their health risks and priorities, and services that they would like to access
- Work with the client to develop a written care management plan and monitor progress in meeting identified goals and priorities
- Maintain proper documentation of all services provided and the challenges and progress made in the implementation of the care management plan
- Provide clients with referrals to additional resources and services (make sure services are culturally appropriate, accurate, up to date, and, if possible, provide a direct contact)
- Maintain client confidentiality as required by law and agency policy
- Work professionally and ethically to provide quality service
- Ask for and obtain the client's permission before releasing information to other providers
- Reinforce health education knowledge and skills
- Maintain contact with clients and monitor and document their progress
- Conduct home visits if appropriate
- Advocate for client needs and priorities
- Participate in conferences with colleagues to discuss care management challenges and successes
- Participate in regular supervision sessions, clearly identifying challenges, concerns, and questions that arise in your work with clients
- Advise others working with your clients about changes within the community that might impact the clinic or program

- *Can you think of other responsibilities for care managers?*

Some CHWs will work as part of a team that includes other service providers such as social workers, psychologists, attorneys, nutritionists, occupational therapists, nurses, physicians, or similar professionals.

In this situation, the roles and responsibilities of all team members should be clearly defined. The team should also develop a process for working together, for identifying and resolving differing opinions or conflicts, and providing appropriate referrals.

If you work as part of a team that includes a health care provider, their responsibilities *may* include the following:

- Provide clinical care, including diagnosis of illness and prescription of treatments in accordance with established protocols
- Establish and maintain communication systems with other team members, departments, hospitals, and community organizations and agencies so that referral systems function smoothly and promote continuity of care
- Work with others to develop referral protocols, entry/exclusion/exit criteria, and clinical management protocols
- Obtain informed consent and necessary releases to share information with other health care providers
- Coordinate medical care services, including referrals for lab work and to specialists, as appropriate
- Maintain appropriate documentation of clinical services
- Participate in conferences with colleagues to discuss care management challenges and successes
- Provide program updates and share outcome data, maintaining client confidentiality

Sometimes you will question whether a certain aspect of care is your responsibility or if it should be provided by another member of the team. Remember to consult with your colleagues to clarify these concerns.

COMMON STAGES OF CARE MANAGEMENT

Care management happens over time. The length of time that you work with an individual client (the number of meetings or sessions or the number of months) may be clearly limited by your agency or the institution that funds your agency. Regardless of the length of time you may work with clients, care management generally consists of several distinct stages, including:

- The initial assessment of strengths, needs, and priorities
- The development of clear goals and steps to achieve those goals
- Implementation of the care management plan and monitoring of progress
- The end or completion of care management (sometimes referred to as discharge or termination)

10.3 Developing the Care Management Plan

Care management plans use slightly different forms and slightly different language among programs and agencies. Some plans will focus on particular issues more than others, such as mental health concerns, substance abuse, or housing. Some care management plans are elaborate and may require ten to fifteen pages or more of documentation, including an extensive assessment. Others are more focused and require fewer details. Again, this will depend on the agency and the program you work for, the funding source for that program, the primary topic or health issue the program is concerned with (such as HIV/AIDS or mental health), and the population you serve. Despite these differences, most care management plans will include the following:

- An assessment of the client's strengths and existing resources
- An assessment of the client's risks and need for additional resources
- The development of one or more goals or objectives to improve the quality of the client's life
- The development of a detailed action plan outlining steps designed to reach identified goals or objectives
- Documentation of who is responsible for putting each step into action (client, care manager, or other professional)
- Documentation of referrals provided and accessed, and outcomes
- Progress notes
- Documentation of the end of care management services (also known as discharge or termination)

A care management plan is a working document to keep everyone focused on desired goals and how to achieve them. After the plan is developed, it is usually signed by the client or family, the care manager, and sometimes by another member of a team who you may be working with, such as a nurse or social worker. The client keeps a copy of the plan, and another copy goes into the file. As a working document, the plan can and is likely to be revised and updated over time, based on the experience and needs of the client.

> **Andrew Ciscel:** I work as a Peer Care Manager or PCM at City College of San Francisco,—supporting students who are in the CHW Program or the Drug and Alcohol Counseling, or Community Mental Health Worker Programs. These students come to talk with me about a wide variety of issues. Sometimes they are related to systems navigation, such as getting help with accessing services on campus like financial aid or academic counseling or the Disabled Students program. Sometimes students just want to check in and get support about the stress or anxiety that they have about being in college, and I can try to help them with study skills and time management. I remember one student was feeling a lot of anxiety because she had to facilitate a group in class, and she'd never done it before, and she was really nervous. So I talked with her about her feelings and helped her come up with a detailed plan for how she would approach her presentation. She came to see me afterwards, and she was elated with how well her presentation had gone. I reflected back on how she had named this challenge, come up with a plan, and handled the stress. I just kind of helped her take in the moment of her success.

THE FIRST MEETING BETWEEN CLIENT AND CARE MANAGER

Before starting to conduct an assessment or to develop a care management plan, apply the skills you learned in Chapter 8 to:

- Welcome the client and assist the person to feel comfortable in your agency
- Build rapport and a trusting relationship with the client
- Explain the nature and the extent of the services that you can provide as a care manager
- Describe any program restrictions and/or costs
- Explain the limits of client confidentiality and other essential program policies
- Answer the client's questions and concerns
- Obtain informed consent (and HIPAA if working in a health care setting) to proceed with the assessment process

Take time to clearly explain your role as care manager, the types of questions you will ask as part of the assessment, and the purpose of asking such questions, as in the example that follows.

CASE STUDY   **Simone** *(continued)*

> Simone, I'd like to start our assessment today. If you agree, we'll talk about some of the resources that you already have, some of your priority concerns and goals, and resources and services that you hope to access. This information will guide us in coming up with a plan to improve the quality of your life and your health in the ways that you care about most. My role is to help you develop and implement this plan. Some of the questions I'll ask—you can see them here on the care management form (CHW hands Simone a copy of the form)— are very personal, and I just want to be clear that you are the one who decides what we talk about together. If I ask you something about your life and you don't want to talk about it with me, or talk about it right then, just let me know, and I'll respect that, okay?

CONDUCTING AN ASSESSMENT

The purpose of an assessment is to establish a clear common understanding of the client's primary concerns, strengths, and needs. This information is then used to guide the development of a care management plan designed to address the client's concerns and promote their health.

Assessments take place in a variety of places, including the care manager's office or at other agencies or locations such as a hospital or juvenile hall. Sometimes care managers may conduct home visits (see Chapter 11) to develop a deeper understanding of their clients' home lives and the resources and risks affecting their health and their goals.

The assessment typically consists of gathering three types of information from clients:

1. Basic demographic information
2. Their strengths (or internal and external resources)
3. Their current risks and needs (including needs for additional resources)

In Chapter 8 we discussed how asking for demographic information—the client's date of birth, address, family status, employment status and income, gender, ethnicity, and so forth—can create an uncomfortable distance between you and a client at the very moment when you are trying to establish a positive professional connection. For this reason, we suggest that you don't begin the assessment by gathering all the required demographic data. Instead, start with questions that are more likely to put clients at ease and may be most important to them, such as: "What do you hope to get out of care management?"

When Forms Don't Recognize People's Identities

Review the forms at your agency. Are they inclusive of all people? Do they provide options other than single, married, and divorced to document relationship status? Do the forms recognize gender identities other than female and male? Do they recognize multiracial identities or instead force people to identify with just one ethnic category? If the questions we ask and the forms we use to document information aren't inclusive of the diverse identities of the clients we serve, we risk offending them and undermining our ability to work together successfully.

How Do I Learn about a Client's Identity?

Try not to make assumptions about a client's identity. Understand that some clients may wish to share their gender identity with you, and others will not. As always, use client-centered practices to follow the client's lead.

When you are working with clients to document specific information on agency forms, and this includes information about sex or gender identity, you may simply provide the client with a form and ask them to fill out the relevant information (Name, Address, Date of Birth, etc.), or you may ask questions like "How do you identify?", "What identities are important to you?" As you get to know a client, provide them with opportunities to share key information about who you are, and express your interest and desire to learn more. Often, transgender and gender variant individuals are told who they are by others. Your welcoming and nonjudgmental attitude will present an opportunity for them to narrate their own stories and define themselves on their terms.

At the same time, CHWs also have a responsibility to do their homework about gender identity and explore some best practices for working with transgender clients. CHWs use cultural humility and client-centered strength-based skills in working with all communities. It is an ethical and critical responsibility to act with respect and understanding. Not doing so can be harmful and damaging to transgender and gender variant clients—and to your reputation as a CHW in the community.

(continues)

How Do I Learn about a Client's Identity?
(continued)

Gender Identity Is Different from Sexual Orientation

A common misconception is that gender identity and sexual orientation are related, but they are distinct and separate aspects of who we are. While gender identity refers to your internal sense of gender (some examples might be male, female, transgender, femme, etc.), sexual orientation refers to who you are sexually and romantically attracted to (some examples of sexual orientations are gay, lesbian, heterosexual, queer, bisexual, etc.). Someone can be a transgender gay man, a bisexual cisgender woman, a genderqueer panromantic, or any combination of the above identities.

CASE STUDY **Simone** *(continued)*

In working with Simone, gathering demographic information may be challenging. Don't make assumptions about Simone's identity: She may identify as a woman, as a transgender woman, as gender queer, or some other identity not listed here. Questions about name, income, address, and phone number may be difficult for Simone to answer, particularly if she does not have a stable address and if Simone is not her legally recognized name.

We recommend that you don't begin your assessment with Simone by asking for detailed demographic information. You may want to gather this data over two or more meetings, once you have established a positive connection. You may also want to talk about this with her directly, at the end of your first session. You might say something like: "Simone, here is a copy of the care management form to fill out as we continue to work together. As you can see, it asks for lots of personal information, including name, ethnicity, age, income, gender, and relationship status. I'd like to gather as much of this as possible as the more information I have from you, the better we can tailor our work together. As always, you decide what we talk about here and what you want to tell me. Can we start to fill out part of this together?"

ASSESSING THE CLIENT'S STRENGTHS AND AVAILABLE RESOURCES

As we have discussed here and in earlier chapters, client-centered practice emphasizes the importance of assessing, valuing, and building on a client's strengths. Starting from client strengths means that you recognize, and assist clients to recognize, what they have, rather than what they don't have; what they can do, rather than what they can't do; and what they've accomplished, rather than their perceived failures. Focusing on strengths allows you and your clients to identify *all* of the resources available to them and aid in building their confidence, capacity, and autonomy.

Assessment typically doesn't happen all at once during one interview in an office setting. Rather, you will learn more about the client's strengths as you establish your working relationship.

TG: I don't always start with a big assessment. I'll ask a few questions, but come back to the rest later as I get to know the client. Generally, I want to listen first to what is on their mind. They almost always have an idea of something they want, or want to change, or some resource that they need. If I can start by learning about that, and working to help them out—like helping them find a good doc (doctor) or some clean clothes or something to eat—then they're more likely to open up and answer all the questions I have to ask.

We encourage you to use a combination of open-ended and closed-ended questions to conduct your assessment of both strengths and needs, as explained in Chapters 8 and 9. The program you work for and the policies, protocols, and forms they ask you to use will provide a certain degree of guidance about how to conduct your assessment and how to identify the client's strengths. In addition, please review the lists of common internal and external resources provided in Chapter 12.

Over time, you will gain a deeper understanding of the client's strengths. One of the pleasures of care management is that you will often have the opportunity to witness clients developing new strengths along the way.

ASSESSING THE CLIENT'S RISKS AND NEED FOR ADDITIONAL RESOURCES

The care manager also asks questions to guide the client in identifying current life challenges, risks, and the need for additional resources. The client's needs and interest in accessing resources such as housing, interpretation services, drug or alcohol treatment, employment, legal assistance, and health care is also addressed.

Specific risks may also be assessed. For example, if you are conducting HIV prevention care management, you will be asked to assess the following types of risks:

- Current substance use
- Risks for exposure during injection drug use (sharing needles or works)
- Current sexual behaviors and risks for unprotected or condomless vaginal or anal sex
- Infection with hepatitis C or tuberculosis
- Not being under the care of a physician with advanced training in HIV/AIDS (for clients who are HIV positive)
- Difficulty adhering to treatment guidelines, including the use of medications for the prevention or treatment of HIV

Open-ended questions are particularly helpful because they provide the client with an opportunity to identify needs that you may not ask about. Open-ended questions might include: "What are you most concerned about right now?" "What is the biggest challenge that you face right now?" "What do you most want to change about your life?" "What resources do you most need in your life?" "What are the biggest risks to your health right now?" "What puts you at risk for HIV transmission?"

Finally, the client is asked to prioritize the risks and needs identified during the assessment. The care manager asks which of these issues or problems the client is most concerned about and what resources they most want to access. For example, Simone might say that a steady job and safe place to live are her highest priorities. She might also talk about her desire for community and a sense of belonging.

Please watch the following video interview .

ESTABLISHING CLIENT PRIORITIES: FACULTY INTERVIEW

http://youtu.be/ isOQoAF4kAA

IDENTIFYING CARE MANAGEMENT GOALS

Martha Shearer: Each individual comes with so many different issues. I had a 72-year old patient who was gone [incarcerated] for 30 years. His parents died while he was gone. He needed food stamps, medication, housing, help with reintegration into society, and clothes. At first I thought "This is more than I should take on," but then I realized, "Who else will do it?" It takes a lot for a person to be reintegrated—they may need help advocating with family, with parole, and with housing, and that is the perfect job for a CHW!

Based on the assessment, you will support the client in identifying one or more specific goals for the care management plan. While it is often meaningful for clients to talk about their ultimate life goals (working as a counselor, reuniting with and living near children or grandchildren, owning their own home, finding a sense of peace), the purpose of care management is to address more immediate concerns. The goals should come from the client, not the care manager, and should be specific and realistic. For example, while a client may not be able to purchase their own home in the next six to twelve months, the client may be able to find stable housing or a place in a transitional housing program. If goals are too unrealistic, this may set the client up for disappointment or a sense of failure. A key task of the care manager is to guide and support clients to develop goals that they can realistically work toward in a reasonable time frame. Other goals may include, for example: securing a part-time or full-time job; entering a drug treatment program, reducing risks for sexual transmission of HIV and other STIs; getting school clothes for their children; reducing blood pressure; or working to re-establish contact with family members.

CASE STUDY **Simone** (*continued*)

As a care manager, you might ask Simone: "What is your first priority for your care management plan? What do you most want to accomplish or change?"

Simone's goals might include:

- Finding a safe and stable place to live
- Connecting with a spiritual community
- Developing a support network of people who aren't using drugs
- Getting treatment for depression
- Reducing drug and/or alcohol use
- Developing new friendships within and outside of the transgender community
- Working with a job counselor to identify career and employment options

---

ESTABLISHING CARE MANAGEMENT PRIORITIES: THE CLIENT'S PLAN

When you provide care management services and work with a client to develop and implement a care management plan, you will establish priority issues or goals to work on. The issues that you as a care manager may view as priorities may be different from those of the client. *Keep in mind that this is* the client's plan, *not yours,* and the client is the one who should establish the priorities. At the same time, you will provide information, referrals, and guidance regarding priorities and actions for enhancing their health and well-being. As always, the client will decide whether to accept or reject this guidance. While you will offer referrals and information appropriate to the client, make sure to continue to prioritize the client's plan, not yours. For example, do not assume Simone wants to attend a transgender support group, if her immediate need is housing. Be mindful and self-reflective if you are focusing on issues around identity and missing the client's real priorities.

You will often be employed to focus on specific health outcomes. For example, you may be working for a prenatal program with the goal of promoting the safe delivery and health of infants and mothers. You may want to focus on your client being able to have access to regular and ongoing prenatal care and to arrange for trained professionals, such as nurses, midwives, and doulas (labor coaches), during the delivery. While the health of her children will be a priority for the client, she may be struggling with other life challenges that pose significant obstacles to her health and ability to access prenatal care. She may be homeless or lack money for food or rent. She may be in a relationship characterized by domestic violence or have immigration concerns. These issues may be her top concerns.

Sergio Matos: Part of the problem is that CHWs often have to work for programs, and the program goals are not in sync with the family's goals. Programs impose themselves on communities and often have different priorities. So you may go into a family's home to talk about asthma. But asthma might not be their real problem, even if they have asthma. They might be hungry or they might be experiencing violence or they might be worried about losing their home or unemployment or living underground with all this immigration hysteria. So asthma might not be at the front of their consciousness right now. But these programs impose these very rigid deliverables and actions that CHWs have to take. On the first visit, you have to talk about this, this, and this. And the second visit, you've gotta complete these five forms. And the third visit, programs can get very rigid and not respectful of what a family is experiencing or wanting. But the CHW is not at liberty to ignore the family's needs and wants, and so they have to negotiate that tension, that conflict. They have to find a way to serve the family to the best of their ability, sometimes in spite of the program they work for.

It is essential to respect the client's priorities. If a mother is most worried about getting school clothes for her children, finding a solution to this problem is the best place to begin your work together. Addressing one issue at a time, and accomplishing some sort of meaningful change—such as finding a place for free or low-cost school clothes for their children—will make it that much easier to establish trust and to move forward to address the next priority issue. Keep harm reduction in mind: anything that the client accomplishes that reduces risks for themselves and their family is a good thing. Make sure to acknowledge and celebrate the progress that your clients make.

TG: My clients wouldn't need care management if everything was working out for them. But they are dealing with big problems like HIV disease and on top of that maybe they're homeless, or they lost their job, or they relapsed and started using drugs again, or their boyfriend beats them up and sometimes all of this combined together. And sometimes what I'm paid to do—like get them to follow through with their antiretroviral therapy—may not be a big concern to them. They almost always have other priorities—like being safe, or getting something to eat, or finding a place to stay. If I don't listen to what they want, then why should they listen to me? And if I'm not listening in the first place, then why am I working as a CHW?

DEVELOPING AN ACTION PLAN

The next step is to work together to develop a detailed action plan to reach the client's care management goal or goals. The plan will identify who is responsible for each action and will provide a timeline for completing these actions.

Care managers are generally responsible for the following types of actions: researching referral resources, preparing release forms at the client's request so that the service providers she works with can exchange information, providing health education or client-centered counseling services (such as risk-reduction or medication/treatment adherence counseling related to HIV disease), and advocating on behalf of clients (with their permission) with another service provider.

Clients may be responsible for the following types of actions: changing patterns of diet or exercise; practicing a new stress management technique; reducing their use of alcohol or other drugs; not sharing syringes or works to inject drugs; carrying important medications with them throughout the day to make it easier to take them on time; attending support groups; scheduling and making an appointment with a new service provider such as a physical therapist or mental health counselor; applying for a new job; enrolling in a community college class; or calling or writing letters to their mothers, grandchildren, nephews, or sisters.

The time frame for each intervention will depend on the issues, how difficult the steps in the action plan are, and the individual or family's strengths and risks. Include some action items that are scheduled for the next few days, week, and month. If the timeline is too long, it increases the likelihood that the actions won't be accomplished. Start with steps that are less intimidating and seem most possible.

CASE STUDY **Simone (*continued*)**

Actions that Simone may take include:

- Drop by the office of the employment counseling agency, pick up a brochure, and look at some of the job listings by the end of the week.
- Make an appointment to meet with a job counselor by next Tuesday.
- Start a list of her strengths, including difficult situations that she has handled in the past, before her next care management appointment.
- Walk by the Temple of Refuge, the church that she heard about, anytime during the week and possibly on Sunday.
- Ask her friend, Terry, about the transgender women's group she goes to.

Actions that the care manager may take include:

- Before the next appointment with Simone, research and identify local resources, including culturally competent mental health counselors, agencies, and services that focus on working with transgender and gender-variant clients.
- At the next appointment, talk with Simone about preparing a release of information to talk with other service providers about how best to coordinate efforts.
- Provide advocacy—if Simone agrees—with the agencies that Simone is referred to, to help prevent further discrimination based on her gender identity.
- Identify opportunities to participate in additional trainings offered by members of the transgender community about issues related to gender identity, transgender health, and transphobia (prejudice and discrimination against transgender or gender-variant people). Sign up for a training or workshop.

Please watch the following video, ▶ which shows a CHW working with a client.

Note that in this role play, the CHW *does not* demonstrate strong client-centered skills.

- What mistakes does the CHW make in this role play?
- How might this approach affect the client?

What would you do differently if you were the CHW working with this client?

Figure 10.1 is a sample care management plan and represents one of many ways to create a care management plan.

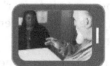

ESTABLISHING PRIORITIES FOR AN ACTION PLAN, ROLE PLAY, COUNTER

∞ *http://youtu.be/ uX65IjyHV6k*

COORDINATE WITH OTHER CARE MANAGEMENT TEAM MEMBERS

If you are working as part of a professional team, the care management plan should be developed collaboratively. The action plan will clearly detail which team member and service provider is responsible for which steps. All team members should attend regular meetings to monitor progress and any need to revise the care management plan.

Date:

Client Name:

Client ID:

CHW Name:

Date of Initial Meeting: _____

Client's Primary Goal(s):

1.

2.

Action/s to take to reach the health Goal are:

1. _____

    Will do this _____ times/week for _____

    Will do this (when, where, for how long, and with whom)

    On a scale of 1–10, confidence in completing this plan is _____

(OPTIONAL):

2. _____

    Will do this _____ times/week for _____

    Will do this (when, where, for how long, and with whom)

    On a scale of 1–10, confidence in completing this plan is _____

Resources (internal and external) that will help to reach the goal are:

Challenges that may get in the way are:

Ways to overcome or resist these challenges are:

Referrals provided (housing, mental health care, etc.):

Next Meeting (date/time/location):

Figure 10.1 Care Management Plan

Care Management Plan, Progress Notes

Date:

Progress Notes (document the client's progress in implementing their Action Plan, including successes and challenges)

The client made the following progress in implementing their Action Plan (include actions taken, when and where):

The client faced the following challenges:

The client wants to make the following changes to their Action Plan:

Referrals provided:

On a scale from 0-10 the client rates their confidence for moving forward with their Action Plan at _____

Other Notes:

Figure 10.1 (*Continued*)

PLANS CAN AND DO CHANGE

Sometimes clients will feel that some (or all) of the care management services are not working. Clients have the right to ask for changes to their action plans, and to withdraw at any time from any services or programs that they feel are not working for them. Sometimes new needs will emerge that are more important to address than the issues identified in the original plan. For example, a client may become homeless, be arrested, or relapse and start using drugs again. These circumstances will cause the immediate focus of care management to shift. When a client is not making progress with the plan, it is time to reassess. Perhaps the action plan or the goals should be revised. Perhaps the care manager should assume new responsibilities, such as advocating with other service providers on behalf of the client. You don't want a client to change the plan so often that no progress can be made (if this happens, it is important to assess why). At the same time, you don't want the care management plan to become so rigid that the client wastes times on actions that are not promoting the client's health or welfare.

PREPARING A RELEASE OF INFORMATION

You cannot divulge confidential client information to another service provider unless they are part of the care management team or the client has given you permission to do so. It may be helpful for the care manager to talk with other service providers in order to better coordinate care and to learn more effective ways to support the client. For example, you might refer a client to a physician to treat their HIV disease, to a drug treatment program, or to an immigration attorney. If you and the client agree that it would be helpful for you as the care manager to be able to talk with the other service provider, you must all sign a release of information form. These forms will clearly identify the client, the service providers, the agency they work for, and the nature of the services that they provide. The form will state that the client authorizes these service providers to share information with each other and why. Most forms will detail what kinds of information can be shared between providers and give a timeline for when the agreement will expire or end. All parties must sign the form. Remember protecting a client's confidential information is extremely important and is the law.

PROVIDING HEALTH EDUCATION AND CLIENT-CENTERED COUNSELING

Some care managers also provide health education and client-centered counseling. For example, a care manager working with a client newly diagnosed with diabetes may assess the client's knowledge about their health condition. Depending on the assessment and the extent of the client's knowledge and interest, the care manager may provide additional health education and information to assist the client in better understanding the condition and knowing how to adhere to treatments, reduce symptoms, and enhance their overall health.

CHW

TG: I provide a lot of risk-reduction counseling to my clients. We talk about how to reduce risks for HIV and other STIs, or transmitting HIV to others. If clients are using drugs, then we talk about what they can and are willing to do to reduce their use or to change it so that they are less likely to be harmed—like going to the syringe exchange to get new syringes and not sharing works with other people. To the extent that I can, I want to help clients look at what may be getting in the way of changing behavior and taking care of their health. Many clients have issues with self-esteem and depression or trauma experiences that get in the way. If they are willing to talk about any of that with me, that is a great opportunity. Of course, if I need to, I always make a referral—like I would try to link them up with a therapist if they are talking about really deep stuff that I know I'm not qualified to handle.

Practicing Cultural Humility

There are many ways to demonstrate cultural humility when working with transgender and gender variant clients and communities, such as:

1. Refer to clients using their preferred names and gender pronouns (pronouns could be he, she, or emerging gender neutral pronoun categories including s/he, they, ze, zie, and many more).

   o If you don't know a client's preferred gender pronoun, just ask. You can say something like "What pronoun do you prefer?" or "How do you like to be called?"

   o For example, a client's file may have the name "Fred" listed for the client, but "Fred" has told you she prefers to be called "Sheila." It is important to continue to call Sheila by her preferred name and pronoun, despite what the paperwork says. If you have to call Sheila by the other name listed for whatever reason (such as calling an agency on behalf of her), ask permission to do so, as this is a delicate and personal situation.

2. Know the local laws and federal policies regarding gender identity discrimination to support clients in navigating these systems. The Transgender Law Center (transgenderlawcenter.org) is a great resource for this information.

3. Advocate for gender neutral (or unisex) bathrooms in your agency. Having a safe place to use the restroom can help clients to feel more comfortable working with you and your agency.

4. Understand that hormone replacement therapy (HRT) and surgeries or body modifications may be choices that some transgender clients make, but not others. Don't assume a client has done or would like to make any of these body changes. If they have made body changes, consider how these changes may impact other aspects of their health.

5. Don't ask invasive questions—if you need to know something about body modification, use respect and ask permission to ask. As yourself, is this relevant for me to know to better support my client?

6. Know that there are very real and potentially detrimental ramifications of daily discrimination and threats of violence and harassment for transgender communities. Chronic stress, depression, anxiety, substance use, and so on, may show up as a natural response to dealing with this level of hostility and transphobia in the world.

Here are some additional suggestions for you to consider:

- The process of learning about gender identity—and transgender identities in particular—may be new for you. Be patient with yourself as you seek to ask questions, learn information, and take time to reflect on your own feelings and reactions.

- Transphobia has a great impact on transgender communities and can lead to violence, harassment, depression, suicide, and other challenges that CHWs must consider. For these reasons it is imperative that CHWs take time to learn about trans communities, ask questions, and become better informed so that they may be stronger advocates for their clients. This also helps conceptualize the many barriers transgender communities face in terms of employment, accessing services, and so on.

- Work with all communities from a client centered perspective, taking time to build rapport and prioritize the client's needs and goals, not your own. Just because a client may be transgender or gender variant, does not necessarily mean they are seeking your help because of these identities. At the same time, don't ignore these aspects of who they are.

- Practice asking "What pronouns do you use?" and remember that gender identity is a continuum. Some people identify outside of the gender binary and use gender-neutral pronouns such as "they."

- Pronouns and names can change over the course of your work together. You don't have to be the expert on this topic, which is why it's important to ask! If you make a mistake (calling someone by the wrong name or pronoun), its okay. Just take time to acknowledge and repair the mistake right away.

- Consult with your supervisor and other colleagues to get the support you need to best help transgender clients.

DOCUMENTING PROGRESS

Document or write down each contact you have with the client or other service provider who is working with the client. This will include in-person meetings with the client, phone and online conversations, and correspondence by mail. Document all relevant developments, including accomplishments and any further challenges to implementing the care management plan.

CASE STUDY   Simone *(continued)*

From Simone's File

- **11/03/2015:** Simone missed her appointment. Did not call. Don't have cell phone/contact information for her.

- **11/11/15:** Saw Simone at Raskins Park. Said hello. She did not respond. 30 minutes later she sat down beside me on a bench. She looked dirty and tired. No makeup. Bruised eye. Said she had heard from her brother. First time in 6 years. He was coming to town on business. He said he would meet her for coffee and would call back to schedule (she does have a cell phone), but never called again. He isn't returning her calls. She went out and "partied" and did crystal meth. Ended up getting in a fight and fell down some stairs. She started to cry. Sat with her for 45 minutes. Gave her my business card again, a voucher to the grocery store, and made an appointment for tomorrow. She gave me her cell phone number (333-555-7777).

- **11/12/15:** Simone was 15 minutes late, but she made it. Said: "I'm wearing my makeup today, so you better not make me cry!" Good to see her sense of humor back in action. She didn't want to talk about her brother today. She wants to start working on a plan. Said her priorities are to get a steady job so she can rent her own room in an apartment. She has been cleaning houses for money, and paying someone to sleep on their couch ("It's a dump, but it's better than staying in shelters or on the street.").

- Simone said she would think about meeting a job counselor from Rise Up, but only if I talked with a counselor first to see if they would treat her with respect as a transgender woman. She agreed for me to call Rise Up from the office, and she would listen in on the call. I reached a counselor named Bev. Said I had a client that I wanted to send her for employment counseling. I told her that the client is transgender, has experienced a lot of discrimination, and wants to be sure that she will be treated with dignity. Thankfully, Bev was wonderful, and I could see that Simone sort of lit up—a big smile. I put Bev on hold and asked Simone if she wanted to talk with her, and she did. They made an appointment for Friday. Also talked with Simone about what she could do if she experienced discrimination on the job again, and if she might talk with me or Bev or someone else about learning new ways to respond so she wouldn't lose her job. She said she'd think about it.

- **11/20/15—office:** (partial notes) Simone looked good. Has met with Bev at Rise Up twice. Progress is slower than she wants, but she is working on her resume, and is going to a workshop on interviewing and to talk with someone about getting some professional clothes. Simone and I signed a release of information. She will bring it to Bev to sign so that we can talk.

Challenges for Transgender and Gender Variant Communities

Discrimination, Harassment, and Violence

Transgender and gender variant individuals face discrimination, harassment, and violence on a daily basis. In January and February 2015 alone, six transgender women were murdered in the United States (Mock, 2015).

(continues)

Challenges for Transgender and Gender Variant Communities
(continued)

These are the murders that we know of; many more transgender folks are violently assaulted and killed every day and it never gets reported in the news. In 2014 an Oakland, California, genderqueer teenager Sasha Fleischmann was set on fire and suffered second- and third-degree burns on the bus by another student because they were wearing a skirt to school. Threats of street violence and murder are a daily reality for many transgender communities.

Employment Barriers

In 2012, the Equal Employment Opportunity Commission (EEOC) announced that the "Title VII federal sex discrimination law protects employees who are discriminated against because they are transgender or gender non-conforming" (Beyer & Weiss, 2014). While trans communities may have this protection legally, they may still face extreme barriers getting hired, or while on the job due to transphobia. Some transgender communities may then find themselves doing survival work (such as selling drugs or doing sex work), which may in turn put them at higher risk for HIV and other chronic health conditions as well as incarceration.

Other factors that impact transgender health include:

- Lack of access to culturally competent health care services (with transgender providers or transgender competent care)
- Discriminatory treatment from providers
- Denial of appropriate medical screening and treatment
- Denial of services based on gender identity (including mental health, drug rehabilitation, and so on)
- Higher rates of depression and suicide than non transgender communities
- Daily harassment including verbal harassment, street violence, and even murder for being transgender
- Employment barriers due to gender identity including being fired for gender transition while on the job
- Barriers to accessing education
- Challenges finding safe restrooms to use at public institutions
- Challenges finding housing
- Lack of culturally congruent mental health services to support transgender communities
- Chronic stress, anxiety, substance use, homelessness, poverty

TG: I can't live my client's life for them . . . but sometimes I fight the urge to tell them what to do. It gets so frustrating sometimes watching someone make the same mistake over and over again. When I start to feel this way, it is a sign that I need to take care of myself—and I usually talk with another CHW or my supervisor to get myself back on track. It also helps me to focus on the positive things, no matter how small they may seem. And every once in a while you get to focus on the truly big positive things. I was on the bus going home and this guy kept calling my name, and at first I couldn't tell who it was. It was a client from way back, someone I never thought would make it 'cause he was so caught up in using, and in and out of jail and prison, and really sick with AIDS. He looked so good. He had gained weight, his eyes were clear. He sat down and told me he was back in college studying to be a drug and alcohol counselor, and he had two years clean and sober. And when he was getting off the bus, he grabbed my shoulder and he said: "You never gave up on me, and that helped me to stop giving up on myself." I just sat there and cried—and I'm not someone who really cries—because nothing will ever feel as good as that moment. That's when I know that what I do is worth it.

SELF-ASSESSMENT

As a care manager, remember that your job is to support clients to develop clear goals and a plan to improve the quality of their lives and that of their families. Always keep in mind that *it is the client's plan, not yours.* To make sure that you are doing client-centered work, we recommend that you regularly ask yourself the following questions:

- Did the client actively establish the goals for the care management plan?
- Does this plan recognize the client's strengths and resources?
- Does it address their priority concerns?
- Did the client determine the list of actions to take to reach these goals?
- Does the client understand, and are they interested in, the referrals provided?
- Does the plan support the client's empowerment? Does it reinforce dependency on others?

ENDING CARE MANAGEMENT SERVICES

Ending care management services may also be referred to as *discharge* or *termination*. Ideally, the decision about when to end care management services will be made by both the client and the care manager, but clients can always decide whether or not to continue services.

Ideally, care management will come to an end when clients have successfully implemented key elements of their action plans and enhanced their health or well-being. Care management also strives to assist clients in developing knowledge and skills that will aid them to stay independent and to successfully manage future challenges on their own.

Ending care management, like ending any professional relationship with a client, shouldn't happen suddenly, and should include making plans to support the transition and independence of the client. In preparation for completing care management, the team may talk about the following issues:

- What has been learned and accomplished through care management
- The client's internal and external resources
- Relapse prevention, if relevant:

    Supporting clients in learning skills to prevent relapsing to old behaviors or patterns they want to avoid, such as drug use or relationships characterized by domestic violence

- What the client can do when faced with challenges or crises in the future

As a care manager, be sure to thank clients for the opportunity of working with them, and congratulate them on the accomplishments that they have made.

Ending can be difficult for both the client and the care manager. If the work has been successful and the team has established a trusting professional relationship, it can be hard to say good-bye. If you find yourself hesitating in bringing your work to a close, reflect on what is happening and seek consultation with your supervisor. You want to be as certain as possible that you are neither prolonging nor rushing to end care management because of your own feelings and needs. Care management should be completed because it is in the best interest of the clients, when they have accomplished key aspects of their plans and gained confidence and skills in promoting their own health and well-being.

TG: I have terminated [ended] my work with some clients, but then started all over again if things got worse for them—like they relapse and start using drugs or go off their AIDS medications or whatever. Expect this to happen. On the one hand, it can get discouraging because a client who worked really hard to take care of themselves and get their life under control has slipped back— usually because something bad happened to them. On the other hand, I am always happy when a client reaches out to me and asks to work together again.

(continued)

Sometimes clients terminate working with me. Sometimes they tell me why and sometimes they don't, and I just need to respect that. Sometimes they terminate me because they're mad at something I said, and then they come back and start working with me again. I had one client that must have fired me five or six times. I actually get more worried about the clients that don't want to terminate even when they've made good progress on their plan—it's like they get attached at the hip. I always worry—am I doing something to make them dependent on me?

10.4 Other Suggestions for Effective Care Management

KEEPING IN TOUCH WITH CLIENTS

Give your business card to clients, including your phone number and email address, and let them know the best way and time to reach you. Let people know how to leave a message for you and about how long, in general, it will take you to return the message.

Maintain professional boundaries, however, and don't give out your personal or home telephone number. This is a mistake that CHWs might be tempted to make with clients. It is rarely appropriate to extend your accessibility beyond the workplace, no matter how much you may want to provide aid to a client.

Ask clients what the best way is to contact them. If they don't have a phone, ask for the number of a neighbor or relative, or the number of the shelter where they're staying, or the number of the agency they are working with for housing. Write down the information and make sure it gets into their file.

Be as flexible as you can, and as your agency and safety require, in scheduling appointments. You may meet with clients at your agency, in their home, in jail or the hospital, or at a homeless shelter or other agency. If clients are uncomfortable or incapable of coming to you, see if you can go to them.

KEY TIMES TO OFFER GUIDANCE

One of the most important concepts of client-centered practice is to respect the clients' right to make their own decisions. *However, this doesn't mean that you will or should always agree with or quietly accept the clients' ideas, plans, or actions. There are key moments when it is important to speak up, gently confront or challenge your clients, and to offer them guidance.* These *may* include moments such as the following.

Clients Establish Unrealistic Goals or Expectations of Themselves

Some clients develop care management plans that are overly ambitious. For example, a client who has diabetes or high blood pressure, a long history of dieting and no history of sustained physical activity, may decide to work out for an hour every morning at a local gym. The concern is that they may be setting themselves up for failure, and if they don't follow through with their plans, they may feel bad about themselves, relapse to behaviors that put their health at risk, or drop out of care management. If you think this may be happening, say something. Assist your clients to remember that lasting change usually happens incrementally—with small steps—rather than all at once. For example, you might say something like: "Kahlil, it is great to see you so motivated to start working out and incorporating exercise in your life! I'm also aware as we have discussed that this is a challenging goal that will take some time to accomplish. Let's discuss some more realistic immediate steps toward this larger goal, that will help you feel a sense of accomplishment." With further discussion, Kahlil may change his goal and start with something that is more realistic, such as meeting with a staff member at the gym to talk about options for beginning to work out. It may be beneficial to use language that is from the client and culturally appropriate body language in these discussions. Also be aware of the words and body language that the client is expressing while engaged. If Kahlil appears to feel disappointed, investigate this response and collaboratively brainstorm other ideas together.

Clients Have Unrealistic Expectations of You or Others

Be wary of clients who put all of their expectations or hopes on you or others to ensure that they succeed in their care management plan. Some clients may pin all their hopes on getting access to a particular resource: "When my Section 8 [a housing benefit] comes through and I have a permanent place again, then I'll be able to focus on getting a job." Some clients place high expectations on winning justice through the criminal justice system: "Once this case is settled, and the judge gives me back custody of my children, then I can think about all this other stuff." Sometimes your role as a care manager is to work with clients to make plans for continuing to move forward in spite of big disappointments or setbacks: "Have you thought about what you will do if . . . (you don't get Section 8 housing, the courts don't award you custody of your daughter)? How will you continue to improve your life and your health, for yourself and for her?"

Clients Engage in Unsafe or Harmful Behaviors or Choices

If you are working with clients who are considering harming or are actively harming themselves or another person, you will need to confront these behaviors and take action to prevent further harm. Let them know that you have a responsibility to report potential harm to your supervisor or to legal authorities. For further discussion, please see Chapters 7 and 18.

- *Have you had to confront clients before?*

- *What was this like for you?*

- *If you haven't done this yet, what are your concerns?*

- *Can you think of other moments when you would consider stepping in to offer more direct guidance to a client?*

WHEN TO ADVOCATE FOR A CLIENT

Sometimes, clients are not successful in accessing the resources they have been referred to, and may benefit from some advocacy from you. For example, you might contact a drug treatment program, domestic violence shelter, or primary care physician and ask them to provide services for one of your clients.

However, the goal of care management is to support clients in managing their own lives and health, and in learning how to effectively advocate for themselves with service providers and others. If you step in too regularly to advocate on behalf of your clients, you are likely to increase their dependency on you and other caregivers and to undermine their own autonomy. To the extent possible, support your clients in developing the skills and the confidence to advocate for themselves. You might try making a call to a referral source together and asking the client to do most of the talking. If you decide to step in and talk with the other provider directly, debrief this afterward with the client: ask the client what this experience was like, and if they would like to do it differently the next time. If they make the contact on their own, follow up with them to find out how it went, if they were able to access services, and what their experience was like with the other agency or service provider. As with many aspects of your work as a CHW, the challenge here is to strike the proper balance between supporting the client's independence and autonomy and stepping in as needed to try to prevent unnecessary harm.

CASE STUDY   **Simone** *(continued)*

As a transgender woman, Simone has experienced ongoing prejudice, harassment, and discrimination. While you can support her in learning new ways of responding when this occurs, you can also advocate for her—with her permission—to try to prevent further discrimination within your own agency and by the service providers you refer her to. This is a human rights issue: all people deserve to be treated fairly and with respect.

10.5 Common Care Management Challenges

CHALLENGING MOMENTS WITH CLIENTS

You will work with clients facing serious health problems and other life challenges. They may be scared, frustrated, angry, or in despair. They may be suspicious of your efforts to assist. They may not always be honest with you. They may complain about you to your supervisor. They may have diagnosed or undiagnosed mental health issues and may or may not be under treatment, be using alcohol or drugs, or have difficulty communicating their needs.

> ### A Note on the Language We Use
>
> Some service providers use the phrase "difficult clients" to describe the challenges they face in working with clients. This language can be used to judge, stigmatize, and discriminate against people who are different from us, who we don't understand, and who may most need our compassion and care management skills. We prefer to consider the many reasons why working with people can be challenging, and to use instead consumer-driven positive language of empowerment and encouragement for all clients.

Try to keep in mind that the clients wouldn't require your assistance if everything were going well in their lives. Try to understand that anxiety, frustration, and anger are likely responses to difficult circumstances. Don't take the client's behavior personally. With time, you may be able to support them in learning more effective ways of handling difficult emotions. Refer to Chapter 13 to review conflict resolution concepts and skills.

CASE STUDY   Simone (*continued*)

> Consider some of the reasons why Simone may exhibit argumentative behaviors (toward other members of her residential drug treatment program) and perhaps towards you. Simone is justifiably angry about her history of discriminatory treatment and the recent experiences that motivated her to see you. Simply as a consequence of who she is—her identity as a transgender woman—Simone was rejected by her family and church; she lost her job, her career, and her home. In addition, Simone faces the daily experience of discrimination and harassment based on her gender identity. This ranges from mean looks to verbal harassment to a very real threat of violence.
>
> In working with Simone, leave space for her to talk about these experiences, if she wishes to, and to express her emotions. Listen with compassion and draw upon your client-centered skills.

> **TG:** Sometimes, when a client is acting out and making a scene or yelling or something, I just get so frustrated. I might have had a really hard day already, or maybe a client died recently or I had a fight with my boyfriend—whatever—and I worry that I'm going to lose it. Sometimes I just have to remind myself, "This isn't about me. This is their life, not mine." It's not like I don't know this, but sometimes I just have to remind myself so that I can take a step back and find a way to be patient and calm.

BEING HONEST AND SETTING BOUNDARIES

From the very beginning, be clear with clients about what you can and cannot do to assist them in your role as care manager. Make sure the individual client or family understands your program's guidelines. For instance, as a CHW you may be able to assist a family to get groceries from a food bank and refer them to WIC or food stamp programs if they are not already enrolled, but you cannot lend them money for groceries.

Lee Jackson: When it comes to loaning money to clients, no way. I explain my job to them and tell them that I have boundaries. Sometimes they'll ask you to lend them money and say they'll pay you back double or something like that. So I tell them: "No, I'm not a loan shark. I'm a health worker. I'm here to get you to your appointments and make sure you're okay and get you back on your feet, and if you need housing we'll help get you housing, but I can't loan you money."

Honesty and healthy boundaries enable your clients to trust you (please see Chapter 7). Healthy boundaries protect your clients from unrealistic expectations and the disappointments that are inevitable when those expectations aren't met. Just as important, honesty and good boundaries protect you. Doing community health work can be very stressful. It can be draining to witness the hardships that your clients face. Nobody gains if you give clients unrealistic expectations that you can't meet. And nobody gains if you overextend yourself, burn out, and quit community health work altogether.

Ramona: I worked with a young lady and visited her at her apartment. When she and her partner got high, he sometimes beat her up. She told me this when I did the initial intake. So, I went to her house several times, and I was trying to help her to leave and go into a safe women's shelter. It was a learning experience for me because I knew about the resource [the shelter] and I just thought all it took was to call them up and get a space and help the lady to move over there. But I needed to understand how much more complicated that kind of situation is and how hard it can be to leave. I didn't really think about or understand that there was danger there for me, too, that I wasn't invincible to that danger, until her partner threatened me also. I just wanted to help her get away from the domestic violence. But rather than going back to the home to see if she was ready to leave, I gave her my number and I made a call to her, and later we met outside and she decided that she did want to go to the shelter. So, for me, it was a learning experience about danger, as well, and about how much I can take on—or what I can do for a client. But I'm still glad that this lady got out. Even for a while, it made her see and think differently about how her life could be.

A REMINDER ABOUT SELF CARE

If you don't learn to take care of yourself with the same dedication you show in working with your clients, you may harm your own health and your ability to provide high-quality, culturally competent services to others. For more information about self care, see Chapter 12.

10.6 Working with Families

As a Community Health Worker, you are likely to work closely with families as well as individual clients. While in many ways, working with a family as the client is similar to working with an individual, there are also key differences to consider. As we don't address the topic of working with families in depth in this textbook, we encourage you to seek out additional opportunities for further training and professional development for understanding family systems and supporting the health of diverse family units.

The types of settings in which CHWs may work with families include both clinical and community-based settings, and you may address a wide variety of health, mental health, and social issues and challenges. CHWs may work independently with families, or in close collaboration with other colleagues or as a member of a team.

A person's life, their personality, and sense of self are informed by their experience in a family system. The influence of the families who raised us may have both positive and negative (or harmful) impacts. Our families of origin show us how and who to be, and along with many other factors (including economic factors, divorce or separation, conflict or abuse, etc.), create the structure for our understanding of the world.

It is important to know and be prepared to accept and respect every family that that comes to you for support in your role as a CHW. This is both an ethical obligation, and an opportunity to demonstrate your cultural humility.

You may work with a family who has a child living with asthma, a person who is caring for an older relative with Alzheimer's, a gay couple, a multigenerational household, and many other forms of families. Family structures are highly diverse and may vary in many ways, including:

- **Age and generation**: Some families include members of more than one or several generations.
- **Partnership and parenting status**: Some families include people who are married or divorced as well as couples who were never married or who have a domestic partner status. Some families are characterized by one or two parents or more. In some families, parenting duties are shared by many different family members.
- **Status of children**: Some children are biologically related, others are adopted or part of a foster care system.
- **Ethnicity**: Many families include people of more than one (or many) ethnicities.
- **Gender and gender identity**
- **Sexual orientation**
- **Immigration status, religious or political affiliation, and so forth**

What Do YOU? Think!

- *How do you define family?*

- *What type of family system did you grow up in?*

- *Who do you consider to be part of your family system today?*

- *What other types of family systems are you familiar with?*

Some family systems and structures may be unfamiliar to you. This will change over time as you work with more families. Along the way, remember to examine your own biases and assumptions about families, identify challenges that you may face, and seek additional training or consultation to enhance your knowledge and ability to demonstrate cultural humility. Apply client-centered skills, including motivational interviewing skills, to learn from the family you are working with about their experiences, identity, values, strengths, and priority concerns.

When working with family systems, it is important to remember that ". . . in any system each part is related to all other parts . . . [so that] . . . a change in any part of the system will bring about changes in all other parts" (Center for Substance Abuse Treatment, 2004). Using a strength-based, client-centered model or approach to care management is a foundation to empower the individuals in the family system as well as the system itself. The idea is that if one person changes a behavior or pattern of communication, the family as a whole may experience a change or shift in their dynamic and an opportunity for change. Keep in mind that if you are working with a family, then the entire family is the client. Care management plans, goals, and actions should reflect the interests of the entire family system, not just one person.

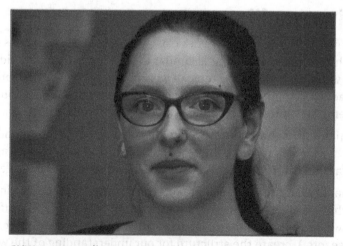

CHWs support clients to set goals and to take action to meet those goals.

Sometimes families seek services related to an "Identified Patient/Client" or the family member who appears to be causing distress to other members. This could be the 14-year-old son who is bullying other children at school, the elderly grandmother who has moved into the house and requires full-time health care, or the husband who is unemployed and suffering from depression. Other family members may feel that they have identified their "problem," and they may not realize how other family members contribute to the challenges they are facing. When this occurs, a care management goal is to reframe the idea and the focus of an "Identified Patient," and to shift the focus of the conversation to examine the larger family system as a whole.

One of the main aspects of working with families is to achieve what is referred to as **homeostasis**, or balance within the family system. For example, a CHW working a family with the 14-year-old boy who is bullying at school, may consider the role of the parents, the role of the school, other factors and stressors that impact the boy, and how all of these elements can throw the whole system off balance. Restoring the balance (or homeostasis) over time will mean addressing all of these factors, not just the boy's bullying behavior.

There are some major differences and similarities between working with an individual versus working with a family. Some of the key differences include:

KEY SIMILARITIES IN WORKING WITH INDIVIDUALS AND FAMILIES

There are also many similarities to working with individuals and families (see Table 10.1). These similarities include:

- **An ecological framework**: Keep an ecological system (see Chapter 3) in mind, looking beyond the individual or family system to consider how broader neighborhood, social and economic factors may influence health and wellness.

- **A systems perspective**: Keep in mind that both individuals and families are part of multiple systems that influence their health (including relationships at school and work, in the community, etc.).

- **Ethics**: The same ethical considerations guide a CHW's work with individuals and families, including issues such as maintaining confidentiality, scope of practice and healthy professional boundaries.

- **Cultural humility**: CHW's should practice cultural humility, recognizing the individual or family as the expert regarding their own cultural values and beliefs.

- **Use of client-centered skills**: CHWs will draw upon the same client-centered concepts and skills, including a strength-based approach, harm reduction, and techniques such as motivational interviewing.

- **Action planning:** With both individuals and families, CHWs will support them to develop action plans including key goals that they wish to reach, and the realistic actions or steps that they can take to reach those goals.

- *Can you identity other similarities regarding how CHWs work with individuals and families?*

What Do YOU Think?

Table 10.1 Key Differences between Working with Individuals and Families

INDIVIDUALS	FAMILIES
Working with one person. The individual is the client.	Working with two or more people. The family is the client.
Prioritizes the health goals and concerns of an individual	Prioritizes the health goals and concerns of a family system
Focuses on supporting an individual to take action to create change and promote health	Focuses on supporting the family system to take actions to create change and promote the health of the family system as whole
Strives for individual "homeostasis" or balance	Strives for family system "homeostasis" or balance
What other differences can you think of?	

10.7 Identifying Community Resources and Providing Referrals

A key part of your job as a care manager is to become familiar with the local resources that your clients may need, including housing, legal assistance, employment training and job counseling, education, child care, health care and mental health care, drug treatment resources, and more. In some cities and counties, local government or private agencies develop and regularly update a list of such resources. Increasingly, these detailed guides to local resources are available online.

If you don't have access to a comprehensive guide to local resources, you and your colleagues may need to develop one. This takes a lot of time, so make sure to talk with your supervisor and ask for support for this task. It will involve undertaking research to identify key resources that are most important to promoting the community's health. You can do this by conducting research on the Internet, going to the local library, reviewing local papers, including free papers, and talking with colleagues to create a list of the full range of resources that you want to assist your clients to access. Most important, don't forget to talk with your clients: they often have extensive knowledge about a wide range of available services, and strong opinions about which ones are the most and least beneficial.

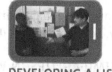

DEVELOPING A LIST OF REFERRALS: CHW INTERVIEW

⬤ *http://youtu.be/ xKJQo6HExq4*

We want to recognize that identifying resources can be particularly challenging when you are working in rural areas or in a large county where services may be spread out geographically and difficult for your clients to reach, particularly if there isn't a good public transportation system.

Please watch the following video ▶ interview with a CHW.

Developing a Guide to Resources

If you need to develop your own resource guide, we recommend organizing resources by category—such as housing resources—and to update them regularly by replacing outdated items with new information. For each agency, gather as much of the following information if available:

- Name, address, and website of the agency. If the agency has a presence on social media sites, such as Facebook, include that information as well.
- A list of the services they provide (support groups, counseling, community organizing, legal or medical services, and so on)
- The cost of services
- Eligibility requirements (such as income limits, age limits, services for families without immigration papers, and so on)
- Email addresses and phone numbers for key personnel (if available)
- Hours of operation
- How to get there: directions, public transportation, parking
- Can clients drop in, or do they need to make an appointment?
- Whom to ask for, if possible (you might want to include the business cards of individual service providers)
- What the client or family should bring to the first appointment

Your up-to-date list of referrals is one of the best ways you can guide clients to the care and assistance they need. However, not all referrals are good referrals. Many people have had the experience of receiving a referral and calling the number only to discover that the line has been disconnected, or they aren't eligible for services. Worse yet is when clients make the effort to go to the agency or program, only to find that the office is closed, that they should have brought certain identification or paperwork, or that they don't meet the eligibility guidelines. To avoid sending your clients or their families on a wild goose chase, provide up-to-date and thorough information about where you're sending them. Once you have gathered one or more resource guides for your area, call the numbers and find out from the agency how to refer clients. If it is a resource you will often refer clients to, build a relationship with a contact person(s) there. Get to know them by name, so that when you send someone there, you can call your contact person and let them know one of your clients is coming.

Be aware that some organizations that provide important services are funded by grants. When the grants end, the program or service may also end or change. Personnel at agencies and organizations also change along with phone numbers and addresses. In order to make sure you provide clients with good referrals, try to update your resource list every month or two. And, remember to reciprocate with other agencies. If your program experiences changes, get the word out to other agencies so that they can update their resource listings. This way, other agencies will also be able to make effective referrals to your program.

Whether a wonderful guide to local resources already exists or you have to create one, you should make time to network and establish professional relationships with local organizations and programs. In many cities there are regular meetings of service providers that you can attend. Bring your business card, and take time before and after the meeting, and during breaks, to introduce yourself to other providers, talk about your work, and learn about the services that they provide. Collect their business cards. If possible, make a time to visit the key resources that you most frequently recommend to clients. While you visit, pick up brochures and other information that will assist you in making effective referrals to the agency in the future. File them in your resource binder, if you keep one.

> **Lee:** Since I've been doing this job, I've become friends with people in different agencies. If I need some help or a referral, I can just call these people and say, "Look, I have this client and they need to come in for detox. Do you have any beds?" Then they might say, "Well, we have maybe two beds, but we'll hold one for your client."

The longer you work as a CHW, the more you will know about existing resources, the quality of services they provide, and the professionals who work there. Getting to know a competent provider at another organization is invaluable. When you can provide a client not only with a referral to quality services they are interested in, but also with the name and phone number of a staff member whom you know and trust, you greatly increase the chance that your client will follow through with the referral, and that they will be received and treated with the respect and attention they deserve. Remember that at the same time, you will become a trusted and valued resource for colleagues at other agencies. Receive the clients they refer to you in the same manner that you would like them to treat your clients.

> **TG:** The longer I do this work, the more I know about the resources that exist out there, even though they are always changing. And I have learned from experience what agencies I can trust to provide good service to my clients. Mostly, it is the same five to six resources that I refer my clients to: places to eat, decent shelters, mental health care, residential or day drug treatment programs, good primary health care—there is a great program at the public hospital, and legal assistance. It has been really hard to find good legal help about immigration issues. My clients have had some horrible experiences. Now I send them to a nonprofit center and let them provide the legal referrals because they are the experts in this area and I'm not. I go to a couple of meetings with different types of service providers so that I can get to know people. I like to know the person that I'm calling—or that my client is calling; it definitely makes a difference in terms of getting a quick response.

- *What types of services have you or your family used in the past that you would recommend to clients?*

- *What types of services do you think would be most important for clients from your own community?*

- *What types of services or resources do you think will be hardest to find in your community?*

PROVIDING EFFECTIVE REFERRALS

Providing an effective referral is harder than it sounds. Some providers assume that all they need to do is to pass on information to a client, and the client will quickly and successfully access this new service. But clients may face many obstacles on the way to accessing a new program or service. For example, the referral may not be a priority or relevant to the client. The client may not understand the nature of the referral and the services provided or be eligible for those services. The client may be hesitant to contact the agency, forget about the referral, or lose the business card or note you provided. The agency you refer them to may or may not provide services that are culturally or linguistically appropriate or accessible to the client.

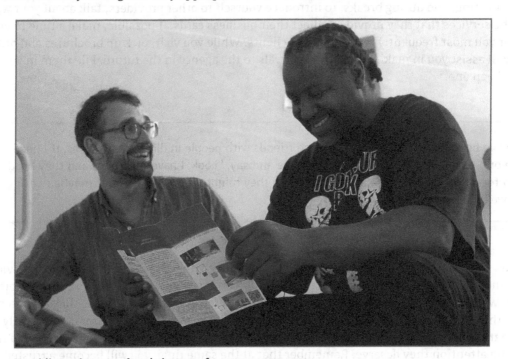

Providing relevant referrals is part of care management.

> **TG:** The thing I always hated when I was a client was when someone would hand me a slip of paper with the name of some organization I never asked them for and tell me that I should call up such-and-such agency and they could help me with such-and-such problem. Then they would just change the topic or leave and act as if they had done me some kind of favor. First of all, don't tell me to go somewhere without even asking me if I'm interested—that drives me crazy! Second, even if I was interested, do you think some paper with an address or a phone number or even a business card is going to help me down the road if I don't really understand what the place is or what they do or who to talk to or anything? That's not a referral, that's an insult!

The goal of providing referrals is to successfully link clients with key resources that they are interested in and may receive services from. To fulfill this goal, we recommend the following:

- The referral should be to a service that is of strong interest to the client.

- Clearly explain the referral, including the name of the agency or provider, the services they provide, and how these may be relevant to the client's identified priorities and needs. To be absolutely certain that the client understands this information, ask the client to repeat it back to you ("Claire, I want to make sure that I am communicating clearly. Can you tell me what you understand about this program I am recommending and how it might benefit you?").

- Check the eligibility requirements of the agencies and their programs to be certain that they still exist and can indeed serve your clients (some programs have requirements based on income, gender, nationality, citizenship, age, language, disability, diagnosis with a specific health condition, length of time in recovery from drug or alcohol addiction, or other eligibility requirements).

- Provide clear and specific guidance about how, when, and where to access the agency or program. Where is it located? How can the client get there? When is it open? If you know and trust someone who works there and may provide services to your clients, give them this professional's name. If you need to make a call to ask for further information, ask the client if she would like to make the call, or if she would like to make the call with you.

- If your client does not speak English (or the dominant language where you work), check to see whether the agency provides services in your client's primary language or will provide interpretation services.

- Write down information about referrals so that clients can remember what you have told them. If you are working with clients who cannot read easily, it is still important to write the information down so that they can show it to family members or friends if they need assistance.

- Contact the referral agency to let them know that you have made the referral.

- Check in with your clients to see if they followed up with the referrals, if they accessed services, and what their experiences were like. Document this in the client's case files. Following up with your clients is particularly important. Taking the initiative to find out what happened allows you to ensure that your clients actually get the services they need.

What Do YOU Think?

- *What has your experience been with referrals?*

- *Have you received helpful or unhelpful referrals?*

- *What else can CHWs do to provide effective referrals?*

Martha Shearer: I explain the program I work for, what clients can expect, and tell them I am there to assist them. I say, "You tell me what you need and let me see how I can help. If I can't do it, I know someone else who can." I know my clients' standard needs are medications, housing, food stamps, clothing, and food. I know all the organizations in and around Birmingham [Alabama] that can provide assistance, so when these issues come up, I am ready to provide a referral to the client. Of course, a lot of the time, with my clients, we go visit the agency or program together the first time. I want to make a personal introduction and make sure I leave them in good hands.

Please watch the following short videos, 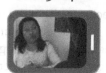 which show a CHW working with a client and providing a referral.

The first video is a counter role play, highlighting a common mistake that helping professionals may make.

The second video shows a CHW who is applying client-centered skills to provide the referral.

- What mistake(s) does the CHW make in the counter role play, and how may this impact the client?
- What did the CHW do well in the demonstration role play?
- What else would you do—or do differently—to provide a client-centered referral in this situation?

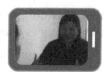

PROVIDING A CLIENT-CENTERED REFERRAL: ROLE PLAY, COUNTER

http://youtu.be/SzYoL5tA4DU

PROVIDING A CLIENT-CENTERED REFERRAL: ROLE PLAY, DEMO

http://youtu.be/2GoI8gJGSZg

Scarce Resources

It is often difficult to find resources for clients. Certain types of services may not exist in your community or nearby. Services may exclude your clients for one reason or another, such as their gender, gender identity, immigration or health insurance status, income, family size, or other factors. Health care, legal assistance, and housing are often among the most difficult types of referrals to locate for your clients. Keep building relationships and networking with other health and social services providers to learn about available resources. And be honest with your clients about the limited availability of certain resources.

10.8 Organizing and Documenting Your Work

MAKE A SCHEDULE AND KEEP IT

Care management is a challenging job, and no two days are likely to be the same. There is no way to accurately predict the times when clients will experience crises, or when your case load or the number of clients you work with will increase. Create a schedule that shows the time and location of care management sessions, team meetings, case conferences, and other responsibilities each week. Be sure to include time to take a break, eat lunch, and to document the services you provide.

Time management is key to avoiding your own burnout as well as maintaining positive professional relationships with your clients.

MANAGING CASE FILES

Documenting the services you provide and managing your case files is an ethical duty and part of your responsibility to clients and your agency. Forms are used to track the services your clients have received in order to evaluate the program and to provide reports to the institution that funds it. These files may be electronic or paper, or both. Accurate documentation and maintenance of case files are essential for ongoing funding.

Your clear records provide insight into the depth and quality of your work and assist supervisors in evaluating your performance. These records can also clear up misunderstandings that may arise.

Most importantly, these records are useful for understanding a client's progress and provide essential information for improving the quality of services that clients receive.

Basic guidelines for managing your case files include:

- **Explain note taking to clients**: Please take time to clearly explain to clients how and why you are taking notes. Let them know that you are taking careful note of what they tell you so that you can remember this information and provide quality services. Provide clients with a copy of the form that you will be using to take notes, so that they can see for themselves the type of information you will be documenting. It may also be helpful to explain to clients that if you are looking down as you take notes, you are still listening to them.

- **Keep all files confidential**: Clients will share personal information with you. In order to maintain your clients' trust, you must protect that information. As a provider, you are also legally required to protect their confidentiality. Don't leave forms or folders lying around where other people might see them. Put files in a file cabinet or other location that you can lock at the end of the day. Treat the information with care and respect. Don't share personal information with other service providers unless you get the client's written permission first. Learn your program's confidentiality guidelines. If you have questions, ask your supervisor.

- **Alphabetize**: Make a file folder for each client or family and keep the folders in alphabetical order by last name. Keep these files in safe place—such as a locked file cabinet or a file drawer in your desk.

- **Use appropriate forms**: Use the forms that your agency provides to document client information and the delivery of services. It will be much easier to keep track of information and share it with other members of your team if everyone is using the same forms. If you don't like something about a form, talk to your supervisor. Perhaps the forms can be changed to improve the quality of your work.

- **Write clearly**: Write clearly when you complete forms and document progress notes. If your handwriting is hard for others to read, print. Write not only for yourself, but for others who will need to read your notes, including others who may work with this client in the future.

- **Keep data in a consistent order**: Keep all the information in each client's folder in the same order: This will make it easier to tell if anything is missing or incomplete. You might even want to use or make a checklist of what is supposed to be in the folder. You may come up with your own system to remind you of things you have promised to do for someone, but be sure that other people can understand it too.

- **Keep files up-to-date**: Update your active case folders periodically, such as every week or month, as appropriate to the program you work for. Jot down case notes every time you have completed a session with a client. Be sure to put down the date of the session, what was discussed, referrals you provided, and any agreements on future actions to be taken. Case notes are very important, but they work for you only if you can understand them when you read them later.

Lee Jackson: For documentation I have a client contact sheet, and each time I come into contact with a client, I document it. I make time every day just to do my notes, or I'd never be able to keep up. There's definitely a lot of paperwork with this job. I write down how much time I spend with the client, and the care management and health education plans we develop, and their progress. At the end of the month, I have to tally up all of my contacts, and we fax a report to the state health department.

TAKING SOAP NOTES

There are many different systems for documenting care management and other client or patient services. SOAP notes is one documentation system that is sometimes used by CHWs and other providers (SOAP notes may or may not be used by the agency you work for). SOAP stands for: **S**ubjective, **O**bjective, **A**ssessment, and **P**lan. Below is an example of SOAP notes based on an interview with a family about the management of their child's asthma.

Subjective

The subjective part of the notes includes *what clients report to you* regarding their knowledge, feelings, attitudes, and behaviors. For example, this might include what a client tells you about their child's asthma, including what they say they do to aid in managing it, things that happened in the past, how they understand the issue, and how they feel about it. Subjective notes provide a picture of the client's experience and perspective. To gather this information, you will need to ask a number of specific questions designed to draw out specific details.

CASE STUDY | **Christa**

Christa's mom reports that her asthma has been under good control. Last week, on her second day of kindergarten, Christa had her first flare-up in months. Christa says she got wheezy on the playground. Her mother thinks the episode may have been brought on by exercise. The teacher did have a copy of Christa's asthma action plan and sent her to the office for medication. Christa says she felt fine after that, but her mother is worried that there may be asthma triggers in the school.

SOAP Notes Should Be

- Brief, to the point
- Based on observations, not judgments
- Strength-based approach

Objective

The objective information that you document includes *what you directly observe and hear during your meetings and conversations with clients.* These notes will simply describe who did what and who said what, without any interpretation, judgment, or analysis from you.

CASE STUDY | **Christa** (*continued*)

When I visited the apartment on June 6, 2008, I saw Christa's asthma action plan taped to the refrigerator. Her medications were in her medication box in the bathroom. The neighbor's cat came into the back kitchen while we were talking and rubbed against the furniture. Christa petted the cat. Her mother said: "I told you not to touch him!" The cat wandered down the hall into their apartment. Christa's mother told me that nobody smokes in the house. I saw an ashtray with several cigarette butts on the kitchen counter by the back door.

Assessment

The assessment is the place where you can document *your own thoughts, interpretations, and analysis (subjective opinion) about what you observed and heard* from the clients (objective information). You want to be careful about making judgments that the objective evidence does not support, particularly allegations that could potentially harm the client. Remember that you may be asked to explain or to defend any assessments that you make regarding your clients. When writing an assessment, be as detailed and as clear as possible about the situation you are describing.

CASE STUDY | **Christa** (*continued*)

Mrs. Lee seems to be more focused on Christa's asthma symptoms at school and in other environments outside the home. She does a good job keeping track of Christa's action plan and medications. She did not seem as worried about trying to control Christa's exposure to asthma triggers at home, such as smoke and the neighbor's cat.

Plan

This is the place to document *what you and the client plan to do in the future.* You will want to include actions that the client plans to take, any special requests the client may make, services you will provide, referrals, and reminders for the next home visit or appointment.

CASE STUDY | **Christa** (*continued*)

Mrs. Lee says she will make notes if Christa has another episode at school. She will also call the school nurse to ask for more information. I will check on Christa's asthma medications at the next visit, and talk with Mrs. Lee about smoking in the house. Will try to determine who is smoking and how to stop or reduce smoking in the apartment. Will bring Mrs. Lee a pamphlet on the risks of secondhand smoke, and some referrals for free smoking cessation programs. Will ask more questions about the neighbor's cat: Does Christa have symptoms when the cat is around? Has she been tested for allergies to cats (there is no note in the file)?

10.9 Participating in Case Conferences

Case or client conferences bring together members of a team who work with common clients, or colleagues who work with similar clients. The purpose of a case conference is to:

- Improve the quality of services provided to clients
- Improve coordination between service providers and service teams
- Enhance the professional skills of service providers

During a case conference, one team member may be asked to present information about a particular client or care. If the meeting is taking place only among team members who have permission from the client to share confidential information with each other, then any of this information may be discussed. If not, then the care is discussed in more general terms, keeping the identity of the client confidential.

Often priority is given to a CHW or other colleague who is working with a client in crisis or who is facing one or more notable challenges. The CHW provides background information (maintaining confidentiality), including the client's care management goals and progress made thus far, and describes current challenges, questions, or concerns. The group discusses the care with the goal of identifying strategies for working with the client and referrals that may promote the client's progress and well-being. Sometimes another colleague will have information about the client that can shed light on the situation. In this way, participants share information and skills with each other, enhancing their own. Most important, clients benefit from new insights and suggestions that may arise.

If you have been asked to present at a case conference, make sure to prepare by updating and reviewing the case files, including the client's goals, strengths, accomplishments, and outstanding risks, needs, or concerns.

What are your questions or concerns? Do you have questions about available resources for the client? What do you want to ask your colleagues? How might they be supportive of your work? What important information about the client should you share with the team, to enable them to provide the best possible care?

Strive to provide your colleagues with the same type of support that you would most benefit from. Let them know about the referrals that have been most beneficial to your clients. Share any suggestions that you might have based on your own experiences working with similar clients and challenges.

Chapter Review

To review care management practices, let's also review the case study about the client named Simone that was presented throughout this chapter. After reviewing the case study, do your best to answer the questions provided, and to consider how you would provide care management services to Simone.

Based on the information in the case study, do your best to answer the following questions:

- What are some of Simone's strengths (internal and external resources)?
- What may be some of her outstanding risks and needs?
- What specific strengths, risks, and needs would you want to assess? What questions will you ask Simone in order to assess these?
- What types of referrals might you want to suggest to Simone?
- What challenges might you face in working with Simone?
- How might you evaluate whether or not you are providing client-centered care management?
- When and how will you document care management services?
- What questions might you pose to the group if you were presenting your work with Simone at a case conference? What types of suggestions or support might assist you to provide more effective care management services to Simone?
- How can you be an advocate for Simone in collaboration with her coordination of care? Within your agency?
- What are some things that are important to remember when providing services to and with transgender communities?

References

Beyer, Dana, & Weiss, Jillian T., with Riki Wilchins. (2014). *New Title VII and EEOC rulings protect transgender employees.* Retrieved from *http://transgenderlawcenter.org/issues/employment/titlevii*

Brownstein, J. N., & Allen, C. (2015). *Addressing chronic disease through community health workers: a policy and systems-level approach* (2nd ed.). Retrieved from *www.cdc.gov/dhdsp/docs/chw_brief.pdf*

Center for Health Care Strategies. (n.d.). *Care management definition and framework.* Retrieved from *www.chcs. org/media/Care_Management_Framework.pdf*

Center for Substance Abuse Treatment. (2004). *Substance abuse treatment and family therapy.* (Treatment Improvement Protocol (TIP) Series, No. 39.) Rockville, MD. Retrieved from *www.ncbi.nlm.nih.gov/books/NBK64265/*

Findley, S., Matos, S., Hicks, A., Chang, J., & Reich, D. (2014). Community health worker integration into the health care team accomplishes the triple aim in a patient-centered medical home: A Bronx tale. *Journal of Ambulatory Care Management, 37,* 82–91.

Mock, J. (2015). *A note on visibility in the wake of 6 trans women's murders in 2015.* Retrieved from *http://janetmock.com/2015/02/16/six-trans-women-killed-this-year/*

Sausa, L. A. (2008). Gender diversity project: Resources for education. City College of San Francisco. Retrieved from *http://www.ccsf.edu/Departments/Health_Education_and_Community_Health_Studies/HIV/GDP%20 binder%20v5%20with%20cover%202.24.09.pdf*

Trappenburg, J. C. A., Monninkhof, E. M., Bourbeau, J., Troosters, T., Schrijvers, A. J. P., Verheij, T. J. M., & Lammers, J. J. (2011). Chronic obstructive pulmonary disease: Effect of an action plan with ongoing support by a case manager on exacerbation-related outcome in patients with COPD: A multicentre randomised controlled trial. *Thorax, 66,* 977–984. Retrieved from *http://thorax.bmj.com/content/66/11/977.long*

Additional Resources

Case Management Society of America. (2010). *Standards of practice for case management.* Retrieved from *www. cmsa.org/portals/0/pdf/memberonly/StandardsOfPractice.pdf*

Center for Human Resources, Brandeis University. (n.d.). Case management with at-risk youth. Retrieved from *http://smhp.psych.ucla.edu/qf/case_mgmt_qt/Case_Management_with_At-risk_Youth.pdf*

Gender Diversity Project at City College of San Francisco. (n.d.) Retrieved from *http://www.ccsf.edu/en/ educational-programs/school-and-departments/school-of-health-and-physical-education/health-education-and-community-health-studieso/LinkCtr/gender_diversity_project.html*

NYC Department of Youth and Community Development, Case Management Standards Toolkit. (2001). Retrieved from *www.nyc.gov/html/dycd/downloads/pdf/NYC_DYCD_Case_Management_Toolkit-2011.pdf*

The Transgender Law and Policy Institute. (n.d.). Retrieved from *www.transgenderlaw.org*

Youth-Centered Referrals, the UFO Model Intervention Replication Manual. (2013). Retrieved from *http://ufomodel.com/referrals*

Selected Resources on Gender Identity

Center of Excellence for Transgender Health. (n.d.).Retrieved from *http://www.transhealth.ucsf.edu*

Gender Bread. (n.d.). Retrieved April 9, 2015, from *www.thegenderbreadkit.com*

Gender Spectrum. (n.d.). Retrieved from *www.genderspectrum.org*

Intersex Society of North America. (n.d.). Retrieved from *www.isna.org*

National Center for Transgender Equality. (n.d.). Retrieved from *www.transequality.org*

Transgender Law Center. (n.d.). Retrieved from *www.transgenderlawcenter.org*

World Professional Association for Transgender Health. (n.d.). Retrieved from *www.wpath.org/*

Home Visiting

11

Craig Wenzl, Tim Berthold, and Emily Marinelli

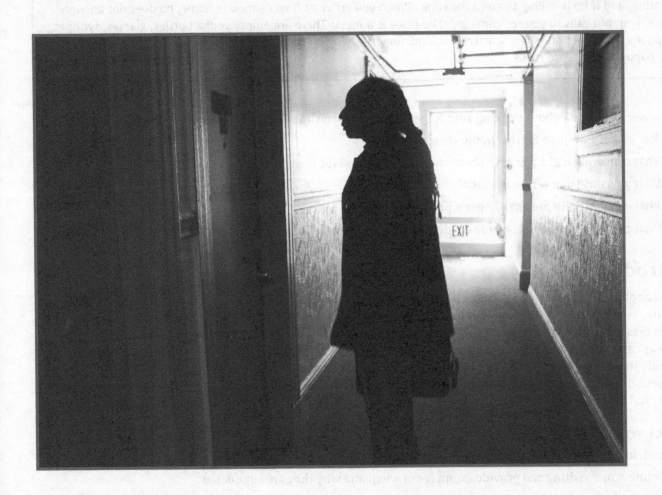

CASE STUDY Roger

Roger is 44 years old and living with HIV and hepatitis C. You provide him with case management services. Recently, Roger missed two appointments with his doctor. He has not been to your agency for over a month. You called Roger this morning and were able to get him on the phone. He sounds very weak and very ill. You set up a time to visit him this afternoon. You want to see how he's doing, if he's taking his meds, if he's eating, and if he is willing to go to the clinic. When you arrive at Roger's mobile home, he does not answer the door, but calls to you to "come in." The place is a mess: There are empty vodka bottles, glasses, syringes, spoons, and other drug gear scattered around. Roger is lying on the couch. When he sees you, he smiles: He is happy that you are there.

If you were the CHW who is working with Roger, how would you answer the following questions:

- How will you prepare for this home visit?
- What concerns might you have about the home visit and for Roger?
- What goals will you set for the visit?
- What will you do to preserve Roger's privacy?
- What type of assessment can you conduct during the home visit, and how?

Introduction

This chapter addresses how to conduct home visits to clients. Home visits are a valuable way to reach some clients, especially those who find it difficult to leave home due to illness, disability, family responsibilities, or other reasons. Home visits are often an extension of the kinds of services that you provide in other settings—such as case management or client-centered counseling and health education. The key difference is that you provide these services in someone's home and have a duty to respect that setting. Meeting clients in their homes can also provide you with an increased understanding of their lives, including their strengths, resources, risks, and needs.

WHAT YOU WILL LEARN

By studying the information in this chapter, you will be able to:

- Define home visiting and provide examples of when and why they are conducted
- Prepare for home visits
- Identify key safety concerns and plan for ways to address them
- Discuss what to do (and what not to do) when you arrive at a client's home
- Conduct a subtle assessment of the home environment, and explain why this is important
- Identify and respond to common challenges related to home visiting

11.1 An Overview of Home Visiting

Home visiting, as the name suggests, involves meeting with clients where they live. This may be an apartment, home, trailer, single-room occupancy (SRO) hotel, a shelter, jail, homeless encampment, on the streets, in the park—any number of possibilities. Home visiting is one of the most direct and personal ways to work with clients.

You will conduct home visits to clients who find it difficult, for one reason or another, to meet with you elsewhere, or because visiting clients at home will be helpful in terms of promoting their health. For example, visiting a client with asthma or a newborn infant can provide you with an opportunity to assess the home environment and explore options for reducing health risks and promoting wellness.

You may visit people you have never met before to encourage them to come to your agency for testing, health screening, counseling, or other services. You may follow up with an existing client who is unable to come to your office because of severe disability, injury, major health concerns, fear, or other barriers. Whether you have met the clients before or not, visiting them in their homes can assist you to better understand the context they live in and certain health risks, needs, and strengths. But visiting clients in their homes requires the utmost respect from you. They are inviting you into their lives, and sometimes their families. Remember that you are a guest, and be as respectful as you would want a visitor to your home to be.

TG: I worked with clients in all kinds of places, including SROs [single-room occupancy hotels], apartments, shelters, group homes, tents in the park—you name it. No matter what kind of place I was visiting, I always remember that this is where the client lives, this is their space, and I respect that. And I always get a better understanding of my client, of how they live and what they may be up against. Also, I think because I am on their turf and not in my office—sometimes we are able to have the most personal or the deepest conversations. They might talk about experiences and feelings they never shared before.

WHY MAKE HOME VISITS?

There are many reasons why CHWs conduct home visits, including:

- To visit clients who are unable to come to your office or to easily leave their homes
- To follow up with clients who recently received services from your program
- To contact clients who have not kept in touch, to see whether they are all right and interested in participating in services again
- To see clients who have recently experienced a decline in health
- Because family members or friends of a client contact you out of concern for the client and ask you to visit that person
- To encourage clients to come to your agency for important services that cannot be delivered at their homes
- To support new parents or guardians
- To enable clients to assess their home environments and possible health risks, such as exposure to mold, dust, or other allergens that cause asthma
- To provide support and guidance to clients regarding how to take medications properly
- To notify clients that they may have been exposed to an infectious disease and to encourage them to get screened
- To meet with clients who are in the hospital, jail, or other institutions

- *Can you think of other reasons to conduct home visits?*

Alvaro Morales: I did partner notification for the health department. When people tested positive for HIV, we asked them if they would like us to contact people—anonymously—who could have been exposed by having unprotected sex or sharing syringes or works with them. Not everybody wanted us to do this, but some did. My job was to visit these partners, to tell them that they might have been exposed to HIV, offer information and counseling, and ask them if they would like to be tested for HIV antibodies. I never knew what to expect. I called them first to see if we had the right contact information for them, to see if they were at home, and to ask them to meet with me. I'd say that I was calling from the health department, and I had some news to tell them, but I needed to tell them in person. It was awkward, but that was the policy. Talking with them on the phone gave me an idea of what kind of visit it might be. On the way to their home, I reviewed what I was going to say and prepared for the kinds of questions they might ask. I wanted to be prepared, and not to do anything that would make a difficult situation any worse. I was kind of surprised, but most people actually took time to talk with me, and some of them asked me to test them for HIV antibodies. I drew their blood—that was back when we still drew blood—and I would follow up to give them their results at their home or at one of our clinics—I let them decide.

THE CHALLENGES OF HOME VISITING

Home visits can be challenging for a number of reasons:

- Clients may not want you to visit or may not want to talk with you right then.
- Clients may be embarrassed about their living conditions.
- Clients may be concerned about their privacy.
- Clients may worry that you will judge them if they live in nontraditional families, or they may have other cultural concerns.
- They may worry that you will learn about or expose their immigration status, or worry that they could lose certain health, housing, or social benefits.
- Clients may have had bad experiences with home visits from child welfare, social workers, the police, or other authorities.
- You may witness or learn about drug use, neglect, or abuse.
- You may face risks to your personal safety.
- Your clients may be very ill or facing death.

- *Can you think of other challenges that you may face when conducting home visits?*

Ramona Benson: I've gone on home visits to new clients—and they won't open the door because they don't really know me yet. I have clients who for whatever reason think "Oh, no. She's gonna judge me when she comes in here." So until they get to know me and know that I'm not going to judge them, the doors are going to stay shut. But if I do my job right, down the road, they'll open up for me. I just need to be patient.

11.2 Preparing to Conduct a Home Visit

The nature of a home visit will be determined by the type of agency and program you work for and the context or situation in which the client lives. Careful preparation will assist you in providing quality services once you reach the client.

PUT YOURSELF IN THE CLIENT'S SHOES

Imagine that you have been living with a life-threatening health condition for several years, and a CHW from a local agency is going to be visiting you for the first time. How might it feel to have a stranger come into your home? What concerns might you have about the visit? What would you want from the CHW? How would you want them to behave? What would you *not* want them to do, see, or ask?

RESPECT A CLIENT'S RIGHT TO PRIVACY—DISCREET HOME VISITS

Some clients will have concerns about privacy or confidentiality. They may not want others to know that they are working with you or your agency, or that they have a certain health issue such as HIV disease, cancer, or post-traumatic stress. How do you protect their privacy during home visits?

> **Craig Wenzl:** Many years ago, I was working with an HIV/AIDS service organization in the central United States. There was a lot of stigma affecting people who were living with AIDS. When conducting home visits, I noticed how some of the neighbors would look out their windows or look over from their yards to see who was visiting. Fortunately, I tucked all of my documents and materials discreetly into a backpack. I made sure that there was nothing on the backpack, my car, or my clothing that would indicate the agency I worked for. I learned to be as discreet as possible.

If you schedule the home visit in advance, ask the client how you can best preserve privacy. For example, if others are present, how should you introduce yourself? Will others be present with whom the client *does* want you to speak? Has the client disclosed their health condition to others?

If the visit was not arranged in advance, use extra discretion upon arrival at the client's home: don't say or do anything that could reveal the client's private information to others. For example, don't introduce yourself by saying: "Hi, I'm Tranh, and I work for the AIDS Support Center." If you aren't sure what you can and cannot say in front of others, don't say it! If others are present when you arrive at your client's home, you might say something like: "Hey, Bernadette, good to see you today. Is this a good time for a visit?" Or, if possible, speak with the client in private to ask whether you should continue with the visit or reschedule.

> **TG:** Yeah, I've worked with clients who didn't share their HIV status with the people they lived with, like their parents, or children, or sometimes their lovers. I need to be careful not to say something that will break this confidentiality. In private, of course, I will ask the client about this. And if they are shooting drugs or having sex with someone, I'll talk to them about taking precautions or disclosing their status. But it is their health, their decision. If I pressure them, or break their trust, my chance to help them is pretty much over.

START THINGS OFF RIGHT

Shadow Another CHW

If you haven't conducted home visits before, we strongly recommend that you spend time learning from an experienced CHW. Ask your supervisor if it is possible for you to accompany or shadow another CHW who works for your program or agency, or another program, on one or more home visits. Be sure the CHW also checks with the client beforehand to ask if they will be comfortable having more than one CHW attend the home visit. If the CHW agrees for you to shadow them, closely observe what they do and how they interact with clients and their families. After the visits, ask questions about anything you want to learn more about. Incorporate what you have learned into your own work as you begin to conduct home visits.

Review and Prepare Client Files

Remember that your client has set aside time for the home visit. Being well prepared demonstrates respect. If you are going to visit a client you are already working with, review the client's file and key strengths, risks, needs, and any health conditions. The file may include a care management plan or action plan and goals (see Chapters 9, 10, and 16). Check to see if referrals were provided. Is the client working with other service providers? Does the file include permissions to release information (or to share information about the client) with other providers? Bring copies of blank release forms in case you need them.

If the client does not have a file at your agency, create a blank one and complete any forms that can be done in advance of your visit. Bring blank copies of any additional forms you may need, such as informed consent forms, referral forms, and home visit assessment forms.

Organize and Pack Resources to Bring on the Visit

Pack everything you may need during the home visit, and review it carefully to be sure that you haven't forgotten anything. Develop a standardized checklist of materials (your agency may already have one) to guide you in preparing these resources. Some of the resources you might include are:

- Your identification badge and business card
- Written information (in the appropriate language or languages) about your agency, your program, and key policies and protocols, including confidentiality and its limits, and any costs associated with the services provided
- Client files, blank new client files, and other forms
- Copies of any test results that you are authorized to review with the client
- Any medications or tests that you are authorized to bring and administer, such as daily observed therapy (DOT) for clients with tuberculosis, or HIV antibody tests
- Educational materials to use to explain something more clearly (videos, pamphlets, booklets, and so forth)
- Risk-reduction or other health materials such as condoms, lubricants, hygiene kits, nutritional supplements, food or transportation vouchers, phone cards, and so on
- A list of other resources that you may want to share with the client, such as resources for food, housing, health care and mental health services, or legal assistance
- A map, phone, or GPS service in case you get lost while trying to find the client's home
- A folding chair or stool to ensure that you have a place to sit during a long visit
- A flashlight, in case you are visiting the client after dark
- A communication device (cell phone in case of emergency or in case you can't locate the client) and a list of emergency numbers

- *Can you think of anything else that might be important for you to bring with you on the visit?*

Organize all of these items into some sort of bag or case to take with you on the visit, such as a backpack, duffle bag, or large briefcase. A backpack with several compartments works well, with places for files and different types of resources. Backpacks are also one of the most discreet ways to bring items with you to the home visit.

> **Francis Julian Montgomery:** I have a folding, portable "travel chair" that I carry with me everywhere I go. I have bad knees, so it is important for me to have a place to sit. But the chair also helps my clients maintain their dignity by allowing me to be respectful while in their home environment. . . . Many of the homes I visit are small single-room occupancy (SRO) units. There is really not much in each room besides a bed for a person to sit on. But I believe a person's bed is a private and sacred space, just for them, and I wouldn't want to be disrespectful of that by sitting on it. At the same time, it would be odd to stand for 20–30 minutes while I am conducting an assessment. So I pull out my chair, which makes it more comfortable for both of us. And people get a kick out of seeing me in my chair!

PLAN HOW YOU WILL TRAVEL TO THE CLIENT'S HOME

Review your contact information for the client. Do you have the proper address? If possible, verify this by calling the client. You'll want to know *exactly* where you will be going. Look at a map or GPS coordinates if you're unfamiliar with the area, to locate the following information:

- Client's address
- Landmarks nearby. You might try looking the location up online or GPS on your phone if you have that capability. A paper map is also fine.
- Public transportation or parking availability
- Anything you might need to know for your safety (see the section on safety below)

If you have an appointment and can talk with the client in advance, try to determine:

- If there is a house, apartment, or room number clearly marked
- If the client has a dog or other pets
- If there is a gate or intercom at the home or building and what you will need to do to get in
- Any possible problems you may encounter, getting to or entering the home

Make sure you have the client's phone number with you (if the client has one), in case you get lost or have trouble getting into the building. If the client does not have a phone, ask if another household member or neighbor has a phone and if it is okay to call them if necessary. If so, make sure you have that number with you if you need it.

IDENTIFY KEY OBJECTIVES

Write down what you hope to accomplish during the home visit. Be as specific as possible. For example, are you visiting to determine whether families are eligible and interested in enrolling in government programs that offer health insurance for children in low-income families? Do you want to check in with a client with asthma to see if the person is experiencing symptoms and taking the medication properly? Don't set too many goals for a single visit. While it is important to identify the purpose of your visit, you also need to stay flexible. Talk with the client to learn about their current health status, needs, and priorities.

PREPARING TO CONDUCT A FIRST VISIT TO A NEW CLIENT

If you are visiting someone you have not met before, please review Chapter 8: it provides basic concepts and skills for introducing yourself and the services that you provide, and obtaining informed consent from a prospective client. You must obtain informed consent before you conduct an initial assessment. If you are working for a health care organization, you should also check to see that the client has recently signed a HIPAA form, and bring one with you if necessary.

Your primary goals for a first visit will be to establish a positive connection with the client, to assess the client's resources and needs, and to determine whether the person is interested in the services that you can provide and would like to begin to work together.

PREPARING FOR FOLLOW-UP VISITS

You will also visit clients with whom you are already working. You may visit established clients because their health has deteriorated or they are unable to leave their homes. Try to prepare yourself for what you may see and learn. It is always difficult to witness a client who is in crisis, whose health is deteriorating, or who is facing the end of life. Yet, these are the very times when clients may need your support the most, particularly if they don't have a strong social support network.

Even if you have worked with the client before, and are visiting to follow up on a specific issue that you have discussed in the past, don't expect that you will both have the same memory of what occurred in the past. For any number of reasons, including depression, deteriorating health, or other life challenges, the client may not remember the nature of your work together, including previous conversations and agreements, or care very much about it at the moment. As always, be patient and compassionate, and be prepared to take time to reintroduce yourself, to review your previous work together, and sometimes to start all over at the beginning. The essence of client-centered work is meeting clients where they are—don't assume that you know where they will "be" when you conduct a follow-up home visit.

Possible goals for follow-up visits may include to:

- Reintroduce yourself and the purpose of your visit
- Review your program's services and key policies, including confidentiality
- Answer the client's questions and concerns
- Obtain informed consent, again, to continue with your visit and to provide services
- Ask what the client remembers about your previous work together
- Review any decisions, agreements, or accomplishments that the client previously made
- Assess their current concerns, needs, and priorities—what do they want to accomplish?
- Establish new goals that the client wants to work on, and let these guide your work
- Provide health education, client-centered counseling, and referrals, as appropriate
- Bring medications and assist clients with medications management (see Chapter 16)
- Provide additional supplies as needed (for example, nutritional supplements, safer sex supplies, bandages, bedding, or clothing, and so forth)
- Set a date and time for your next visit

- *What other goals might you have for these home visits?*

11.3 Common Courtesies and Guidelines

RESPECT THE CLIENT'S TIME

If the client is expecting you, it is important to show up on time. If something unforeseen happens and you are running late, call or text the client to inform them and to apologize. If you make a practice of being late, you risk losing the client's trust and respect: the client's time is just as valuable as your own.

If you schedule a home visit in advance, discuss how much time you both have for the visit. If you really need an hour, ask for it, but respect the client's limits and needs: "I'd like to visit for about an hour, will that work for you?" When you arrive, ask the client if it is still a good time to visit, and how much time the person will be able to spend with you. Stay aware, throughout the visit, of signs that the client may want the visit to end. Perhaps a family member is calling the client to go somewhere, or the client has to make a call, or go to the store, or rest. Be respectful: it is the client's home, the client's time, and the client's life. If you don't accomplish all of your goals during this visit, schedule a follow-up appointment in the home, at your agency, or at another location that works for both you and the client.

ANNOUNCE YOURSELF

When you arrive at the client's home—wherever it is—announce yourself. Use your name, but not the name of your agency in order to protect the client's privacy. You might say something like: "Hello, Sam? It's Sunil Gupta. We spoke earlier about meeting today. Is this still a good time?"

> **Francis Julian Montgomery:** For safety, security, or other reasons, people often don't feel comfortable having a stranger in their home. As a result, when I am trying to conduct a home visit, sometimes I end up talking to someone from outside the door to their room. I might sit in my portable chair in the hallway of the SRO [single-room occupancy hotel], and I make sure I am speaking in a low tone so that no one else can hear. Once a person sees that I am committed to respecting their comfort and their space, they often decide to invite me inside. In order to build trust, I have even spoken to clients on my cell phone while standing right outside their building.

INTRODUCE YOURSELF

Once you're inside the home, introduce yourself again: "Hello, Sam. I'm Sunil Gupta. We spoke on the phone earlier. It's nice to meet you." Be sure you have proper identification with you when you arrive, and show it to the client or family if requested.

If you provide services related to sensitive and highly personal issues, and you are not confident that you are alone with the client, be careful about saying the name of your organization or the issue you are working for. If other people are around, follow the client's lead. If you aren't sure how to proceed, ask the client: "Sam, is this a good time to talk or would you rather reschedule our appointment?"

IF THE CLIENT IS NOT AT HOME

If no one answers, follow up with the client later. If someone other than the client answers, and the client isn't home, leave a simple message that preserves the client's confidentiality such as: "Could you tell him that Sunil dropped by to say hello?"

DRESS FOR THE OCCASION

Make sure to wear clothing that is appropriate for the setting. Consider comfort, and what is culturally respectful to the community you are visiting, as well as the safety guidelines discussed below. Some situations call for slightly more professional clothing, and others for more casual wear. If you're visiting someone who is incarcerated, be sure to find out beforehand what the dress code is for visitors to the institution. If you are visiting a family with young children, wear comfortable clothes that will allow you to engage with the children. Ask your colleagues, particularly other CHWs who conduct outreach and home visits, what they would wear, and use your own best judgment.

DEMONSTRATE RESPECT AND ESTABLISH A POSITIVE CONNECTION

During a home visit, you are entering a client's private space. Observe common courtesies when you are in the home: introduce yourself to others, ask people how they are doing, and thank them for inviting you into their home. Many of the clients you visit won't have much money and may live in housing of very poor quality, with many family members or roommates sharing a small space. Clients are likely to be struggling with other challenges as well, such as chronic illness, mental illness, addiction, disability, and interpersonal conflicts.

Ramona Benson: Sometimes, a client's family has had a bad experience with home visits in the past, and based on that, they ask me: "Why you want to come to my house?" So I always say to people, "I don't have to come to your house. I'll meet you anywhere you want me to meet you at." I don't push myself on anybody—that's not going to do anyone any good. Sometimes they want to have the home visit at a McDonald's because home life is not fine, you know? Or they might want to have the home visit at the doctor's office, and so we meet there, but any public place where I'm meeting, I have to make sure that what we are saying is not being heard, because of confidentiality.

Your warmth, honesty, and kindness will assist in making the visits a success. Let your work be guided by respect for your clients' identities, cultures, and right to self-determination.

Lee Jackson: Sometimes I go out to check on a client to see if they are okay. Some people you have to treat very delicately because they are living right on the edge. I always build rapport with clients, and this takes time. But by taking time to know them, and letting them know me, we establish a basis for our work together. I always acknowledge them when I see them in the community, and treat them as human beings. That way they don't look at me only as their health worker, but as a human being as well. It goes both ways.

PRACTICE CULTURAL HUMILITY

Home visits are a critical time to practice cultural humility (see Chapter 6). The cultures, values, and traditions of the clients and families you visit will be reflected in their homes. The furnishings and art, the foods and smells in the homes, the religious symbols or lack of them, the makeup of the families, and their customs may be different from what you are familiar with. View home visiting as an opportunity to learn more about the cultures of others. Abide by the rules in place in their homes, as you would expect in yours, and ask questions if you are unsure about what to do.

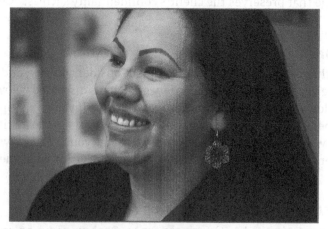

When conducting home visits, CHWs draw upon cultural humility to demonstrate respect.

What Makes a Family?

As you visit people in their homes, remember that there are many different kinds of families. Some families include people who are not related by blood. Don't assume that a family with children includes both a mother and a father. Children may have one or more parents or guardians, and this could include aunts, grandparents, a mom and a dad, two moms, or two dads. In some families, many people take an active role in raising the children. Put your assumptions aside, be respectful, and learn about the family you are visiting.

SPEAK CLEARLY

People often talk quickly and loudly when they are nervous. Your calm voice can serve to relax others as well as yourself. If people are living on the streets, in shelters, at the hospital, in SROs or apartments with thin walls or a large family, your voice may be overheard. Speak loudly enough for the client or clients to hear you, but not so loudly that you broadcast private information to others. If you can't hear or understand what a client tells you, ask them to tell you again: you don't want to miss important information.

Try to determine beforehand if the client is hearing impaired or if they have language requirements that may require culturally appropriate accommodations (such as interpreters or another CHW who can speak their language).

Please watch the following video interview 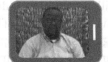. In this interview, a CHW shares tips for conducting successful home visits.

- What information did the CHW share that you would like to put into practice as you conduct home visits?

CONDUCTING HOME VISITS: CHW INTERVIEW

http://youtu.be/ BSgqpdyvZ5w

MAINTAIN HEALTHY BOUNDARIES

To aid in preventing potentially dangerous or harmful situations, maintain healthy boundaries with clients. Be cautious about disclosing personal information (home or cell phone number or address) or private details about your life. If a client asks you personal questions that you do not feel comfortable answering, be ready to explain and clarify your role as a CHW and why you won't answer these questions. You might say something like, "My role is to be here for *you*, to support you to improve your health. I don't talk about my private life when I'm at work, because that will distract us—this is *your time*." Be clear and kind as you assert these boundaries. If a client starts to say things that are not acceptable (such as sexual innuendos), interrupt or stop the conversation. If the client continues to push at your boundaries you may have to leave. For more information about boundary setting, see Chapters 7 and 10.

STAY ON-TOPIC

Plan for how you will disengage from conversations that are taking too much time and attention away from the primary purpose of your visit. At the same time, be prepared to do some casual visiting. This is a customary part of most visits to another person's home. The client may show you personal belongings, such as family photographs, or want to introduce you to family members who will engage you in discussions about a range of issues, from politics to the latest ball game.

While you hope that clients will feel comfortable enough to open up and talk with you about the personal issues that are influencing their health and well-being, some clients will want to talk with you for a very long time about their lives, their families, their hopes, and their dreams. For some clients, this may be a sign of their isolation and loneliness, or of fears related to their health and mortality. Develop your own kind and polite way to interrupt clients and remind them of the time and main purpose for the visit.

Craig Wenzl: When I first began providing home visits, I discovered that some clients hadn't had another visitor in their home for a long time. They were lonely and starving for companionship. At first, I didn't know what to do when a client began telling me everything about their life. I didn't want to be rude or hurtful by cutting off the conversation, so I found myself in situations where a client would talk to me for a long time and I would run out of time to do other home visits. With experience, I became better at gently expressing that my time was limited. I also learned how to express to a client that the conversation was getting out of hand or too long. I might say something like: "Marty—here we go again, talking about other interesting things. I wish I had the time to talk about this today, but I don't. Let's get back to talking about the case management plan—all right?"

Whenever you are working with a client who likes to talk excessively, figure out a way to calm the person down or slow down the discussion. A lot of times, a client who is talking nonstop is doing so because of a combination of nervousness, loneliness, and other feelings. Be mindful of these feelings when you try to curtail excessive talking, and be prepared to talk a little bit about things that may be off-topic—this is often part of the process of building rapport with clients and showing them respect in their homes.

OVERCOMING DISTRACTIONS

You will encounter a wide range of distractions that may keep you and your client from communicating and working well together. The telephone may ring. People may be sharing a meal, watching television, or playing video games. Other people or pets may make it difficult to focus on the purpose of the visit. This goes with the territory when conducting a home visit—unexpected things will happen. As you become more accustomed to doing home visits, you will learn how to handle different experiences. Allow yourself time to adjust and learn.

Media: To handle distractions such as the telephone, television, radio, or video games, ask the client if it would possible to turn these off or down so that you can focus on their needs and concerns. Be patient and polite. Always keep in mind that this is the client's home, not your office, and it is up to the client to make these decisions.

Pets: If there is a pet such as a large dog that makes you uncomfortable, ask if it would possible to put it in another room or area of the room. Describe this as *your* need. Explain that it will help you to better focus on the task at hand. But keep in mind that for many people, pets are family: they may not understand your request, or may be most at ease with the animal beside them.

Other People: If other people prove to be a distraction, find an opportunity to ask the primary client if it would be possible to talk privately. Perhaps you can move into another room or onto a porch or balcony to talk about confidential matters.

Drug and Alcohol Use: You may visit a client who is drinking or using drugs. Clarify your agency's policy about this. Some programs may limit your ability to work with people who are currently high on drugs or alcohol. A key concern is the ability of people to give informed consent when they are using substances. However, you may work with clients who are often or usually using substances, and it isn't realistic to wait until they are sober. Do your best to talk with the client, to provide the services you are authorized to provide, and to be sensitive to informed consent issues, and don't ask a client to make big life-changing decisions when high. Evaluate if, how, and when you may be able to meet with the client when the person is not using. If the client has a history of being abusive or violent while high, don't attempt to work under these circumstances: this is a safety issue for you and the client, and leaving is probably the best policy.

Cluttering or Hoarding: You may enter a home that is filled with items that take over or block the space. You may find it difficult to walk or move in these areas, and this may get in the way of your ability to work with the client in this space. Furthermore, the clutter or hoarding sometimes creates health hazards from factors like mold, shifting piles of contents, or structural damage. Issues related to hoarding should be handled with great sensitivity. CHWs don't want to offend or stigmatize clients by making critical or negative comments about the clutter, or attempt to move anything, as this could be severely disruptive and upsetting to the client.

We recommend bringing a portable stool to sit on when you conduct home visits, and to find a less cluttered area where you can talk with the client. If the clutter creates a safety issue (such as mentioned above), you may express your concerns to the client, provide education about the safety issue, and explore finding a different and mutually convenient location to meet. This could be a local park or public library, for example.

- *What are some other distractions that you might encounter?*

- *Which types of distractions may be most challenging for you?*

What Do YOU Think?

11.4 Safety Guidelines for Home Visits

Whenever you are meeting people in the community—especially when you are entering their homes—pay attention to safety. Some of the communities you serve experience high rates of poverty, homelessness, drug use, police intervention, and gang activity. You need to balance your commitment to serving the client with the need to protect your own safety.

Safety concerns for home visiting may include witnessing violence and other illegal activity; observing signs of neglect or abuse; the need to report harmful or abusive conduct; damage to your car (if you drive); unintentional involvement in police actions; witnessing arguments or domestic violence; threats and assault; or encountering someone who is angry or aggressive.

Sometimes our own biases and/or lack of knowledge influence our assessment of safety. Try not to let your bias guide or distort the way that you assess safety risks or result in discriminating against communities that already experience high rates of prejudice, stigma, and discrimination. Remember that safety issues are present in any work setting and with clients of all backgrounds.

Some members of the community may see you as an outsider or intruder, and may view you with suspicion or fear. This is one of many reasons why it is so essential to take time to get to know the community you will be working in, and to build respectful relationships with key opinion leaders. Knowing as much as possible about the neighborhoods and areas where you do home visits allows you to be prepared, and to keep yourself safe.

Listen to your instincts. When you arrive at the location for the home visit, evaluate the current situation. Is there anything unusual going on at this time? Your instincts will develop over time. Pay attention to them when you feel particularly ill at ease, anxious, or unsafe—they may be tipping you off to a dangerous situation. If you are concerned that the situation is not safe, consider talking to your client about rescheduling the visit for another time.

> **Lee Jackson:** When you do home visits, you're going into the trenches. Think about how to mentally prepare for your visits. You may not run into any problems, but be prepared in case you do. Be aware of what you're wearing. You want to be sure to wear slacks or jeans and comfortable shoes. Don't wear anything too expensive like nice jewelry or a watch—someone there might really need a fix that day.

CHW

SAFETY TIPS

Many of the following tips also apply to conducting health outreach, which you will learn about in Chapter 19. Additional tips specific to street outreach will be covered in that chapter.

Be Prepared

- Find out as much information as you can about the client you will visit (for example, have they reported domestic violence, do they live alone, do they have any pets that might be dangerous?).

- Find out what type of housing the client lives in and where.

- Find out detailed information about the locations you will be visiting, including the reputation of the areas and recent events such as homicides, assaults, or burglaries.

- If you are working in areas that the community itself considers risky, have a plan and be prepared. Consider working with a partner. Talk with your supervisor about the situation and what you can do to minimize risks to yourself and your clients.

- Let your supervisor know whom you will be visiting, where you will be going, and when.

- Dress appropriately.

- Avoid agency logos or signage on your car, clothing, or anywhere else that might draw attention.

- If you have a cell phone, bring it with you in case you encounter a safety concern or an emergency. If you do not have a cell phone and will be doing home visits, ask if your agency can provide one for safety purposes.

- If you are going to be visiting clients after dark, be sure to carry a flashlight with you.

Pay Attention, and Be Discreet

- Be discreet when visiting a new location. Try not to draw attention to yourself.

- Carry yourself with secure body language.

- The risks to women are different from those to men. Be aware of these risks, and make decisions that preserve your safety.

- Be aware of your surroundings at all times.

- Be ready to think on your feet—to make quick evaluations and decisions about situations as they develop.

If Conflict or Danger Arises

- *De-escalate conflict and work to calm the person involved:* see Chapter 13 to learn skills for handling conflict effectively. Keep your own voice calm when interacting with someone who is angry.

- *Apologize:* You may have unintentionally done something that provoked the person's anger.

- Leave *if you don't feel safe* and don't feel confident that you can de-escalate the conflict.

- *Report and document:* If you witness violence or other reportable incidents related to your clients, report them to your supervisor immediately, and document them in your field notes. Debrief the incidents with someone you trust.

- *Only call the police if it is absolutely required.* Most situations do not require such a drastic measure. If you feel you *must* contact the police in order to preserve your safety, then do so. However, consider the effect this might have on your work with this community. Be cautious about calling the police into a community that has a history of tensions with the law; you might lose the community's trust and respect, and hence your ability to continue to work with the community.

- *Can you think of other safety tips?*

- *What are your biggest safety concerns?*

- *How will you address them and keep yourself safe as you work in the community?*

11.5 How to Conduct a Home Visit

Once you have introduced yourself and been invited into the home, confirm that you are talking to the client, or the primary caregiver in case of a child. You may have already met the client at your agency, on the street or elsewhere, or spoken with them by phone. If you have never met the client in person before, you might say something such as: "Hi, I'm Sunil Gupta, are you Mrs. Ramirez?"

If other people such as family members are present, be friendly and patient. Once you are talking with the client or primary caregiver, explain again why you have come and see if the two of you can find a quiet spot to work. Say something like: "Mrs. Ramirez, it's a pleasure to meet you. I'm Sunil. Is this still a good time for us to visit? Is there a private place where we can sit down together to talk?"

Clearly explain why you are conducting the home visit, and ask what the client would like to accomplish.

> **LaTonya Rogers:** On my first home visit, I tell the families, I'm here to help you get what you need to handle your child's asthma. What would you like to talk about today?

CONDUCT AN ASSESSMENT

During each home visit you will conduct some type of an assessment, such as:

- A client's knowledge about and interest in a particular service
- A client's strengths, risks, and needs in order to develop a case management or risk-reduction plan
- A client's current health status and needs for additional services
- Adherence to specific treatments such as taking daily medications for diabetes or HIV disease
- A client's progress with a risk-reduction or case management plan
- Exposure to environmental health risks

> **Francis Julian Montgomery:** I know I am asking for a lot of personal information during an intake or assessment, so I try to make it a conversation instead of an interrogation. I don't just read questions off of an intake list. And I make sure to really listen, because clients will often tell me things in response to one question that fills in answers to other questions as well.

CHWs often conduct home visits to clients who are living with chronic illnesses (See Chapter 16). In these circumstances the assessment may also address:

- The client's current understanding of the health condition. For example, does the client understand the risks of high blood pressure and strategies to reduce it?
- Current signs and symptoms. While CHWs are not clinicians and must not work outside of their scope of practice (see Chapter 7), they are often trained and authorized to check and report on specific symptoms and to communicate their findings to clinicians. This may include current asthma symptoms or complications from HIV disease.
- Recent test results. Occasionally CHWs will be trained, certified, and authorized to perform certain tests, such as HIV antibody tests, or to teach clients how to understand the meaning of recent tests, such as blood pressure readings.
- Support with self care (see Chapter 16) and implementation of a personalized action plan.
- Medications management (see Chapter 16).
- Scheduling and reminders about upcoming appointments, such as well-baby exams, and showing clients how to plan to keep the appointment.

Jason Stanford: I also do in-home case management [with the Black Infant Health Program], which means that if a client is pregnant, I visit them at home. I provide referrals but also educational information about pregnancy. I focus on talking to the dad about parenting practices. But not just that, it's also helping him with issues that may be stopping him from being the best dad he can be. It may be a legal issue, it may be education, it may be getting a job, or changing some of his behaviors. It may be domestic violence, it may be anger management issues, just a whole host of things that I try to assist him with.

CONDUCTING AN ENVIRONMENTAL ASSESSMENT

During your visit, you will observe the home environment. What you observe may provide you with a better understanding of the client's strengths, risks, and needs. For example, you may observe:

- The client's level of stress at home
- Basic living conditions, including access to clean sheets, clothing, and resources for hygiene (toilet paper, running water, soap, shampoo, toothpaste, and so on)
- Availability of food
- Environmental risks such as mold, dust, insect or rodent issues, or safety hazards for young children
- The presence or absence of friends, family, roommates, and the quality of those relationships (Do they seem close? Attentive? Are they arguing?)
- Challenges with mobility within or outside of the home
- Exposure to safety risks such as abuse or neglect

- *What else might you observe during a home visit that could inform you about your client's health and well-being?*

Occasionally, you will be asked to conduct a more thorough environmental assessment during a home visit—with the client's participation and permission. For example, if you are working with a client living with diabetes, heart disease, cancer, or HIV disease, you may assess:

- Needs for immediate assistance or referral to a medical provider
- The status of medications. Are they up-to-date? Does the client have enough medication for the next few days, week, or month? Is the client taking the medications? Are the medications clearly labeled and organized? If the client takes multiple medications in a day, is there a schedule or system to remind the person to do this?
- Exposure to environmental factors that may trigger illness. In the case of asthma, this might include assessing exposure to excessive dust, mold, animals, secondhand smoke, and diesel emissions from a nearby street or highway.
- Access to food. Is there food in the house? Is it nutritious and in keeping with the diet prescribed by the person's health care provider? What did the client eat this morning or last night?
- Access to clean sheets and clothes, or a laundry
- Signs of alcohol and/or drug use. Do they understand how street drugs and alcohol may interact with their medications and impact their health condition?

You can conduct an environmental assessment by observing what is in sight and asking the client's permission to look at other parts of the home. For example, you might ask: "Roger, where do you keep your medications? Do you mind if I check to see that they are up-to-date?" or "Do you mind if I look in the kitchen to see what you have to eat?" *Never* start to look around a client's home without the person's knowledge or permission. Be sensitive in the way that you ask, the way that you look, and the comments you make as you learn more about the home: This type of assessment can be difficult for clients who may be acutely embarrassed by the current state of their living conditions.

> **TG:** I had a client who always wanted me to help him check up on his medications. He took so many that it was confusing and difficult to manage. I'd do what I could to help him organize them—and sometimes this would take us 20 or 30 minutes. But he never wanted me to look in his fridge or cabinets. He used to own his own home, but after he got sick, he lost everything: he lived in one small room. I think he was really embarrassed. I always respected his wishes, and his pride. But I also brought grocery vouchers or a bag of groceries from the food bank with me if I could.

Your goal is always to assist clients to identify any barriers or risks to their health, and to work with them to identify changes that they can and want to make to their environment that will reduce these risks. This may mean assisting clients to organize their medications, to report mold to the landlord or housing authority, or to make changes in the types of food that they prepare and eat at home.

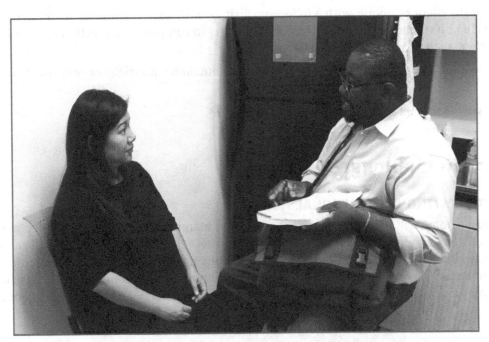

A CHW meets with a client in her kitchen to talk about healthy eating.

PROVIDING CASE MANAGEMENT, CLIENT-CENTERED COUNSELING, AND HEALTH EDUCATION

Depending on the client's needs, your skills, and your existing relationship, you may provide additional services such as client-centered counseling, health education, or case management. Please note that these topics are addressed in depth in other chapters of the *Foundations* textbook. You may continue to work with the client at their home, your office, or in other locations.

For example, you may provide health education about a specific condition—hypertension or heart disease—to clients who are at risk and interested. This may include assessing their levels of knowledge, providing information, and supporting them in thinking about relevant behavior changes such as changes to diet or patterns of exercise. You may also provide client-centered counseling or coaching (see Chapter 9) about any number of issues, including parenting, domestic violence, or depression, and support clients in identifying their own risks and developing personalized risk-reduction plans.

EXPLAIN THE NEXT STEPS

Take time to clarify and document what the next steps will be for you and the client. This plan should address each of the concerns and priorities that the client discussed with you. Confirm the date and location of your next appointment. Write down the plan and leave it for the client. If the client can't read, ask if there is someone who can review the plan with them.

GOOD-BYE AND THANK-YOU

Tell the client (and other family members) good-bye. Thank them again for their time and hospitality. If you need directions or assistance getting out of the building, ask before you leave.

11.6 After the Visit

Depending on your program and your relationship with the client you just visited, you will have several things to do after your visit:

- Complete paperwork documenting the visit, any assessment you conducted, information you learned, services provided, and agreements made. The longer you wait to document your work, the less you will remember.

- Write down future appointments or visits in your planner or calendar.

- Find out information you needed during your visit but did not have, such as the name of an agency that provides hot meals to people unable to leave their homes.

- Check in with the client by phone, with a follow-up visit, or with an appointment at another location. Check to see if the client has followed through or faced challenges in completing the action steps that you discussed together, such as a plan to see the doctor.

- Talk with your supervisor or another colleague about any remaining questions or concerns that you may have.

- *What else would you want to do to follow up on a home visit?*

What Do YOU ? Think

11.7 Common Challenges

VISITS TO PEOPLE WITHOUT TRADITIONAL HOMES

When you conduct a home visit to someone who is homeless or marginally housed, it may take place on the street, in a doorway, under an overpass, or in the park or parking lot where they spend time or sleep. Be as respectful of this space as you would any other home. All the same rules apply. If clients express that they don't want you there through words or actions, leave. Do your utmost to keep your communication confidential. Keep your voice low. If others are nearby and may be listening, don't discuss confidential matters, and follow your client's lead.

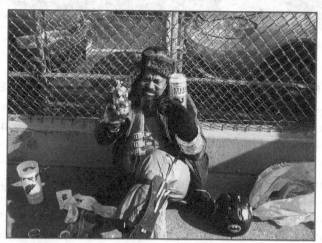

Home visits are also conducted to clients who live on the streets.

Lee Jackson: To work with clients who are homeless, I'll ask them for three locations where they tend to hang out. This is a big help when I am trying to check in with them later on.

WHEN CLIENTS ARE ANGRY

Expect to work with clients who are sometimes in a "bad" mood, frustrated, or angry. You would likely experience these same emotions if you were walking in their shoes. While their anger may sometimes be about you—related to something you or someone else from your agency said or did—generally it is about other issues they are confronting, such as experiences of discrimination, violence, mental health conditions, separation or conflict with family members; the loss of jobs, homes, or relationships; a relapse to drug or alcohol use; the deterioration of their health; or confronting the possibility of their own death.

As discussed in Chapter 13, be patient and stay calm. Keep in mind that you don't want to do anything that will harm the client or your professional relationship and reputation. Stay respectful, professional, and polite. However, if the client is acting in ways that are threatening or physically aggressive, and you are unable to de-escalate their anger, leave the situation immediately.

Lee Jackson: Lots of times a client will be upset. Sometimes they'll be verbally aggressive. If you treat everyone like a human being and don't act judgmental, they'll usually come around. Always remember it's not personal. I will talk with them calmly and see if that helps. I might explain: "I'm here today to escort you to your appointment. If we need to, we can schedule you for a different time." If the client refuses to go, then rescheduling is a good way to go. If they can, maybe we go for coffee or a pastry. If I can't calm them down, I leave. I don't argue.

WORKING WITH CLIENTS WHO ARE INCARCERATED

Your program may work with clients who are incarcerated, or one of your ongoing clients may be sent to the local jail or juvenile hall. There are several things to consider when working in corrections facilities. You will need to gain a security clearance: contact the jail or prison in advance to apply for one. The facility will provide you with guidelines for your visit, including what to wear.

Even if you are uncomfortable working in a corrections facility, do your utmost to establish and maintain positive and professional relationships with the staff. Doing so will enable you to continue to have access to your clients.

Most clients will deeply appreciate your visit and understand that you had to jump through some hoops to see them. They may also be in a mood to reflect and talk about their lives and to make plans for when they are released. This may be especially true for clients who are caught up in street life and drug use. If possible, assist them in making plans for what to do in the very first hours and days when they are released. Clients with substance-use issues are at risk of using as soon as they are released. If they want to make changes, assist them to figure out what they can do that will reduce their risks of using. You might ask them to call you when they know that they will be released or after they have been released, to schedule a time to meet as soon as possible. As always, these choices are up to the client.

TG: The clients who I visit in jail are usually really glad to see me, and in a mood to talk. They are motivated to make changes, because they never want to go back. They are missing their family and their freedom. I try to help them make a realistic plan for the near future—not something that sounds more like a dream. I try to talk to them about what they might face when they get out. Like if I know that they have been in and out of jail and prison, and they usually go right back to using as soon as they are released, I'll say: "You know, you told me that the last time you got out of jail, you fixed right away. What will help you to do it differently this time?" And I also let them know that if they don't follow through, I still want to hear from them: "Whatever happens, you know I'll still be there for you, right?"

Chapter Review

Review the case study presented at the beginning of this chapter. You will conduct a home visit to Roger, who is living with HIV and hepatitis C. Please answer the following questions:

- What are your goals for the home visit?
- What challenges might you face?
- What safety concerns might you have, and how will you address these?
- How will you greet Roger?
- What do you want to assess during the home visit? What questions will you ask?
- How might you conduct an environmental assessment? What might you learn that would be helpful in guiding your work with Roger?
- How will you follow up with Roger about his case management plan and actions that he can take to improve his health?
- What referrals will you provide?

Additional Resources

The Center for Home Visiting. (n.d). Retrieved from *www.unc.edu/~uncchv/*

Community Health Worker Initiative of Sonoma County. (n.d.). *SRJC Community health worker home visiting program.* Retrieved from *http://chwisc.org/SRJC_Home_Visiting.html*

Garcia, C., Hermann, D., Bartels, A., Matamoros, P., Dick-Olson, L., & Guerra de Patino, J. (2013). Development of Project Wings home visits, a mental health intervention for latino families using community-based participatory research. *Health Promotion Practice, 13,* 755–762.

Health Resources and Services Administration, U.S. Department of Health and Human Services. (2011). *Community health workers evidence-based models toolbox.* Retrieved from *www.hrsa.gov/ruralhealth2/pdf/chwtoolkit.pdf*

Nelson, T. M., & Gunderson, J. M. (2014). *Health care home spotlight: Early lessons and results from CHW integration promoting patient-centered care and community health* [Slide presentation]. Minnesota Community Health Worker Alliance Statewide Meeting. Retrieved from *http://mnchwalliance.org/ get-powerpoints-from-our-conference/*

Oklahoma State Department of Health. (2007). *Safety guideline manual for home visitors.* Retrieved from *http:// friendsnrc.org/cbcap-priority-areas/home-visitation/oklahoma-home-visitor-training*

Vanderbilt Kennedy Center for Excellence in Developmental Disabilities. (n.d.). *Home visits: Tips and resources for making safe and effective home visits.* Retrieved from *kc.vanderbilt.edu/kennedy_files/HomeVisitsTipsandResources June2011.pdf*

ENHANCING PROFESSIONAL SKILLS

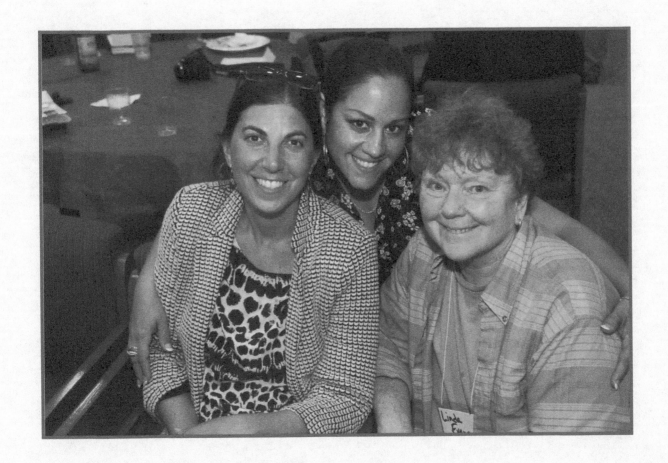

Stress Management and Self Care

12

Joani Marinoff, Tim Berthold, and Sal Núñez

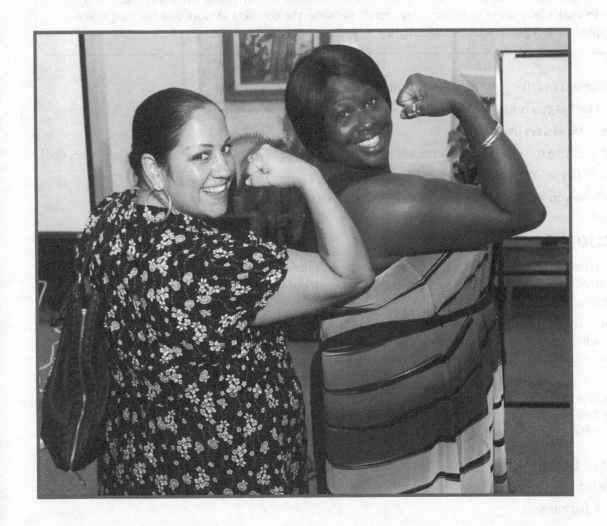

CASE STUDY	Mamphela

Mamphela's daughter is sick, and was dropped off at an aunt's house for the day. Mamphela was recently promoted to supervisor of a team of outreach workers, something she has been working towards for many years. She is happy about the promotion, but has inherited a team that does not work well together. Last night, one of the senior members of the team called Mamphela at home to say that she was thinking about quitting unless "You do something to get P.'s attitude under control. It is affecting the entire team, and I don't want to work under these conditions any more!" Between the conflicts at work and her daughter's illness, Mamphela didn't get much sleep last night.

Please take a moment to reflect on the following questions:

- What do you feel as you read the case study about Mamphela?
- Have you ever faced days like this?
- How do stressors like this—a sick family member, conflict at work, a new promotion, lack of sleep—affect you?
- What happens to you when you are feeling "stressed out"?
- What skills have you learned for coping with or managing stress?

Introduction

Everyone experiences stress; it is a natural and inevitable part of life. It keeps us alive, gives us energy, and stimulates creativity. Stress can also have a significant impact on our health, including increased risks for chronic health conditions.

CHWs often face significant stress on the job. It is important for both your professional success, and your personal well-being, to develop skills in managing stress. This chapter is designed to assist you in identifying signs of stress and burnout in yourself, and to make a realistic plan to manage stress and promote your wellness.

While we recognize that CHWs also support clients in better managing stress, the focus of this chapter is on promoting self care skills among caregivers. Once we learn how to better manage the stress in our own lives, we can be more effective in supporting others to do the same.

WHAT YOU WILL LEARN

By studying the information presented in this chapter, you will be able to:

- Define stress *and* burnout
- Recognize common sources of stress (stressors) and stress responses
- Assess personal signs of stress
- Better manage your stress and prevent burnout
- Develop an action plan for self care
- Support a client with stress reduction planning

WORDS TO KNOW

Burnout	Stress
Post-Traumatic Stress	Stressor

12.1 Defining Stress and Burnout

Stress is defined as the way we respond to and are affected by events or situations that place a demand on our internal and external resources. The event or circumstance that places demands on us is called a **stressor**. As we will describe in greater detail below, stress may be characterized by physiological responses (responses in your body), including increased blood pressure, heart, and respiration rates, as well as by emotional, cognitive (thoughts and how the mind functions), behavioral, and spiritual responses.

STRESSORS

Stressors include everyday events, such as juggling work and family responsibilities, driving in heavy traffic or depending on public transportation, as well as more dramatic events, such as the death of a loved one, homelessness, or exposure to war as a soldier or civilian. Stressors include events that may be characterized as positive, such as competing in sports, graduation from school, or falling in love. Stressors also include more negative events or dynamics such as poverty, incarceration, divorce or separation from family, receiving a failing grade, illness, or death. Common stressors may include:

- Moving
- Starting a new job
- Loss of a job
- Rushing to meet deadlines
- Planning a celebration or vacation
- Taking care of children
- Driving or taking public transportation during rush hour
- Financial difficulties
- Illness and disability
- Joining a new community or social group
- Family conflicts
- Immigration
- Experiences of prejudice or discrimination

- *What are common "positive" and "negative" stressors in your life?*

What Do
YOU?
Think

CHWs will also encounter stressors on the job, such as:

- A heavy caseload (too many clients to serve and not enough time to provide quality services to all of them)
- Working with a client who is facing particularly difficult life circumstances or challenges
- Conflict with a coworker or supervisor
- Starting a new job or earning a promotion
- Supervising others
- Managing paperwork and meeting deadlines
- Speaking before a large audience
- Lack of local resources for your clients such as housing, drug treatment, or health care
- Insufficient training and skills to perform a particular duty, such as facilitating a training or support group
- Ethical challenges

- Witnessing a client:
  - With declining health
  - Facing the end of life
  - Struggling with depression or suicidal thoughts
  - In an abusive relationship
  - Continuing to engage in harmful behaviors
  - Experiencing prejudice and discrimination based on their identity or history
- Low rates of pay or benefits
- Ending a successful professional relationship with an ongoing client
- Government policies reducing or eliminating access to essential services for your clients
- Lack of status and recognition for the role and contributions of CHWs
- Lack of stable funding for CHW positions or programs

- *Can you think of other on-the-job stressors?*

- *What types of client situations might be particularly stressful for you to face as a working CHW?*

12.2 Internal and External Resources

People respond in different ways to stressors. For example, two individuals who are exposed to the same event, such as an earthquake or hurricane, may be affected in very different ways. To a great extent, our response to stress depends on our access to internal and external resources—the same resources that we encourage our clients to identify and enhance.

INTERNAL RESOURCES

Internal resources are located within each of us and may include:

- A sense of humor
- Patience
- The ability to put events in perspective
- Good health, particularly a healthy immune system
- The ability to achieve a calm and relaxed state of mind and body
- The ability to connect in meaningful ways with other people
- A sense of pride in your professional contributions
- An understanding that facing stress is a natural part of life
- Healthy self-esteem (what you think and how you feel about yourself)
- Confidence in your ability to face adversity
- History of successfully coping with stressful life events
- Knowledge of stress management techniques
- Love of music, reading, writing, or other pastimes
- Healthy eating habits
- The ability to reach out and ask for support when you need it

- Engaging in regular exercise
- Faith, including religious or spiritual faith

- *What are your most important internal resources?*

EXTERNAL RESOURCES

External resources are located outside of us, and may include:

- Close and supportive relationships with family
- Strong friendships
- A sense of belonging to a particular community or communities
- Safety (including home, neighborhood, and society free from violence)
- A strong sense of cultural identity
- Supportive coworkers
- A skilled and respectful supervisor at work
- Pets
- Trust in and respect for a CHW, social worker, physician, teacher, or other helping professional
- Access to quality education, stable housing, good nutrition
- Access to parks and other recreational facilities
- Employment benefits including health care, sick pay, and vacation leave
- Government-provided disability benefits
- Respect for and enforcement of your civil and human rights

- *What are your most important external resources?*

It is important to understand our complex relationship to stress. For example, with sufficient internal and external resources at hand, meeting and overcoming a stressful situation or challenge can have positive effects and promote a sense of resiliency and capacity to deal with future challenges. In contrast, the damaging effects of stress are more likely to occur when the stress is ongoing or chronic and we have fewer internal and external resources to rely upon.

12.3 Stress Responses

Stress may provoke physical, emotional, cognitive, behavioral, and spiritual responses. There is no way to predict how any individual will respond to a specific stressor. Please note that the following lists do not include every possible response to stress.

The lists emphasize "negative" responses, as these tend to present the most difficult challenges. Remember that stressors can also include positive events, and that "negative" stressors, handled well, can sometimes result in positive experiences. Stress responses can compel us to new awareness and actions that create positive changes.

COMMON PHYSICAL RESPONSES

Stress is sometimes thought of primarily as a physiological (bodily) phenomenon. When confronted with a crisis or emergency, or significant new challenges or demands, our body responds by releasing hormones, such as adrenaline, which speed up our heart and respiration rates (breathing), blood pressure, and metabolism. These hormones deliver more oxygen and blood sugar to our large muscles, and dilate our pupils to improve vision. This physiological stress response is sometimes referred to as the "fight-or-flight" response, and it prepares us to take action during emergencies in order to avoid harm. Animals experience the same type of stress response in nature, which enables them, for example, to escape predators.

While this type of stress response prepares us to take action and to avoid harm during an emergency situation, in other situations, and over time, it can be harmful to our health. For example, when you experience this type of stress response as a consequence of a conflict at work, the release of hormones may leave you feeling jumpy, nervous, or overstimulated. You may be less able to focus on the situation at hand and to take calm, measured, and effective action. When we are exposed to stressors on a more frequent or chronic basis, the stress response can also suppress our immune system and contribute to illness, including chronic health conditions such as cardiovascular disease.

Other physical responses to acute (short-term) or chronic (ongoing) stress may include:

- Fatigue
- Changes in sleeping patterns, including insomnia and nightmares
- Chest pain, palpitations, or tightness
- Breathlessness
- Pain, including headaches, stomachaches, backaches
- Anxiety
- Impairment to concentration and memory
- Increased risks for developing a wide range of chronic health conditions including depression, cardiovascular disease, and diabetes
- Increased risk of preterm delivery (before 37 weeks of pregnancy)
- Nausea, digestive tract problems, ulcers
- Changes in menstrual cycles
- Rashes
- Freezing or the inability to move or take physical action
- A surge of energy
- Quick reactions in moments of crisis

- *Can you think of other physical stress responses to add to the list?*

What Do YOU Think?

Stress and Chronic Health Conditions

As we discuss in Chapter 16, there is a connection between exposure to stress and the risks of developing chronic health conditions such as depression, cardiovascular disease, and diabetes. Research also indicates that exposure to chronic stress early in life can impair the body's ability to manage stress in the future (Egerter, Braveman, & Barclay, 2011).

COMMON EMOTIONAL RESPONSES

- Frustration and anger, including anger directed at yourself
- Embarrassment or shame

- Guilt
- Anxiety or fear
- Sadness, sorrow, or despair
- Numbness or lack of emotion
- A feeling of hopelessness
- Elation, joy, satisfaction (particularly when we respond to crisis in effective ways)

COMMON COGNITIVE RESPONSES (THOUGHTS)

- Worrying (about the stressor)
- Thinking about the stressors or events over and over again
- Difficulty concentrating
- Trying to avoid thinking about the stressful situation
- Memories about other similar experiences
- Doubting your own abilities and value
- Thoughts about escaping your current situation by quitting your job, dropping out of school, ending a relationship, or moving
- Thoughts that life is no longer worth living, or thoughts of suicide
- Thoughts or fantasies of revenge
- Thoughts of gratitude for escaping harm

COMMON BEHAVIORAL RESPONSES

- Withdrawing from family, friends, or community
- Building community by working with others to confront common challenges or stressors
- Avoiding locations or activities that are stressful, including work, school, and home
- Snapping at or yelling at others, including people who have not had a part in causing the stress
- Changing patterns of eating, drinking, smoking, drug use, hygiene, or dress
- Engaging in behaviors that may seem to relieve or escape the stress, but that are harmful, especially smoking, drinking alcohol, overspending, or using drugs
- Stopping behaviors that used to give you pleasure
- Developing behaviors that enable you to better manage stress, including exercise, meditation, talking with friends, reading or writing, going to support groups, spiritual practices, playing an instrument, or making music

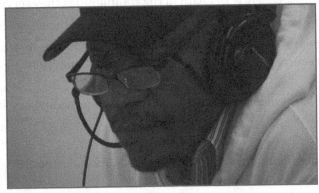

Music can help to manage and reduce stress.

> **Ramona Benson:** I was hearing things from my daughter and my husband, who were saying, "What's wrong with you?" I just wasn't acting like myself because of all the stress I was facing at work. It was a wake-up call for me to find a better way of handling it.

COMMON SPIRITUAL RESPONSES

- Loss or weakening of religious, spiritual, or metaphysical faith or beliefs
- Loss of a sense of meaning or purpose
- A sense of hopelessness or despair
- A sense of alienation from others
- Anger at god, creator, human kind, fate, or luck
- Finding or strengthening religious, spiritual, or metaphysical faith, beliefs, and practices
- A sense of connectedness to others, the world, god, or creator

BURNOUT

Burnout presents a very real risk for CHWs and other service providers. A resource developed to train CHWs working in HIV/AIDS in Zimbabwe provides the following definition of **burnout**:

> *Burnout is often difficult to conceptualize. It can be thought of as the point a person reaches when the demands made on her/him over an extended period of time are too great for the resources she or he possess[es]. Burnout has been described as a physical, emotional, psychological and spiritual phenomenon—an experience of personal fatigue, alienation and failure—or a progressive loss of idealism, energy and purpose sometimes experienced by people working in helping professions. (International Training and Education Center on HIV [I-TECH], 2005)*

The I-TECH curriculum refers to the Stage Theory of Burnout, as follows:

First Stage: The initial stage includes physical warning signs, such as the inability to shake off a lingering cold or fever, frequent headaches, and sleeplessness. The thought of going to work loses its appeal.

Second Stage: The middle stage involves such emotional and behavioral signs as angry outbursts, obvious impatience or irritability, or treating people with contempt. An attitude of suspicion often intensifies at this stage.

Third Stage: The last stage is critical and severe, and it occurs when someone becomes sour on one's self, humanity, everybody. Intense feelings of loneliness and alienation are characteristic.

For CHWs, when the high level of commitment to clients and communities is combined with stress on the job and the lack of adequate professional support, it can lead to burnout. Situations that CHWs face can aggravate and increase the likelihood of burnout, such as:

- Witnessing widespread illness, violence, or death in the communities they serve.
- Witnessing clients relapse to previous behaviors that are harmful to their health (such as drug use).
- Inability to assist your client to access local resources such as shelter, safety, food, or health care. Many communities lack these resources, or there are waiting lines, or eligibility requirements that exclude some of the clients you work with.
- Lack of adequate training, supervision, and support necessary to providing quality services to clients and communities.

- *Can you think of other circumstances that could contribute to burnout among CHWs?*

Because burnout may happen gradually, or over a series of stages, it can be difficult to recognize in ourselves or in others. When we are burned out, we are often incapable of providing services well. In the worst circumstances, we can actually do harm to our clients. A CHW who is "burned out" may:

- Not show up to work on time or keep appointments with clients
- Not complete necessary paperwork accurately or in a timely fashion
- Fail to listen deeply to clients
- Act as if they don't particularly care about the client's situation
- Bring their own issues and feelings into their work with clients
- Act out their frustration on clients or coworkers
- Fail to pay attention to details and miss opportunities to make effective referrals that could prevent poor health outcomes for clients

- *Have you ever received services from a CHW, nurse, social worker, teacher, or other aid professional who you think may have been burned out?*

- *What did you observe?*

- *What was this experience like for you?*

- *Have you ever experienced any of these stages of burnout? What signs did you experience and when did you recognize them?*

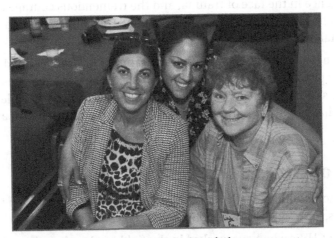

Positive relationships with coworkers helps to prevent burnout.

Andrew Ciscel: Avoiding burnout means having an awareness of when you might be at risk. The work that we do as CHWs is difficult. We witness clients going through overwhelming experiences. In order to be able to help them, we need to be grounded and well-rested and taking care of ourselves. We need to "walk the walk" when it comes to self care, taking care of our own wellness just like we hope that our clients will. This is really an important part of being a CHW.

POST-TRAUMATIC STRESS

Post-traumatic stress is a special kind of stress response that may occur when people are exposed to war, torture, child abuse, sexual assault, incarceration, natural disasters, and other traumatic experiences characterized by intense fear, horror, or a sense of helplessness (for more information about post-traumatic stress, please read Chapter 18). These events often involve the loss of control and a threat of bodily harm or death.

Traumatic experiences are sometimes considered to be rare or unusual occurrences. However, as Judith Herman writes, quite the reverse is true:

> *Rape, battery, and other forms of sexual and domestic violence are so common a part of women's lives that they can hardly be described as outside the range of ordinary experience. And in the view of the number of people killed in war over the past century, military trauma, too, must be considered a common part of human experience: only the fortunate find it unusual. (Herman, 1997)*

The impact of traumatic experience on survivors may be similar to the list of stress responses provided above. However, trauma responses are generally more severe and long-lasting. Because traumatic events are so common, it is likely that some of you, and many of your clients, may experience signs of post-traumatic stress. *Please note:* If you are working with a client who informs you that they are a survivor of trauma, or who appears to be suffering from post-traumatic symptoms, we encourage you to provide the client with a referral to a local program or provider who specializes in working with survivors of trauma.

CHWs are also at risk for a phenomenon known as secondary or vicarious trauma. This refers to the impact on helping professionals who work with survivors of traumatic events including war, rape, and child abuse. Sometimes, as a result of their work, helping professionals may develop their own symptoms of traumatic stress. Developing strong skills in self care is essential to preventing secondary trauma among CHWs.

Just as CHWs and other caregivers may experience secondary trauma, they may also experience secondary or vicarious resilience. This happens when caregivers who work with survivors of trauma are affected and inspired by the survivor's own resilience in the face of trauma, and the tremendous courage and other resources they bring to their own process of healing or recovery (the concepts of secondary trauma and secondary resilience are discussed in greater detail in Chapter 18).

We encourage you to seek out additional opportunities for training on issues related to trauma. These may be available at local colleges or public health, mental health, or social services agencies. For example, many cities and counties have rape crisis centers, suicide prevention centers, and domestic violence agencies that provide outstanding training in exchange for a volunteer commitment. These trainings are an asset to your work as a CHW.

12.4 Assessing for Stress and Burnout

Sometimes, we become so accustomed to stress in our personal lives and on the job that we lose sight of how it affects us. When this occurs, we may be at risk for burnout.

We can all learn from senior CHWs who have worked in the field for decades without experiencing burnout. They have accomplished this by developing stress management skills and a regular practice of self care. Ongoing self care is only made possible, however, by developing self-awareness and skills in assessing your exposure to stressors and their impact in your life. To do so, consider the following three methods.

1. **Reflect upon your exposure to stress and its impact in your life:** The following questions may assist to guide your reflection. Consider writing down your responses.

- What types of stressors are most difficult for you?
- What event or circumstance was particularly stressful for you today, this week, and in the past year?
- In general, how do you know when you are under stress?
- How does stress impact your body? Your thoughts? Your emotions? Your behavior? Your spirituality or beliefs?
- How do these stress responses impact your personal life, work, or experience in school?
- What have you learned that helps you to better manage stress?

2. **Ask some to provide feedback about your stress level**: We don't always have a clear picture of how stress affects us. Consider asking someone who knows you well to share any observations they may have about how you are affected by stress. Be sure to ask for this feedback at a time when you are truly prepared to listen to whatever your friend, family member, or colleague may have to share with you. Be prepared to be surprised, and to learn something new about yourself. Don't try to respond to what they say, or to defend yourself. Ask questions that will assist you to clarify the feedback you receive (for example: "Can you share a couple of examples with me? Do you notice anything about the type of situation when I may be more likely to respond in this way?").

Continue to reflect on what you hear from others. What else would you like to know? How might this information be useful in your life?

3. **Take a stress self-assessment**: There are many stress self-assessment tools available on the Web and elsewhere. Many assessments will provide you with a "score" that is designed to tell you something about your stress responses and risk for burnout. As you will see below, we have decided not to quantify or score these self-assessments. Because much of our experience and response to stressors is highly personal and subjective, we find it difficult to quantify or assign a numeric value to the range of our responses. Some people may be exposed to multiple stressors in a short period of time, but not experience strong or harmful stress responses. Others may experience profound stress responses after a single exposure. While some people find that physical stress responses are most problematic in their lives, others are more impacted by emotional or spiritual stress responses. Please use the assessment below to identify the stresses you might be facing, your access to resources for dealing with stress (internal and external), and your symptoms (stress responses).

We have included questions not only about recent exposure to stressors, but also about lifetime exposure to traumatic events and your risks for secondary trauma. We do this because exposure to traumatic events, and witnessing the trauma experiences of others, can affect us in profound and enduring ways that call out for support and recovery.

Take this self-assessment. Reflect on your answers. Feel free to use this self-assessment as a resource, share it with coworkers and clients, and revise or rewrite it.

STRESS SELF-ASSESSMENT

Stress Self-Assessment

1. Exposure to Stressors

Have you *recently* experienced the following stressors (define *recently* for yourself)? Many self-assessments use the timeframe of six months or a year.

Yes	No	
____	____	The death of a family member or close friend?
____	____	A serious injury or illness?
____	____	The end of a long-term relationship?
____	____	The beginning of new relationship or marriage?
____	____	Birth or adoption?
____	____	Serious argument or conflict with family members or close friends?
____	____	Financial or legal difficulties?
____	____	Significant changes in your sleeping or eating patterns?

(continues)

Stress Self-Assessment

(continued)

____	____	Depression (lack of feeling or persistent and overwhelming sadness)?
____	____	Violence or witnessing violence?
____	____	Loss of housing or employment?
____	____	Beginning school, a new job, or moving to a new home?
____	____	Jail or prison or incarceration of a close family member?
____	____	Discrimination in school, employment, housing, or other contexts based on your identity?
____	____	Other (fill in events that you think are significant stressors)
____	____	Other
____	____	Other

Have you *ever* experienced the following types of traumatic events:

Yes	No	
____	____	Incarceration
____	____	Armed conflict or war
____	____	Physical abuse or assault
____	____	Intimate partner violence
____	____	Sexual abuse
____	____	Fleeing your country of origin
____	____	Other
____	____	Other
____	____	Other

Work related stressors:

____	____	Received a professional evaluation that you felt was not fair?
____	____	Changed jobs or received a promotion or demotion?
____	____	Missed work because you felt too stressed to go in?
____	____	Conflict with a coworker?
____	____	Conflict with your supervisor?
____	____	Witnessing the decline of a client's health or related circumstances?
____	____	Worked closely with a client who shares their trauma experiences with you?
____	____	Other

Stress Self-Assessment
(continued)

____	____	Other
____	____	Other

For the following questions, we suggest using a Likert Scale. Rank your response to each question on a scale from 0–5.

Strongly Disagree   Strongly Agree

0	1	2	3	4	5

My input is valued by my employer	0 | 1 | 2 | 3 | 4 | 5
I can rely on guidance and support when I need it at work	0 | 1 | 2 | 3 | 4 | 5
Workplace policies are implemented in a fair manner	0 | 1 | 2 | 3 | 4 | 5
My contributions are recognized and valued	0 | 1 | 2 | 3 | 4 | 5
I feel safe at all times on the job	0 | 1 | 2 | 3 | 4 | 5
I am isolated in my job	0 | 1 | 2 | 3 | 4 | 5
I receive the resources I need to perform my job	0 | 1 | 2 | 3 | 4 | 5
I have at least one colleague at my workplace who I feel values and connects with me as a person and an individual	0 | 1 | 2 | 3 | 4 | 5

2. Stress Responses

Please circle yes or no if you have recently experienced the following stress responses:

Yes	No	
____	____	Difficulty sleeping
____	____	Smoking or drinking more frequently/more than I want to
____	____	Being more irritable with family and friends
____	____	Difficulty getting out of bed in the morning, going to work, keeping social commitments
____	____	Withdrawal from valued family, friends, community, activities
____	____	Muscle tension and chronic pain or nausea
____	____	Increased blood pressure
____	____	Difficulty sleeping, including insomnia and nightmares
____	____	Significant changes in diet
____	____	Difficulty breathing or panic attacks
____	____	Increased symptoms of depression

(continues)

Stress Self-Assessment
(continued)

_____	_____	Critical thoughts about my own value, intelligence, or abilities
_____	_____	Thoughts of not wanting to be alive or thoughts of suicide
_____	_____	Significant changes in spiritual life or faith
_____	_____	Other

Have you experienced the following at work?

_____	_____	Tuning out when listening to a client
_____	_____	Talking more than your clients during sessions
_____	_____	Increased anxiety about work
_____	_____	Increased irritation with clients or colleagues
_____	_____	Less satisfaction from professional contributions
_____	_____	A lack of hope related to my work or the prospects of my clients
_____	_____	I take it personally when clients fail to progress and achieve their goals
_____	_____	I spend a lot of time worrying about my clients or other aspects of my job when I am not working
_____	_____	I have difficulty creating a strong boundary between my work and the rest of my life
_____	_____	Other

3. Inventory of Internal and External Resources

For the following questions, we suggest using a Likert Scale. Rank your response to each question on a scale from 0–5.

Strongly Disagree   Strongly Agree

0   1   2   3   4   5

I exercise on a regular basis	0 | 1 | 2 | 3 | 4 | 5
I regularly experience restful and uninterrupted sleep	0 | 1 | 2 | 3 | 4 | 5
I eat a healthy diet	0 | 1 | 2 | 3 | 4 | 5
I drink too much coffee	0 | 1 | 2 | 3 | 4 | 5
I smoke cigarettes	0 | 1 | 2 | 3 | 4 | 5
I rely on alcohol or drugs to help me relax	0 | 1 | 2 | 3 | 4 | 5
I do something fun on a regular basis	0 | 1 | 2 | 3 | 4 | 5

Stress Self-Assessment

(continued)

I have one or more close friendships	0 | 1 | 2 | 3 | 4 | 5
I enjoy close positive relationships with family	0 | 1 | 2 | 3 | 4 | 5
I have a faith, religion, or set of beliefs that provide me with a sense of purpose and comfort	0 | 1 | 2 | 3 | 4 | 5
I am able to express my emotions, including feelings of frustration and anger	0 | 1 | 2 | 3 | 4 | 5
I do something that helps me relax when I am experiencing stress	0 | 1 | 2 | 3 | 4 | 5
I do not have a major health condition	0 | 1 | 2 | 3 | 4 | 5
I am able to pay my bills on time	0 | 1 | 2 | 3 | 4 | 5
Based on previous experiences, I am confident that I can handle most life challenges	0 | 1 | 2 | 3 | 4 | 5
I have stable housing and health benefits	0 | 1 | 2 | 3 | 4 | 5
I like my job	0 | 1 | 2 | 3 | 4 | 5
I respect my employer	0 | 1 | 2 | 3 | 4 | 5
I am a valued member of a work team	0 | 1 | 2 | 3 | 4 | 5
I know that I make a positive difference in the lives of the clients and communities with whom I work	0 | 1 | 2 | 3 | 4 | 5
I am prepared and confident in my ability to witness the trauma experiences of clients	0 | 1 | 2 | 3 | 4 | 5

Analyze Your Responses

Notice how many times you indicated that you are exposed to stressors or signs of stress responses.

- What have you learned about your exposure to stressors?
- What do you notice about your response to stress?
- How do you assess your level of access to internal and external resources?
- Are you prepared to enhance your skills in managing stress and preventing burnout?

12.5 Enhancing Stress Management Skills

Don't become disheartened if you face a lot of stressors in your life. Most of us do. The *good news* is that we can each cultivate positive, life-affirming, and health-sustaining skills and habits. We can use these activities or practices to counter the stressors in our lives. Despite our neurological programming, and the challenges inherent in our society and in our professional and personal lives, relaxation is possible. When we develop good skills and habits for caring for ourselves, we are better able to deal with the negative experiences we face and are more confident about our ability to handle positive challenges and opportunities.

How Do You Relax?

Many of us already participate in practices that are relaxing and stress relieving. There are many simple activities that we use to alleviate stress, such as:

- Getting adequate rest and sleep
- Eating a well-balanced and nutritious diet
- Spending meaningful time with family, friends, and pets
- Spending some quiet time alone
- Listening to or playing music
- Taking a hot bath
- Playing games
- Physical activities including walking and playing sports
- Journaling, writing, poetry
- Painting, drawing, sculpting
- Cooking
- Gardening
- Walking on the beach or in the woods, parks, or other natural settings

What are you already doing to relax and refresh yourself and to alleviate stress?

Lee Jackson: I meditate and relax, go to the gym, listen to jazz. Basically, I take care of myself.

Please watch the following video interview ▶ about stress management.

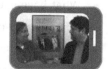

STRESS MANAGEMENT: FACULTY INTERVIEW
🔗 *http://youtu.be/ YH2na2xuuuo*

MOTIVATION FOR STRESS MANAGEMENT

What about those of us who have a hard time making the activities that reduce stress into a regular part of our lives? Sometimes, just trying to find the time to do stress-reduction activities can create even more stress. In addition, we often do things that may seem like stress reduction or taking care of ourselves in the moment, but over the long term they actual damage our health and well-being. Examples include smoking cigarettes; using drugs or alcohol; being lulled into a stupor by the television, Internet, or digital gadgets; and shopping or "retail therapy" that overspends our budget.

How can we be motivated to participate in healthful stress-reduction practices? One definition of motivation is to impart courage, inspiration, or resolution. It takes courage to step back and take care of ourselves in skillful and health-promoting ways, in the midst of a consumer culture media frenzy that is trying to sell us so many ways to distract ourselves and escape.

This may be where courage and resolution come into play. CHWs are courageous, inspired, and resolute in so many ways. You work for the benefit of others, often through great obstacles and challenges. You must also step up and work for the benefit of yourselves, in order to continue to be able to provide services of the very highest quality to the clients and communities you work with.

Please don't wait for motivation to "just happen" in order to do something good for yourself. Motivation often will result through experiencing the direct benefits of the practice. One of our colleagues keeps images that motivate him posted around his office. These include photographs of family, artwork made by clients, and posters of inspirational heroes.

- *Where does your motivation come from?*

- *What does motivation mean to you?*

- *How can you sustain it?*

- *Why do you reward yourself?*

- *How do you choose what to use as your reward?*

- *How can self care and respect be put into practice every day?*

First, we'll look at some of the key areas for self care. Then we will look in depth at one very easy and effective activity that some people engage in to reduce stress, with instructions for how to get started.

12.6 Self Care

There are many different strategies for taking care of our physical, emotional, and spiritual health. Strategies and approaches commonly employed by CHWs and other working professionals are highlighted here.

HEALTHY EATING

What we eat and drink can have a significant impact on our health and wellness. Chapter 17 provides guidelines for healthy eating that are grounded in research. As you will see, these guidelines encourage us to develop a daily diet that features a lot of vegetables and fruits (with a variety of colors) and whole grains whenever possible (such as whole-wheat pasta or brown rice). Try to reduce your consumption of processed foods that often include saturated and trans fats, cholesterol, corn syrup or other added sugars, salts, or alcohol. It is also important to drink plenty of water and avoid soda (often described as liquid candy), which have been recently identified as an important factor in the rise of chronic health conditions. Take time to review the guidelines presented in Chapter 17 and to consider what steps you can take to improve the quality of your diet.

- *Do you have a favorite healthy meal that you truly enjoy?*

- *Can you make time this week to prepare and savor a healthy meal (on your own or with family or friends)?*

- *What will you do to improve the quality of your daily diet?*

PHYSICAL ACTIVITY

Engaging in physical activity is another effective strategy to reduce stress. A regular program (in consultation with your health provider) of physical activity such as walking or running, swimming, dancing, playing soccer, and many sports activities can have healthful benefits, including the alleviation of many of the physical and emotional symptoms of stress. Walking is a great form of physical activity. It has the advantage of being free, something that you can do with others, and is relatively accessible to people of all ages and fitness levels. In some workplaces, people have begun holding walking meetings, or have created walking clubs that walk during the lunch hour or during breaks. For more information about physical activity, please see Chapter 17.

Tai Chi and yoga are examples of physical activities that are becoming more widespread in the United States. Both are particularly good stress-busters, because they include a focus on relaxation and peaceful concentration as part of the exercise itself. For both of these, initial instruction is recommended for beginners and can usually be found at your local community college, a neighborhood center, or private settings. With more advanced and ongoing instruction you may develop a deeper practice.

Tai Chi is a practice from China and is thousands of years old. The focus of Tai Chi is on concentration and simple flowing movements to balance the energy called Chi (pronounced "chee") in the body.

Yoga is a practice from India and is also thousands of years old. The focus is to encourage an individual feel whole. Yoga teachings include physical, mental, and spiritual dimensions. In the West, a yoga practice of physical poses or *asana* is the most common, and can strengthen muscles and increase flexibility, coordination, and balance. A central teaching is to simply be present and accepting of the action of the body in any given moment or pose. Yoga is not a competitive sport. A teacher once explained that progress is measured not by increasing strength or flexibility, but by the big heart of compassion for what *is*, right now.

- *Do you engage in some form of physical activity that allows you to relax?*

- *How can you enhance your level of physical activity?*

- *Can you make time to engage in physical activity, even briefly, this week?*

What Do YOU Think?

Jerry Smart: I am not exempt from stress. I am a working, single father who is also in school. It's important for me to have quiet times when I can turn off the TV or take a walk. I like to take really long walks, to be by myself, and to stay away from drama or negative environments. Doing this helps me to get myself back; I can be restored.

STRESS REDUCTION BY PROFESSIONALS

There are a wide range of professional services that are helpful in managing stress and preventing burnout. These include the following examples.

Acupuncture works by correcting the balance of energy known as *Qi* (pronounced "chee"). It involves inserting hair-fine needles into specific anatomic points in the body to stimulate the flow of energy. Practitioners also apply pressure, suction, electromagnetic stimulation, or heat to the acupuncture points.

Coaching and psychotherapy are overlapping models. Coaching generally focuses on the here and now, problem solving, and assisting individuals in developing new skills to cope and adjust to present life situations. Psychotherapy focuses on evaluating, diagnosing, and treating emotional problems and severe psychological conditions. Although talking about your sense of distress with a friend, family member, or peer may be effective, seeking professional support is recommended if the level of stress becomes high and ongoing. Professional support is also particularly valuable if you are experiencing post-traumatic stress.

Massage is the systematic and intentional manipulation of soft body tissue and may include joint movements and stretching. The goal is to assist the body to achieve well-being while alleviating distress and specific disease-related symptoms. Different systems of massage include Swedish, deep tissue, neuromuscular, Chinese, Indian, Thai, Japanese, Indigenous American, and Caribbean (such as *Sobadoras)*. Practitioners usually use their hands to apply fixed and movable pressure to the body.

Sweat lodges and *temexcales* are sacred and spiritual healing spaces created and utilized by the indigenous peoples of North and South America, respectively. The lodge or *temexcal* is often seen as a womb that gives birth and life, and also serves for communing with the Creator. The sweat lodge ceremony is complex and traditionally led by an experienced elder. The etiquette varies according to the lodge leader and may include singing, chanting, and drumming, all of which is considered prayer. The lodge ceremony provides cleansing of the spirit, heart, mind, and body, and has been successful in treating certain conditions.

- *Can you think of other professional services and traditions that may be helpful in reducing stress?*

What Do YOU Think?

SIMPLE DEEP BREATHING

One of the most basic and effective relaxation methods is diaphragmatic breathing or deep breathing (the diaphragm is a dome-shaped muscle located between the lungs and abdominal cavity). This involves taking a deep breath while flexing the diaphragm, and is marked by the expansion of the abdomen (belly) rather than the chest. Usually individuals inhale slowly through the nose until the lungs are filled and follow by slowly exhaling through pursed lips to regulate the release of air. Practicing diaphragmatic breathing for five to ten minutes three or four times a day may significantly reduce your level of stress.

A Deep Breathing Activity

If you wish, take a few minutes to try this simple deep breathing activity.

Place the tip of your tongue against the roof of your mouth just behind your front teeth, and keep it there throughout this activity. Exhale through your mouth (feel free to make noise when you do this!).

1. Close your mouth and breathe in through your nose, letting your belly expand, for a count of 1-2-3.

2. Hold your breath for a count of 1-2-3.

3. Exhale and push all your breath out through your mouth to a count of 1-2-3.

Repeat this breathing rhythm three to five times as you wish. If you continue to do this activity, try to hold your breath for longer counts, as long as it is comfortable for you to do so.

- What was this activity like for you?
- What changes, if any, do you notice to your body, your thoughts or feelings, your level of stress?

PRAYER, FAITH, AND SPIRITUALITY

Research indicates that the states of consciousness often produced by deep faith or prayer can provide relief from worries and difficulties and lead to enduring physical, emotional, and mental change. Religious or spiritual practices vary significantly. Some individuals attend a church, temple, mosque, or other center, while others prefer to practice independently, in community, or by communing with nature.

- *Is prayer, faith, or spirituality an important resource in your life?*

- *How can you enhance your ability to access these resources in ways that will serve to relieve stress?*

What Do YOU Think?

Lee Jackson: I'm spiritually grounded. To me that's number one. That's the key in my life. I don't push it off on anyone else, but that's what works for me: a firm belief in a supreme being or a force greater than me that's a power unseen. That's God to me.

MEDITATION

Meditation is a term that covers a wide range of practices that generally involve awareness or contemplation. Almost all cultures have some set of practices that assist people to develop awareness of the present moment. There are many forms of meditation practice including relaxation, visualization, concentration, chanting, and prayer. Yoga and Tai Chi are often considered examples of movement-based meditation.

Meditation is used to quiet the mind and calm the body. It eases some of the symptoms of stress, such as the racing heart or repeated thoughts about a stressful event. It creates breathing room and some distance from and perspective about the situations and challenges we face. Meditation has also been found to help manage health conditions such as depression, anxiety disorders, asthma, cancer, high blood pressure, and chronic pain (NCCIH, n.d.).

MINDFULNESS MEDITATION

Mindfulness is a meditation practice growing in popularity that focuses attention on the present moment. Mindfulness meditation, often in the form of "Mindfulness-Based Stress Reduction" (MBSR), is taught in many settings across the country, including health care organizations, the high-tech industry, and the U.S. military, to promote stress reduction and general well-being.

Mindfulness cultivates the ability to be more present in and with our lives, a willingness to be with what is without judgment. Mindfulness meditation is a way to explore waking up from or coming out of an "automatic pilot" way of living. We are often so preoccupied with either rehearsing a possible future or rehashing something in the past that we move through our lives without noticing the moments that are significant right now. By rushing through and over the present, we miss out on possibilities for knowledge and transformation, or making different choices.

When people begin to practice mindfulness meditation, they are often surprised at how active their minds actually are—jumping around from thought to thought, rehearsing for the future or rehashing the past, spinning all kinds of stories and making judgments. Sometimes this is referred to as the "Monkey Mind" because our many thoughts are like a monkey jumping from tree to tree. In mindfulness meditation the focus is on this present moment because it is the only time we have to perceive, grow, learn, or actually change to answer the challenges and opportunities arising in our lives. We cannot learn, grow or change in the past or the future, only in the present moment.

A Mini Mindfulness Moment—Stop

This is a practice often used in Mindfulness-Based Stress Reduction. It is a reminder to help us to stop for a moment to become more aware of our body and thoughts. Here is how it goes:

S: Remind yourself to STOP whatever you are doing in this moment.

T: TAKE a breath. This reconnects you to your breathing and your body *right now.*

O: OBSERVE what is happening *in this moment.* What do you notice in your body? You may become aware of posture, sensations, or your breath. You may notice your thoughts, perhaps memories or plans, a mood or emotion.

P: PROCEED with what were doing before you came to a stop.

It's just that simple.

12.7 A Mindfulness Meditation Practice

Mindfulness meditation uses a variety of things as the focus for meditation. Often the focus is our breath. Breathing is always happening; our breath is always present and available to us as a point of concentration. It is always changing, allowing our attention to become ever more subtle to enable us to follow the tiny changes in sensation of the breath. This attention to sensations takes us away from the ever-present verbal chatter in the mind, our own internal dialog. Any time we notice we are distracted by thought, feelings, or emotions we can, simply and without any judgment, note what has distracted us, and gently allow our awareness to return to the breath.

Through this process of focusing the attention, meditation quiets the mind. And as we concentrate, we experience how our mind continually shifts from thought to thought, sensation to sensation, memory to memory, and plan to plan. Remember, our neurobiology is wired to notice what is around us and figure out if it represents a threat to our safety or survival. Thus, it takes a good deal of patience, commitment, and a heart full of loving-kindness to continue on this path of practice. An important way to be kind to yourself in developing a mediation practice is to start with what you can do right now. Five minutes a day, every day is great. You can gradually increase your time in meditation as your interest and situation allow. By doing an Internet search for "meditation," you will be able to find many resources and local centers and teachers for support and community.

Here are instructions for a simple sitting mindfulness meditation. If you choose to give it a try, set aside at least 20 minutes.

A Sitting Meditation

Let Your Mind Settle Like a Clear Forest Pool

To begin this meditation, select a quiet time and place. Sit on a cushion or chair, taking an upright yet relaxed posture. Let yourself sit with quiet dignity. Close your eyes gently and begin by bringing a full, present attention to whatever you feel within you and around you. Let your mind be spacious and your heart be kind and soft.

As you sit, feel the sensations of your body. Then notice what sounds and feelings, thoughts, and expectations are present. Allow them all to come and go, rise and fall like the waves of the ocean. Be aware of the waves and rest seated in the midst of them. Allow yourself to become more and more still.

In the center of all these waves, feel your breathing, your life-breath. Let your attention feel the in-and-out breathing wherever you notice it, as coolness or tingling in the nose or throat, as a rising or falling of your chest or abdomen. Relax and softly rest your attention on each breath, feeling the movement in a steady easy way. Let the breath breathe itself in any rhythm, long or short, soft or deep. As you feel each breath, concentrate and settle into each movement. Let all other sounds and sensations, thoughts and feelings continue to come and go like waves in the background.

After a few breaths, your attention may be carried away by one of the waves of thoughts or memories, by body sensations or sounds. Whenever you notice you have been carried away for a time, acknowledge the wave that has done so by softly giving it a name such as "planning," "remembering," "itching," "restless." Then let it pass and gently return to the breath. Sometimes waves will take a long time to pass, others will be short. Certain thoughts or feelings will be painful, others will be pleasurable. Whatever they are, let them be.

At some sittings you will be able to return to your breath easily. At other times in your meditation you will mostly be aware of body sensations or of thoughts and plans. Either way is fine. No matter what you experience, be aware of it, let it come and go, and rest at ease in the midst of it all. After you have sat for 20 or 30 minutes in this way, open your eyes and look around before you get up. Then as you move try to allow the same spirit of awareness or mindfulness to go with you into the activities of your day.

The art of meditation is simple but not always easy. It thrives on practice and a kind and spacious heart. If you do this simple practice of sitting with mindfulness or awareness every day, you will gradually grow in centeredness and understanding.

(Kornfield, 1994. Additional meditations on walking, eating, loving-kindness, and forgiveness are also presented in this book.)

12.8 Working with Clients on Stress Reduction

As a CHW, you have an important role to play in supporting clients to better manage stress. Start by listening to your client. Facilitate dialogue using client-centered concepts and skills such as motivational interviewing and OARS (see Chapter 9), and provide clients with an opportunity to talk about the stress they face in their life, how it affects them, and the skills they already have for stress management. As you support clients to enhance their skills for stress management, keep the following six principles in mind:

1. **Maintain a neutral stance**: Keep an open mind and heart as you listen to the client's experience. Keep any thoughts or judgments about the client to yourself (or better yet, try to let any judging thoughts or assumptions go altogether). *You probably know from your own personal experience how it feels when you sense that you are being judged and how it is not useful in developing trust or encouraging you to make any changes.*

2. **Be client-centered**: Let the client's experience, culture, knowledge, skills, and beliefs guide the discussion, and form the basis of any plan for stress management.

3. **Use a strength-based approach**: Focus on the strengths that the client already possesses. Sometimes clients doubt or have a difficult time noticing their own strengths. By acknowledging their positive attributes, you can support the client to gain confidence in their own abilities, and to enhance their own skills and self-esteem.

4. **Apply harm reduction**: Keep the principles of harm reduction in mind: Any actions that reduce potential harms to the client or their loved ones are a positive step towards promoting their health and wellness.

5. **Develop a realistic action plan**: Support clients to develop a practical action plan for stress management that they have a good chance of implementing. Remember that behavior change is hard, and often begins with a small step forward. Check in regularly, if possible, to support clients to implement their action plan and to revise it over time.

6. **Use positive reinforcement**: Provide positive feedback and encouragement for the actions and decisions that clients take to better manage stress and promote their own wellness.

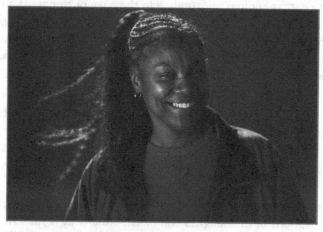

CHWs support clients to enhance skills for stress reduction.

Please watch the following video 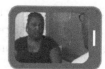 of a CHW supporting a client to better manage her stress.

- How did the CHW use the principles explained above to support this client to better manager her stress?

- What did the CHW do well in supporting this client?

- What else would you do as a CHW to support this client with stress management?

ACTION PLANNING AND STRESS MANAGEMENT: ROLE PLAY, DEMO

⊂⊃ *http://youtu.be/ H_62Cbm5W_c*

> **Ramona Benson:** One of the things that I love to do is to help women get empowered so they can eliminate barriers in their life and live a healthy lifestyle. Our program is 18 months. I have seen a lot of ladies leave out of here like a blossomed flower, moving to environments that they never dreamed they could ever move into.

Chapter Review

DEVELOP YOUR ACTION PLAN FOR STRESS REDUCTION

Please consider developing a simple plan for self care and stress reduction. Write down your answers to the following questions and keep the page in a place where you can easily refer to it in the future.

1. Two ways that stress is currently affecting me that I want to change are: _____

2. The reasons why I want to address and handle this stress effectively include: _____

3. Three realistic actions or steps that I can take to help relieve stress and take better care of myself are:
   a. What I will do, when I will begin, and how frequently I will do it: _____
   b. What I will do, when I will begin, and how frequently I will do it: _____
   c. What I will do, when I will begin, and how frequently I will do it: _____

4. Internal resources (my personal qualities, strengths, knowledge, and skills) that will assist me to achieve my self care action plan include: _____

5. External resources and sources of support that will assist me to achieve my self care action plan include: _____

6. A professional colleague (such as a classmate or other CHW) whom I will talk with about my self care action plan is: _____.

7. A meaningful source of motivation that will assist me to achieve my plan is: _____

8. Something productive and positive that I will do if I face challenges or setbacks in implementing my self care action plan is: _____

Signature: _____

Date: _____

References

Egerter, S., Braveman, P., & Barclay, C. (2011). How social factors shape health: Stress and health. Princeton, NJ: Robert Wood Johnson Foundation. Retrieved from *www.rwfj.org/en/research-publications/find-rwjf-research/2011/03/how-social-factors-shape-health.html*

Herman, J. (1997). *Trauma and recovery: The aftermath of violence from domestic abuse to political terror.* New York, NY: Basic Books.

International Training and Education Center on HIV (I-TECH) and the Ministry of Health and Child Welfare, Zimbabwe. (2005). *Integrated counselling for HIV and AIDS prevention and care: Training for HIV primary care counsellors.* Unpublished training manual.

Kornfield, J. (1994). *Buddha's little instruction book.* New York, NY: Bantam Books.

National Center for Complementary and Integrative Health (NCCIH). (n.d.). *National institutions of health.* Retrieved from *https://nccih.nih.gov/health/meditation/overview.htm*

Additional Resources

Bays, J. C. (2011). *How to train a wild elephant & other adventures in mindfulness*. Boston, MA: Shambhala.

Braveman, P., Egerter, S. & Barclay, C. (2011). *What shapes health related behaviors?* Princeton, NJ: Robert Wood Johnson Foundation. Retrieved from *www.rwjf.org/en/research-publications/find-rwjf-research/2011/03/what-shapes-health-related-behaviors---.html*

CBS (2014). Mindfulness. 60 Minutes. Retrieved from *www.cbsnews.com/news/mindfulness-anderson-cooper-60-minutes/*

International Society for Traumatic Stress Studies. (n.d.). Retrieved from *www.istss.org/resources/index.cfm*

Kabat-Zinn, J. (n.d.). *Guided mindfulness meditation practices with Jon Kabat-Zinn*. Retrieved from *http://www.mindfulnesscds.com/*

This is the link to the website for Jon Kabat-Zinn, founder of Mindfulness-Based Stress Reduction (MBSR). Internet searches on Mindfulness will reveal multiple listings for books and other resources such as guided meditations.

Perry, B. (2003). *The cost of caring: Secondary traumatic stress and the impact of working with high-risk children and families* [Booklet]. The Child Trauma Academy. Retrieved from *https://childtrauma.org/wp-content/uploads/2014/01/Cost_of_Caring_Secondary_Traumatic_Stress_Perry_s.pdf*

This booklet is for parents, teachers, and various professionals working with traumatized children.

Sidran Foundation (n.d.). *Traumatic stress education and advocacy*. Retrieved from *www.sidran.org/*

Sood, A. (2013). *The Mayo Clinic guide to stress free living*. Philadelphia, PA: Da Capo Press.

Stahl, B., & Goldstein, E. (2010). *A mindfulness-based stress reduction workbook*. Oakland, CA: New Harbinger.

Book includes a CD with many guided mindfulness meditations.

University of California, Los Angeles, Mindful Awareness Research Center. (n.d.). Free guided meditations. Retrieved from *http://marc.ucla.edu/*

UCLA also has a mindfulness training program.

University of Massachusetts, Center for Mindfulness. (n.d.). Retrieved from *www.umassmed.edu/cfm/*

University of Massachusetts has a training program for learning to facilitate mindfulness and host a national annual conference.

Van Dernoot Lipsky, L., with Burk, C. (2007). *Trauma stewardship: An everyday guide to caring for self while caring for others*. Seattle, WA: Las Olas Press.

Conflict Resolution Skills

13

Darlene Weide, Joani Marinoff, and Tim Berthold

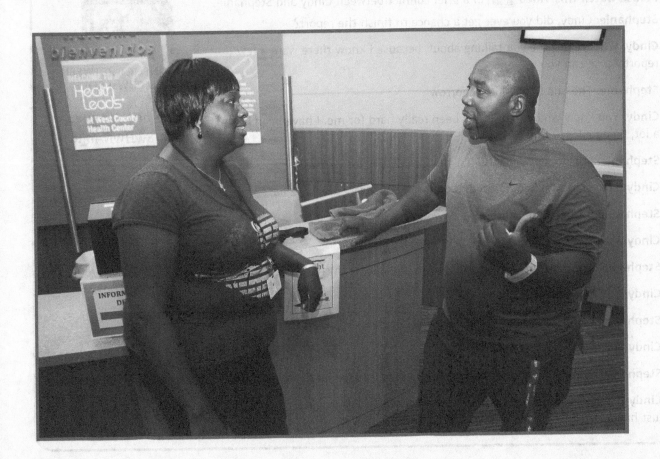

CASE STUDY Cindy and Stephanie

Cindy and Stephanie are CHWs at a busy urban community health center serving formerly incarcerated clients. They have been assigned a report to complete together, and the deadline is coming right up. Cindy takes the lead and asks Stephanie for her contribution to the report. Stephanie responds that she has been too busy to do it, and their interaction escalates.

Please watch this video ▶ of a brief conflict between Cindy and Stephanie.

Stephanie: Cindy, did you ever get a chance to finish the report?

Cindy: What report are you talking about, because I know there were a few reports ... so can you tell me?

Stephanie: The one that's due tomorrow

Cindy: You know what, I didn't. It's been really hard for me. I have been in the field a lot, doing a lot of outreach.

Stephanie: I mean, I understand but this deadline is tomorrow!

Cindy: I haven't even had no time to do it . . . I'm barely touching base here!

Stephanie: It's been on your desk for two weeks.

Cindy: Wait, hold on, who put you in charge?

Stephanie: The deadline that's due tomorrow made me in charge.

Cindy: You're my equal!

Stephanie: I understand that, but we have a deadline, and I've been . . .

Cindy: But who made you in charge?

Stephanie: But I have to keep us on task and stay focused on deadlines. Deadlines can't be pushed back.

Cindy: Then why don't you do some of the outreach? I'm dealing with this guy, one of our patients, who just had a stroke . . . and I've been working with him every day.

CONFLICT BETWEEN TWO CHWs: ROLE PLAY

🔗 *http://youtu. be/8wHwNAnhC1Y*

How might you answer the following questions about the conflict between Cindy and Stephanie?

- What is the conflict between Cindy and Stephanie really about?
- How might this conflict impact each of them and their work?
- What conflict styles are Cindy and Stephanie using?
- If you were Cindy, how would you deal with the issue of Stephanie's missing report?
- If you were Stephanie, how would you respond to Cindy?
- What could Cindy and Stephanie have done differently to resolve this conflict?

Introduction

CHWs are often employed by agencies that lack sufficient financial resources and provide services to low-income communities with long histories of discrimination. Given this context, it is not surprising that CHWs are likely to encounter conflict over the course of their career, including conflicts with coworkers, supervisors, and clients.

CHWs are not alone in experiencing conflict at work: it is part of every healthy workplace and all human relationships. When people work closely together, differences inevitably arise. If addressed productively, these conflicts present opportunities for greater understanding and stronger relationships. However, conflicts that go unresolved can be harmful to clients, CHWs, and the organizations that employ them.

This chapter is designed to help you better understand the sources of workplace conflicts, increase awareness of your own styles of engaging in or responding to conflict, and support you in learning skills to resolve conflicts and enhance the quality of your working relationships.

This is an introductory chapter, and we encourage you to look for additional opportunities for training in conflict resolution. Resources for learning more about conflict resolution are provided at the end of this chapter.

WHAT YOU WILL LEARN

By studying the material in this chapter, you should be able to:

- Define the terms *conflict* and *conflict resolution*
- Identify common sources of conflict in the workplace
- Discuss the importance of understanding personal and cultural conflict styles and become more familiar with your own conflict style
- Discuss how power and anger can affect conflict resolution
- Implement steps to take to handle your own anger professionally and to de-escalate the anger of others
- Negotiate a common framework and process for resolving conflict and explain why this is so important
- Apply essential listening skills during conflict, and discuss their importance for conflict resolution
- Explore and apply a conflict resolution model that you can adapt to your situation

WORDS TO KNOW

Mediation

13.1 Conflict Resolution Skills Are Essential for CHWs

Saul Alinsky (1969) says, "Life is conflict and in conflict you're alive." For CHWs, learning how to manage and respond to conflict is an essential job qualification: a survey conducted in the San Francisco Bay Area with employers of CHWs identified communication and conflict resolution skills as one of the most important qualifications for employment (Cowans, 2005). Why is it so important to have conflict management skills? Let's face it, being a CHW is a stressful job and work-based conflicts are bound to happen. CHWs often work with people who have experienced racism, poverty, exposure to violence, and a lack of access to safe housing or healthy food. Research has shown that when communities are under stress, conflict is more likely to occur (Cohen, Davis, & Aboelata, 1998). If CHWs do not learn how to effectively resolve conflicts, they are likely to miss out on opportunities for career advancement and promotion and may lose their job altogether.

Few CHWs have received training in the skills and techniques for successfully managing conflicts. Role models for productive communication, teamwork, and effective negotiation are often few and far between. As a result, CHWs may find that their work environment is one of quick fixes, hot tempers, avoidance tactics, and at times, deep frustration.

The good news is that conflict prevention and resolution skills can be learned. Resolving conflict requires courage, commitment, and compassion—traits that CHWs have in abundance. The goal is not to eliminate conflict, but to find ways to enhance its positive contributions to the workplace. When approached constructively, conflicts lead to insights and opportunities that might not have been seen otherwise. By developing conflict resolution skills, CHWs and their organizations can deepen their capacity for collaboration and creativity.

What Do YOU Think?

- *What words, feelings, and images come to mind when you think of conflict?*

- *As a child, how were you taught to deal with conflict? In your experience, what contributes to successful conflict resolution?*

13.2 Understanding Conflict

There are many ways to define conflict. The Office of Human Resource Development (OHRD) at the University of Wisconsin defines *conflict* as "a disagreement through which the parties involved perceive a threat to their needs, interests or concerns" (Academic Leadership Support: Office of Quality Improvement, 2007).

Let's look closely at this definition. For conflict to exist there must be a disagreement, which is some kind of difference in the position of two or more people. Often the people involved in a conflict have very different perceptions about the cause or nature of the disagreement. When people experience a disagreement, they are responding to their own perception of a threat or demand.

Our first thoughts about a disagreement don't always go to the heart of what the conflict is about. Workplace conflicts are often very emotional and complicated. Learning to understand the core issues of a conflict is key to resolving it.

In addition, there is often a basic disagreement about who is involved in a conflict. A supervisor may be surprised to learn that everyone on her team is upset about a new policy. One coworker may express feeling burned out only to learn that others feel the same way. A coworker may be oblivious to the fact that his actions have upset another. An office mate may take sides without knowing the whole picture. Clients may be outraged that they don't qualify for services and take their anger out on staff members. When conflicts occur at work, it is necessary to take time to figure out who is involved in the conflict and who needs to be a part of the resolution process. Sometimes, two parties initially meet to discuss the issue. As the core issues are explored, it may be necessary to invite coworkers or a work team to discuss the issues and find solutions.

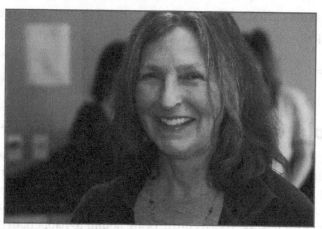

CHWs learn to view conflict as natural and as an opportunity for positive change.

Conflicts are inevitable and may be both productive and destructive in the work environment.

Conflict is destructive when it:

- Diverts energy from more important issues and tasks
- Deepens differences in values
- Polarizes groups so that cooperation is reduced
- Results in bias or discrimination
- Destroys the morale of people or reinforces poor self-concepts
- Harms the quality of services provided to clients and communities

Conflict is constructive when it:

- Promotes new understandings of self, others, and working relationships
- Creates possibilities for positive change and transformation

- Enhances working relationships and the cohesiveness of work teams
- Reduces stress
- Results in better-quality services for clients and communities

  - *Can you think of other ways that conflict may be destructive or constructive?*

13.3 Common Sources of Workplace Conflict

The first step in learning how to resolve conflicts is to understand common sources of conflict, as well as your own reactions to and feelings about conflict. Conflicts between employees can spring from a variety of sources. They may have a single cause or multiple causes. If left unaddressed, workplace conflicts can escalate from small annoyances to more serious issues.

Common sources of conflicts that occur at work may include the following examples (adapted from Gaitlin, Wysocki, & Kepner, 2007):

1. **Insufficient resources**: Everyone requires sufficient resources to do their job well. Yet workers often compete for scarce resources. CHWs often feel frustrated about the lack of supplies, supervision time, space, adequate pay and benefits, administrative and technical support, and resources to share with clients. Funding from year to year may be tentative. When teams or individuals have less than they require, especially if they perceive others as having more, conflicts are quick to arise.

2. **Conflicting personalities and work styles**: Personality clashes occur in all work environments. People have different work styles: one coworker may prefer to chat and talk loudly throughout the day, while another may need a closed-door setting. When these differences are brushed aside, over time, people's tempers can flare.

3. **Delegation of power and authority**: Some organizational leaders welcome input into decision making, while others are very hierarchical and place the power in the hands of a few. People in higher-status positions may be more free to engage in conflict and less likely to avoid confrontation. People new to the job or in lower-status or lower-paid positions may feel uncomfortable questioning authority and leadership decisions for fear of being fired.

4. **Conflicting values**: It is common for workers in the public health and nonprofit sectors to share similar values such as commitment to diversity, social justice, equality, and community ownership of programming. Indeed, these values are often what motivates us to work in the field of public health in the first place. At the same time, when differences in values emerge, staff may feel tremendous tensions that can lead to conflict.

5. **Lack of acknowledgment for one's contributions**: Everyone wants to be acknowledged for one's hard work and contributions. Yet, not everyone needs the same type of acknowledgment. Some people like to be praised publicly, while others prefer a special lunch out with their boss, a bouquet of flowers, or time off. When a supervisor fails to acknowledge someone's work, or fails to acknowledge everyone in the same way, she may create frustration. For volunteer CHWs who are contributing their time and talent without getting paid, lack of acknowledgment for their work can be especially frustrating.

6. **Disagreements over roles and responsibilities**: Coworkers may disagree about who should do what and how things should be done. Some employees may be unaware or misinformed about the job duties of others. When new programs are developed, or when there is staff turnover or downsizing, questions about roles need to be reviewed. Unrealistic work expectations or different perceptions about how the work should be done can easily result in conflict between individuals and between teams and leadership.

7. **Intercultural misunderstandings**: People from different cultural backgrounds may have different expectations, verbal and nonverbal habits, assumptions, and beliefs. Workplace conflicts between parties from different cultural backgrounds can often be traced to cultural miscommunication, stereotypes, prejudices, or lack of understanding.

8. **Poor communication**: Without clear procedures for handling conflict, workers may end up talking about their challenges in unproductive ways, such as venting problems behind people's backs. This type of

indirect communication almost always increases tensions. Workers who gossip often lack skills to take more productive actions.

9. **Poor leadership and unpredictable policies**: When employees feel that the leadership is not responding to the changing needs of an organization or team, staff can feel demoralized and frustrated. When low performance is allowed for some people and not others, the staff feel frustrated. When leadership values one department over another, resentments intensify. When leadership, at any level, avoids conflict, employees experience low morale. In the absence of clear workplace policies, uncertainty and conflict may arise (Hart, 2002).

10. **Conflicting pressures**: Conflicting pressures occur when two or more staff members are responsible for completing different tasks with the same deadline. In this situation, the deadline of the person with more authority often takes precedence, putting pressure on other workers. For example, a program director needs to finish a report for a funder and needs some information from a CHW. The program director interrupts the CHW when she is busy organizing supplies for the night's work. The CHW feels upset that she is asked to stop what she needs to get done to provide information for the report.

11. **Perceived threat to one's identity**: The Harvard Negotiation Project emphasizes how conflicts may threaten our identity. For example, conflicts may provoke concern about whether we are valued, trusted, respected, and perceived to be intelligent, competent, hardworking, or ethical. When conflicts touch on these core concepts and feelings about our identity and worth, they are likely to trigger strong emotions and may be particularly challenging to address (Stone, Patton, & Heen, 2010).

Keep in mind that conflicts and disputes seldom have a simple cause and are typically influenced by a number of factors.

- *Think about a conflict you have experienced at work. What were your initial perceptions of the cause of the conflict?*

- *Referring to the list above, what else may have contributed to the conflict?*

- *How could knowing about the causes of the conflict assist you in addressing it?*

Signs and Symptoms of Unresolved Conflict in the Workplace

Common signs of conflict in the workplace include:

- Absenteeism
- Turnover
- Accidents
- Poor teamwork
- "Us versus them" attitudes
- Open bickering
- Low productivity
- Excessive competition
- Gossip
- Aggression or hostility
- Blaming
- High stress
- Sabotage

Signs and Symptoms of Unresolved Conflict in the Workplace

(continued)

- o   Poor job satisfaction
- o   Low creativity
- o   Tardiness
- o   Alcoholism or substance use
- o   Prejudice, such as homophobia, sexism, or racism

Source: **Sharon and Clark, 1989.**

13.4 Common Sources of Conflict for Clients

CHWs often witness conflicts between clients, and will also experience direct conflicts with clients themselves. The following list identifies some of the common sources for these conflicts (adapted from Sadalla, Henriquez, Holmberg, & Halligan, 1998).

1. **Conflicts over resources**: These conflicts occur when two people want the same thing, and there is not enough to go around. These are often the easiest types of conflict to identify.

A client in a drop-in shelter for youth may be upset that there aren't enough beds in the shelter, enough food to eat, taxi vouchers, comfortable chairs or sofas to sit in, or enough time with a case manager. The client may act angry or aggressive. For example, he may yell at another client to get off the couch so he can sit down.

2. **Conflicts over psychological needs**: We all have the same needs for food, shelter, health care, friendship, love, belonging, accomplishment, safety, stability, and control. Clashes over these needs may be played out in conflicts about material things or seemingly trivial matters. Often, the real psychological motivations for conflict are harder to understand and to resolve: the client in the homeless shelter who starts a fight may be feeling powerless. If the underlying issue isn't attended to, these conflicts are likely to reoccur.

A homeless Japanese-American woman is hostile to the Caucasian staff at a women's shelter. She often says, "You're not the boss of me!" During a conversation, her case manager learns that as a child she was taken to an internment camp in Utah. Learning this allows her case manager to have a greater understanding of and compassion for her behavior.

3. **Conflicts involving values and identity**: Values are the basis of our belief systems. Challenges to our values may also be experienced as challenges about our identity and worth, and may stimulate strong emotions and dramatic interactions. Keep in mind that for most people, and particularly people without a lot of material resources, our values and identities are our most important resources.

A transgender youth at a homeless drop-in center is continuing to engage in survival sex and is buying hormones on the street. A CHW raises concerns about the client's behavior and associated health risks. The client is used to people judging their identity and to adults trying to control their behavior. The client is frustrated and angry and says to the CHW: "You don't understand the first thing about what it is like to walk in my shoes!"

- *Can you think of other common sources of conflict for clients?*

What Do YOU Think?

13.5 Common Responses to Conflict

How we perceive and react to conflict varies greatly from one person to another. It is often surprising to learn that coworkers feel differently about an important conflict. These differences are influenced by personal and cultural conflict styles.

Becoming aware of your own conflict style is an essential first step in learning how to successfully resolve conflict. An awareness of your own approach to conflict allows you to see what your strengths are as well as the areas in which you can improve. Awareness of what influences other people's approaches to conflict can assist you to create a common framework for resolving conflicts that arise.

Remember that none of us is born knowing how to resolve conflicts. These skills, like all social skills, are influenced by one's own temperament; family examples; past experiences; peer influences; social, economic, and political context and dynamics; and cultural factors such as gender roles and ethnic socialization (Figure 13.1). However, new skills for dealing with conflict can be learned and put into practice.

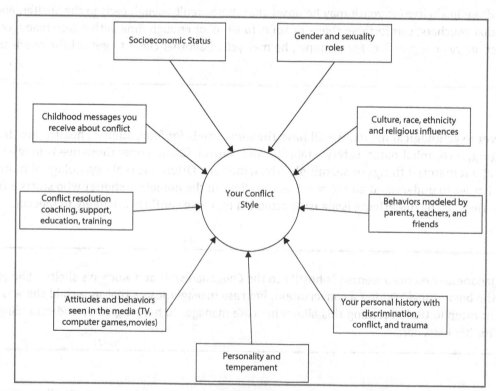

Figure 13.1 Influences That Contribute to an Individual's Approach to Conflict

- *Can you think of other factors that influence the way you handle or respond to conflict?*

THE INFLUENCE OF CULTURE

Culture influences how we understand, communicate about, and react to conflict. For example, some cultures are more likely to value the needs of the group over the needs of the individual. These cultures may emphasize harmony and compromise in the face of conflict in contrast to cultures that encourage people to stand up for their individual rights (Ting-Toomey & Oetzel, 2001).

Continue to develop and practice cultural humility as you face conflict. Always keep in mind that *your way* of dealing with conflict, informed by your own culture or cultures, is just one way, not *The Way* of thinking about and responding to conflict. Don't make assumptions about the conflict styles of coworkers or clients. Use your client-centered counseling skills: ask open-ended questions, observe, and listen closely to learn how others understand and respond to conflicts.

- *Have you experienced conflicts that were influenced by cultural differences?*

- *How do your cultural identities influence your approach to conflict?*

PERSONAL CONFLICT STYLES

Your conflict style has been shaped not only by culture, but also by your personality and life experiences. Taking a conflict style inventory allows people to be aware of their own style of dealing with conflict, and provides a resource to talk about patterns of conflict resolution. Discussing one's style in a team or group setting can aid in developing a greater tolerance and patience for each other's styles.

Keep in mind that each of us probably uses several of these styles, depending on the context or type of conflict we face. Five common ways that people deal with conflict are detailed in this section (Araiz-Iverson et al., 2006; see also Community Boards at the end of the chapter).

1. **Avoiding**: The person may simply ignore the conflict, pretend it does not exist, or decide that the risk of an argument is not worth any further effort on their part. The person withdraws and shuts down. When a conflict occurs, an avoider might say, "Leave well enough alone" or "It's someone else's responsibility." Because issues are not addressed, over time, this approach generally results in more conflict. There are times, however, when it may be the best approach.

2. **Accommodating**: The person sacrifices or compromises their own point of view by allowing the other party to have their way. Over time, the accommodator may become resentful of both the other party and of themselves for continually yielding their own interests.

3. **Competing**: This is the opposite of accommodating. The person works hard to get her own way at the expense of the other party's interests. The underlying interests of both sides are not clarified or addressed. A person with a competing style might think: "My way or the highway."

4. **Compromising**: The person works to find a mutually acceptable solution that partially satisfies all parties. Issues are addressed, although sometimes not fully or deeply. There is some mutual give and take that may result in "splitting the difference" or "finding the middle ground."

5. **Collaborating**: The person focuses on talking, listening, and working with the other party in an attempt to find solutions that satisfy all concerns. Spending time exploring, clarifying, and discussing the conflict often results in both parties' understanding each other's perceptions and finding creative solutions without feeling that anyone gave in or conceded their interests. A collaborator values the relationship with the conflicting parties and tries to produce a win/win, respected, trustworthy solution. You might hear a collaborator say, "Everyone can win if we work together."

Different situations require using different styles. From time to time, each of the styles identified here can be a valuable resource.

- *What are the pros and cons of each of these styles?*

- *Can you identify situations where it might be valuable to use these different styles?*

- *What problems can arise from using each style?*

- *What do you think is your dominant style?*

THE VALUE OF COMPROMISE

Many people approach conflicts with a win/lose mentality. They feel that they are mostly (or completely) in the right, and other parties are completely (or mostly) in the wrong. They seek a resolution to the conflict that will affirm their own position and compel the other party or parties to concede and make changes.

An unwillingness to compromise is problematic for many reasons, including:

1. Conflicts are rarely so simplistic that one party is 100 percent correct and the other party is 100 percent wrong.

2. Even if you are completely right, holding out for a "win/lose" solution in which the other party has to give in is likely to become a "lose/lose" solution in the long run. This mentality often leads to resentment and continued conflict that undermines your sense of comfort at work, and it is likely to create an environment that negatively affects clients and coworkers.

3. Being right is not the most important thing! Ultimately, it is much more important to find a way to work peacefully, professionally, and respectfully with coworkers and clients so that you can effectively promote community health.

4. Holding on to the need to be right is likely to create a lasting perception that you are rigid, controlling, or worse (insert your own adjective here!). It may undermine your career advancement.

5. It isn't good for your health. Always needing to be right is stressful and likely to be harmful to your physical and mental health. Learning to accept responsibility for your own contributions to conflict, and to compromise, can be deeply rewarding in and of itself and promote your well-being. These skills are likely to be useful in your personal and family relationships as well, especially if you are a parent.

- *Have you ever interacted with someone who had a compelling need to be right?*

- *Did you enjoy this experience?*

- *Would you like to be in an ongoing professional relationship with someone like this?*

- *What gets in the way of your ability to compromise?*

- *What assists you in seeking a win/win solution to a conflict?*

IDENTIFY YOUR OWN CONFLICT STYLE

Try this activity on your own, with classmates, or with coworkers to learn more about your personal conflict styles. If you do this activity alone, place an X next to the statements you feel best describe your conflict style. If a facilitator is leading this exercise, have participants respond to each statement by raising their hands and stating, "That's me!" and voluntarily describe the circumstances when these statements apply.

That's *Me!*

_____ I actively participate in conflict when it arises.

_____ I avoid conflicts and controversy at all costs.

_____ I always believe there is a middle ground.

_____ I feel very uncomfortable with conflict.

_____ I feel skilled at handling most conflict.

_____ I like to assist others when they are in conflict.

_____ Open discussion is the best way to address problems.

_____ I lose my cool when I experience conflict.

_____ I have to win at all costs when I am in conflict.

_____ I feel depressed or anxious when I am experiencing a conflict.

_____ It is better to keep friendships than get involved in conflicts.

_____ I'm afraid the other person will be mad at me, so I avoid conflict.

_____ I work for what I believe in.

_____ I enjoy coming up with new, creative solutions to conflicts.

_____ I had negative experiences with conflicts in the past and try to avoid them at all costs.

_____ I will give up some of my interests in order to win other more important interests.

_____ I take the lead in resolving conflicts.

Source: **Adapted from Sharon and Clark, 1989.**

13.6 The Challenge of Anger

As we discussed above, conflicts in the workplace are often connected to important issues such as fairness, justice, respect, and values. Not surprisingly, such conflicts are often accompanied by strong emotions, including anger. We make a point of addressing the challenge of anger here because it is a difficult emotion for people to handle well, and it can significantly undermine attempts to resolve conflicts.

Everyone experiences anger from time to time. It is a natural and powerful emotion with the potential to be both beneficial and harmful to our health and well-being. Anger can mobilize an individual, a team of workers, or a community to make positive change.

Anger becomes a problem when it is used in a way that is threatening, harmful, or insulting to oneself or others. Chronic anger may be turned inward toward the self, resulting in depression. When chronic anger is turned outward, it may be expressed as hostility. When you find yourself alienating those whom you need to work with, then you know that your approach to conflict is destructive and needs to be changed.

Kevin

Kevin works for a nonprofit agency. When he perceives that his skills are being questioned, he is easily angered. He recognizes that he inappropriately vents his anger in the workplace, but he has a hard time changing his behavior. He just can't control getting angry. Kevin has the habit of sending out angry emails when he feels upset. Several times, he has stormed into a coworker's office to make rude and insulting comments. Once he releases his anger, he feels better and gets back to work, and later apologizes. When he is not angry, most people on staff think Kevin is a nice, funny, creative, and hardworking guy. But his rude and angry emails and name-calling episodes have upset most of the people he needs support from: his supervisor, most of his team members, and some of his volunteers. He has been written up for his behavior and has been given two warnings. He is on the edge of being fired.

Learning how to better manage your anger starts with being aware of what pushes your buttons and upsets you the most. There are many situations that can trigger someone's anger. It differs from person to person and from situation to situation.

HOW TO HANDLE YOUR ANGER PROFESSIONALLY

Knowing how to stay in bounds with your anger is an essential life skill and crucial for keeping your job. Here are six tips to stay in bounds with anger.

1. **Be aware**: Become familiar with what triggers your anger. Do you get mad when someone questions your abilities or skills? When you feel excluded from a group, event, or committee? When you feel your autonomy or independence is threatened? When you feel your value as a person or coworker is questioned? What triggers your anger?

2. **Stop**: When you feel angry, *stop* and stay in bounds with your behavior. Take time away from the source of conflict. Breathe, write, walk, repeat a relaxing phrase such as "I can take it easy." Don't engage with others when you feel angry. Take time away to cool down. What works for you to interrupt your anger?

3. **Think**: Think about the consequences of taking action when you feel angry. Try to figure out what made you so upset. Try not to engage the person with whom you feel angry while you are still angry. Find an appropriate time to engage with the other person. How can you safely vent or express your emotion and return to the situation ready to take positive actions toward resolution?

4. **Choose**: Choose behaviors that stay in bounds, that are safe, and that do not hurt you or others. If you need assistance, talk to someone who can support you—a friend, coach, supervisor, or counselor. You are responsible for all the choices that you make.

5. **Understand**: Try to see the issue from the other person's point of view. Try to find a way to hold respect for the other person, even if you disagree with them or feel hurt by their actions.

6. **Take Action**: Do at least one thing that reduces the potential for harm and makes a positive contribution to improving the situation.

- *Think of a situation that made you really angry. What happened that contributed to your anger?*

- *How did you act or react in the moment?*

- *What result did it lead to?*

- *What would you like to do differently the next time?*

What Do YOU? Think?

Please watch the following videos [▶] that show a CHW who, at first, does not respond well when a client expresses her anger (counter role play). The second role play (demo) shows the same scenario, but this time the CHW does a much better job of responding to the client's anger.

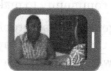

RESPONDING TO ANGER: ROLE PLAY, COUNTER

🔗 *http://youtu.be/ kOZWxisLm5s*

- What mistakes did the CHW make in the counter role play? How might these mistakes impact the relationship between the CHW and the client?

- What did the CHW do differently in the demo role play?

- What did the CHW do well in this role play, and what else could she have done or said in responding to the client's anger?

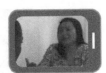

RESPONDING TO ANGER: ROLE PLAY, DEMO

🔗 *http://youtu.be/ lMxXFufpHFc*

SUGGESTIONS FOR DE-ESCALATING THE ANGER OF OTHERS

Alvaro Morales: I was called out to the front room at the drop-in center [for clients who are homeless] because there was this client there who was insulting employees. He had a long history of causing trouble at the center, so he was looking at a suspension [meaning that he couldn't return to the center for a period of time]. I was in charge of the suspensions, so I had to ask him to leave.

I started by reaching out to shake his hand and saying "Good afternoon, R_____ [calling the client by name]." I was talking with him as clearly and respectfully as I could, keeping my voice down. He kept raising his voice. I tried to calm him down. This was happening by the reception area in front of two other employees that I supervise, so I wasn't just dealing with the client, but also kind of teaching the staff how to deal with these situations. I felt the pressure, you know, that I really had to do it right. We have a plan for these situations at the center because it happens a lot. If the client gets more out of control and threatens anyone or does something physical, then one of the staff pushes a panic button and everyone comes to help out.

So I started talking with R_____, and he was insulting a staff person. I reminded him that it wasn't acceptable to call people names like that, and that he needed to leave the center. Then he started insulting me, too. I kept talking with him respectfully, but also more firmly. I just keep saying: "No, you have to leave now." We had to go through a hall full of clients to leave the agency, and he kept insulting me as we walked. I knew he was leaving, but he was still saying all these disrespectful things, and he wanted to stay because he knew that lunch was coming soon. So I just kept saying: "No, you have to leave and come back another day. We'll talk. Right now you're not able to talk calmly."

Then he spit on me. The whole room went "Ooooooh!" It isn't unusual for fights to break out at the drop-in center. Fights about things like—somebody took my chair, or somebody looked at me wrong—things like that. So for people to see somebody spitting on somebody—I am sure they thought we would start fighting. But I kept my cool, even though I was boiling inside. I escorted him outside, and other staff went to stand by the door. He left, cursing us, but he left. I just went into my office and kind of exploded internally. I didn't want to do it in front of the clients or my staff. On the bright side, R_____ returned to the center a week later and apologized, and we ate lunch together.

Alvaro handled this difficult situation calmly and professionally and took action to diminish the risks of harm to the clients, staff, and to himself.

Anger and aggression are often the products of feeling frustrated and powerless. Given the many challenges clients face in their lives, it is no wonder that they sometimes approach you or each other in anger. Before it is possible to work effectively to meet their needs, it will often be necessary to calm them first or defuse their anger. Remember that it is not always possible to calm an angry person. Taking actions to maintain safety may

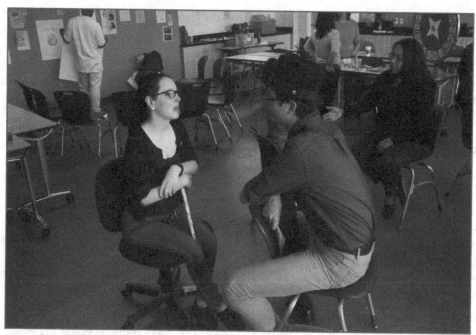

CHWs practice conflict resolution skills.

be necessary. When a client is really angry, the most important job you will have is to avoid escalation. Here are some recommendations for reducing anger in others while keeping yourself safe:

- **Listening skills are crucial to defusing anger.** The first element in defusing anger is to communicate your respect using nonaggressive body language and appropriate listening skills. Try to understand their concern. Avoid judging their behavior.

- **Offer reassurance and space for big emotions to settle.** Use a calm voice, ask them to take a deep breath, and acknowledge their emotions positively: "I can see that you are upset. Can you take a few minutes to catch your breath?"

- **Express your desire to understand the other party,** and encourage them to communicate with you in a way that will best make this possible. For example: "I'd like to hear about what is going on. Please take your time—and can you lower your voice? It's hard for me to listen and understand when you are speaking so loudly and quickly."

- **Asserting your own needs and agency policies is essential** for managing the potential crisis and will give your client a sense of boundaries and limits, too. Statements such as, "I am really glad that we can talk about this, but I want to remind you that we can't yell or disturb other clients. It's expected that everyone here, even when we're angry, will treat each other with respect. Are you able to follow these ground rules right now?" If the client does something that feels threatening, remember to use I-messages.

- **Everyone wants to feel understood and listened to.** Try not to interrupt or correct the person who is angry. When people are under stress, there is potential for miscommunication. Use active listening skills such as restating and paraphrasing, clarifying, validating, and gathering information. You don't have to agree with the person who is angry, but demonstrate that you are listening ("It sounds like you were really disappointed when your family didn't invite you . . . "). Show your curiosity. Use open-ended questions (for example, "Is there anything else that is going on in your life that is contributing to this?" "What would you like to see happen now?" "What helps when you experience feelings like this?" "How can I be supportive?").

- **Reframing will allow you to redirect aggression into a nonthreatening discussion** of the person's underlying needs. Reframing changes direction and can clarify the positive attributes of the person in anger.

- **Safety should always be of utmost important to you and your organization.** Your workplace should have a prearranged safety plan. When escalation cannot be prevented, it is important to stay calm. Use a prearranged warning signal to alert others and to get backup. Talk slowly and calmly. At one clinic, the signal was to call out loudly for "Doctor Strong." When staff heard this, they came quickly to offer support.

- **Knowing when to disengage is essential.** If you feel yourself getting angry and unable to communicate professionally, it is time to disengage. Sometimes, a short break to get a drink of water or take a walk can allow the client to calm down. You can always recommend that you reconvene later when they have had some time to think over the situation. Perhaps someone else at the organization is better suited to this session. Let your client know this.

If you are unsuccessful in de-escalating the situation and are still concerned about your own safety or the safety of others, disengagement may require you to leave the situation or to ask the other party to leave. If you ask the other party to leave, do so in a calm manner. If you determine that safety is an issue, request assistance from a coworker or call 911 immediately. If the situation calls on you to leave, make an excuse, leave immediately, and get assistance.

When the situation has been resolved, debrief with coworkers. Discuss what you and your coworkers did well and how to improve the response to similar situations in the future.

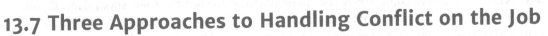

- *Have you ever had to de-escalate the anger of another?*

- *What did it feel like to face this challenge?*

- *What did you do in the situation, and what was the outcome?*

- *What recommendations do you have for others who face similar challenges?*

13.7 Three Approaches to Handling Conflict on the Job

There is no magic formula or method that can effectively resolve all conflicts. In conflict management, context is everything. There are many factors that influence a conflict, and many situation-specific approaches to managing them. In this section we will look at a few different contexts and some new interventions for managing conflict. Three common approaches to conflict are: prevention, early intervention, and third-party intervention (often called mediation).

PREVENTION
Because conflicts are natural and inevitable, leadership in organizational settings should develop clear policies and protocols to address conflicts in their early stages. Supervision meetings where challenging issues are discussed, team meetings where staff talk about what is not working well, and conflict resolution trainings for staff are just a few examples of how organizations can work to prevent the development or escalation of conflicts. On a personal level, CHWs can begin to identify disagreements and misunderstandings in their early stages and address them using productive communication skills in a one-on-one or group setting. A CHW can approach a conflict by presenting their concerns specifically, clearly, and positively.

EARLY INTERVENTION
If the people engaged in conflict are still able to talk to each other, using a one-on-one approach is useful. A CHW may say, "I've been really affected by our lack of communication lately. It seems to be causing some serious problems between us. I'd really like it if we could sit down sometime soon and discuss what is at the root of our communication problems. It's getting in the way of my ability to focus on my work, and I imagine it's affecting you, too. Would you be willing to talk with me so we can try to find a solution?" We will address skills for doing this later in this chapter.

THIRD-PARTY INTERVENTION
Sometimes, it isn't possible for two individuals or groups to resolve a conflict on their own. The issues may be too complex to be adequately identified by the people involved. Feelings may be too strong. In these situations,

asking for assistance from someone with strong conflict resolution skills may be necessary. There are a number of well-tested third-party processes (Sadalla, Henriquez, Holmberg, & Halligan, 1998), including mediation. In **mediation**, a neutral person (someone who doesn't favor one side or the other) is asked to facilitate communication between the disputants as they express their feelings and needs and identify issues. After actively listening to both sides equally, the mediator assists the participants in identifying their own solutions to the conflict and coming up with action steps. Sometimes, a mediator might facilitate the rebuilding or repair of the relationship between the participants.

THE INFLUENCE OF POWER

What happens when the people in conflict don't have equal status or power? Over the course of your career, you are likely to experience conflict with a coworker who is your equal, with a supervisor who has power over you, and with a client whom you have power over. How will these differences in power affect your approach to conflict resolution?

Conflict with a supervisor can be particularly challenging. People often worry that addressing these conflicts will place their job at risk. Ideally, we want supervisors to invite and encourage us to speak freely about our concerns and challenges. However, supervisors often face competing pressures and may not have the time or the ability to listen or communicate well. If you are experiencing a conflict with a supervisor, reflect before you speak. Not all supervisors are skilled in conflict resolution. Sometimes silence and avoidance are prudent choices. Based on prior experience, do you trust that your supervisor will be able to work constructively and respectfully with you to resolve the conflict? If not, consider what the possible consequences of keeping silent or speaking up may be for yourself, your program, and your clients (please see Chapter 14 for more information about working with a supervisor).

If you decide to address the conflict directly, be sure to follow your organization's "chain of command" and speak first to your supervisor rather than going above that person's head to speak to their supervisor. If your supervisor discovers that you have spoken to others about a mutual conflict before speaking directly with them, it may undermine your working relationship and your career at the agency. There are very few exceptions to this rule. However, if the conflict involves issues that are as serious as allegations of sexual harassment or corruption, it is often best to speak to someone who is higher up in the chain of command at the agency you work for.

It is helpful to know your workplace policies in advance, in case your conversation with your supervisor doesn't go well. Find out if your human resource manual outlines a grievance procedure. Do you have an employee assistance program in place that will allow you to talk to a counselor? Do you have a union representative who can advise you?

When you have a conflict with someone you have power over, whether that is someone you supervise, someone who volunteers with your program, or a client, you have responsibility to take leadership in resolving the conflict and in creating an environment in which the other party can honestly communicate their concerns. Recognize that by communicating about a conflict they have with you, they are taking a risk. Clients may be afraid to approach you about a conflict for fear of creating negative feelings, or harming their ability to access services with you or your agency. You may need to take the lead in assuring your clients that you welcome input and appreciate their honesty in sharing concerns. Strive to model active communication skills.

13.8 Communication Skills for Conflict Resolution

CHANGING THE WAY WE VIEW CONFLICT

We want to emphasize three concepts from the Harvard Negotiation Project (Stone, Patton, & Heen, 2010) designed to shift the way we view conflict and promote resolution.

Moving from Certainty to Curiosity

We have a tendency to make assumptions and judgments about conflicts, including what *really* happened and what the other parties did, thought, and felt. When we bring these assumptions to a conversation designed to resolve the conflict, we are likely to undermine the process and outcome. Try shifting your perspective from one of certainty about the situation ("I know what really happened") to one of curiosity ("What happened?

What was going on for _____ [the other party]?"). When you can set aside your prejudices and assumptions, you are likely to discover new ways of understanding yourself, the other party, the conflict itself, and possibilities for its successful resolution.

Disentangling Intent from Impact

During conflicts, we often make assumptions about the intentions of others. When we are hurt or harmed by the conflict, we may assume that the other party intended this result. Once again, these assumptions can keep us from seeing the true nature of the conflict and moving forward toward its resolution.

For example, Simon and Latanya get into a conflict. Simon says or does something that offends Latanya.

- Because Latanya is offended does not mean that Simon intended to offend her.
- Because Simon didn't intend to offend her doesn't mean that Latanya is not offended.

Give the benefit of the doubt to the other party. When we are able to separate the impact of actions from their intentions, we often diminish the emotional charge of the conflict and reduce its potential for escalation.

Distinguishing Blame from Contribution

It is easy for people in conflicts to become caught up in accusations and blame. Trying to prove who is to blame can easily derail us from being able to listen, to learn, to find solutions, and to build new working relationships and alliances.

Rather than focusing on what the other did wrong, focus on understanding the contributions that each party made to the conflict, *with an emphasis on trying to understand our own contributions first.* You are likely to find that both or all parties did or said something that contributed to the conflict. Understanding this can support you in identifying solutions and in preventing similar conflicts in the future.

The shift in focus from blame to contribution may seem subtle, but it can powerfully transform your efforts to resolve the conflict.

DEVELOPING A COMMON FRAMEWORK AND PROCESS FOR RESOLVING CONFLICT

We strongly recommend that you talk about the process you will use to resolve the conflict before you start to talk about the conflict itself. Many attempts to resolve conflicts are undermined because the parties don't take time to develop a common understanding of the process and ground rules that will guide their conversation. They may jump right into the heart of the conflict, making accusations and stirring up strong emotions. This can escalate the conflict and make it more difficult for parties to communicate effectively in the future.

Take the time to have a preconversation to discuss the process you wish to put in place and develop mutually agreed upon ground rules before you begin to discuss the actual conflict situation.

Consider the following guidelines for initiating a conversation designed to resolve a conflict:

1. Express your commitment to resolving the conflict.
2. Express your desire to establish a positive working relationship.
3. Acknowledge the value of the other party or parties. Find something positive to say about who they are, the work that they do, and a time when you worked well together.
4. Identify and acknowledge your common values, such as your commitment to providing quality services to clients or to advocating for social justice.
5. Be prepared to move from certainty to curiosity. Express your desire to listen and learn about their experience and perspective.
6. Negotiate common ground rules for your discussion that use the active listening skills described later on in this chapter. Ground rules may include, for example:
   a. Agree not to yell at each other, insult each other, use disrespectful words, or otherwise escalate the conflict.
   b. Use I-statements (described later on in this chapter) and emphasize your own experience rather than your assumptions or judgments about the other party.

c. Take turns talking and listening to each other's personal experience of the conflict, using active listening skills. It is amazing how deeply listening, without making judgments, can often transform our understanding of the other party's intentions and feelings, and of the conflict itself.

7. Work to disentangle impact from intention.

8. Focus the discussion not on assigning blame (discovering who was wrong), but on understanding what contributed to the conflict and on identifying how you can transform your relationship to avoid similar problems in the future.

9. If you mean it, apologize and take responsibility for something you said or did that may have contributed to the conflict or been hurtful to the other party.

10. If things get heated and it seems as if the conflict might escalate, agree to take a break. Continuing to talk with each other when you are unable to control your emotions and statements may do lasting damage to the relationship, your career, and the important work that you do with clients and communities.

11. After you have talked about what contributed to the conflict, agree to focus on what you can do now to improve the situation and your ability to work well together in the future.

ESSENTIAL LISTENING SKILLS

The following set of skills will assist you to learn how to communicate so that both you and the other party experience the safety and support necessary to engage with the issues and feelings at the heart of the conflict.

Regardless of who is involved in a conflict, strong communication skills can enable the parties to move from tension to resolution. These communication skills include **essential listening**, which can be defined as deeply listening with the specific intention to fully understand what is being expressed both in content, emotion, and meaning. An important component of essential listening is the ability to convey what is understood back to the speaker. When we are engaged in essential listening we are not simply waiting for our turn to speak, but instead really paying close attention to all the details of the content and emotion of what another is expressing to us. Essential listening demonstrates awareness of and respect for the other person's experiences, thoughts, and feelings and is an essential skill for CHWs; it is an example of client-centered counseling.

A person who is practicing essential listening doesn't have to agree with the other party, but demonstrates that the other person deserves to be heard and understood. Essential listening aids in breaking the cycle of conflict. When you show respect and empathy and reserve judgment, people are more likely to express themselves and to get to the heart of the conflict.

Essential listening is difficult because it requires the listener to provide focused attention in situations that often involve strong opinions, emotions, and judgments. It requires respect for and attention to the other's values, needs, and feelings. And it requires you to express this respect and reflect what you hear. If all a speaker hears back from the party who is listening is silence or an occasional "uh-huh," they can't tell if they are successfully communicating about vulnerable feelings and issues. We don't want people in conflict to clam up. We want them to participate so that the conflicts can be resolved.

Here is a set of core listening skills (Sadalla, Henriquez, Holmberg, & Halligan, 1998) that are very similar to the skills for client-centered counseling presented in Chapter 9. Not everyone uses all of these techniques in each conversation, and how they are used varies from culture to culture. With practice, you discover which listening skills work best for you.

Encourage

This technique uses neutral words and respectful body language to convey interest and to encourage the speaker to continue talking. To be effective, encouragement must be based on the listener's genuine interest in hearing and understanding what is being said by others. For example, "I really want to learn about your experience and your point of view. Will you tell me more about it?"

Clarify

Clarifying involves the gathering of information in order to understand what the other party is saying. This is especially important when we find ourselves drawing swift conclusions about circumstances or other people based on our own experiences. Clarifying questions should be open-ended and phrased respectfully, so that people don't feel challenged or judged. For example, "Would you tell me more about what happened on the day of the incident?" or "I want to understand better. Did this happen before or after your meeting with Yana?"

Restate

Restating is to use your own words to express the main thoughts and ideas that the other party has communicated to you. This demonstrates that you have heard what is being shared, and allows you to check your understanding. People rarely feel understood in a conflict situation. Restating is a powerful way to show that you are listening. A common restating phrase may begin with: "Help me understand. If I hear you right, you are saying that you were frustrated during the training and felt like you weren't given enough opportunity to respond to the questions from the participants. Is that right?"

Reflect

Reflecting shows that you understand the feelings behind what is being expressed. Reflecting can assist the speaker to clarify what she is feeling and acknowledge these feelings. For example, "What I'm hearing is that you felt frustrated and disrespected when I showed up late to the training."

Summarize

By pulling all the information together, summarizing allows the speaker to know that he or she has given you all the information. Summarizing may also give the speaker a chance to correct or add some more information. For example, "Overall, what I'm hearing you say is that you weren't happy with the way that we worked together during the training, and you want to make sure that we do it differently next time."

Validate

A validation is a statement that acknowledges the speaker's worth, efforts, and feelings. When we validate, we show empathy toward the speaker by acknowledging the importance of their experiences. For example, "I appreciate that you took a risk and shared this with me" and "It sounds like it was a really frustrating experience for you."

"I" Messages

Whether you are doing the talking or the listening, there are a few other essential communication skills you'll need in your tool bag. When we are angry or upset, it is easy to blame others for what has happened, "You can't keep anything to yourself!" or "You never listen!" These types of messages blame the other person and rarely bring people together to resolve the problem. With an I-message, however, the speaker describes her feelings about the other's behavior and how this behavior affected her. For example: Angela might say to Peter, "I felt angry that you told John that I didn't think he was a good counselor. I don't feel like I can share my thoughts with you in the future."

I-messages focus on the speaker's wants, needs, or concerns. The listener is less likely to feel judged and more willing to listen. A formal I-message has three parts:

1. **"When** you . . ."** Describe the specific behavior.

2. **State** the feeling "I feel . . ..

3. **"Because . . ."** Describe the effect of the other person's behavior on you.

Here are some examples: "I feel frustrated when you borrow my outreach bag and don't return it on time, I feel frustrated because I can't get ready for my own shift." "When you turn on the radio loudly, I feel distracted because I need to get a lot of work done and I work better when it's quiet."

Using I-messages take a lot of practice. Think of something that someone is doing at work, at school, or at home that is bothering you. How can you let them know what is on your mind using an I-message? Practice and see what happens.

Turning a You-Message into an I-Message

Practice turning these statements into I-messages.

Example:

You-message: "You always avoid me when I'm in the room."

I-message: "I feel ignored when you don't acknowledge me when we're in a room together. We used to work so well together, and I worry that you may be upset with me about something."

"Once again, you are taking credit for my work and ideas."

I _____

"You always expect me to do more work than others on this team."

I _____

"You are just looking for ways to push your work off onto others."

I _____

"You never carry through on the suggestions I offer you."

I _____

"You keep forgetting your commitments. These are your responsibility, not anyone else's!"

I _____

THE POWER OF APOLOGY

None of us is perfect. We *all* make mistakes. We have all said or done something that contributed to a conflict and may have been be hurtful to others.

We strongly believe in the power of an apology to transform relationships. This is true with coworkers, supervisors, and clients. We view making an apology, like compromising, as a demonstration of generosity, humility, and strength of character. Be prepared to take responsibility for actions that may have contributed to the conflict and unintentionally hurt or harmed the situation, or the other party.

Some examples are:

- "I hear that when I was late, it felt disrespectful to you. I want you to know that I really did try my best, and I am sorry that I was late."

- "I wish I had remembered to invite you to the meeting. I apologize. I'll make sure to put you on the email list serve as soon as I get back to the office."

- "I didn't mean to insult you. I apologize. I truly respect you and enjoy working with you."

Unfortunately, some people seem to think that making an apology is the same thing as saying, "I am a bad person who is 100 percent wrong and deserves to be punished for the rest of my life!" However, if you can't learn to take responsibility for your own mistakes, and to provide an honest apology when appropriate, you will undermine the success of your career.

- *What are your thoughts and feelings about making an apology?*

- *Is it hard for you to apologize to others? If so, why?*

- *What would support you to provide an apology to a client, coworker, or supervisor?*

Please watch the following video interview, 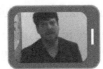 which addresses the importance of learning to provide a timely and authentic apology to a client or coworker.

13.9 Models of Conflict Resolution

THE ART OF APOLOGY, FACULTY INTERVIEW

http://youtu.be/ obtQn3fdGOY

These are several key steps to consider when thinking about how to approach a conflict resolution process. We encourage you to address each of these steps as you develop a process designed to promote a resolution of a conflict and stronger relationships among key parties. The information presented here is informed by the work of the Harvard Negotiation Project's *Difficult Conversations* (Stone, Patton, & Heen, 2010) and *Getting to Yes* (Fisher, Ury, & Patton, 2011).

STEP 1: INVESTIGATE AND PLAN

Unfortunately, many people skip this critical step and jump straight in to address a conflict without stopping to reflect. Take time to consider the key elements of the conflict, such as the sources of conflict, issues of culture, power, and authority. Let this information guide you in planning to resolve a conflict in which you are directly involved or when you are acting as a third party to try to facilitate or guide a conflict resolution process.

Take time to investigate:

- What is the story of each person involved in the conflict?
- What are the feelings involved?
- What is at stake in this conflict? Are resources or roles on the line?

Consider the following questions as you set up a time and place to talk:

- Is it a good time for all parties to meet?
- Is it a safe setting for all involved?
- Has everyone agreed to discuss the issue and try to reach a positive solution?

STEP 2: CREATE A SAFE SPACE

Set a tone and create an environment that is respectful and supportive for everyone involved. Incorporate key elements for a successful pre-conversation such as:

- Express your commitment to resolving the conflict
- Express your desire to establish positive working relationships
- Develop and negotiate guidelines for your conflict resolution process
- Share common professional values such as commitment to providing care for clients

STEP 3: INVESTIGATE THE CONFLICT ISSUES TOGETHER

Now is the time to investigate and describe the issues involved in the conflict. Remember to avoid judgments during this step. Create an opportunity for each person to share their experience and feelings, and to express what is at stake for them.

Here are some tips to keep in mind during this state of the process:

- Don't present your experiences as "The Truth" (*remember to use "I" statements*)
- Don't exaggerate the situation by using words such as "always" and "never"
- Be curious about the experience of others, and inquire about them
- Apply your client-centered skills, including essential listening skills, Motivational Interviewing, and OARS (see Chapter 9)

- Emphasize mindful listening (really listen to what is being said, don't just wait for your turn to speak)

If you are in a position to facilitate or guide this process, here are some sample questions that may encourage people to share their experience:

- Can you say a little bit more about how you see/experience things?
- What information do you have that others don't have?
- How do you see this situation differently?
- How are you feeling?
- And then what happened?
- Can you tell me more about why this is important to you?

When you are the facilitator for others during a conflict resolution process, it can be helpful to pause after one person has the chance to speak and to ask the other person to "repeat back" what they heard. Ask the original speaker if what was just repeated is correct. This gives both people the opportunity to clarify what is being said, and an experience of being heard. This process alone can often reveal what the core of a conflict really is.

Summarize along the way and *emphasize any progress made*, no matter how small. Acknowledging each person's efforts, and any progress made, can help the parties in a conflict to find a workable solution.

STEP 4: EXPLORE SOLUTIONS: IS THERE THE POSSIBILITY FOR A WIN–WIN?

Conflicts may involve a single issue or multiple issues. Similarly, solutions to conflicts may be simple or complex. Ideally, solutions should be:

- *Acceptable to all parties*
- *Specific, including clear statements of what all parties are expected to do, and when*
- *Balanced, so that all parties contribute to the solution*

STEP 5: FOLLOW-UP AND EVALUATION

Agree to a follow-up meeting to check in after the conflict has been resolved. Unexpected issues may arise, so it is helpful to schedule a time for all parties to meet and discuss how well the conflict situation has been resolved. This is an opportunity to assess if the agreements that were made are being honored, or if they require further discussion and adjustments. It is also an opportunity to reinforce the importance of professional relationships and maintaining a positive working environment.

Because conflicts often follow cyclical patterns and may reoccur, sometimes in a slightly different manner, we also recommend setting a later date to check-in, several months after the original conflict situation was resolved. This is an opportunity to prevent flare-ups or new conflicts from developing and, again, to assert intentions for maintaining positive working relationships. It is particularly important for you to take responsibility for scheduling a follow-up meeting if the conflict was with someone whom you hold power over (such as someone who you supervise).

- *What would you do to follow up with R., the client who was so angry at the drop-in center?*

Each of these five steps is important to the successful resolution of a conflict. Often Steps 1 and 2 are overlooked, and people jump right into a conversation without adequate investigation of the issues or attention to creating a safe space, including the development of mutually agreed-upon guidelines for the process. This can often escalate a conflict. The final check-in after some time has passed is also often skipped, but it may be key to preventing further conflict.

Chapter Review

Apply conflict resolution concepts and skills to the scenario between Cindy and Stephanie that was introduced at the beginning of the chapter. Answer the following questions:

- What may be some of the sources of this conflict?
- What may be some of the underlying issues?
- What conflict styles are the two parties using?

If you were Cindy or Stephanie, how might you answer the following questions?

- How might you try to shift the way that you view this conflict, using the suggestions from the Harvard Negotiation Project?
- How would you talk with your colleague to set up a process for communicating about your conflict?
- What would you want to communicate to your colleague at the very start of your conversation?
- What ground rules would you want to negotiate?
- What type of compromise might you be willing to make?
- What will you do to follow up on the resolution that you reach about the conflict?
- How might you apply the five-step model for conflict resolution presented in this chapter? Using this model, what would you say to your colleague?
- What other resources might be helpful to you in resolving this conflict?

References

Academic Leadership Support. (2007). *About conflict.* Office of Quality Improvement & Office of Human Resource Development. Madison, WI: University of Wisconsin–Madison. Retrieved from *www.ohrd.wisc.edu/onlinetraining/resolution/aboutwhatisit.htm*

Alinsky, S. D. (1969). *Reveille for radicals.* New York, NY: Vintage.

Araiz-Iverson, R., Blagsvelt, K., Hoburg, M., Hopson, N., Lanctot, K., Lindbeck, L., . . . Volante, H. (2006). *The basics of mediation: Community boards' mediation training guide.* San Francisco, CA: Community Boards.

Cohen, L., Davis, R., & Aboelata, M. (1998). Conflict resolution and violence prevention: From misunderstanding to understanding. *The Fourth R, 84,* 3–8, 20–15.

Cowans, S. (2005). *Bay area community health worker study* [HED 892—Final Report]. San Francisco, CA: San Francisco State University.

Fisher, R., Ury, W., & Patton, B. (2011). *Getting to yes: Negotiating agreement without giving in.* New York, NY: Penguin Books.

Gaitlin, J., Wysocki, A., & Kepner, K. (2007). *Understanding conflict in the workplace.* Gainesville, FL: University of Florida, Institute of Food and Agriculture Sciences Extension. Retrieved from *http://edis.ifas.ufl.edu/HR024*

Hart, B. (2002). *Conflict in the workplace.* Retrieved from *http://www.excelatlife.com/articles/conflict_at_work.htm*

Sadalla, G., Henriquez, M., Holmberg, M., & Halligan, J. (1998). *Conflict resolution: A middle and high school curriculum.* San Francisco, CA: Community Boards.

Sharon, R., & Clark, L. (1989). *Conflict: A way to peace—the AFDA model: A guidebook for personal and professional development of peaceful conflict resolution skills.* Englewood, CO: AFDA Group.

Stone, D., Patton, B., & Heen, S. (2010). *Difficult conversations: How to discuss what matters most.* New York, NY: Penguin Books.

Ting-Toomey, S., & Oetzel, J. G. (2001). *Managing intercultural conflicts effectively.* Thousand Oaks, CA: Sage.

Additional Resources

Association for Conflict Resolution. (n.d.). Retrieved from *www.acrnet.org/*

This is a professional organization dedicated to enhancing the practice and public understanding of conflict resolution.

Center for Nonviolent Communication. (n.d.). Retrieved from *www.cnvc.org*

The Center for Nonviolent Communication is a global organization that supports the learning and sharing of NVC, and helps people peacefully and effectively resolve conflicts in personal, organizational, and political settings. The website has many free resources.

The Conflict Resolution Information Source (CR Info). (n.d.). Retrieved from *www.crinfo.org/*

This is a free service that maintains a keyword-coded catalog of over twenty thousand Web, print, organizational, and other conflict resolution–related resources. These core catalogs are supplemented with thousands of additional links to Web-based news stories, feature articles, cultural background information, documents describing ongoing conflicts, and government dispute resolution–related Web pages.

Cornelius, H., & Faire, S. (2011). *Everyone can win.* New York, NY: Simon & Schuster.

Hamilton, D. (2013). *Everything is workable: A Zen approach to conflict resolution.* Boston, MA: Shambhala Publications.

National Association for Community Mediation. (n.d.). Retrieved from *www.nafcm.org/*

Community mediation offers constructive processes for resolving differences and conflicts between individuals, groups, and organizations.

Rosenberg, M. (2012). *Nonviolent communication: A language of life.* Encinitas, CA: PuddleDancer Press.

Sande, K., & Johnson, K. (2011). *Resolving everyday conflict.* Grand Rapids, MI: Baker Books.

Community Boards

Based in San Francisco, Community Boards operates the longest-running, no-cost neighborhood mediation program in the United States. Community Boards is a local and national provider of training and training materials in dispute resolution, mediation, and facilitation and a national leader in youth-to-youth peer mediation through the Conflict Manager Program. *www.communityboards.org/*

Professional Skills

Getting a Job, Keeping a Job, and Growing on the Job

Amber Straus, Rhonella C. Owens, Tim Berthold, and Jeni Miller

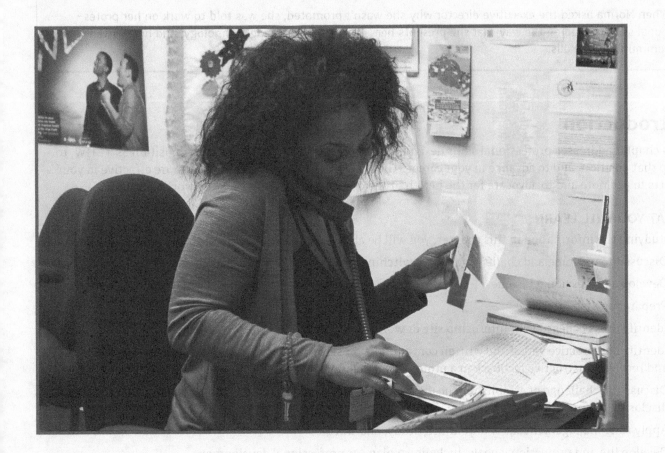

CASE STUDY	Norma

Norma has worked for five years as a CHW at a large nonprofit agency that provides services to girls and women. Norma is highly respected by coworkers and by the clients and communities she serves. Six months ago, Norma was honored as *Outreach Worker of the Year* at an agency fundraiser.

Recently, Norma applied for a job at her agency as the supervisor of a team of six CHWs. Norma was not offered the position: A younger woman with much less experience and a college degree was hired. Norma met the other candidate on the day of their interviews. Norma was dressed as she does each day to conduct outreach, and brought flip-chart paper to make a presentation to the hiring committee. The woman who was hired wore a suit and brought a laptop computer and a projector to make a PowerPoint presentation.

When Norma asked the executive director why she wasn't promoted, she was told to work on her professional skills, including the way that she presents herself, her skills in using technology, and her written communication skills.

Introduction

This chapter addresses professional skills designed to help you to get a job or volunteer position as a CHW, to keep that position, and to advance in your career. These skills will also assist you to be more effective in your efforts to promote and to advocate for the health of the clients and communities you work with.

WHAT YOU WILL LEARN

By studying the information in this chapter, you will be able to:

- Discuss the meaning and challenge of code switching
- Develop a professional resume
- Prepare for a job interview
- Identify dress codes at your internship site or workplace
- Identify and practice verbal and written communication skills relevant for CHWs, including how to provide and receive constructive feedback in a professional manner
- Discuss the challenge of establishing healthy professional boundaries and making sound choices regarding disclosure of personal information
- Apply time management skills to your life, study, and work
- Develop life and professional goals, including a plan for professional development

WORDS TO KNOW

Code Switching

Resume

Supportive and Corrective Feedback

14.1 The Challenges and Benefits of Code Switching

All workplaces have written or unwritten codes of conduct that guide standards for dress, time management, professional boundaries, written and spoken communication, and giving and receiving constructive feedback. Adapting to the professional environment and codes of conduct can be challenging. This challenge is sometimes called **code switching** (or moving between one or more sets of expectations and guidelines for conduct or behavior).

There are different codes of conduct—or rules of the road—for different contexts, communities, cultures, and employment settings. The codes that we learn from our families and in our communities are sometimes different from the codes that guide employment settings. When we move from our family to the community and to the workplace, we may not understand the new codes of conduct and why they matter. As a consequence, like Norma, we may miss out on opportunities for employment or promotion.

> **Alvaro Morales:** I had to learn that there were different ways for me to dress and to talk—different words to use—when I was conducting street outreach versus counseling in the clinic versus making a presentation to the City Council. Sometimes I dressed up—even though I'm not really all that used to wearing a suit or tie—so that my message would be better heard by a professional audience. And I would use different kinds of language to talk about the same things—like sexual behaviors—with my supervisor versus my clients, or adults versus youth. It is kind of a balancing act—switching between different cultures without losing who you are. As an immigrant to the United States, I'm used to that kind of balancing act—I have to do it all the time.

Most of us have had experience with code switching, though we probably didn't think of it in these terms. We act or speak differently with our family and friends, at school, at work, or in church or other religious or spiritual places.

What Do YOU Think?

- *Can you think of places where you switch codes?*

- *Have you ever been in a new environment and not known what the codes of conduct or rules of the road were? What was this like?*

- *How did you begin to identify and adapt to the new codes of conduct?*

Code switching is a valuable skill for CHWs. The ability to adapt to different settings, and to build positive working relationships with diverse communities is a tremendous asset for building a long and successful career.

However, it is also important to note that institutional codes can be biased, and may represent and promote a particular cultural standard for dress, speech and conduct. At their worst, professional codes may discriminate against people from different educational or cultural backgrounds or identities, such as people who look, dress, and speak differently from those in authority.

For example, consider the following quotes from City College of San Francisco students who encountered bias in an educational or workplace setting:

A graduate of the CCSF CHW program reports: "I finally made it to graduate school, but it wasn't always a very supportive place. I was the only Black woman in my cohort. During my first week, the only Black female professor at the school pulled me aside to tell me that I needed to straighten my hair and buy a suit if I wanted to succeed. It may have been meant kindly, but it didn't come across that way. It made me feel like I didn't belong. Even if I had the money, I wasn't going to straighten my hair. But on top of working full-time and raising my family, I made sure that no one ever had a reason to challenge the quality of my work. And I want people to know that I *did* earn my master's degree!"

A student who was completing his internship with a local agency reports: "You know that I read, write, and speak English very well. It is my third language. At a staff meeting [at the agency where the student is doing their internship], I spoke up a couple of times, and it felt good to be participating, you know? After the meeting, one of the managers thanked me for participating, but he also told me that I needed to work harder to "lose my accent."

But I don't know if that is even possible. And is it okay for them to say that to me? If I work well with the clients, and they accept me, isn't that good enough?"

- *What is your reaction to these testimonies?*

- *Have you or your coworkers ever encountered challenges like this in the workplace (or at school)?*

- *How can you adapt to new codes while retaining your own identity, language, and culture?*

While the codes that guide conduct in employment settings should be clearly presented to all employees and volunteers, often they are not. The codes should be used to promote the organization's mission and goals, as well as respectful communication among colleagues and between staff and the clients and communities they serve. The codes of conduct in workplace settings shouldn't require us to abandon our own cultures or identities, including identities that are related to ethnicity, nationality, religion or faith, disability, sexual orientation, or gender identity.

The decision about whether or not you will switch codes to adapt to a professional setting is up to you. We would rather that you had an opportunity to make an informed choice about code switching, however, instead of losing job opportunities for failing to meet a professional standard that you didn't know existed.

Code switching is also a relevant concept for the clients you work with. They may not know about or want to follow the codes of conduct at the various agencies and institutions they turn to for assistance with legal, medical, public benefits, housing, or social services. Unfortunately, the professionals in these agencies may sometimes judge or discriminate against clients who do not adapt to their codes of conduct. *We hope that as CHWs, you will always do your best to make clients feel welcomed and respected regardless of their identity, background, desire, or ability to "switch codes."*

Helping Agencies and Programs to Update Their Codes

While employees are asked to adapt to the codes of the organizations they work for, agencies and programs are also asked to adapt their codes in order to better serve clients and communities. In other words, the challenge of code switching goes both ways.

Consider the following example. A public health department in the San Francisco Bay Area funded a support group for Latino men who have sex with men. However, Latino men were not attending the group. Finally, a representative from the health department met with the local agency and two CHWs. When the representative asked "Why aren't men coming to the support group?", the CHWs explained that the idea of a support group wasn't culturally relevant for Latino men. The CHWs advocated to change the program from a support group to something else that would be a better fit for men in their community. They facilitated a couple of focus groups with Latino men who have sex with men and, as a result, started a new program that invited men to cook and share a meal together one night a week. With this change, the group took off, and the men were able to form a community and to support each other to promote their health in a natural and culturally relevant way. The CHWs guided the agency they worked for and the local health department to shift their codes and their funding priorities in order to better serve the community.

14.2 Getting a Job

Getting a job often requires these key steps:

1. Finding out about available jobs

2. Applying for jobs

3. Interviewing for jobs

FINDING JOB OPPORTUNITIES

There are many ways to find out about jobs in your community:

- Search online job sites on your own or with the help of a career counselor (generally available for free at a community-based or community college career center)

- Look at the websites of employers in your community for job openings, including local health departments (or departments of public health)

- Call or visit agencies that you are interested in working for to see if and when they may have job openings

- Network and talk with CHWs and other public health providers to see if they are aware of any job openings with their own agencies or other organizations

Once you hear of a job opening, request the job description and read it carefully to learn whether this is an opportunity you are truly interested in and qualified for. Job descriptions also provide information to guide you in writing your application, including which experience and skills to highlight.

Sample Job Description

Community Health Worker with the Center City Clinic

This position will conduct outreach and provide health education and case management services to patients living with chronic health conditions. Duties include promoting Center City Clinic and recruiting patients into care. The CHW will also support patients with the self-management of health conditions such as cardiovascular disease, depression, diabetes, and cancer. CHWs provide services at the clinic and in community settings, and provide home visits as necessary. Qualified candidates will have skills for providing client-centered health education and case management services, strong oral and written communication skills, and the ability to work effectively with people from diverse backgrounds.

Additional Qualifications

Spanish speaking preferred. High school diploma or GED required.

How to Apply

Send cover letter, resume, and the names and contact information of three professional references to Center City Clinic, Attention Audra Laing, NP, 3000 Hamilton St., Suite 505, Philadelphia, PA 19130. Email: ALaing@centercityclinic.org. Fax: 215-982-8266.

- *If you were interested in the job as a CHW with the Center City Clinic, which of your skills and work or life experiences would you highlight in your application?*

APPLYING FOR JOBS: APPLICATIONS, COVER LETTERS, RESUMES, AND REFERENCES

Applications

For most jobs, you will be asked to fill out an application. The employer will review all applications received. You want yours to stand out in a positive way. If possible, type the application, or fill it out on a computer. If the application can only be filled out by hand, use a black or blue pen and fill out the application clearly and neatly. Check your resume to correct any spelling or grammatical errors.

Some job applications ask you if you are a U.S. citizen and if you have ever been convicted of a crime (Chapter 15 discusses Ban the Box initiatives across the country that aim to prevent employment discrimination against people with histories of incarceration). It is important to answer these questions truthfully. Citizenship or permanent resident status may not be a requirement, and the agency may distinguish between misdemeanor and felony convictions, between long-past and recent convictions, and understand concepts of recovery and rehabilitation.

Cover Letter

You should include a cover letter with every job application. The letter should be simple and include your contact information at the top, the date, the person to whom you are submitting the application (by name if possible), and a formal salutation (Dear Ms. Laing). In a couple of brief sentences, identify the job you are applying for (its exact title and job number if there is one), how you learned about the job, and why you are qualified for the position.

Sample Cover Letter

Jane Q. Doe
P.O. Box 14567
Centerville, PA, 19876
February 9, 2015

Audra Laing, NP
Center City Clinic
3000 Hamilton St., Suite 505
Philadelphia, PA 19130

Dear Ms. Laing:

Attached please find my resume and application for the job of Community Health Worker with the Center City Clinic. I am a certified Community Health Worker and bilingual in English and Spanish. I have two years' experience working as CHW in urban settings, and one year of experience as a volunteer with the Philadelphia Suicide Prevention Center.

I am dedicated to promoting the health of low-income communities, and interested in working in a primary health care setting. I have skills in providing health education, client-centered counseling, and case management, and would love the opportunity to apply these skills in working with the patients at Center City Clinic.

Thank you for your attention to my application. My resume includes three professional references.

Sincerely,

Jane Q. Doe

Attached: application; resume

Resumes

When you apply for a job, employers will usually ask to see a **resume**, a formal document listing your work experience and education. The goal of a resume is to engage a potential employer's interest at a glance. Please note that these types of documents are sometimes called a CV or a curriculum vitae.

Your resume makes a first impression; it is key to getting the job you want. Your local library, community college, or employment development department may hold free resume writing classes. You can also review sample resumes on the Internet and in books at your local library.

Resumes follow standard style guidelines, although there are a variety of accepted styles. Take a look at the sample resume below. Notice the order of the words, the type of information the applicant provides, and how easy she makes it for potential employers to:

- Identify the applicant's experiences
- Review the applicant's skills
- Know exactly where to call or email the applicant to discuss the job

Writing a Resume

There are a number of ways to organize a resume, as you will see if you look for samples online, at the library, or in a career counselor's office. One example of a resume is shown in Figure 14.1. However you organize your resume, it should include the following information, on one to two pages, organized in a way that is easy to read at a glance.

Name and Contact Information

Your name and up-to-date contact information should be at the top of the resume. Make sure that all of your contact information is current, including your mailing and email address and phone number. If you do not have a reliable phone with voice mail, you may provide only an email address. Make sure your email address is appropriate to share with a potential employer.

Education

List your education and training, beginning with your current or most recent educational experiences. Be sure to list any certificates, degrees, scholarships, or honors. Include the name of educational or training institution, and the city and state (or country) where it is located. Identify the type of certificate or degree you earned, and the date when you completed your training.

Work and Volunteer Experience

Clearly present information about your employment history, starting with your most recent job and going back in time. Include the name of the company or organization, the city where it is located, your job title, and the dates you worked. Don't use any acronyms in your resume, such as the initials used for an agency or coalition instead of the full name of that agency or coalition. List your professional responsibilities, the skills you used on the job, and your key accomplishments. Use positive action words as described in the text box. Use the present tense (such as "Conduct outreach") for current positions, and the past tense (such as "Conducted outreach") for any jobs that you had in the past. Do the same for any volunteer experiences that may highlight key skills and accomplishments.

Always be 100 percent truthful about the information you include on your resume: Any inaccurate statements may be cause for termination and could seriously damage your reputation in the community.

> **Action words:** When you list your experiences, use action words to explain your responsibilities and accomplishments. These words show an employer the skills you have to offer. Be sure to use the past tense for past experiences and the present tense for your current work. Describe briefly how you led, demonstrated, coordinated, accomplished, created, managed, organized, repaired . . . you get the idea.

"I don't have any work experience! What do I put on my resume?"

Even if you have never had a full-time job, you have had life experiences and had an impact on the world around you. Focus on what you have learned by working in your community or family, and use action words to present your skills to employers.

References

On your resume or in your cover letter, list at least three people who can tell a potential employer about your qualifications for the job. Don't forget to ask each person in advance if they are willing and able to provide a reference for you to a prospective employer. If your present employer knows you are looking for a job and can be expected to give you a good reference, that should be the first reference you list. Teachers and neighborhood or community leaders are also good references; family members are not. Ask potential candidates if they would be

Cassie Adanya
409 Andover Street
New Orleans, LA 70183
(614) 222-5555
cassieadanya@email.com

PROFESSIONAL EXPERIENCE

Counselor and Program Coordinator   **New Orleans Safe House, New Orleans, LA**

October 2014–Present. Work with developmentally disabled children ages 6–12. Facilitate small group activities and provide individual counseling as required. Coordinate the Safe House Summer Camp Program. Organize daily activities, manage work assignments, and supervise 3 staff and 8 volunteers.

Assistant Teacher   **Jubilee Camp, Elbert, LA**

January 2011–September 2014. Provided daycare services for infants and children ages 0–36 months. Responsible for creating and implementing a daily activity plan, and facilitating small groups of three to six children.

VOLUNTEER EXPERIENCE

Food Pantry   **First Methodist Church, New Orleans Parish, LA**

2010–Present. Assist staff with the inventory of food items, packaging food and delivering food to shut-in clients twice each month.

Youth Summer Camp   **New Orleans Regional YMCA, New Orleans, LA**

Summer 2008 to 2010. Assisted with managing activities for youth with special needs, ages 8–12. Designed and facilitated arts and sports projects, and group trips to local New Orleans attractions.

EDUCATION

Carlton Community College, New Orleans, LA

Community Health Worker Certificate, 2013

Associates of Science Degree, 2015

Ceder Cliff High School, New Orleans, LA

Graduated, 2010

TRAINING AND ACHIEVEMENTS

- First Aid and CPR certification. American Heart Association. Renewed June, 2016
- Awarded Gabriela Munoz Family Scholarship, Carlton Community College, September 2014
- Recognized by the New Orleans Regional YMCA with the Youth Leadership Award, August 2009

REFERENCES

Precious Mamphele, Director, New Orleans Safe House

(123) 456-7890

Dr. Alberto Reyes, Director, Jubilee Camp

(234) 567-8901

Lucky Martinez, Instructor, CHW Certificate Program, Carlton Community College

(345) 678-9012

Figure 14.1 Sample Resume

willing to provide a reference, and tell them about the job you are applying for so they can be as helpful as possible when they talk about your strengths and skills. You can also ask them if they will write you a letter of reference for CHW jobs. You can include copies of these letters of reference with your resume and application, or bring them with you to interviews.

What Do YOU Think?

- *Who will you ask to be your references?*

- *Which of your skills, personal qualities, and job experiences will they be able to talk about with potential employers?*

- *How are these relevant to employment as a CHW?*

INTERVIEWING FOR A JOB, INTERNSHIP, OR VOLUNTEER POSITION

You sent in your application with a cover letter and a resume, and you've been called for an interview. Now what do you do? Relax; interviewing is a skill. It can be practiced and learned.

Job interviews are about finding out whether there is a good 'fit' between the interviewee, the job, and the agency. The interviewer asks questions to learn whether you would be the best employee for the position they are trying to fill. You can also ask questions to see whether this organization is one that you would like to work for. In other words, they are interviewing you, but you are also interviewing them. If you know how to conduct a good client interview, you can learn to do a good job interview.

What Employers Want

- Skills and abilities that fit the job
- Good communication skills and the ability to answer all questions satisfactorily
- A strong work ethic and emotional maturity (including the ability to prevent and manage disagreements on the job)
- The ability to manage time efficiently
- Interest in the agency and the position
- Enthusiasm
- Confidence

Preparing for the Interview

Know the Agency

Learn as much as you can about the agency you are applying to. You can often find out much of what you want to know from an organization's website:

- What is the agency's mission?
- Which communities do they serve?
- What services do they provide?
- What have they accomplished?

Practice Interviewing with a Career Counselor or Friend

We encourage you to practice or rehearse what you will say in the interview. You might do this with a trusted friend or family member, a colleague or classmate, or a professional at a local employment or career counseling center.

Practice responding to common interview questions such as:

- Why are you interested in this position?
- Please describe your qualifications for this position.

- What are your professional goals?
- What experiences have prepared you for this position?
- Why are you considering changing jobs?
- Please describe your educational background and accomplishments.
- Please briefly describe your skills in (topics and areas such as outreach, case management, group facilitation or health education)
- Why are you the best candidate for this position?
- What are your greatest accomplishments or successes?
- What are your greatest strengths? Your greatest weaknesses?

Do your best to stay on topic when answering an interview question. It is also important to respond to each question briefly, prioritizing the most important points only. A common mistake is to spend 10 or even 15 minutes answering a question when speaking for two to three minutes would have provided sufficient information to the employer and demonstrated your ability to manage time well.

Ask for feedback from your friend or colleague, and consider how you might improve or clarify your responses to these interview questions. Be prepared to address or explain gaps in your employment history, and reasons for leaving previous jobs.

What to Take with You to the Interview

- Copies of your resume, a list of professional references or letters of recommendation
- Driver's license or other form of identification
- Samples of your professional work, such as flyers, brochures, reports, or articles that you personally developed.

Dressing for the Interview

Dress in a professional manner, and more formally than you will on the job. A suit, or suit jacket over dress pants or a skirt is almost always considered appropriate for an interview, even for places with a much more casual daily work culture. Don't wear jeans, T-shirts, shorts, or other casual clothes.

The Interview

Greet each of the people who are interviewing you. Speak slowly and clearly, and look your interviewer in the eye often. Prepare questions to ask about the job and agency during the interview. Use the interview to find out how you could fit into the organization and as an opportunity to share your skills with a potential employer.

The interviewer will generally break the ice and make an introduction. He or she may ask for general information about you, your background, or your goals, such as:

- "Tell me about yourself."
- "Why are you interested in our organization?"
- "What are your goals for the next year? Next five years?"
- "Why did you enter this field?"

Then the interviewer will probably share general information about the organization and the job position before asking you specific questions.

Strategies for Responding Effectively to Interview Questions

1. Listen carefully to the question and answer it as specifically as possible.
2. Honesty is always the best policy—don't exaggerate or provide false information to the employer.
3. Ask clarifying questions when necessary.

4. Speak clearly, but don't talk too much. Try not to repeat yourself. Interviewers don't want candidates to take up too much of their time.

5. Focus on the job you are applying for.

6. Present yourself and your skills, abilities, and qualifications and demonstrate how you are a match for the job.

7. Focus on your accomplishments and successes.

8. Answer questions in a way that supports your strengths (don't answer with "yes" or "no" remarks, but state your strengths).

9. Clearly demonstrate your interest in the position.

10. Don't forget to be yourself. Allow your authentic voice and personality to shine through.

Engage the Interviewer

Instead of seeing the interview as an exam you must pass, try to view it as a conversation in which you have valuable information to share with the employer, and they have valuable information about their organization to share with you. Be prepared to ask the interviewer one or more (but not too many!) questions, such as: "Please describe a typical day in this position." "What communities does your agency serve?" "What do you like best about working here?"

Closing

This is a time to ask any remaining questions that you may have *but, again, be conscious of time and don't ask too many questions.* These questions might include, for example: "Is there anything else I can tell you about my qualifications or experience?" "I have copies of my letters of recommendation. May I leave them with you?" "When may I expect to hear from you?"

Remember to thank the interviewer for the opportunity to meet with them.

After the Interview

Reflect upon and evaluate your performance. What did you do well? How might you improve your performance in future interviews?

Thank the interviewer in a follow-up letter or email:

- State your interest in the position again
- Summarize how you qualify for the position

14.3 Keeping the Job

Keeping your position as a CHW will depend to great extent on your interpersonal skills. The most important part of your job is how well you build and maintain positive relationships with clients as well as your coworkers and supervisor. The ability to get along well with colleagues in other agencies, clinics, or organizations, and with the communities you serve is also key to your long-term success. In addition to the other skills you are learning as a CHW, mastering the skills addressed in this chapter will help to create a positive first impression and to inspire trust and confidence from the people your agency serves.

DRESS CODE: WHAT YOU WEAR MATTERS

What people wear is like a language. It is often the first information that someone you meet in person has about who you are. The doctor's white coat, the mechanic's overalls, and the team uniform are obvious examples of clothing that communicate to others something important about who someone is or what they do. You dress up for a job interview as a signal to a potential employer that you understand the codes of the professional world. Codes are cultural, too: someone's ethnic, national, or religious background may influence what they wear and how they perceive what you wear. Before getting dressed for your interview or workday, consider where you are going and who you will be meeting with, and the message that you hope to convey with what you are wearing.

Phuong An Doan Billings: For the Vietnamese community, our culture is very formal. I have to wear my best clothes when I go out to the community. To me it's very natural. That's the way we are. As a teacher in Vietnam, I had to stand in front of a few hundred students every day. Before I left the house, I always had to dress up, even going to the market, because I might meet my students there.

When you work with the community, you have to know how to present yourself. I don't dare to go out to do presentations if I don't have on good clothes. If I didn't dress formally, they wouldn't listen to me. I have to be formal and in a style appropriate to my age and my status.

If I have some staff that I feel do not dress appropriately, we talk about it. I say to them, "You know, this is how our community is. We are formal. That's the reality we have to accept."

The dress code at your job may be different from the dress codes in the community you are working with. When you work in the community, consider these questions about what you wear:

- Will it put my clients at ease? Will it alienate them?
- Will it show respect to the community I'm working with?
- Will it give people the confidence that I have the skills and knowledge to assist them?

In most of the situations you will face at work, a helpful guideline is to dress a half to one step above how your clients dress. Wearing jeans and T-shirts may not be appropriate, but if your clients typically dress in jeans and T-shirts, dressing a half to one step above their clothing may translate into you wearing khakis or cotton dress pants and a button-down shirt, polo-style shirt, or a sweater. As we saw above, however, some communities may expect you to dress much more formally as a sign of respect or to gain their confidence.

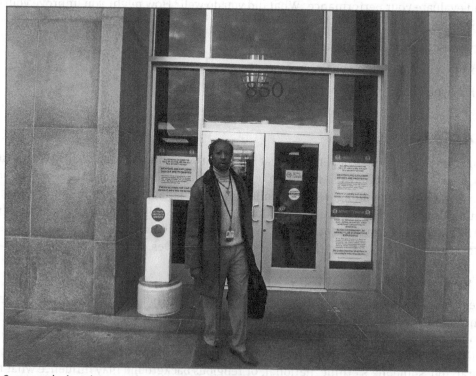

Some work situations require more formal dress. A CHW prepares to attend a court hearing with a client.

As a CHW, how would you dress to meet with the following groups?

- Homeless youth
- Program managers and the board of directors
- The women's auxiliary at the local mosque or temple

In order to for you and your work to be welcomed and respected, you may need to alter your appearance to fit the context (for example, wearing a jacket, dress, or tie to talk with the local Health Commission). These adjustments may assist people to focus on your message, rather than getting distracted by what they think about your appearance.

VERBAL COMMUNICATION AND BODY LANGUAGE

How you present yourself verbally and through body language makes a difference in how people hear you.

Do you stay focused on the topic when others are speaking, asking clarifying questions? Is your voice friendly, assertive, and clear? Do you find yourself telling people what to do? How loudly are you speaking?

Do you stand or sit very close or far away from others? Do you fail to engage in eye contact or insist upon it? When others speak, do you cross your arms, frown, or roll your eyes? How might these or other types of body language be perceived by others?

Some types of communication are not welcome in the workplace:

- **Sexist, racist, homophobic, and other types of prejudicial language** are never appropriate. It is illegal and could get you fired.
- **Profane language**: You should never use curse words under any circumstances. Some words might not be curse words, but are still rude or distasteful.
- **Talking or gossiping** about your coworkers or supervisors negatively is unacceptable. Use the appropriate outlets to get your concerns heard constructively. See the section on giving and receiving constructive feedback further on.
- **Repeating the same information** over and over, constantly interrupting others, or taking time away from a common agenda to talk about other topics can be perceived by others as rude or disrespectful.

Talking on the Telephone

You are likely to spend a lot of time on the phone, contacting clients about their appointments, talking with representatives from other agencies who can provide services for your clients, or contacting local businesses to ask for donations or support for events in your community.

Here are six tips for professional phone calls:

1. Start with a friendly, time-appropriate greeting such as "Good morning."
2. Identify yourself and your agency.
3. State the reason for your call, and ask whether it is a good time to talk, giving an indication of how long the call might be.
4. Write down any key information that other callers provide you, such as names and phone numbers, and read them back to make sure they are accurate.
5. If you will need to call again, say so and ask when you might do so.
6. End the call with "thank you" and "good-bye."

If you leave a message:

1. Begin with a greeting such as "Good morning" or "Good afternoon" followed by the person's name. Deliver these words in a friendly voice.
2. Follow the greeting by identifying yourself and your agency.

3. Briefly state the reason for your call.

4. Repeat your name and give your phone number again, speaking clearly and slowly enough for others to understand.

5. End the call with "thank you" and "good-bye."

Preserve confidentiality: Do not leave any sensitive or confidential information in a message.

Cell Phones and Other Digital Technology

Depending upon the time and place, receiving cell phone calls or text messages can be distracting in the workplace. Be sure that your digital technology is turned off during meetings and do not check digital technology while talking to others (checking for text messages makes you seem distracted and uninterested).

Be aware of your surroundings. If you are working in the community and need to make a call concerning a client, find an appropriate place to speak quietly on the phone without disclosing confidential information in public.

Written Communication

How well you write makes a lasting impression on the people who receive your written communications. Written communications pose particular code-switching challenges. The emphasis in school on spelling, punctuation, and grammar was basically teaching you a "professional" (white, middle-class, English-speaking) code. The way we were taught, and the way that we were judged, can leave us feeling inadequate and intimidated when we have to write letters, memos, emails, and reports.

If writing in English is a challenge for you, consider an adult education class at your high school or community college. Here are some commonsense tips to make your written communications reflect your skills as a successful CHW.

Why are you writing? Depending upon the length and scope of what you write, you may want to jot down a brief outline of what you really want to say before writing. What are your main points? Think of questions your reader may have, and answer them.

Put yourself in your reader's place: Read your message aloud. How would you feel reading this letter or email? Remember: once it has been sent, you cannot take it back. Is your message short, clear, and easy to read? Is there any slang that may not be understood by everyone or may not be appropriate? Is the information accurate? Did you double-check your facts? Is your tone professional and courteous?

Use a simple structure: Start with an introduction. Give the details. Summarize or conclude.

Use clear language: Don't use too many abbreviations, acronyms, or jargon used only at your agency or only in your profession. Keep the language simple and at a level you know all people will understand.

Spell-check is your friend: When you have completed the message, be sure to use spell-check on your computer before you send it.

Email

Increasingly, professional communication is conducted by email. Because it is so easy to write and send, we can be tempted to think of email as less formal or less important than mail that's printed out on paper. *Email is professional communication just like any other form of written communication.* Everything about written communication discussed previously applies to email, and there are a few tips that apply to email in particular.

Subject line: The subject line is like the headline of a news story. Be sure that what you write in the subject line is short and accurate. Some busy people will not open email if the subject line doesn't grab their attention.

Replying: Sometimes you will get an email that is addressed to an entire group of people. Be careful to reply only to the sender of the message; it is unprofessional to reply to everyone unless you have a clear reason for doing so.

Don't hit the send button when you're mad! We've all done it; someone sends you an email message that upsets you, and you respond from your anger. If you're upset, don't send the email: wait until you are in a calmer state and can think more clearly about the potential impact. You might want to check out some of the conflict resolution tips in Chapter 13.

GIVING AND RECEIVING CONSTRUCTIVE FEEDBACK

Part of being a CHW is learning to receive constructive feedback about the quality of your work from clients and community members, coworkers and supervisors. You will also have a duty to provide feedback to others.

Your ability to provide and receive feedback in a respectful and professional manner is key to the long-term success of your career. The inability to handle feedback is a common reason why employees miss out on opportunities for promotion, face disciplinary action, or lose their jobs.

The purpose of constructive feedback is, ultimately, to improve the quality of the services provided to clients and communities. For CHWs, the purpose of constructive feedback is to assist you in enhancing your knowledge and skills, and the quality of your professional relationships with coworkers and clients alike.

Constructive feedback may be supportive or corrective. ***Supportive feedback*** reinforces current behaviors and skills by identifying what is being done well or right. ***Corrective feedback*** indicates desired changes in behavior, by explaining what didn't work, is unacceptable in the workplace, or needs improvement. In both cases, the goal should be to improve performance and effectiveness.

Challenges with Receiving or Providing Feedback

Most of us have had difficulty, at some point in life, with receiving or providing feedback in a calm and professional manner. Some of the factors that get in our way include:

- Past negative experiences with feedback or verbal abuse
- Learning from poor role models that the way to provide feedback is through conflict or accusation, with anger or sarcasm
- Prior disagreements or conflicts with the same person that have eroded trust or respect
- Bias, prejudice, or discriminatory treatment or policies
- Anxiety or fear, such as the fear of losing your job
- Emotions such as anger or frustration that may result in defensiveness, sarcasm or attack
- The desire to be right, and related difficulties accepting accountability or negotiating compromise
- A lack of self-awareness and acknowledgment of our own limitations and areas for personal and professional growth and development
- Difficulty providing a sincere apology

- *What is your experience with feedback?*
- *Have you faced challenges in providing or receiving feedback to colleagues or coworkers?*
- *What lessons have you learned that help you in providing and receiving feedback?*

Guidelines for Giving and Receiving Feedback

We encourage you to reframe the way that you view feedback. Try to consider it as a resource and an opportunity to learn and improve your skills, especially when the nature of the feedback provided is difficult to hear.

We will share brief guidelines for giving and receiving constructive feedback. We also encourage you to seek out professional development opportunities to enhance your skills, and to learn from experienced and respected colleagues. The information provided in Chapter 13 on conflict resolution may also be helpful.

Giving Feedback

When providing others with feedback, we recommend sandwiching corrective feedback between substantive supportive feedback. In other words, start and end your conversation by sharing positive feedback with your colleague. Everyone we work with has strengths. Let them know you what you appreciate about their attitude, knowledge, skills, and contributions.

Other guidelines include:

- Express what you value about the other person and your working relationship.
- Don't provide feedback when you are feeling angry or unable to focus on supporting your colleague.
- Speak in a respectful tone of voice. Don't raise the level of your voice.
- Provide detailed and specific feedback (what, where, when) about the person's behavior or conduct. What did they do—or not do—that you want to draw to their attention to?
- Explain what you think the impact of a specific decision, behavior, or policy may be on others such as yourself, your colleagues, or the clients and community you serve. Use "I statements" when focusing on your own reactions (see Chapter 13).
- Provide *practical and realistic* suggestions for what your colleague could do differently the next time they face a similar situation. If relevant, refer to your agency or program standards, goals, or policies.
- Don't hold back on sharing important corrective feedback. When we do this, we deprive a colleague of the opportunity to learn how to enhance their skills and performance.
- Feedback should be timely: Share it in the moment it occurs or as soon afterward as possible.
- Invite the person or group to ask questions to clarify the feedback you provide and to respond.
- Invite your colleague to talk with you and to identify concrete steps they can take to improve their skills and performance.
- Whether the person agrees or doesn't agree with the feedback you provide, express your appreciation for their listening to you.

- *What else would you want to do when providing constructive feedback to a colleague?*

What Do YOU Think?

Receiving Feedback

Suggested guidelines include:

- Breathe! Try to center yourself, remain calm, and strive to listen and understand the information that is being shared with you.
- Assume that the person who is providing you with feedback is doing so with a positive intention (such as improving the quality of services and working relationships).
- Listen for key content such as feedback about specific behaviors or decisions, and any suggestions for what you could do differently.
- Ask questions to clarify the information your colleague (or a client or community member) is providing. If the feedback is vague or unclear, ask them to provide you with a specific example.
- Maintain a calm and conversational tone and voice level.
- Paraphrase or summarize the feedback to make sure you have heard it correctly.
- Notice if you are feeling defensive. Don't react in the moment with anger, or try to defend yourself, especially if the person providing the feedback is a client, your supervisor, or another leader at your agency or in the community.
- Ask for a break if you need one, and only return to the conversation when you are truly prepared to listen to what your colleague has to say. Vent any strong emotions later, away from the workplace. You can always respond to your colleague at a later date, when you are calm and prepared for a respectful and productive conversation.
- Honestly reflect on the feedback provided, and decide if and how you wish to incorporate what you have learned into your future work. What did you learn that might help you to improve your skills and performance?

- Clearly and respectfully communicate any specific requests you have for the other party to make changes to their own conduct (or to policies).

- Don't forget to end with sharing additional supportive feedback to the other party.

- Regardless of how you feel in the moment, express your appreciation to the other party for taking time to provide you with feedback.

- If it is relevant and desirable, schedule a future meeting to follow up on the issues discussed at this meeting.

- *What else would you want to do when receiving constructive feedback from a colleague?*

Please watch this video interview 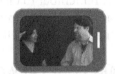 with CCSF faculty about the challenge of providing and receiving constructive feedback in the classroom and beyond.

PROVIDING & RECEIVING CONSTRUCTIVE FEEDBACK: FACULTY INTERVIEW
http://youtu.be/ 7NqVUo-foEw

COMMUNICATE WITH YOUR SUPERVISOR

In an ideal work situation, communication with your supervisor is frequent, clear, straightforward, respectful, and effortless. Unfortunately, most of us are likely to face challenges in working with supervisors over the course of our careers. Some of these challenges will arise from unwritten codes raising their heads again: does your supervisor have certain expectations that they have not clearly explained? Do you get the feeling your supervisor doesn't want you to raise your concerns in staff meetings or at a case conference? And some of the challenges may arise because of the limitations of the supervisor: they may lack some of the key skills and attributes necessary for effectively leading and supporting others in the workplace.

Supervisors are responsible for helping you and the program you work for to be successful. They are looking for employees who are reliable, consistent, and who can learn and grow on the job. Do your utmost to forge and sustain a positive working relationship with your supervisor, especially during times when you have different perspectives, needs, or values. Try to find common ground. Look for opportunities, or create them, to work together in a focused way on a common task in which you each have valuable expertise to offer.

Express Your Concerns

If you face difficulties or challenges in your relationship with your supervisor, consider taking the initiative by asking to talk about your concerns. Keep in mind that the supervisor may not already be aware of your concerns or perspective. *Draw upon your client-centered skills!* Be respectful and patient. Ask open-ended questions to help clarify your understanding of the supervisor's perspective and position. Summarize key information in order to confirm that you have understood it correctly. Listen calmly. Don't do or say anything in the heat of moment (if you are frustrated, angry or hurt) that might undermine your employment status or career. And don't talk negatively about your supervisor—or other colleagues—behind their back. This is a powerful way to damage trust and the quality of professional relationships.

Accept Limitations

Keep in mind that it may not be possible to work out every difference of opinion or conflict with your supervisor. *Part of work is accepting constraints or conditions determined by our employers and supervisors.* This includes accepting policies and protocols that we don't like or agree with. Try to distinguish between differences or disagreements that you are able to accept and live with, and those that you feel so strongly about that you are willing to take a risk to advocate for.

Speak Directly to Your Supervisor

Always try to speak directly with your supervisor about any complaint that you have about their performance. Going around your supervisor to speak to another administrator may be perceived as "going behind their back," and further damage your working relationship (note that there are a few exceptions to this rule, such as complaints of sexual harassment or other charges of illegal conduct). If you have difficulties with a supervisor that you cannot resolve, you may need to turn to your union or human resources department for assistance in mediating the communication.

Weigh Your Options

Despite the problems you encounter, continue to bring your best self to your interactions with your supervisor. Work to improve the relationship. At some point, if the changes that you desire do not occur, you may need to reconsider your strategy. You may decide to seek employment elsewhere, either within the organization you currently work for, or with a different agency. If you decide to stay in your current position, find a way to focus on the aspects of your job where you have greater autonomy, as well as those that bring you satisfaction and meaning.

And please remember to take care of yourself along the way. Disharmony or conflicts with supervisors can take a significant toll on our professional life and on our physical, mental, and spiritual health. Apply your skills for stress management and self care, and engage in life affirming activities outside of work.

BOUNDARY ISSUES AT WORK: DISCLOSURE OF PERSONAL INFORMATION

You will spend a lot of time with your coworkers. You may wish to develop closer personal relationships with some coworkers, or to talk with them about personal issues.

You may find yourself trying to decide whether or not to disclose or share certain information about yourself on the job. For example, this might include your recovery from drug and alcohol use; living with a health condition such as cancer, diabetes, hepatitis C, or a mental health condition; your identity as a lesbian, gay, bisexual or transgender person; or a history of incarceration. Sharing this information may be perfectly natural and common at the agency where you work as a CHW. It is common, for example, for people in recovery from drug and alcohol use to work with programs addressing these issues, and so on. But you don't have to share personal information at work. Before you do, we encourage you to consider the potential consequences. Are you someone who is completely comfortable with other people knowing these details of your life? Do you have a good reason to trust that your employer and coworkers will understand and be supportive when you share this information? Are you working in a context where this information could be used to harass or discriminate against you?

On the other hand, some of the value you bring to the community you serve may be as a role model. If you have overcome challenges that are similar to those that clients are facing, hearing about your experience may give them hope that they, too, can achieve meaningful changes in their own lives. Please refer to the guidelines for determining if, when and how to self-disclose personal information to a client provided in Chapters 7 and 21.

MANAGE YOUR TIME

As a CHW, you will have a lot of key tasks and deadlines to manage, as well as the challenge of balancing work and your personal life. Time management can make the difference between success and failure at work and in life. It provides resources to make conscious decisions about how to address competing demands.

Some people resist the idea of time management because they like the idea of being spontaneous. But having a plan for each day can free you from the stress of remembering what to do and when, or being backed into a corner when you forgot to do something and a deadline is fast approaching. Managing your time also helps you to free up time for the things you most want to do.

Plan Your Week

If you don't use one already, start to use a portable print or electronic calendar or planner. It is a valuable tool for keeping track of your busy schedule.

Write down your appointments, meetings, deadlines, family obligations and activities, and so forth.

Make a "to-do list" of all the other tasks you need to accomplish that don't have a specific date and time commitment. Mark those tasks that are the highest priority for the upcoming week.

Don't schedule every minute of each day: leave room for new demands on your time that will come up, and for ongoing activities that always take time, such completing case notes and other forms of documentation. Review your calendar and your to-do list to make sure that you have scheduled all key tasks and obligations.

Review Tomorrow's Schedule

At the end of each day, take 10 minutes to review tomorrow's schedule. Identify one or two priorities, and make sure you have set aside enough time to complete them. Look at appointments you have, and think about whether you need to prepare anything in advance. Review your personal and family needs for the day, to see if you need to do errands on the way to or home from work, if you need to make phone calls, or do any urgent tasks at home. This one simple habit, if you do it each evening at the end of the work day, or at home before you go to bed, will help you feel prepared to manage your responsibilities at work and at home.

Set Priorities

Most of us have more things to do than we can actually accomplish. Part of managing your time involves making conscious decisions about what your priorities are—what you will do right now, what you will postpone, and what you won't do. There will be times when you have to say "No" to certain activities and responsibilities and stick to your original plan in order to accomplish your tasks. At work, your commitment to your clients should always be your number one priority. Don't fill up your calendar with other activities that make it difficult for you to fulfill your commitment to the community.

When you start managing your time, you may find yourself frustrated or feeling as though keeping a planner and maintaining a daily to-do list is taking up too much time. Don't give up! In the long run, this kind of planning will give you more control over your busy days. It will help you make sure you get the most important tasks done. And it will help you balance your work demands with taking care of yourself and your family.

14.4 Professional Development and Career Advancement

Ramona Benson: I came from the community and my highest education was the twelfth grade. I had some life experiences that weren't so great, and because of those experiences, my confidence level wasn't high. So when I first became a CHW, I struggled with having the professional people see me as genuine or respect my suggestions or ideas, or just respect me. What helped me was the CHW certification program. It validated my knowledge and skills. I was able to do the work and that said to me, "You are college material." That helped boost my confidence. It also made me more comfortable interviewing for jobs and telling employers all the knowledge and skills that I would bring to their agency. I also decided to stay in school. I completed my Associate's Degree at Berkeley City College, and went on to earn my Bachelor's Degree In Liberal Studies and Health Education. Now I am thinking about applying to graduate school!

Imagine that you are working successfully as a CHW. You've settled into your current position and you're doing a great job. Now is the time to think about professional development to enhance skills for your present job, and to help you to advance to new positions with more responsibility (and better pay and benefits).

PROFESSIONAL DEVELOPMENT

Professional development is seeking out opportunities to enhance your knowledge and skills in key areas related to your work as a CHW. This might include, for example, knowledge about:

- Specific health issues such as depression, post-traumatic stress, substance use, or diabetes
- Local resources such as mental health services
- The history, resources, and health concerns of specific populations or communities
- Statistics or epidemiology

It may also include skills in areas such as:

- Public speaking
- Crisis intervention and suicide prevention

- Program planning and evaluation
- Research or community diagnosis
- Grant writing
- Media advocacy
- Conflict resolution
- Cultural humility
- Supervising and managing others
- Leadership

- *What other skills or knowledge do you think would assist you to advance in your career as a CHW?*

Professional development opportunities include participating in free or low-cost trainings at a nonprofit agency or the local health department; enrolling in a class (including online classes); attending a lecture at a local college or university; conducting research; and reading articles and books or watching a documentary by yourself or with others.

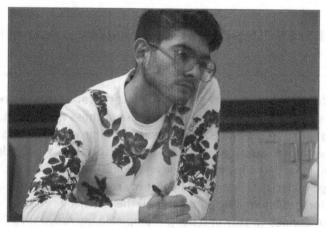

CHWs engage in ongoing professional development opportunities to enhance their knowledge and skills.

Case Conferences

If you work in a team setting, you may have the opportunity to participate in case conferences (see Chapter 10) and to discuss your work with colleagues. This is a wonderful opportunity for professional development: You receive immediate feedback from peers and other professionals on an urgent problem such as working with a suicidal client or a pregnant 13-year-old. Whether you're getting the advice or assisting a colleague, case conferences can be a great opportunity for continuing education.

Support and Mentoring

Mentoring by an experienced CHW may be the best form of professional development you can hope for. You may work surrounded by doctors, nurses, or social workers who want to know, or think they know, what it takes to be a great CHW: but only an experienced CHW can really know this. Ask to meet regularly with an experienced CHW. Share your questions and concerns, and listen to their guidance. If you are fortunate enough to work near a CHW network, take advantage of it. If you are more isolated, you may find support through regional or national networks such as the Community Health Worker Section of the American Public Health Association (*www.apha.org/apha-communities/member-sections/community-health-workers*). And in 10 years, you will be the experienced CHW who supports a new CHW in establishing their career.

> **Andrew Ciscel:** I learn so much from my colleagues—other Peer Specialists and CHWs. There is such a wide range of tools and approaches that CHWs use to work in different communities. By building connections with other CHWs, we can share our resources and skills. We also vent and laugh together and provide mutual support and inspiration to keep going. This is really important for me because there are so many challenges that come in the work, and sometimes it is hard to keep going. For me, building that community with other CHWs is a key part of my professional development and self care.

Chapter Review

Please practice and apply the information covered in this chapter. For example, consider the following questions and suggestions:

- What advise might you share with Norma, the CHW from the Case Study presented at the beginning of this chapter? What else might Norma do—if anything—to adapt to the codes of her workplace?

- How can you enhance your own skills for code switching while maintaining your own identity and culture?

- Develop or update your resume

- Rehearse what you might say in a job interview about your experience, knowledge, and skills as a CHW

- Create a prioritized to-do list—including professional and personal responsibilities—for next week, and schedule these activities in a planner

- In the next month, practice giving or receiving professional feedback. Reflect on your performance using the guidelines presented in this chapter.

- Identify two or more skills or areas of knowledge that you would like to learn or enhance that will assist in advancing your career. Identify professional development opportunities to enhance your knowledge and skills.

- Identify a peer support network or an experienced CHW who might serve as a mentor to you. How do you feel about contacting these resources? What type of support will you ask for? What questions do you have?

Additional Resources

American Public Health Association. (n.d.). Community Health Worker Section. Retrieved from *www.apha.org/apha-communities/member-sections/community-health-workers*.

Daily Writing Tips. (n.d.). Retrieved from *www.dailywritingtips.com/email-etiquette/*

Decker, D. C., Hoevemeyer, V. A., & Rowe-Dimas, M. (2006). *First-job survival guide: How to thrive and advance in your new career.* Indianapolis, IN: JIST Works.

Inc. Magazine. (2010). *25 tips for perfecting your email etiquette.* Retrieved from *www.inc.com/guides/2010/06/email-etiquette.html*

Kissane, S. F. (1997). *Career success for people with physical disabilities.* Chicago, IL: VGM Career Horizons.

Mind Tools. (2015). *Essential skills for an excellent career.* Retrieved from *www.mindtools.com/*

National Association of Social Workers. (2011). *Setting and maintaining professional boundaries.* Retrieved from *http://careers.socialworkers.org/documents/Professional%20Boundaries.pdf*

The Productivity Institute. (n.d.). Time management articles. Retrieved from *www.balancetime.com/articles_online.php*

Red Earth Software. (n.d.) *Email etiquette*. Retrieved from *http://emailreplies.com/*

Remshardt, M. A. (2012). Do you know your professional boundaries? *Nursing Made Incredibly Easy!*, *10*, 5–6. Retrieved from *http://journals.lww.com/nursingmadeincrediblyeasy/Fulltext/2012/01000/Do_you_know_your_professional_boundaries_.3.aspx#*

Skills You Need. (n.d.) Retrieved from *www.skillsyouneed.com*

Wennerstrom, A., Johnson, L., Gibson, K., Batta, S. E., & Springgate, B. F. (2014). Community health workers leading the charge on workforce development: Lessons from New Orleans. *Journal of Community Health, 39,* 1140–1149.

APPLYING CORE COMPETENCIES TO KEY HEALTH ISSUES

PART
4

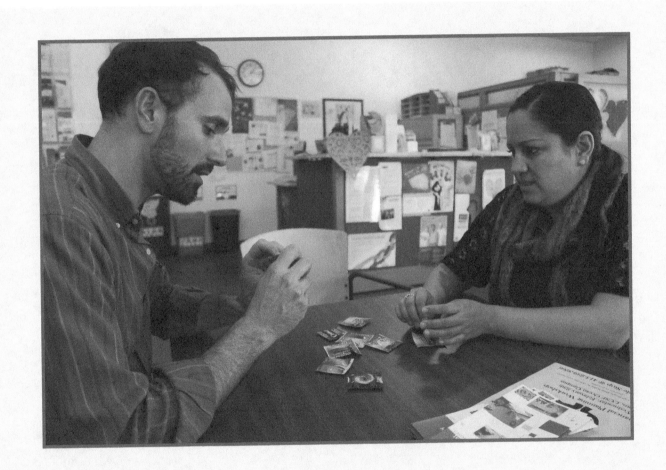

Promoting the Health of Formerly Incarcerated People

15

Donna Willmott

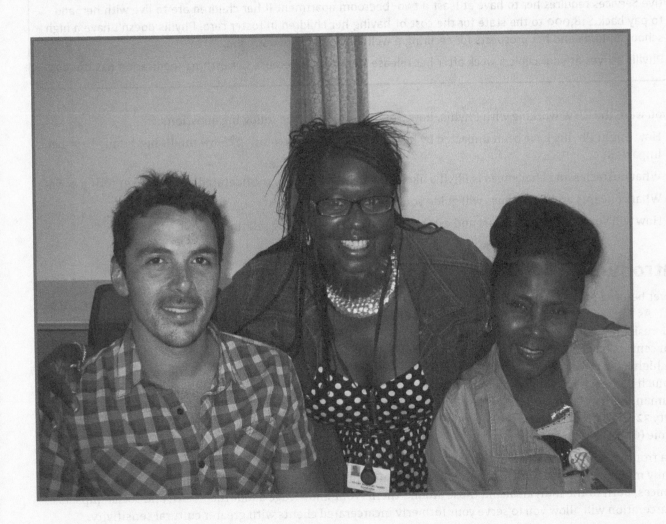

CASE STUDY   Phyllis

You are a CHW with a community-based clinic. Today you are meeting with Phyllis, a new client. She is a 32-year-old woman and the mother of two young children. Phyllis was just released from prison after serving three years for a drug-related offense. She has asthma, recently tested positive for hepatitis C, and wants to work on substance-use issues, but received no treatment while in prison. She is a survivor of sexual abuse from an early age, but has never had mental health counseling for the trauma she experienced.

Phyllis wants to reunite with her children. They were initially cared for by her mother, and eventually placed in foster care. Phyllis used to live in public housing but can't return because of her conviction. Child Protective Services requires her to have at least a two-bedroom apartment if her children are to live with her, and to pay back $18,000 to the state for the cost of having her children in foster care. Phyllis doesn't have a high school diploma and her prospects for securing a well-paying job are not good.

Phyllis arrives at your clinic a week after her release from prison because her asthma medication has run out.

If you were the CHW working with Phyllis, how would you answer the following questions:

- How might Phyllis have been impacted by her experience of incarceration? How might her family have been impacted?
- What obstacles and challenges is Phyllis likely to face as a formerly incarcerated woman re-entering society?
- What concepts and techniques will guide your work with Phyllis?
- How will you work to build trust and establish a supportive working relationship with Phyllis?

Introduction

Never before in the history of the United States have so many lives been affected by the experience of incarceration. As the War on Drugs, "tough on crime" policies, and harsh immigration laws have criminalized millions of U.S. residents in the past three decades, our county jails, juvenile halls, state prisons, and immigration detention centers have become overcrowded. In 2008, the United States held 2.3 million people behind bars, giving it the highest incarceration rate in the world—762 per 100,000 residents (Human Rights Watch, 2009). This rate is much higher than that of other democracies like Great Britain (152 per 100,000), Canada (116), and Japan (63) (Human Rights Watch, 2009). It is also estimated that over 7.2 million adults in the United States—1 out of every 32—is currently under the control of the criminal justice system through incarceration, probation, or parole (Glaze, 2010).

As a frontline community health worker, you are likely to have clients who have been incarcerated or have a family member who has been incarcerated. Imprisonment is a traumatic experience with far-reaching consequences, both to the individual and those around them. Your knowledge about the health and social impacts of incarceration will allow you to serve your formerly incarcerated clients with greater cultural sensitivity.

This chapter analyzes the ways in which mass incarceration contributes to higher rates of illness, particularly within poor communities and communities of color. You will learn about the many laws and regulations that make it more difficult for your formerly incarcerated clients to re-enter society. This chapter draws on the experience of some of the country's first CHWs whose practice is focused on post prison health and wellness. We hope that it will enhance your understanding of the many ways that imprisonment shapes the health of individuals, families, and communities.

Prisoners are severely stigmatized within our society and often face fractured relationships and a sense of dislocation when returning home. Many doors will be closed to them as they work to rebuild their lives. Frontline health and social services workers in communities most affected by incarceration have a critical role to play in supporting former prisoners in their re-entry. By approaching formerly incarcerated clients in a nonjudgmental way, linking them with appropriate resources, fostering social support, and promoting social change, you will be in a position to challenge some of the worst collateral effects of incarceration and contribute to building healthier communities.

WHAT YOU WILL LEARN

By studying the information in this chapter, you will be able to:

- Analyze the ways that incarceration influences the health of individuals, families, and communities
- Identify common health issues faced by formerly incarcerated people
- Explain the stigma and the systemic barriers to reintegration faced by newly released prisoners
- Discuss the role of CHWs in promoting the health and well-being of formerly incarcerated clients
- Examine best practices and emerging models for promoting the health of formerly incarcerated people
- Identify areas of potential policy change and the role of CHWs as advocates for change
- Learn about resources for successful re-entry

WORDS TO KNOW

Recidivism

Re-entry

Basic Terms and a Note on Language

JAILS VERSUS PRISONS

While people sometimes use these terms interchangeably, *jails* are different from *prisons*. Jails are run by the county sheriff's department and hold people who are awaiting trial, and people who are sentenced for a short term, usually less than a year. Prisons are run either by a state or federal correctional department; they hold people who have been convicted of a crime, and usually those sentenced for more than a year.

DETENTION CENTERS

Detention facilities hold people suspected of a crime, awaiting trial or sentencing, or found to be an undocumented immigrant. Young people are often held in juvenile detention centers, in secure residential facilities for young people awaiting court hearings and/or in long-term care facilities and programs. Immigrants who are in custody for more than 72 hours are held in detention centers overseen by the Department of Homeland Security (DHS).

PROBATION AND PAROLE

Many people who are found guilty of less serious offenses are placed on probation instead of being sent to prison, allowing them to serve their sentence in the community. While on probation, a person must avoid further contact with the law and must fulfill certain requirements, such as periodic drug testing or attendance in specific classes or programs. Travel is generally restricted to the immediate district where the probationer lives. Probationers are placed under the supervision of a probation officer and must report on a regular basis. If the probationer violates a condition of probation, the court may place additional restrictions on the probationer or order the probationer to serve a term of imprisonment.

A judge can also order probation in addition to a period of incarceration. For example, a sentence might consist of a jail term and, after release, probation for a specified period of months or years. Probation is generally reserved for persons sentenced to short terms in jail: it is not combined with a long prison sentence.

If a person is subjected to supervision after a stay in prison, a parole officer will conduct this supervision. Both probation and parole involve the supervision of people who have been convicted of crimes, but the systems are distinct. Probation is ordered by a judge; parole is granted by a parole board. Probation is an alternative to prison; parole is the early release from prison. Probation is reserved for persons convicted of less serious offenses; parole is given to persons convicted of serious offenses.

THE SIGNIFICANCE OF THE LANGUAGE WE USE

The language we use for people who are in or have been in jail or prison is critically important because of the stigma our society places on a history of incarceration and the risk of alienating the very clients and communities we are pledged to serve. Societies often label groups of people and in the process undermine their identity and status as human beings. When we refer to people as homeless or addicts or mentally ill or illegal aliens or convicted felons, we set them apart from others and diminish their worth. One of the quickest ways to undermine your ability to work with any client is to call them out of their name (or call a person by a name that they do not want you to use), perhaps by assigning them an unwelcome label such as those referenced above.

The language that many institutions and helping professionals use to refer to formerly incarcerated people is highly stigmatizing and a barrier to developing effective professional relationships based on respect. This includes the use of terms such as "offenders" or "convicts" or "felons" or "convicted criminals" or "inmates." In this chapter and in our work we use the terms "incarcerated person" or "formerly incarcerated person" which is consistent with the language many people use to self-identify.

15.1 Incarceration Policies in the United States

How did the wealthiest nation in history come to use imprisonment more than any other society?

In the 1980s, inner cities were undergoing an economic collapse due to a number of factors including globalization (the exporting of jobs to countries with lower-paid workers and little regulation) and deindustrialization (the shift from blue-collar to service-sector jobs). The bold changes brought by the Civil Rights Movement and other social movements of the 1960s were met with a backlash of new law-and-order rhetoric that appealed to racial fears. Ronald Reagan's highly racialized appeals to the insecurities of poor and working-class whites are exemplified in his false but often-repeated story of a "Chicago welfare queen with 80 names, 30 addresses, and a tax-free income of $150,000" (Alexander, 2010). His campaign rhetoric was very effective, as large numbers of Democrats abandoned their party to vote for him. At the top of his agenda was the "War on Drugs," a war "that had little to do with public concern about drugs and everything to do with public concern about race" (Alexander, 2010). Under Reagan's tenure, the Anti-Drug Abuse Act was signed, instituting harsh penalties and "mandatory minimums," which required judges to sentence defendants using a prescribed formula according to the weight of the drugs involved, thus denying judges any discretion in sentencing.

George Bush Sr.'s most famous racial appeal, the Willie Horton ad, featured an African-American convict who raped and murdered a white woman after he escaped from prison during a work furlough. The ad blamed his opponent, Michael Dukakis, for the woman's death because he had endorsed the work furlough program. That ad was the end of Dukakis' political career. Bush's victory ushered in a tough-on-crime agenda, with the War on Drugs taking center stage. Under his leadership law enforcement budgets were higher than ever and the prison population exploded.

Bill Clinton escalated what his Republican predecessors began, with a $30 billion crime bill that "resulted in the largest increase in federal and state prison inmates of any president in American history" (Guard, 2008). The bill mandated life sentences for some three-time offenders ("three-strikes" laws) and created a number of new federal crimes that carried the death penalty. Clinton also "ended welfare as we know it" by imposing a five-year lifetime limit on welfare assistance. President Clinton replaced President Johnson's "war on poverty," which increased the social safety net, with a war on the poor.

While politicians built support for these fear-based policies, the vast majority of the new admissions to state prisons have been convicted of nonviolent offenses, primarily drug-related. Most dramatically, four out of every five drug prisoners were African-American (56 percent) and Hispanic (23 percent), well above their respective rates (13 percent and 9 percent) of drug use (King & Mauer, 2002). While some policy makers and stakeholders have tried to convince us that mass incarceration is inevitable, this is not a common practice in other parts of the world.

The United States locks up hundreds of thousands of people each year for drug law violations that would not warrant imprisonment in many European or Latin American countries (Drug Policy Alliance, 2011). In contrast, policies in Canada and Great Britain promote access to drug treatment, counseling, and employment training and result in significantly lower rates of incarceration. For many decades in Great Britain, heroin was dispensed to addicts under legal supervision; this model was adopted in other countries, and nowhere was there any indication that these policies led to higher rates of addiction (Maté, 2008). In the 1990s, Portugal stopped actively prosecuting drug use to focus on other criminal justice issues, and provides community-based access to clean syringes and works, drug treatment, and other services. As a result, incarceration rates declined dramatically.

- *How has the War on Drugs affected communities you belong to and/or work with?*

- *What percentage of people who are incarcerated in your city, county, or state are serving time for drug-related crimes?*

The War on Drugs has been the single greatest force driving racial inequalities in imprisonment. Despite the fact that rates of drug use do not differ significantly by race, the burden of incarceration falls disproportionately on members of racial and ethnic minorities, a disparity which cannot be accounted for solely by differences in criminal conduct. One in 10 Black males aged 25–29 were in prison or jail in 2009; for Hispanic males the figure was 1 in 25; for White males the figure was 1 in 64 (Human Rights Watch, 2009). Blacks constitute 34 percent of drug arrests, 44 percent of persons convicted of drug felonies in state court, and 37 percent of people sent to state prison on drug charges, even though they constitute only 13 percent of the U.S. population, and Blacks and Whites engage in drug offenses at equivalent rates (Human Rights Watch, 2009).

The American prison system has developed into a system of social control unparalleled in history (Alexander, 2010). People of color face systematic discrimination across the criminal justice spectrum and are disproportionately more likely to be searched, prosecuted, convicted, and sentenced to longer periods of incarceration (Donohoe, 2006). While African Americans represent 13 percent of the U.S population, they comprise more than 48 percent of the overall prison population. Latinos represent 11 percent of the U.S. population, but make up 22 percent of prisoners serving time for drug-related crimes. This pattern of systematic discrimination is similar to patterns discussed in Chapter 4 that highlight the ways in which people of color are denied equal access to safe housing, quality education, employment, civil rights, and other essential resources and rights.

While women of all races use drugs at approximately the same rate, African American women are 6 times more likely than White women to be imprisoned. The lifetime chance of incarceration for Black men is 1 in 3, for Latino men it is 1 in 6, for White men it is 1 in 17 (U.S. Department of Justice, 2003). Imprisonment on this scale is creating an undercaste of people who are locked up, and then locked out of mainstream society upon their return. In her groundbreaking book *The New Jim Crow*, Michelle Alexander describes the politics driving this phenomenon:

> *The law and order perspective, first introduced during the peak of the Civil Rights movement by rabid segregationists, had become nearly hegemonic nearly two decades later. . . . More than two million people found themselves behind bars at the turn of the twenty-first century, and millions more were relegated to the margins of mainstream society, banished to a political and social space not unlike Jim Crow, where discrimination in employment, housing and access to education was perfectly legal, and they could be denied the right to vote.* (Alexander, 2010)

15.2 The Health Impacts of Incarceration

As discussed in Chapters 3 and 4, public health research demonstrates that the health status of populations is largely determined by social factors such as access to quality education, safe housing, a living wage, affordable health care, civil rights, and personal safety that are the foundation of good health. We live in a society characterized by social inequalities based on gender identity, race/ethnicity, income, education, immigration status, sexual orientation, and disability. These social inequalities produce health inequalities, which mean that some populations will get sick and die much earlier than others. Mass incarceration is driven by many of the same factors that are the basis for health inequalities in the United States, particularly racism, poverty, and sexism.

Incarceration itself is increasingly recognized as a social determinant of health. As we will see in this chapter, it contributes greatly to poor health outcomes on all levels, from the individual to the family and the community. The policies that drive unprecedented levels of imprisonment are increasingly understood to be health policies as well. They exacerbate health inequalities on a population level, and for this reason the crisis of mass incarceration is increasingly acknowledged as a public health crisis.

As much as prisons are designed to create a literal wall between prisoners and the rest of society, prisoners are nevertheless part of the broader community. More than 11 million people are released from jails and prisons each year, and just as their absence profoundly affects those left behind, their return affects the community as well. This is a population that had a higher rate of chronic disease than the general population before going to prison. Substandard medical care in prisons and jails means that people often return home with deteriorated health (Binswanger, Krueger, & Steiner, 2009). Approximately 70 percent of released prisoners have a chronic disease, mental health, or substance abuse issue, and the vast majority are uninsured and have little access to primary care (Flanagan, 2004; Lincoln et al., 2006). People are usually released from prison without medication prescriptions or adequate referrals, making it difficult to access medical care and continue to take necessary medications. Most important, they come home to a society that, through social stigma and policy, creates nearly insurmountable barriers to a safe return.

Please watch the following video interview ▶ with Donna Willmott, the author of this chapter. She talks about the importance of understanding mass incarceration as a public health issue.

HEALTH CONDITIONS IN JAILS AND PRISONS

INCARCERATION AS A PUBLIC HEALTH ISSUE: FACULTY INTERVIEW

⊕ *http://youtu.be/ 07AdDUAyu54*

People in prison have higher rates of chronic illness, including mental health conditions, than the general population. More than one out of three prisoners has at least one chronic illness, and there is a higher prevalence of hypertension, asthma, cervical cancer, and arthritis in prisons (Binswanger, Krueger, & Steiner, 2009). Lack of proper diet, fresh air, and exercise can exacerbate many chronic illnesses. All prisoners live with a fairly constant level of stress from the prison environment itself, and the emotional stress of separation from loved ones takes an additional toll on their health. As discussed in Chapters 4, 12 and 16, public health researchers have demonstrated that prolonged exposure to stress is a key cause of chronic disease and of inequalities in rates of illness and death among populations.

Rates of human immunodeficiency virus (HIV) disease among incarcerated populations are 5 times higher than in the general population, and rates of infection with the hepatitis C Virus (HCV) are 9 to 10 times higher (Donohoe, 2006). Although risks for HIV and HCV infection occur in prison through the reuse of needles in injection drug use and tattooing, and consensual and nonconsensual sex, the vast majority of men in prison living with HIV disease were infected in community settings (Vlahov, 2006). The high rates of infection in incarcerated populations reflect the fact that the majority of incarcerated people come from impoverished and disenfranchised communities with limited access to prevention, screening, and treatment services. These same communities have the high rates of HIV, HCV, sexually transmitted infections (STIs), and other infections on the outside.

In most prison and jail settings drug use, tattooing, and sexual activity are all punishable offenses, and harm reduction practices such as provision of condoms and clean needles are rarely implemented, thus thwarting attempts to further prevent infection by incarcerated people themselves.

According to Barry Zack and Katie Kramer:

> There is a misconception that incarcerated men are responsible for increasing rates of HIV/STI's. Imprisonment does affect HIV/STI rates in the community, but not from men getting infected on the inside and bringing it out to their female sexual partners once they are released. Instead, incarceration decreases the number of men in the community, which disrupts stable partnerships, changes the male-to-female ratios and promotes higher risk concurrent, or overlapping partnerships. (Zack & Kramer, 2009)

Given the high rates of incarceration of people of color in the United States, particularly African Americans, "the link among race, prison, and HIV is so strong that it almost completely explains the disproportionate impact of HIV in the Black Community" (Johnson & Raphael, 2005).

Overcrowded and unsanitary conditions increase a prisoner's risk of exposure to tuberculosis, including multidrug-resistant TB and to Methicillin-resistant *Staphylococcus aureus* (MRSA) (Donohoe, 2006). MRSA is becoming a major public health concern because it resists newer antibiotics and threatens to exhaust the available treatment options. Crowded conditions such as prisons increase the likelihood of transmission (Malcolm, 2011).

Prison medical care is generally far below the community standard; treatment is often delayed and inadequate, there is very little follow-up and preventative care is almost nonexistent (Donohoe, 2006). Many prison doctors have been found to be incompetent, and the practice of allowing "impaired physicians" facing criminal charges to treat prisoners in lieu of being incarcerated themselves has historically degraded the quality of medical care in some state prisons (Skolnick, 1998). Even though prisoners have a long-established Constitutional right to health care, many institutions are not in compliance with the law. For example, the California Department of Corrections has been under court-ordered receivership that was mandated in 2005 because of "an unconscionable degree of suffering and death" resulting in an average of one needless death per week in its prisons (*Plata v. Schwarzenegger*, 2005). The privatization of medical care in nearly half of U.S. facilities has also contributed to poor quality health care that leaves prisoners with compromised health.

In addition to lack of access to quality medical care, prisoners often experience long delays in receiving treatment and prescribed medications. People who require regular medication for seizures, high blood pressure, heart disease, diabetes, hepatitis C, HIV, and other conditions can find their chronic condition becoming unmanageable.

Frank's Story

In 2008, Frank Lucero, a glaucoma patient [glaucoma can impair eyesight and sometimes causes blindness], was serving time for a parole violation at the California Institution for Men in Chino when he started experiencing nausea and severe headaches. He filed a request to see the doctor, and after four months had still not received his glaucoma medication. The prison eventually approved a visit with an ophthalmologist, then cancelled it. Mr. Lucero appealed, but his appeal was denied by the Chief Medical Officer. His glaucoma became more serious and "his eyeball exploded" according to a lawsuit filed against the prison system for willful neglect. The prison authorities maintain that Mr. Lucero received "appropriate care in a timely manner" (Small, 2010).

Experience with substandard medical care in prison often makes it more difficult for people to access health care services after they have been released. Formerly incarcerated people may expect to be treated poorly by health care professionals in any setting, and this may lead to delaying or avoiding medical attention when in need. A key role of CHWs and other frontline providers is to help ensure that formerly incarcerated clients are supported in their efforts to access quality health care.

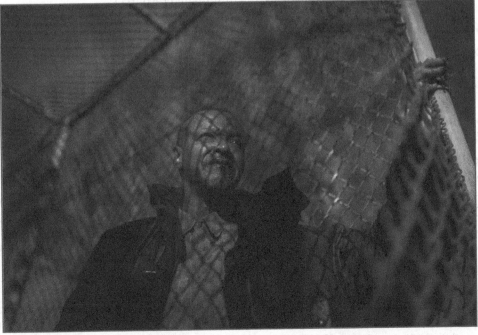

Incarceration continues to impact people's health long after they are released from prison.

IMMIGRATION DETENTION

Approximately 400,000 people are held in immigration detention facilities each year in highly restrictive conditions, even though most have no criminal records (Physicians for Human Rights, 2011). They are confined with little access to their families or outside legal support, and are often subjected to substandard medical and mental health care. As a result, their health can deteriorate very quickly. Medical care in immigration detention centers has come under increased scrutiny in the past several years because of the high number of deaths in U.S. Immigration and Customs Enforcement (ICE) custody (Physicians for Human Rights, 2011).

MENTAL HEALTH

As social services have been cut across the United States, and mental illness and homelessness have become increasingly criminalized, jails and prisons have become the primary psychiatric facilities in the United States. More than 700,000 people with severe mental illnesses are admitted to U.S. jails and prisons every year (James & Glaze, 2006). It is estimated that one in six U.S. prisoners has a mental health condition; and one out of ten state prisoners is on psychotropic drugs (Donohoe, 2006). Approximately three out of four prisoners have a history of substance abuse (James & Glaze, 2006). Mass incarceration is directly linked to our failure to develop sound public policies that provide access to quality and affordable mental health and drug treatment services to those in need.

> *Prisoners are in double jeopardy for posttraumatic stress disorder (PTSD). On average, their preincarceration backgrounds include much more trauma than the average person experiences, and then when they go to prison new traumas await them, possibly including beatings, sexual assault, and/or time spent in segregation. Harsh prison conditions and new traumas that occur behind bars are more difficult to cope with because of the past history of multiple traumas. (Kupers, 2005)*

Prisoners who are survivors of trauma often suffer "breakdowns" or become suicidal while incarcerated. Solitary confinement units, like the sensory deprivation environments that were studied by psychologists in the 1960s, often induce psychosis, especially in prisoners who have histories of mental illness or a predisposition to psychiatric breakdown (Grassian & Friedman, 1986). While those in solitary represent only 5 percent of the prison population, they account for almost half of the suicides in prison (Drucker, 2011).

When treatment services are available in jails and prisons, their quality is often questionable. A community standard of psychological counseling and therapy is virtually unheard of in most jails and prisons, and most people with serious mental health problems who are incarcerated leave prison more damaged than when they entered.

In general, people often leave prison sicker than when they went in, physically and psychologically. They come home needing more help, placing increased demands on their families and communities—communities that often are already struggling with health inequalities and diminished resources.

SOCIAL CONDITIONS IN PRISON

Since the goal of rehabilitation has largely been abandoned in favor of an openly punitive approach in American penal institutions, the culture of prisons is built on control over the prisoner. Prison culture is designed to diminish a prisoner's self-worth. All privacy is denied, as is any control over the most mundane aspects of life: when and what to eat, when to make a phone call or take a shower, when to read a book, when to have a conversation with another person. Extremely overcrowded facilities and budget crises have led to the dismantling of most meaningful educational and vocational programs in prison, including drug treatment programs.

The psychological impacts of incarceration are long-standing and carry over into the re-entry process. In many prisons, fear defines a prisoner's day-to-day existence, leading to a kind of hypervigilance that may continue after they are released to the community. Many prisoners work hard to develop a "prison mask," cultivating an ability to hide their feelings, sometimes at risk of extreme alienation, from themselves and others. Prisoners have to face isolation, literally and psychologically, from family, friends, and community as part of incarceration. The fracturing of these bonds contributes to depression and makes reintegration into the community a significant challenge.

Women prisoners face additional problems. A government study revealed that a majority of women in state prison (57 percent) reported a history of physical or sexual abuse (Harlow, 1999). The environment of most women's prisons extends that history of abuse. Women prisoners are subject to strip searches, pat searches by male guards, and degrading and sexually explicit language from guards on a daily basis. This sexualized environment contributes to worsening mental health and post-traumatic stress disorder (PTSD) for many women, especially for survivors of violence and abuse. In the words of one female prisoner, "the prison just took up where my abusive boyfriend left off" (Harlow, 1999). Very few prisons offer support or treatment for survivors of trauma (Covington, 2003).

Transgender, gender-non-conforming and intersex prisoners are visible targets for homophobic and transphobic discrimination and abuse within prisons by the administration, guards and other prisoners. Prisons are sex-segregated; authorities typically house prisoners according to their birth-assigned sex and/or genitalia, and often refuse to recognize their gender identities. While some transgender prisoners may choose to be isolated in protective custody, many are isolated against their will. Regardless of placement, transgender prisoners report being subjected to humiliation, verbal harassment, sexual and physical assault, and rape. In addition to being subjected to the inadequate medical care suffered by most prisoners, transgender prisoners are often denied hormones and other related treatments that affirm their gender identity (Sylvia Rivera Law Project, 2007).

15.3 The Impact of Incarceration on Families and Communities

The multigenerational impacts of mass incarceration reverberate in our communities, especially communities of color. The war on drugs has taken a particular toll on the health and well-being of whole families as more and more women are removed from the community: The number of incarcerated women has increased by 750 percent between 1980 and 2006 (Thayer, 2004, pp. 10–13). In 2007, 1.7 million children in the United States had a parent in prison, leaving them at risk for entering the foster care system; 70 percent were children of color (Mauer, Nellis, & Schirmir, 2009). The human cost of the war on drugs is beyond calculation: families are torn apart, human potential is wasted, and whole communities are permanently marginalized.

Families are affected financially and emotionally when someone is in prison. As a society, we recognize that children who grow up with safety and stability have a better chance to become healthy adults, but we fail to recognize that the criminal justice system often undermines these outcomes. Children of incarcerated parents suffer humiliation and shame. They often experience feelings of loss, abandonment, and extreme anxiety, and these feelings are more prominent when incarcerated parents are not able to see their children—a situation that holds true for approximately half the women in prison (American Civil Liberties Union, 2005).

Maintaining family ties through phone calls and visiting makes it much less likely that the parent will return to prison and, in most cases, is a benefit to the children's sense of well-being. Malcolm, who was four at the time of his mother's arrest, describes visiting his mother in prison:

> We made the most of each visit that we had. My mom was very special about trying to give time to each little child. Like for my sister, she would sit there and braid her hair while she had her little private time to talk to her.... I remember her pushing me on a swing. Me showing her my muscles, even though I didn't have any. Just me being relaxed and having fun with my mother is what I remember most. And me realizing how much I missed her towards the end of the visit, when someone would tell us we had to say goodbye.

> I couldn't even begin to express to you in words how fulfilling that was to my soul to give my mother a hug. For her to give me a kiss. For me to sit in her lap. If I hadn't been able to do that, I would have felt very empty then, as a child, and maybe now as well....

> Because I didn't have that permanent separation—I always had contact in some form, whether it was writing or phone calls or visits, with my mother—I understand the strength of a family. When it's hard times, you stick together. And that was just a hard time. (San Francisco Children of Incarcerated Parents Partnership, 2005)

Yet many children in Malcolm's situation lose the relationship to their parents forever. The Federal Adoption and Safe Families Act mandates that any parent who has not had custody of their child for 15 out of the previous 22 months can have their parental rights automatically terminated, forever breaking family bonds. The children are subject to placement in foster care if no relative who is judged suitable is able to assume custody while their parent is imprisoned. Because of disproportionate incarceration rates in communities of color, these policies mean that Black and Latino children are much more likely to lose family ties and become wards of the state.

"By taking children from their imprisoned parents on a permanent basis, simply because they are imprisoned, we have effectively transformed parental incarceration into a mechanism for permanent family disintegration and dissolution" (Drucker, 2011). The failure of child protective agencies to protect children whose parents are caught in the system is well publicized. Individuals who were in foster care experience higher rates of physical and mental health problems than the general population and suffer from not being able to trust (McCann, James, Wilson, & Dunn, 1996). This cycle puts children at an increased risk of incarceration themselves; recent studies show that a child with a parent in prison is six times more likely to be imprisoned than his or her peers without an incarcerated parent (Weaver, 2001).

Antonio's Story

When I was four years old, my mother started doing drugs. She used to be in and out of jail, and then she started going to prison when I was seven years old. That's when I first got taken from her. Her friends took me to social services, dropped me off, left me there.

I've been in about 18 different group homes since then, and three or four foster homes. I don't care how bad whatever we were going through, I still wanted to be with my mom. . . . One foster home I was in, I called the lady my grandmother, 'cause she took care of me. She always made sure that I got in touch with my mom. Even if my mom was locked up and tryin' to call collect, she could call there. My grandmother knew that mattered in my life.

The other places, they didn't care. There was only a couple of people that I lived with that actually took me to see my mom.

In the group homes, they knew my mom was in jail and they would just tell me, "Oh, it's gonna be alright." But they don't know how I feel because they're not going through it.

(San Francisco Children of Incarcerated Parents Partnership, 2005)

More and more grandparents are raising grandchildren while their own children are incarcerated, straining their finances and taxing their own health. Relative caregivers often receive less financial support than foster parents who are unrelated; sometimes they receive no support at all. Many seniors live on the edge financially, and assuming full responsibility for their grandchildren can drive the entire family deeper into poverty.

CASE STUDY   Sonia

10-year-old Sonia comes into a community clinic because of severe asthma attacks. Sonia is accompanied by her grandmother. During the intake interview, you learn that Sonia's mother was recently sentenced to four years in prison. Sonia lost her housing and health insurance, and had to transfer to a new school when she came to live with her grandmother.

- How would this information guide your work as a CHW?
- How might Sonia be affected by her mother's incarceration?
- Besides making sure she had her medical needs addressed, what else could you do as a CHW to support Sonia and her grandmother?

Most people coming home from jail or prison return to communities that suffer from the impacts of racism and poverty. They experience a lack of affordable housing and educational opportunities, and high unemployment rates. While all people living in poverty suffer these conditions, formerly incarcerated people face additional challenges, including the stigma of incarceration and the many legal barriers to re-entry. These interlocking barriers have a profound impact on the family and the community at large. They create instability, homelessness, and unemployment; they make family reunification difficult and increase the likelihood that families will remain fractured. For immigrant families, parental incarceration may mean permanent separation with no possibility of direct contact between parents and children in the future. These policies make it harder for people to stay clean and sober, and to resist returning to illegal activity to support themselves. Parents who want to reunify with their children often find themselves caught in a vicious cycle, defeated in their efforts to rebuild their families.

Incarceration impacts the entire community in the form of broad scale economic hardships and destabilization, increased risk of exposure to disease, and weakened social networks. High incarceration rates take an economic toll on the whole community. Imprisonment means a loss of income to the family left behind, and reduces the future earnings of people newly released from prison, whose prospects for employment are diminished. Even a short stay in jail can lead to loss of a job and homelessness (Travis, Solomon, & Waul, 2001). For many years, incarceration was regarded first and foremost as a criminal justice issue. But as the negative social effects of increasingly harsh sentencing policies become more evident, mass incarceration is also recognized as a public health issue, and a significant social determinant of health. Policies that were supposed to create public safety have in fact brought extreme economic hardship and social instability to communities most affected. And they have dramatically increased the existing health inequalities based on race, gender, and socioeconomic status.

- *Can you think of other ways that incarceration harms families and communities?*

- *How has incarceration impacted the communities that you belong to and/or work with?*

15.4 The Challenges of Re-entry or Coming Home

As people return home from prison (**re-entry**) with the intention of rebuilding their lives and reuniting with their families and communities, they face systemic legal barriers. Accessing basic needs such as stable housing, employment, and benefits becomes a major hurdle once a person has been convicted, especially of a drug-related offense. These postconviction penalties are not part of anyone's original sentence; they are additional, enduring discriminatory punishments that often contribute to **recidivism** or return to jail or prison. On the one hand, policy makers urge formerly incarcerated people to reintegrate themselves into society, and on the other hand public policies create significant barriers to successful reintegration.

> *Once you are labeled a felon, the old forms of discrimination—employment discrimination, housing discrimination, denial of the right to vote, denial of educational opportunity, denial of food stamps and other public benefits, and exclusion from jury service are suddenly legal. As a criminal, you have scarcely more rights . . . than a black man living in Alabama at the height of Jim Crow. We have not ended racial caste in America, we have merely redesigned it. (Alexander, 2010)*

HOUSING

People who are released from jail or prison, especially those returning to their communities after a lengthy sentence, face a very basic challenge of where to live. Few programs and services connect those recently released from jail or prison to housing. Public policies discriminate against the formerly incarcerated, making it more difficult for them to find and maintain a stable home.

The federal "one-strike" housing policy bans anyone with a drug-related or violent offense from living in Section 8 or other federally assisted housing, and the entire family can be evicted if a formerly incarcerated family member is found living there. In reality, this means that some people are forced to abandon formerly incarcerated children or partners or risk eviction and homelessness. While public housing authorities can make case-by-case decisions, the threat of losing housing is devastating to families. Many landlords now ask about history of incarceration on housing applications and, because of social stigma, are more likely to choose tenants without prior convictions. Often, homeless shelters will screen out and turn away people with certain types of criminal histories, leaving them no option but to live on the streets. Without the possibility of stable housing, it's very difficult for former prisoners to rebuild their lives.

EMPLOYMENT

Formerly incarcerated people often have difficulty finding work, sometimes because there are legal prohibitions against their employment, and sometimes because employers are reluctant to hire someone with a criminal record.

Most job applications include a "box" on the form that asks if you've ever been convicted of a felony; answering "yes" creates an immediate barrier to being considered for employment. One survey found that over 65 percent of employers said they would not hire someone with a felony conviction (Travis, Solomon, & Waul, 2001).

Many states will not allow someone with a conviction to work in certain jobs; this is especially true in the areas of health care, education, and child care. One study showed that one year after release, approximately 60 percent of former prisoners were not employed in the regular labor market (Travis, Solomon, & Waul, 2001). With diminished access to employment opportunities, formerly incarcerated people face a significant barrier to building a stable and secure life.

BAN ON FINANCIAL AID FOR EDUCATION

In 1998, Congress passed a law banning federal loans to students who were convicted of selling or possessing illegal drugs, further restricting access to education. For people newly released from prison who are trying to further their education, this poses yet another barrier to creating a stable and productive life. Given the disproportionate number of people of color in prisons, this policy has a significant and adverse impact on educational opportunities for low-income students and students of color.

PUBLIC BENEFITS

A person coming home from prison will encounter barriers in accessing public benefits that may be critical to rebuilding their families. The federal government passed a lifetime ban on Temporary Assistance to Needy Families (TANF) and food stamps for people with felony drug convictions regardless of their rehabilitation and recovery. States are permitted to opt out of the ban.

DISENFRANCHISEMENT

Over four million Americans have lost their voting rights due to a felony conviction; 35 states prohibit felons from voting while on probation/parole. This is far from the norm in other countries, like Germany, that actively encourage former prisoners to vote as a strategy for promoting successful reintegration into society.

Michelle Alexander writes:

> *If shackling former prisoners with a lifetime of debt and authorizing discrimination against them in employment, housing, education and public benefits is not enough to send the message that they are not wanted and not considered full citizens, then stripping voting rights from those labeled criminals surely gets the point across. (Alexander, 2010)*

FAMILY REUNIFICATION

Often one of the most important goals for formerly incarcerated people is to rebuild relationships with their family. While many are successful, others struggle to reconnect. The children of incarcerated parents are often deeply affected by the experience and may wrestle with feelings of confusion, anger, fear, and distrust. Formerly incarcerated parents may be affected by lasting guilt and doubts about how to reconnect and rebuild trust with their children.

Parents who go to prison are at risk for losing their children permanently because of the Adoption and Safe Families Act. It's important to remember that both children and parents are harmed when families are torn apart, and that most children want to maintain a relationship with their parents, even under difficult circumstances.

Many parents owe child support to the government for the period of time when their children were in foster care, and newly released parents can find themselves in overwhelming debt. On average, parents leaving prison owe $23,000 or more in back child support payments. Since their wages will be garnished when they find a job, this policy drives many people into the underground economy.

There is a need for community-based services and programs that support families scarred by incarceration to build and sustain healthier relationships.

Please watch the following digital story ▶ about the journey that one man took from prison to establishing a career as a CHW.

- What did you learn from Emory's story?
- How may Emory's story inform or influence your work as a CHW?

EMORY'S STORY: HOPE AND TRANSFORMATION

⌘ *http://youtu.be/ oSx1OPt6r8M*

STIGMA AND DISCRIMINATION

In some ways, the systemic barriers to re-entry after incarceration are not the worst part of coming home from prison. For many, it's the social stigma and discrimination that comes with being labeled "criminal"—a kind of social exile that can become a permanent exclusion from the rest of the community. As a society we are bombarded with negative, highly racialized images of incarcerated people, which creates a pervasive sense of suspicion and automatic distrust of someone who has done prison time. Michelle Alexander describes this with painful accuracy:

> *Criminals, it turns out, are the one social group in America we have permission to hate. In "colorblind" America, criminals are the new whipping boys. They are entitled to no respect and little moral concern. . . . criminals today are deemed a characterless and purposeless people, deserving of our collective scorn and contempt. . . . Hundreds of years ago our nation put those considered less than human in shackles; less than a hundred years ago, we relegated them to the other side of town; today we put them in cages. Once released, they find that a heavy and cruel hand has been laid upon them. (Alexander, 2010)*

Formerly incarcerated people often experience isolation. This feeling of being permanently exiled by housing officials, employers, neighbors, and sometimes family members is described this way:

> *The shame and stigma that follows you for the rest of your life—that is the worst. It is not just the job denial but the look that flashes across the face of a potential employer when he notices that "the box" has been checked— the way he suddenly refuses to look you in the eye. It is not merely the denial of the housing application but the shame of being a grown man who has to beg his grandmother for a place to sleep at night. It is not simply the denial of the right to vote but the shame one feels when a co-worker innocently asks, "Who you gonna vote for on Tuesday?" (Alexander, 2010)*

The stigma and social isolation attached to imprisonment often create a deep sense of shame and self-hatred that is experienced not only by the former prisoner, but by their family as well. Fear of negative stereotypes and judgments can lead to silence and the denial of prison experience. Family members sometimes feel they have to lie about the whereabouts of an incarcerated loved one to avoid the negative judgments of teachers, ministers, friends, and neighbors. This collective silence makes true reintegration and healing nearly impossible.

In this context, the role of a culturally sensitive CHW becomes critical. By refusing to reinforce such stigma, by providing nondiscriminatory care to formerly incarcerated people, CHWs can be part of creating a different, more inclusive culture that does not demonize an entire population and reaffirms the humanity of people who have been to prison.

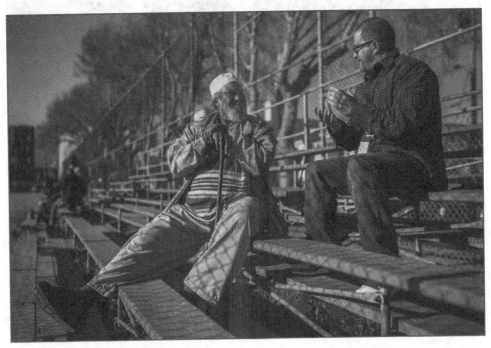

A CHW and a client find a place to talk.

15.5 Best Practices and Emerging Models

POST-RELEASE WELLNESS PROJECT (PRWP)

The Post-Release Wellness Project (PRWP) was developed to meet the health needs of prisoners coming home to the community. Based in San Francisco, the PRWP was a partnership between the Transitions Clinic Network (*www.transitionsclinic.org*), the nonprofit advocacy group Legal Services for Prisoners with Children (*www.prisonerswithchildren.org*), and City College of San Francisco's Health Education Department (*www.ccsf.edu/hlthed*). The partnership integrates primary health care services, case management, advocacy and empowerment opportunities, and access to educational and career preparation for formerly incarcerated individuals in the United States and Puerto Rico. The project developed the nation's first college-based vocational education certificate to train front-line public health providers to work with incarcerated and formerly incarcerated people, the Post Prison Health Worker certificate. The PRWP has a community advisory board that guides their work.

TRANSITIONS CLINIC NETWORK (TCN)

The Transitions Clinic Network (TCN) is a growing network of clinics throughout the U.S. and in Puerto Rico dedicated to providing comprehensive primary and behavioral health care tailored to patients returning home from prison and jail. TCN aims to avoid unnecessary emergency department visits, improve health outcomes, and address patients' social determinants of health to ensure healthy reintegration into the community.

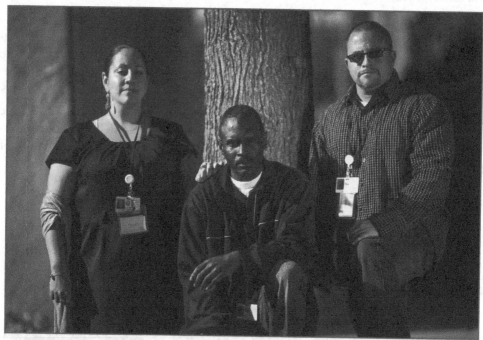

CHWs from the San Francisco Transitions Clinic are dedicated to promoting the health of formerly incarcerated people.

The first Transitions Clinic was established in San Francisco in 2006 and is based in the Southeast Health Center in Bayview Hunter's Point. Since then the TCN model has been adopted in over 14 community clinics across the country in neighborhoods highly impacted by incarceration.

The services at TCN support all aspects of a healthy reintegration in a community-based and patient-centered setting. Patients receive primary care, behavioral health services such as psychotherapy, substance abuse counseling, and opiate addiction treatment with suboxone, connections to housing and employment, and can be referred onsite for dentistry, podiatry, and pharmacy centers.

The TCN also creates jobs for people with histories of incarceration by integrating previously incarcerated CHWs into the clinical team. The CHWs meet newly released prisoners where they are—the parole office, their homes, community centers, and faith-based organizations—to link them into primary care early on and avoid unnecessary emergency department utilization. These CHWs are specially trained to identify the highest risk individuals returning to the community, and then to provide case management and health education as well as referrals to specialty and social services.

Despite pervasive mistrust of the medical system within the re-entry population, the presence of CHWs with a history of incarceration on the clinical team engenders a high level of trust for previously incarcerated patients. Because CHWs are personally familiar with the process of re-entry, Transitions patients know they won't be judged and stereotyped because of their convictions. Similarly, CHWs are invaluable to the clinical team, helping to close the communication gap between patients and their providers. Dr. Emily Wang, one of the clinic's founders, described Ron, their first CHW this way: "He has proven himself over and over to be an excellent guide to the health care system and an excellent liaison to our patients, because he has a deep understanding of what our patients are going through" (Willmott, 2013). Cities around the country are turning to the Transitions Clinic program as a model of successful primary care, integrated behavioral care, and social services that promote the health and well-being of people coming home from prison. CHWs are at the heart of this model.

> *They don't judge you—they treat you like a human being—like you are still a person. That's something that prison, they take away from you and when you get out, society takes that away from you. With Transitions Clinic that doesn't matter, they treat you like a human being. (Transitions patient, quoted in Willmott & Robinson, 2008)*

To read more about the TCN, visit their website at: *www.transitionsclinic.org.*

The following videos ▶ **were created by CHWs working at Transitions Clinics, and by patients.** All CHWs hired by transitions clinics have a history of incarceration. These videos share their stories, and how they came to be CHWs.

As you watch any of these short digital stories, consider the following questions:

- What did you learn from the story?
- How may these stories influence your work as a CHW?

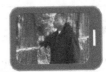

RON'S STORY: A GRANDMOTHER'S LOVE

🔗 *http://youtu.be/ ePDOB5OtjzM*

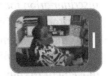

JUANITA'S STORY: EVERYONE HAS PURPOSE IN LIFE

🔗 *http://youtu.be/ _AfVE1DCEVc*

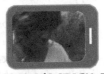

TRACY'S STORY: FROM DELIVERANCE TO RECOVERY

🔗 *http://youtu.be/ KEVRnTTGQlw*

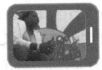

JERMILA'S STORY: A STEP FORWARD

🔗 *http://youtu.be/ vYOsRcrnZ1M*

PROJECT BRIDGE

Project Bridge in Rhode Island is a federally funded program that assists prisoners living with HIV disease in their transition to society through intensive case management. Patients are treated upon release by the same doctors who treat them in prison. Project Bridge offers "continuity of person" by having a social worker connect with clients before their release, develop a discharge plan that includes both medical and social goals, and accompany them to their medical appointments in the community. Again, a strong human relationship is central to this project's success. Evaluations show that this model of co-located doctors and intensive case management can lead to stabilized health, a high rate of medical care engagement, and a decrease in the rate of people returning to prison (Yeung, 2009).

HAMPDEN COUNTY

Hampden County in Massachusetts also uses the co-located model. The project operates a Federal Health Clinic in the jail and then links prisoners who are about to be released to clinics in their neighborhood. As with Project Bridge, the patients see the same doctors and case managers upon release as they saw in jail, thereby having continuity of care (Massachusetts Public Health Association, 2006).

Ban the Box: Preventing Employment Discrimination

One of the most inspiring examples of community organizing to fight the discrimination of formerly incarcerated people is the work of All of Us or None. The "Ban the Box" campaign, described below, has taken root all across the country. For more information, please go to www.prisonerswithchildren.org/our-projects/allofus-or-none/

All of Us or None is a national organizing initiative started by formerly incarcerated people to fight against discrimination faced after release and to fight for the human rights of prisoners. We are determined to win full restoration of our civil and human rights after release from prison. Our goal is to build political power in the communities most affected by mass incarceration and the growth of the Prison Industrial Complex. The emergence of All of Us or None is a concrete manifestation of the people most affected by an issue building a movement to combat it.

Our "Ban the Box" campaign calls for the elimination of the questions about past convictions on initial public employment applications. Our aim is to win policy change through grassroots mobilizations, and to build a political movement of formerly incarcerated activists. This campaign will allow us to target and challenge the many "boxes" on a variety of applications (i.e., employment, housing, social services, etc.) we are required to check that supports structural discrimination against formerly incarcerated people.

Banning the box on public employment applications will contribute to public safety because it will promote stable employment in our communities. Communities of color and poor communities already are targeted by mass imprisonment, racial profiling, school closures, and low employment rates. People coming out of prison or county jails need to be able to feed their families, pay rent, and reunite with their families, and return their lives as productive members of the community. People with jobs and stable community lives are much less likely to return to committing crimes in order to survive.

15.6 The Role of CHWs in Promoting the Health of Formerly Incarcerated Clients and Their Communities

Being released from prison is a highly vulnerable time for most people. A study showed that people newly released from prison are 13 times more likely to die than members of the general public in the first two weeks after release. The principal causes of death include drug overdose, cardiovascular disease, homicide, and suicide (Binswanger, Krueger, & Steiner, 2009).

Ron Sanders: Basically, it's scary getting out. You have nowhere to go, you have $200 if you have that. It's scary. And if they make it to us [The San Francisco Transitions Clinic], we make sure we take care of them. It's a long road between San Quentin Prison and San Francisco, there's a lot in between here and there.

Unemployment, lack of education, poverty, unstable housing, substance abuse, PTSD, depression, and other chronic health conditions are some of the challenges faced by people released from jail or prison. The transition from prison to community can be emotionally overwhelming as people begin to readjust and rebuild relationships, especially with family members. To compound the situation, former prisoners face stigma as well as the multiple systemic barriers to rebuilding their lives. Postconviction penalties create formidable barriers to employment and receipt of supportive services such as food stamps and public housing. For many, the immediate struggle for survival takes precedence over other concerns.

Because they are trusted members of local communities, CHWs play an important role in creating a supportive re-entry process. Many CHWs have first-hand knowledge of the impacts of incarceration, and many are already serving formerly incarcerated people and their families. This experience puts them in a unique position to help someone transitioning from prison to the community. Former prisoners can relate to CHWs as people who have "been there, done that," whose similar life experience and roots in the community help to establish a trust that may not be there otherwise.

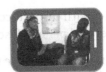

FIRST MEETING BETWEEN A PATIENT AND CHW: INTERVIEW

 http://youtu.be/ OrfXKN8lgxA

Please watch the following video 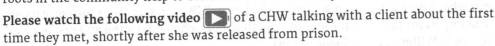 of a CHW talking with a client about the first time they met, shortly after she was released from prison.

Ron Sanders: We know where they come from; we've been there, done that. We also know the barriers, the doors closing on you. . . . We've faced those same barriers, and we've overcome them. [Our clients] respect the realness, they respect the dignity, they're not a number.

Juanita Alvarado: Having that connection [inside and outside prison] is important. We write our patients [before they get out], we have somebody who works inside the prison at San Quentin. Just seeing that friendly face inside the prison, then seeing us here, in the field, that's comforting to them. They see our faces all over the place. They know that we're going to make that appointment for them when they get out, and help them take steps to be successful . . . it makes them feel like they're cared about, truly cared about. They're not just a number, not just another parolee coming out. People make mistakes, it's OK to make mistakes . . . we're not here to judge.

As a CHW, you are likely to be one of the strongest bridges between a client and the social support necessary to rebuild a life after prison. For example, many former prisoners come to the health care system with a great deal of distrust and anxiety. A number have suffered at the hands of an incompetent prison health system, and that history of abuse makes it difficult for them to trust health care providers in the community. By working with a client respectfully and treating them with dignity, you can lay the basis for a relationship of trust with new health care and other service providers.

> *The most help is the listening and the dignity. Sometimes we work with clients who've been in the system so long that they're not treated with respect, and all they need is someone to recognize that they're human beings and they have values and listen to them. Once you give them that, they can take it from there. That first step is self-esteem. (Anonymous Community Health Worker, in Becker, Kpvacj, & Gronseth, 2004)*

Please watch the following video interview 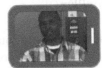 with a CHW who has a history of incarceration talking about his work with clients who are coming home from prison.

CHALLENGING STIGMA

Prisoners are one of the most stigmatized groups in our society; there is a sense of shame associated with incarceration that can be extremely damaging. The experience of incarceration often begins a downward cycle of economic dependence, isolation, homelessness, depression, post-traumatic stress, substance abuse, and other physical and mental health problems.

A CHW WITH A HISTORY OF INCARCERATION: CHW INTERVIEW

http://youtu.be/ PfBJ9GCvkKk

The first steps of acceptance and understanding by a CHW are important for an individual coming home from prison (Willmott & van Olphen, 2005). A culturally aware and competent CHW who approaches a newly released prisoner with respect, compassion, and a nonjudgmental stance can make a significant difference. One formerly incarcerated person described their positive experience with a health provider:

> *Just to have someone who wasn't afraid to be in the same room with me, who wasn't afraid to touch me, who didn't judge me, made me feel like I wanted to come back. The doctor I saw in prison wore a mask and gloves the whole time, even though I wasn't contagious. He sat behind his desk and refused to touch me, even though I had a lump on my breast. (Anonymous, quoted in Willmott & Robinson, 2007)*

A formerly incarcerated patient who visited a health care clinic staffed by a CHW who was also a formerly incarcerated person, remarked: "The important thing for me was to be with people who understand and respect you" (Transitions Clinic patient, quoted in Willmott & Robinson, 2008).

Juanita Alvarado: One [patient] was in the hospital, and we were right there. They didn't have any family, they didn't have anybody. We were there. And we're right there when they go back to jail, we're there visiting them. We're the ones they can call.

Ron Sanders: I have two words [for CHWs working with former prisoners]: *passion* and being *genuine*. If you're not genuine, they'll read you in a heartbeat and turn straight off on you. They won't even deal with you if they feel you're not genuine and you don't care and it's just a job to you. You have to really care, and you have to have passion.

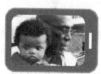

ERNEST'S STORY

🔗 *http://youtu.be/ 2HVB_ZDRs1s*

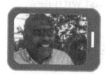

LEE'S STORY: CHANGE

🔗 *http://youtu.be/ VElbOb7BkmQ*

The following videos ▶ highlight the impacts of incarceration on health, and the value for patients of being able to access quality health care services at an agency that truly supports their return from prison.

UNDERSTANDING OUR OWN VALUES AND BELIEFS

Our values and beliefs influence our interactions with others and the services we provide. In order to effectively serve formerly incarcerated clients, it is essential to reflect on our own beliefs about prisoners and the prison system. This is particularly important because we are all constantly exposed to negative, racialized images of prisoners that paint a biased picture of crime and the criminal justice system. Take a few minutes to consider the following questions and reflect upon your answers:

- What images and thoughts come to mind when you think about people who have been to prison?

- Do you have certain expectations about the behavior of people who have been in prison? Where do those expectations come from?

- How do you feel about the idea of working with formerly incarcerated clients? If you knew what your client was in prison for, would that influence your ability to provide compassionate and unbiased service? Would it vary according to the offense they were convicted of? If so, why?

- Do you have personal experience with the prison system (yourself, a friend or family member)? If so, how did this experience impact the person who was incarcerated? How did it impact their family?

- What are your beliefs about the ability of a formerly incarcerated person to create a positive and meaningful life? What are your beliefs about the types of contributions that formerly incarcerated people can make to their community?

- What can you do to increase your knowledge and skills in order to work effectively with formerly incarcerated clients?

RECOGNIZING THE CHALLENGES OF COMING HOME

Keep in mind that the first few weeks after release are the most risky for people coming home from prison. A CHW who understands the tremendous legal barriers for those coming home from prison will be in a position to view her patients' lives in a holistic way. They will recognize the social aspects of the person's situation, be able to offer appropriate resources and, most important, will remain patient and compassionate during the process of the client's long journey home.

Some ex-prisoners and their families may be reluctant to access government agencies for assistance. Using a harm reduction approach, CHWs can effectively support formerly incarcerated clients to address multiple issues, both medical and social, and to navigate complex and sometimes overwhelming systems of services.

Ron Sanders: I didn't put so much emphasis on the health aspect in the beginning, when I was a drug counselor . . . then I started to see that if I got them housing, employment, education, that their health outcomes will be better.

MAKE CONSCIOUS CHOICES ABOUT THE LANGUAGE YOU USE

Many formerly incarcerated clients expect you to be just one more person who judges them as somehow less worthy of respect than people who have not been incarcerated. They may expect you to use the same stigmatizing language that they hear from others on a daily basis: convict, felon, ex-offender, criminal, and so on. Your use of these terms may present a significant and lasting barrier to developing a positive working relationship with a formerly incarcerated client, and may even keep them from accessing essential programs and services.

All of your clients deserve the same respect, including the right not be called out of their name or referred to with language that they find offensive. Ask your client how they would like to be called (such as Thomas or Tom or Mr. Daniels), and honor this request. If it is appropriate to refer to their history of incarceration, we recommend that you use language such as "formerly incarcerated." Most important, if you make a mistake and use a term that you suspect or can tell is uncomfortable or offensive to your client, apologize in a sincere fashion and do your best not to repeat the mistake.

What Do YOU Think?

- *Have you or your family members ever been called names that you find offensive?*

- *Have services providers (physicians, social workers, teachers, outreach workers, etc.) ever used such language with you?*

- *What would it be like if an important service provider constantly refered to you by a name or label that you found offensive?*

A CLIENT-CENTERED APPROACH

Client-centered concepts and skills, including motivational interviewing, should guide your work with *all* clients. Keep in mind that people who have been incarcerated have had personal freedom and control taken away, often for a prolonged period of time. Do your best not to replicate this dynamic by taking control away from your client through your practice. Watch out for any tendencies to undermine a client's control by directing conversations or sessions towards a specific question, topic or outcome or, for example, by trying to influence an action plan or telling a client what you think their priorities and choices should be. Remember that client-centered practice aims to enhance the autonomy and capacity of all clients to better manage their lives and promote their own health and welfare. Use your OARS and other motivational interviewing skills (see Chapter 9) to support clients to explore their own experience, ideas, values, and feeling; to choose what to talk about during your time together and what to keep private; to determine their own health goals and the steps they want to take to reach those goals. Remember the Big Eyes, Big Ears, and Small Mouth of the effective CHW (Chapter 7). Don't dominate conversations and interactions with clients. Listen deeply to what the client chooses to share with you and build from there.

Try to be aware of your own desire to know certain information about the lives of your clients. Remember that we don't have a right to know why someone was incarcerated, how many times they were incarcerated, or for how long they have been incarcerated. Prying into any aspect of a client's life, especially when they have indicated that they wish to keep it private, is only likely to push them away, and has the potential to do them harm.

- *What other aspects of client-centered practice are important when working with formerly incarcerated clients?*

What Do YOU? Think ?

Please watch the following video 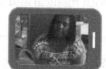 role play of a CHW working with a client who is coming home from prison. In this role play, the CHW does not do a good job in demonstrating client-centered practice.

- What mistakes does the CHW make in this role play?
- How might the CHW's action impact this client?
- What would you do differently to demonstrate client-centered skills in working with this client?

LISTENING TO A CLIENT'S PRIORITIES: ROLE PLAY, COUNTER

⏻ *http://youtu.be/ n96TZKnnhec*

ETHICAL DILEMMAS

Being a formerly incarcerated person can be a real asset for a CHW serving former prisoners, but it can also present some particular ethical challenges. In these circumstances, CHWs need to be able to confidently assert and maintain healthy professional boundaries (see Chapter 7). Ron and Juanita, CHWs at Transitions Clinic, describe their experiences this way:

> **Ron Sanders:** A lot of times you have to watch the ethical things. I have a few clients I actually did time with, I've known them way back. I did time with them, I got high with them. . . . I had to break away from that "prison thing" and focus on what I'm doing now. They'll try to tie me to that, like "You owe me," but I don't owe you. A lot of them have seen me at my worst, so this [seeing me as a professional health worker] is inspiring for them, too.

> **Juanita Alvarado:** A lot of our patients are people I did drugs with, or people I bought drugs from. They'll ask "you got a couple extra dollars" or "will you do a UA (urine analysis) for me?" . . . that's a big no-no, we won't go there. I'm not willing to sacrifice my job; I have children and I'm not willing to lose everything I worked hard for to do a favor. Those are some of the things we run into.

PROMOTING PARTNERSHIPS, ADVOCATING FOR CHANGE

In addition to assisting individuals with re-entry, CHWs are well positioned to shape re-entry programs and promote partnerships that build stronger, safer communities. Communities dramatically impacted by mass incarceration may feel an increased sense of powerlessness in the face of so much loss and instability. Community health workers can play a positive, empowering role by bringing people together to challenge the systemic factors that create ill health, and encourage community organizing to promote health and safety. For example, CHWs from the Transitions Clinic in San Francisco play an important role in the Community Advisory Board of the Post Prison Wellness Project. One of the CHWs also serves on the City's Safe Community Re-entry Council, a body appointed by the Mayor to encourage partnerships in order to better coordinate services for people coming home from prison.

Community health workers can become powerful agents for social change. The crisis of mass incarceration presents us with an opportunity for major policy changes, and frontline health workers have the potential to make a real difference in this movement towards social justice and equity. Again, the CHWs from Transitions offer us examples of the powerful role of frontline health workers in advocating for systems change. They have been vocal advocates for treatment over incarceration, challenging the food stamp ban for those convicted of drug offenses, and have testified about the regulations that make it impossible for people convicted of sex offenses to live within the confines of San Francisco.

Ron Sanders: Watching people turn their lives around, being productive, seeing people working, going to school . . . those are the biggest rewards. When they're housed, taking good care of their health, making their appointments, they're an asset to the community, instead of being against the community.

Juanita Alvarado: Being this role model for this population helps with my personal growth, to stay sober, to stay on track. Everybody around me wants to do the same thing, like "what did you *do*?" Because I was the person who was the addict, who tried to kill myself, who didn't give a damn about anybody. For people who know me, it's "wow, *she's doing it*, she's a professional." It brings tears and it warms my heart.

15.7 Continued Professional Development

Do you want to learn more about incarceration and its effect on our communities? Do you want to increase your knowledge and skills for working with formerly incarcerated clients and their families?

Here are some suggestions for how to enhance your professional skills:

- Become informed about conditions of confinement and the movement challenging mass incarceration.
- Invite a prisoners' rights activist to speak at your organization's function. A comprehensive list of organizations is available from the Prison Activist Resource Center.
- Volunteer with a prisoners' rights organization.
- Read and respond to newspaper stories. Write letters of encouragement for sympathetic editorials and challenge tough-on-crime op-eds.
- Keep informed about relevant bills/laws and contact your representative to voice your opinion.
- Challenge those around you who subscribe to stereotypes about prisoners.
- If you are an employer, consider hiring former prisoners for job vacancies.

This list was adapted from "Ten things you can do to support the struggle for prisoners' rights" compiled by Legal Services for Prisoners with Children (*www.prisonerswithchildren.org*)

And please remember always to listen deeply and learn from what your formerly incarcerated clients tell you. They will be your most important teachers.

- *What else could you do to increase your capacity to provide quality services to formerly incarcerated clients and communities?*

Please see the list of Additional Resources included at the end of this chapter.

Chapter Review

Please review the two case studies presented in this chapter featuring *Phyllis* and *Sonia*. Consider what your goals would be for working with each client. Do your best to answer the questions that accompany each case study.

In addition, please do your best to answer the following questions:

- How does incarceration influence the health of formerly incarcerated individuals? How does it influence the health of their families?

- Why do some professionals say that mass incarceration is a public health issue?

- What health conditions are most common among formerly incarcerated people?

- Why do some formerly incarcerated clients feel distrustful of the medical system? What risks does this pose for their health? How might you work to build the trust of such a client?

- How does stigma influence the health of newly released prisoners?

- What legal barriers to re-entry do newly released prisoners commonly face?

- Describe a best practice model for providing quality health care services to formerly incarcerated clients.

- Identify at least three changes to public policy that could better promote the health of formerly incarcerated people.

- What types of mistakes might CHWs make that could get in the way of establishing and maintaining an effective professional relationship with formerly incarcerated clients?

References

Alexander, M. (2010). *The new Jim Crow*. New York, NY: New Press.American Civil Liberties Union. (2005). *Caught in the Net: The impact of drug policies on women and families.* With The Brennan Center at NYU School of Law. Retrieved from *www.aclu.org/drug-law-reform/caught-net-impact-drug-policies-women-and-families*

Becker, J., Kpvacj, A., & Gronseth, D. (2004). Individual empowerment: How community health workers operationalize self-determination, self-sufficiency, and decision-making abilities of low-income mothers. *Journal of Community Psychology, 32*, 327–342.

Binswanger, I., Krueger, P., & Steiner, J. (2009). Prevalence of chronic medical conditions among jail and prison inmates in the United States compared with the general population. *Journal of Epidemiology and Community Health*. Retrieved from *http://jech.bmj.com/content/early/2009/07/30/jech.2009.090662*

Covington, S. (2003). A woman's journey home: Challenges for female offenders. In J. Tavis & M. Waul (Eds.), *Prisoners once removed: The impact of incarceration and re-entry on children, families, and communities* (pp. 67–103). Washington, DC: The Urban Institute Press.

Donohoe, M. (2006). Incarceration nation: Health and welfare in the prison system in the United States. *Medscape Ob/Gyn & Women's Health, 11*(1).

Drucker, E. (2011). *A plague of prisons: The epidemiology of mass incarceration in America*. New York, NY: New Press.

Drug Policy Alliance. (2011). Retrieved from *www.drugpolicy.org*

Flanagan, N. (2004). Transitional health care for offenders being released from United States prisons. *Canadian Journal of Nursing Research, 36*, 38–58.

Glaze, L. (2010). *Correctional populations in the United States, 2009*. Bureau of Justice Statistics. Washington, DC: U.S. Department of Justice. Retrieved from *http://bjs.ojp.usdoj.gov/index.cfm?ty=pbdetail&iid=2316*

Grassian, S., & Friedman, N. (1986). Effects of sensory deprivation in psychiatric seclusion and solitary confinement. *International Journal of Law and Psychiatry, 8*, 49–65.

Guard, D. (2008). *Clinton crime agenda shortsighted: May hurt poor and minorities, advocates say.* Retrieved from *http://stopthedrugwar.org/trenches/2008/apr/15/clinton_crime_agenda_shortsighte*

Harlow, C. (1999). *Prior abuse reported by inmates and probationers.* Bureau of Justice Statistics Selected Findings. Bureau of Justice Statistics. Washington, DC: U.S. Department of Justice. Retrieved from *www.bjs.gov/content/pub/pdf/parip.pdf*

Human Rights Watch. (2009). *Prison Nation.* Retrieved from *www.hrw.org/print/news/2009/04/09/prison-nation*

James, D., & Glaze, L. (2006). *Mental health problems of prison and jail inmates.* U.S. Department of Justice. Bureau of Justice Statistics Special Report. Washington, DC: Bureau of Justice Statistics. Retrieved from *http://bjs.gov/content/pub/pdf/mhppji.pdf*

Johnson R. C., & Raphael, S. (2005). The effects of male incarceration dynamics on AIDS infection rates among African-American women and men. *Journal of Law and Economics, 52,* 251–293.

King, R., & Mauer, M. (2002). *Distorted priorities: Drug offenders in state prisons.* Washington, DC: The Sentencing Project. Retrieved from *www.sentencingproject.org/doc/publications/dp_distortedpriorities.pdf*

Kupers, T. (2005). Schizophrenia, its treatment, and prisoner adjustment. In S. Stojkovic (Ed.), *Managing special populations in jails and prisons.* Kingston, NJ: Civic Research Institute.

Lincoln, T., Kennedy, S., Tuthill, R., Roberts, C., Conklin, T., & Hammett, T. (2006). Facilitators and barriers to continuing healthcare after jail: A community integrated program. *Journal of Ambulatory Care Management, 29,* 2–16.

Malcolm, B. (2011). The rise of methicillin-resistant Staphylococcus Aurous in United States correctional population. *Journal of Correctional Health Care, 17*(3), 254–265. Retrieved from *http://jcx.sagepub.com/content/17/3/254*

Massachusetts Public Health Association. (2006). *A public health model for correctional health care* [Hampden County]. Jamaica Plain, MA: Massachusetts Public Health Association. Retrieved from *www.mphaweb.org/PublicHealthModelforCorrectionalHealth.htm*

Maté, G. (2008). *In the realm of hungry ghosts.* Berkeley, CA: North Atlantic Books.

Mauer, M., Nellis, A., & Schirmir, S. (2009). *Incarcerated parents and their children—Trends, 1991–2007.* Washington, DC: The Sentencing Project. Retrieved from *www.sentencingproject.org/doc/publications/publications/inc_incarceratedparents.pdf*

McCann, J., James, A, Wilson, S, & Dunn, G. (1996). Prevalence of psychiatric disorders in young people in the care system. *BMJ (Clinical research ed.), 313*(7071), 1529–30.

Physicians for Human Rights. (2011). *Dual loyalties: The challenges of providing professional health care to immigration detainees.* Retrieved from *http://physiciansforhumanrights.org/issues/torture/asylum/dual-loyalties-immigration-detention.html*

Plata v. Schwarzenegger. (2005). *Findings of fact and conclusions of law re: appointment of receiver.* U.S. District Court for the Northern District of California. Retrieved from *www.prisonlaw.com/pdfs/receiver.pdf*

San Francisco Children of Incarcerated Parents Partnership (SFCIPP). (2005). *Children of incarcerated parents: A bill of rights.* San Francisco, CA: SFCIPP. Retrieved from *www.sfcipp.org/rights.html*

Skolnick, A. (1998). Prison deaths spotlight how boards handle impaired, disciplined physicians. *Journal of the American Medical Association, 280*(16), 1387–1390. Retrieved from *http://jama.ama-assn.org/content/280/16/1387*

Small, J. (2010). *California inmates still suffer from lapses in prison medical care.* Retrieved from *www.scpr.org/news/2010/08/25/17497/prisonmed3/*

Sylvia Rivera Law Project. (2007). *It's war in here: A report on the treatment of transgender and intersex people in New York state men's prisons.* Retrieved from *http://srlp.org/files/warinhere.pdf*

Thayer, L. (2004). *Hidden hell: Women in prison.* New York, NY: Amnesty International.

Travis, J., Solomon, A., & Waul, M. (2001). *From prison to home: The dimensions and consequences of prisoner reentry.* Washington, DC: The Urban Institute.

U.S. Department of Justice. (2003). Bureau of Justice statistics: Special report. Prevalence of imprisonment in the U.S. Population, 1974–2001. NCJ 197996. Retrieved from *www.bjs.gov/content/pub/pdf/piuspo1.pdf*

Vlahov, D., & Putnam, S. (2006). From corrections to communities as an HIV priority. *Journal of Urban Health,* 83(3), 339–348.

Weaver, V. (2001). The incarceration generation. *Focus: The Magazine of the Joint Center for Political and Economic Studies,* 29(8), 5–6.

Willmott, D. (2013, October 13). Interview with Emily Wang. (Unpublished). San Francisco, CA.

Willmott, D., & Robinson, S. (2007, March 23). Interviews with frontline health workers. (Unpublished). San Francisco, CA.

Willmott, D., & Robinson, S. (2008, February 8). Interviews with patients of Transitions Clinic. (Unpublished). San Francisco, CA. February 8, 2008.

Willmott, D., & van Olphen, J. (2005). Challenging the health impacts of incarceration: The role for community health workers. *California Journal of Health Promotion,* 3(2), 38–48.

Yeung, B. (2009). *Freeze, you're under examination.* Miller-McCune. Retrieved from *http://www.psmag.com/health-and-behavior/freeze-you-are-under-examination-3611*

Zack, B., & Kramer, K. (2009). What is the role of prisons and Jails in HIV prevention. [Fact Sheet]. Retrieved from *http://caps.ucsf.edu/uploads/pubs/FS/pdf/revincarceratedFS.pdf*

Additional Resources

All of Us or None. (n.d.). Retrieved from *www.prisonerswithchildren.org/our-projects/allofus-or-none/*

Prison sentences for millions of people with felony convictions never really end when prejudice and discrimination based on felony criminal histories persist outside the prison walls. Former prisoners, prisoners, people convicted of felonies and their allies have come together to combat the many forms of life-long discrimination in All of Us or None.

California Coalition for Women Prisoners (CCWP). (n.d.). Retrieved from *http://womenprisoners.org/*

CCWP is a grassroots social justice organization, with members inside and outside prison, that challenges the institutional violence imposed on women, transgender people, and communities of color by the prison industrial complex (PIC).

Campaign for Youth Justice. (n.d.). Retrieved from *www.campaignforyouthjustice.org*

In the 1990s most states passed laws that made it easier to try, sentence, and incarcerate youth in the adult criminal system. Today an estimated 200,000 youth are prosecuted into the adult criminal justice system each year. Research shows that youth incarcerated in adult jails and prisons face an increased risk of being physically, mentally, and sexually assaulted or abused. Prosecuting kids as adults also increases the likelihood that they will stay involved in the criminal justice system. For information, research, and how you can become involved, visit their website.

The Center on Juvenile and Criminal Justice (CJCJ). (n.d.). Retrieved from *www.cjcj.org/*

CJCJ provides services to youth and adults across the country that are facing or transitioning from incarceration. CJCJ's model programs demonstrate how alternatives to incarceration can be successful.

The Council on Crime and Justice. (n.d.). Retrieved from *www.crimeandjustice.org/*

The Council on Crime and Justice is an independent, nonprofit organization integrating research, demonstration projects and advocacy to bring just solutions to the causes and consequences of crime.

Critical Resistance. (n.d.) Retrieved from *www.criticalresistance.org/*

Critical Resistance seeks to build an international movement to end the Prison Industrial Complex. CR's work seeks to demonstrate how providing basic necessities such as food, shelter, and freedom makes our communities secure, not incarceration, prisons, and other forms of social control.

Detention Watch Network. (n.d.). Retrieved from *www.detentionwatchnetwork.org/*

The Detention Watch Network (DWN) is a national coalition of organizations and individuals working to educate the public and policy makers about the U.S. immigration detention and deportation system and advocate for humane reform so that all who come to our shores receive fair and humane treatment.

The Drug Policy Alliance. (n.d.). Retrieved from *www.drugpolicy.org*

The Drug Policy Alliance works to end the war on drugs and promote realistic alternatives. The guiding principle of the Alliance is harm reduction, an alternative approach to drug policy and treatment that focuses on minimizing the adverse effects of both drug use and drug prohibition.

Families Against Mandatory Minimums (FAMM). (n.d.). Retrieved from *www.famm.org*

FAMM is a national nonprofit organization that challenges mandatory sentencing laws. Mandatory minimums can propagate inflexible and excessive penalties. To change the system, FAMM promotes sentencing policies that give judges the discretion to sentence defendants according to their role in the offense, seriousness of the offense, and potential for rehabilitation.

Human Rights Watch Prison Project. (n.d.). Retrieved from *www.hrw.org/*

Working in conjunction with numerous local partners, Human Rights Watch monitors conditions of detention around the world, pressuring governments to bring their treatment of prisoners into compliance with basic human rights standards.

Justice Now. (n.d.). Retrieved from *www.jnow.org/*

Justice Now works to end violence against women and stop their imprisonment. They provide legal services, support prisoner organizing efforts that promote health and justice, and promote alternatives to policing and prisons.

The Justice Policy Institute (JPI). (n.d.). Retrieved from *www.justicepolicy.org/*

JPI is a Washington DC-based think-tank that is committed to reducing society's reliance on incarceration. The policy work of JPI aims to advance the quality and content of public discourse in the ongoing debate around juvenile and criminal justice system reform.

The Real Cost of Prisons Project. (n.d.). Retrieved from *http://realcostofprisons.org/*

The Real Cost of Prisons Project brings together justice activists, artists, justice policy researchers, and people directly experiencing the impact of mass incarceration to create popular education materials and other resources that explore the immediate and long-term costs of incarceration on the individual, her/his family, the community, and the nation.

The Sentencing Project. (n.d.) Retrieved from *www.sentencingproject.org*

The Sentencing Project is one of the nation's leading organizations that develops alternative sentencing programs, conducts policy research on U.S. criminal justice, and advocates for creating meaningful reforms.

The Transitions Clinic Network (TCN). (n.d.). Retrieved from *www.transitionsclinic.org/*

TCN is a patient-centered, primary care medical home for recently released prisoners with chronic diseases. The network is growing and includes clinics in Birmingham, AL; San Francisco and Richmond, CA; Rochester and New York, NY; Boston, MA; Caguas, Puerto Rico; Baltimore, MD; and New Haven, CT.

Introduction to Chronic Disease Management

16

Tim Berthold, Jill Tregor, and David Spero

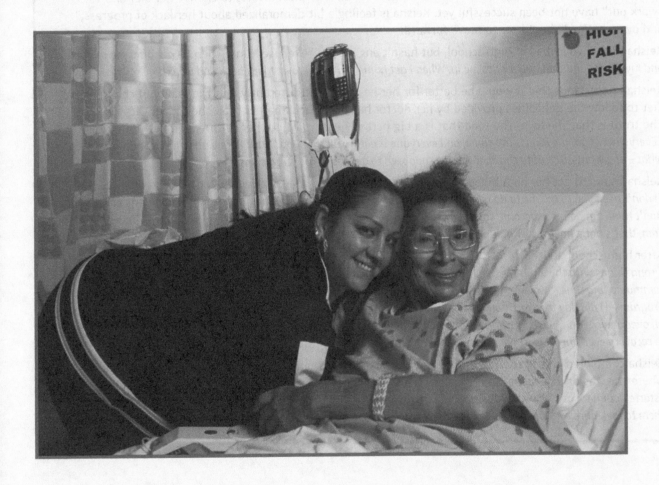

CASE STUDY   Keisha Mitchell

You are a CHW working as part of a primary health care team at a busy neighborhood health center. Today you meet with a new client, Keisha Mitchell, a dedicated single mother with a 9-year-old daughter, Marina. Keisha shares custody of Marina with her ex-husband, and they have a positive relationship as coparents. Keisha works as a drug and alcohol counselor at a local nonprofit agency, and is proud of the work she does to support clients in their recovery. She works long hours for not enough pay, but receives health benefits.

Keisha has high blood pressure that is not yet under control. She is taking two different types of high blood pressure medications, but sometimes forgets to take her pills. Efforts to change her diet and to "work out" have not been successful yet. Keisha is feeling a bit demoralized about her lack of progress, and overwhelmed about how to move forward.

Keisha played volleyball in high school, but hasn't engaged in "exercise" since then. *"I run after my daughter and my clients and that about does me in. When I get home I'm ready to just kick back and relax!"*

Keisha understands that it would be better for her health to eat differently, but the reality of changing her diet to follow the guidelines provided by her doctor has been much harder than she thought it would be. The truth is that she loves the food that is a big part of her family life, her culture, and her community. *"Everywhere I go, the food is the same, and everyone is eating all that good stuff I grew up with and part of me says, what—you want all of us to change? Are we supposed to give up all our traditions?"*

Keisha wants to get her high blood pressure under control, in a way that works for her. She tells you, *"I don't need you to tell me to do a bunch of crazy stuff that won't work for me and that you couldn't do either! Don't think I'm going to become some carrot-eating yoga lady, because that is not going to happen. That's not who I am, that's not who I'm ever going to be."*

After high school, Keisha admits that she became addicted to drugs and alcohol. *"I got caught up doing the wrong things with the wrong people, and it was a bad time to be in the streets. That was when crack was hitting my community big time."* Keisha has been in recovery for over 10 years now. *"It wasn't pretty. I was in and out of programs—I did day treatment and residential treatment, and I'd get clean and then I'd go back out and start using all over again. I burned some bridges with my family in those years but, finally, I got to where I needed to be. I been in recovery ever since. Eleven years next April."*

Keisha completed certification as a drug and alcohol counselor and now works for one of the programs where she was once a client. She tells you: *"I like telling the women, when they first come in to our program— I started out here as a client, I was sitting right where you're sitting! Some of them are surprised at first, but it helps them to feel more comfortable and really, if I can get clean, then so can they."*

If you were the CHW who is working with Keisha Mitchell, how would you answer the following questions?

- What factors in Ms. Mitchell's life pose risks to her health?
- What factors promote her health and wellness?
- Which of the factors that influence Ms. Mitchell's health is she most likely to be able to change, and which factors may be most difficult to change or influence?
- What else would you like to know about Keisha in order to best support her health?
- What is your role, as a CHW, in supporting Ms. Mitchell to self-manage her hypertension and improve her health and wellness?
- What concepts will guide your work with Ms. Mitchell?

Introduction

This chapter addresses chronic health conditions (also referred to as chronic illness or chronic disease), the leading cause of illness and death in the United States. Community Health Workers often work closely with patients like Keisha who live with chronic conditions. The U.S. Centers for Disease Control and Prevention (CDC) has highlighted the important role that CHWs can play in the management of chronic disease (CDC, 2014).

Effective management of chronic conditions should be grounded in the client's life circumstances, their needs and hopes. It should build and support the clients' ability to manage their own conditions and health. This self-management approach has been shown to improve health and wellness (Lorig et al., 2001).

Please note that this chapter does not provide detailed information about specific chronic conditions (such as diabetes, cancers, heart disease, asthma, arthritis and depression). To do so would take up an entire textbook rather than just a chapter! In addition, new research continues to inform and change treatment guidelines, including the list of available and recommended medications. Therefore, we will provide tips for how to research and learn about chronic conditions including causes and consequences, symptoms, and treatment guidelines. With these skills, you should be able to find the information you need to support a client with any chronic condition.

This chapter also builds upon information presented elsewhere in the *Foundations* textbook, and is best studied after reading Chapters 3, 4, and 6–11. We will address how to apply concepts and skills covered in other chapters—including case management and action planning, and the challenge of supporting a patient to more effectively manage a chronic disease.

WHAT YOU WILL LEARN

By studying the information in this chapter, you will be able to:

- Identify some of the most common chronic diseases in the United States, and discuss health inequalities in rates of chronic disease among populations
- Apply the ecological model to analyze the causes and consequences of chronic conditions
- Analyze and discuss the limitations of traditional medical models for the treatment of chronic conditions, and ways to integrate medical and public health approaches
- Discuss team-based approaches to the delivery of primary health care, and the role and scope of practice of CHWs within these teams
- Analyze and explain the concept of patient empowerment and the self-management of chronic conditions
- Discuss the application of client-centered concepts and skills to supporting patients in learning how to effectively manage their own chronic conditions

WORDS TO KNOW

Adherence	Discordance
Chronic Condition	Medication Management
Concordance	Panel Management

16.1 Defining Chronic Conditions

A **chronic condition** is defined as an illness or health condition that lasts for at least three months (and typically much longer), and are generally slow to progress. Chronic conditions become more common as we age: the vast majority of Americans over the age of 65 have one or more.

The illnesses that are categorized as chronic conditions vary depending upon the source. For example, some health organizations are more likely than others to include mental health conditions, such as depression and post-traumatic stress, or chronic disabilities such as muscular dystrophy and multiple sclerosis. We encourage you to develop a comprehensive or inclusive understanding of the illnesses and disabilities that are classified as chronic conditions.

There are hundreds of chronic conditions. Some of the most common chronic conditions in the US and worldwide are:

- Cardiovascular diseases including hypertension (high blood pressure) and coronary heart disease
- Diabetes
- Respiratory diseases including asthma and chronic obstructive pulmonary disease (COPD)
- Cancers
- Depression, post-traumatic stress, schizophrenia, and other mental health conditions
- Substance use
- Arthritis
- HIV Disease, Hepatitis C, tuberculosis, and other communicable chronic conditions
- Chronic kidney disease
- Alzheimer's disease, multiple sclerosis, muscular dystrophy, and other progressive and disabling conditions

HEALTH DATA

Chronic conditions are the leading causes of illness, hospitalization, and death in the United States. The CDC estimates that chronic conditions account for more than 70 percent of all deaths each year. Together, heart disease, strokes, and cancer are the causes of more than 50 percent of all deaths annually (CDC, n.d.-b). Chronic conditions are the leading cause of hospitalization, and account for more than 75 percent of all health care costs in the United States (Ibid).

The CDC estimates that 117 million Americans—or approximately 50 percent of adults—have at least one or more chronic health conditions (CDC, n.d.-c). Risks for developing a chronic condition increase with age. Approximately 39.7 million Americans live with one or more limitations to daily activities (CDC, 2012) due to their chronic conditions. Globally, chronic conditions accounted for approximately 60 percent of all deaths in 2008, or an estimated 36 million of 57 million deaths worldwide (World Health Organization, 2010).

16.2 Chronic Conditions and Inequalities

Chronic conditions are characterized by highly unequal rates of illness and death among populations at both the national and international levels, based on factors including income, ethnicity, age, and sex.

For example, in 2009, the Centers for Disease Control and Prevention estimated the prevalence of asthma in the United States at 8.2 percent (approximately 8 out of every 100 people had asthma). An estimated 7.1 million children under the age of 18 and 17.5 million adults are living with asthma (National Health Statistics Reports, 2011). However, research shows that the prevalence of asthma is quite different among populations. While 7.8 percent of White Americans were estimated to be living with asthma, the prevalence among Black Americans was estimated at 11.1 percent, and the prevalence among Puerto Ricans was estimated at 16.6 percent (more than twice the rate than among Whites). Asthma prevalence for Americans living at 200 percent of the poverty level and above was estimated at 7.3 percent, compared to 11.6 percent for those living below poverty (National Health Statistics Reports, 2011).

To find out more about inequalities in rates of asthma and other chronic conditions where you live and work, investigate your local city or county data. Your local public health department is likely to have a website that includes health statistics. If not, find the website for your state's health department and search there to see if they have data available for your county.

16.3 Factors That Cause and Contribute to Chronic Conditions

We will use the framework of the ecological model (see Chapter 3) to identify factors that cause and contribute to chronic conditions at the levels of the individual patient, their family, immediate neighborhood or community, and the society. This includes factors such as stress, which operate across all four dimensions of the ecological model.

INDIVIDUAL FACTORS

Individual factors that cause or contribute to chronic conditions vary considerably depending upon the disease in question. For example, pathogenic (disease-causing) agents such as bacteria and viruses play a role in certain chronic diseases such as liver and cervical cancer, and HIV disease. Heredity, or our genetic makeup, also plays a role in the development of many chronic conditions including, for example, cancer, cardiovascular disease, depression, arthritis, and diabetes, and disabilities such as muscular dystrophy. The extent to which genetics plays a role depends upon the disease in question. Research points to the interaction between genetics and our environment in determining the development and progression of many chronic conditions. An individual's age and general state of health, including the health of their immune system, nutritional health, and the presence of infectious or chronic conditions, can also play a role in the development of other chronic conditions.

Knowledge, attitude, and behaviors also play a significant role in the development of most chronic conditions. Leading national and international health organizations highlight the role of four key behavioral factors for chronic conditions.

Levels of Physical Activity
- Engaging in physical activity is one of the most profound and effective ways to promote our physical and mental health.
- Regular physical activity has been shown to reduce risks for chronic conditions such as cardiovascular disease, diabetes, some cancers, and depression. **Note:** More detailed information is provided in Chapter 17, Promoting Healthy Eating and Active Living.

Diet and Nutrition
- Hunger and malnutrition is still the leading health concern for many in the United States and around the world. At the same time, many Americans consume too much of certain kinds of foods and drinks. In general, we eat too much fast and processed foods, sugar, salt, refined carbohydrates, saturated and trans-fats. Research demonstrates that these foods increase our risks for cardiovascular disease, cancers, and diabetes.
- Eating a healthy diet that features vegetables, fruits, and whole grains can reduce risks for chronic conditions. **Note:** More detailed information is provided in Chapter 17, Promoting Healthy Eating and Active Living.

Tobacco Use
- Tobacco use—including exposure to second-hand smoke—is considered the most preventable cause of illness and premature death in the United States.
- The World Health Organization estimates that tobacco accounts for 13 percent of all male deaths worldwide (World Health Organization, 2009).
- Tobacco use contributes to cardiovascular disease, cancers, and respiratory conditions. It is a primary cause of lung cancer, the most common cancer in the United States.

Alcohol Consumption
- Excessive alcohol use contributes to chronic conditions including cardiovascular disease, diabetes, cancers, and liver cirrhosis.

What Do
YOU?
Think?

- *Is there a history of chronic disease in your biological family?*

- *To what extent may your diet, patterns of exercise, tobacco, and alcohol use influence your health and risks for chronic disease?*

FACTORS RELATED TO FAMILY AND FRIENDS

Our families and friends often play a critical role in promoting our health and well-being. They also contribute to our risks for illness. For example, family and friends often influence our diet, patterns of alcohol and tobacco use, our level of activity and fitness, and our exposure to stress.

When you are working with an individual client to change behaviors, such as their diet, keep the role and influence of the family in mind. For example, the client's family may influence the types of foods that are available in the household. If the rest of the family eats less healthy foods, this will impact, and may limit, the client's ability to eat a healthier diet.

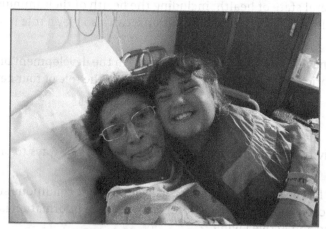

Family relationships play a key role in promoting the health of people living with chronic conditions.

- *To what extent do your family and friends influence your health-related risk factors?*

- *In what ways do they support your health and well-being?*

What Do
YOU?
Think?

NEIGHBORHOOD AND COMMUNITY FACTORS

The neighborhoods and communities where we live and work also influence our health status. This includes the level of access to health-related resources such as quality schools and job-training programs, affordable housing, and grocery stores stocked with affordable fresh fruits and vegetables. Exposure to air pollution and mold contributes significantly to chronic respiratory conditions like asthma.

Health is also influenced by access to after-school and child-care services, affordable and quality health care, parks and opportunities for recreation, community-based services, including those provided by nonprofits and faith-based institutions. Levels of violence in the community, including police and handgun violence, impact levels of stress and risks for chronic conditions (as well as injury and premature death).

- *What health risks are you and your local community exposed to?*

- *What health resources do you have easy access to, and which are lacking?*

What Do
YOU?
Think?

SOCIETAL FACTORS

Social, economic, and political factors have a significant impact on the development of chronic conditions. Throughout the world, populations with the least access to critical health resources—including healthy food, clean drinking water, affordable housing and health care, safe working conditions, a living wage, and meaningful protection of civil and human rights—are most likely to experience higher rates of illness and premature death from chronic conditions. Access to these critical health resources is determined by the interaction of economic and political factors, including actions taken by key policy makers and governments at the local, national, and global levels.

The World Health Organization (WHO) emphasizes the role of social determinants (see Chapter 3) in the causation of chronic disease, and describes a vicious cycle of the interaction between poverty, illness and premature death. For example, the 2010 World Health Report estimates that over 100 million people are forced below the poverty line each year as a consequence of paying for health care treatments (WHO, 2010).

These economic and political factors also influence agricultural and nutritional policies. The development and marketing strategies of food corporations plays a key role in shaping the American diet. Over the course of the 20th century, government and corporate policies promoted an unhealthy diet featuring processed foods high in sugar, salt, fat, and refined carbohydrates (Moss, 2013). This new American diet resulted in increasing rates of chronic conditions including diabetes, cardiovascular disease, and cancer.

There is a rising epidemic of diabetes throughout the world. David Spero, RN, a chronic conditions expert, argues that the political, economic, and social policies in the US facilitate the development of diabetes:

> *Diabetes is not something people do to themselves and it's not a curse. . . . Individuals get the symptoms and pay the price, but the environment is set up to make people sick. It's toxically high in sugar and stress, low in social support, opportunities to exercise or to feel good about ourselves. The unhealthy state of the environment in modern society will give people diabetes if they lack the power to fight it off or change it. (Spero, 2006)*

The Pima Indians

Pima Indians living in Arizona have one of the highest rates of type 2 diabetes in the world. The Pima have been the focus of hundreds of research studies seeking to understand the causes of such a high rate of diabetes. Many of the initial studies focused on identifying a presumed genetic risk factor for diabetes. However, research ultimately revealed that the Pima do not have a uniquely high genetic risk for diabetes, and emphasized that Pima living in Mexico do not have elevated rates of diabetes. High rates of diabetes among Pima in the United States were caused by political—not genetic—factors. The federal government took the Pima's land and water, forcing dramatic changes in their traditional economy and diet, and rendering them dependent upon handouts of processed foods high in salt, sugar, and fats. The inevitable result of these policies was the production of high rates of diabetes, disability, and premature death (Jones, 2011).

THE ROLE OF STRESS IN THE DEVELOPMENT OF CHRONIC CONDITIONS

Stress operates across all four levels of the ecological model and is a major contributor to chronic conditions (to review basic information about stress, please refer to Chapter 12). This is particularly true for communities exposed to chronic stress arising from factors such as living in poverty, food insecurity and hunger, institutionalized discrimination, and exposure to violence. Stress raises heart rates and blood pressure, and causes our bodies to release hormones such as cortisol. In order to save energy, stress takes energy from the immune system, our bodies' long-term healing system, and uses it for fight, flight, or fat storage. Over time, these biological stress responses increase risks for a range of chronic conditions including diabetes, depression, hypertension, coronary heart disease, and stroke.

Post-traumatic Stress and Illness

Please note that Chapter 18 provides more information about trauma. Post-traumatic stress affects people who survive life's most horrifying events, such as war and armed conflict, torture, sexual assault, child abuse, and neglect. Research demonstrates that childhood exposure to trauma increases the risks of developing other chronic conditions including cardiovascular disease, diabetes, depression, and chronic obstructive pulmonary disease (COPD) (CDC, n.d.-a).

16.4 The Consequences of Chronic Conditions

Chronic health conditions have a significant impact on the lives of individual patients as well as their families, and on the communities and the larger society in which they live.

THE CONSEQUENCES FOR INDIVIDUAL PATIENTS

Consequences for individuals living with chronic conditions depend upon the type and number of conditions they are living with, their age, genetics, and family status, their income, and other factors. Common consequences include:

- Fatigue or extreme tiredness
- Chronic pain
- Challenges with daily living and activities. Due to their symptoms, people with chronic conditions may find it hard to study or work, to live independently, and to care for others, including children
- Nausea, bowel or bladder control problems
- Nerve damage
- Disability such as the loss of mobility, eyesight, or limbs
- Increased levels of stress, anxiety, and depression
- Stigma or negative attitudes from others about people who are living with certain chronic conditions such as HIV and hepatitis C disease, addiction, mental illness, and diabetes. Stigma also affects people who are perceived as being "overweight," or who have engaged in certain behaviors, such as drug use
- Shame, isolation, and the loss of career, of relationships or key roles within the family and community, of hope, identity, purpose, or faith
- Symptoms often get worse over time and may result in complications, including long-term hospitalization and premature death

- *Can you think of other consequences for individuals living with chronic conditions?*

What Do YOU Think?

THE CONSEQUENCES FOR FAMILIES

The consequences for families may depend upon how many family members have chronic conditions, which family members are ill, the severity of the illness, and the social and economic circumstances of the household. Consequences include increased costs for the treatment of chronic conditions and, as a result, fewer funds to invest in other resources such as housing, education, transportation, food, or health care.

When one member of the family falls ill, others typically assume increased caretaking responsibilities. Caretaking roles require time and energy, and sometimes prevent family members from taking on other roles within and outside of the household. Both the family member who is ill, and the caretaker(s) may experience a reduction or loss of employment and income and this, in turn, may result in the loss of other assets such as health insurance or housing.

It can be difficult for people to adjust to changing roles within the family. Chronic illness may affect other roles including parenting and other household responsibilities. Witnessing the pain, suffering, and premature death of loved ones affects the rest of the family. They may experience frustration or anger directed towards the person with a chronic condition for getting sick and for not taking better care of themselves. They may feel guilt about these feelings, or about being healthy when a loved one is ill.

- *Have you experienced or witnessed consequences of chronic illness?*

- *Can you think of other consequences for families?*

What Do YOU Think?

THE CONSEQUENCES OF CHRONIC CONDITIONS FOR OUR COMMUNITIES AND SOCIETY

The consequences for communities and our society include increased illness and disability (such as high rates of diabetes, post-traumatic stress, or HIV disease), and increased costs for treating chronic conditions (Chronic conditions account for the majority of all health care costs in the United States). The funding spent on the treatment of preventable chronic conditions could otherwise have been invested in other key public benefits such as housing, education, or job training.

Chronic conditions also result in a devastating loss of human potential when people die prematurely or are too sick or disabled to fully contribute to the community socially, culturally, politically, or economically. The World Health Organization cites high rates of chronic conditions among low-income nations—and the costs and losses associated with illness—as a key factor limiting economic development and the hope of a higher quality of life (WHO, n.d.).

- *Can you think of other consequences at the community and societal levels?*

What Do YOU Think?

Your Experience

As a CHW, it is important for you to be aware of your own experience with chronic conditions. Please take time to reflect on the following questions:

- What is your personal experience with chronic conditions? Are you living with a chronic condition? Do other members of your family have a chronic condition?

- How do chronic conditions impact your life, and the lives of your family members?

- What types of chronic conditions are most common among the communities that you belong to?

- Do people in your community living with chronic conditions—or risk factors for certain chronic conditions—face stigma and prejudice? If so, which health conditions and risk behaviors are stigmatized?

16.5 Treatment Options

If you work directly with patients who have chronic conditions, you will become familiar with the types of treatments that are available in your workplace and in other local hospitals and clinics. Available treatments for chronic conditions depend upon the disease and may include:

- **Changes in behavior to reduce risk factors and manage symptoms**: People with chronic conditions may work on their own, or in partnership with health care providers or other helping professionals, to change risk behaviors. These changes typically include:
  - Increasing activity levels and fitness (See Chapter 17).
  - Dietary changes such as increased consumption of fruits, vegetables, and whole grains (Chapter 17).

- ○ Stopping or reducing tobacco and alcohol consumption.

- ○ Stress management (Chapter 12). People can learn techniques to better manage the effects of stress, and limit the harm that stress causes. Stress management techniques may include exercise, meditation, therapy, art (music, dance, photography, etc.), keeping a journal, participation in social or support groups, spiritual or religious practices, and many more.

- **Medications**: Medications are available that help to reduce the symptoms of certain chronic diseases, and to prevent further progression of the disease. For example, people with asthma may use inhalers to help them breathe more easily and to prevent asthma "attacks" and hospitalization. Medications are frequently used to treat chronic conditions such as hypertension, diabetes, HIV disease, asthma, arthritis, and depression.

- **Physical or occupational therapy**: These treatments help people to regain strength and mobility, and to reduce pain, and can help patients to participate more actively in daily activities such as dressing, walking, cooking, or working.

- **Medical interventions**: For example, some patients may receive chemotherapy or radiation to treat cancer. Patients may undergo procedures such as joint replacement surgery to treat conditions such as arthritis, and laser therapy may help others to keep their vision.

- **Mental health therapies**: These include individual, family, or group counseling to help people better cope with depression, anxiety and loss, and behavior change.

- **Medical equipment**: For example, an oxygen tank to assist with breathing or a wheelchair to assist with mobility.

- **Assistance:** A patient may need someone to help out with daily activities including dressing, cooking, or taking care of a home.

- **Holistic and Integrative therapies** such as acupuncture, herbal remedies, and other practices.

Please keep in mind that the information provided here about treatment may be different from the guidelines followed in the clinic or hospital you are working for. *The policies and procedures of your employer always take priority in guiding your work with clients. When in doubt about the type of health information to share with clients, always talk with your direct supervisor.*

ACCESS TO TREATMENT

The types of treatments that patients actually receive depend upon several factors, such as:

- Whether or not the patient has health insurance, the type of insurance they have, the types of treatments covered, and the cost to the patient (such as fees for deductibles and copayments)

- The health care practice and system that will serve the patient, the level of training and expertise of health care professionals, and the range of services and treatment provided

- Availability of services including mental health services, food, housing and legal assistance, recreational facilities and programs. Access to services can be particularly difficult for rural and low-income communities, and those lacking reliable and affordable transportation

- Cultural identity and health beliefs, such as a distrust in western approaches to medicine versus other cultural approaches to healing

- Trust in health care providers: Trust is in turn influenced by the client's personal history with medical providers, as well as the historical treatment of the client's community by medical providers. Some communities, including Native American, African-American, and formerly incarcerated communities, have experienced significant discrimination and harm from medical providers in the past (and may continue to face such discrimination in the present. For more information, please refer to Chapter 6 of *Foundations* (Practicing Cultural Humility)

- The experience, knowledge, and attitudes of family and friends

- Time and competing priorities and responsibilities (such as employment, child care, or other caretaking responsibilities)

- The stigma associated with the chronic condition and/or risk factors (including issues such as diet, exercise, drug or alcohol use, sexuality, a mental health diagnosis, HIV and hepatitis C, etc.)

- Depression/mental illness. Having depression or any mental health condition can make it much more difficult for patients to seek or maintain services and available treatments for any health condition

- Health literacy, or knowledge about health issues and health care systems

- Disability, mobility, and the availability and cost of transportation to and from health care services

- The client's experience and perception of the severity of symptoms and the degree to which their illness is interfering with their quality of life. Some patients ignore symptoms and delay accessing care for many reasons including fear, depression, stigma, and denial

- Expectations and beliefs about the treatability of their condition, and the extent to which a client believes that their symptoms can be meaningfully reduced

- *Can you think of other factors that might influence a client's access to treatment for a chronic condition?*

- *Have any of these factors affected your own access to treatments (or those of your family)?*

- *How might your awareness of these factors influence your work with clients and communities?*

Understanding Hypertension

While we are unable to provide detailed information about the most common chronic conditions in this brief chapter, we present a basic overview of high blood pressure here to illustrate the type of information that is helpful for CHWs to learn about the most common chronic conditions among the communities they work with.

Definition

"Hypertension" means having high blood pressure. It is diagnosed when our blood pressure is measured consistently over 140/90. Our blood pressure is reported in the form of two numbers: systolic pressure, measured while our heart is beating; and diastolic pressure, measured in between heart beats, while our heart is at rest. In general, a healthy blood pressure is less than 120/80.

Prevalence

Hypertension is one of the most common or prevalent chronic conditions in the United States The U.S. Centers for Disease Control and Prevention estimate that over 67 million Americans, or 1 out of every 3 adults have hypertension (CDC, 2014). Hypertension is more common among men than women, among people aged 65 and older, and among African Americans. Approximately half of adults with hypertension do not have it under control (Ibid).

Key Causes and Contributing Factors

- *Heredity.* Our genes play a role in determining our risk for hypertension.

- *Diet*, or what we eat and drink. Consuming too much sugar, saturated fat, salt, and calories increases risks for hypertension. (For more information, please see Chapter 17, Promoting Healthy Eating and Active Living.)

- *Exercise.* The lack of regular physical activity (including walking) and exercise also increases risks.

- *Stress.* Exposure to chronic stress, including post-traumatic stress, increases the risks for hypertension.

(continues)

Understanding Hypertension

(continued)

- *Substance use.* Tobacco, alcohol, and drug use (especially cocaine and methamphetamines) all increase risks.

Common Consequences

Over time, if high blood pressure continues, it can result in damage and narrowing of the arteries, increasing risks for stroke, heart attack, and death. High blood pressure can damage the kidneys and lead to kidney failure, damage to the eyes and eyesight, and may result in sexual dysfunction (Mayo Clinic, 2014a).

Symptoms

Hypertension is sometimes called a "silent killer" because people generally do not have noticeable symptoms for many years. When symptoms do occur, they may include chest pain, blurred vision, memory loss, headaches, and blood in the urine (Mayo Clinic, 2014b).

Treatments

Hypertension is typically treated by a combination of medications and changes to diet, exercise, and other behaviors or habits.

- Medications: There are a wide range of medications used to help control blood pressure. Some clients respond better to certain types of medications, and some may be treated by more than one medication. For information about the different types of medications commonly used to treat hypertension, please review the following information from The Mayo Clinic at: www.mayoclinic.org/diseases-conditions/high-blood-pressure/basics/treatment/con-20019580

- Tobacco, alcohol, and drug use: Patients are encouraged to stop or reduce their use of tobacco, drugs, and alcohol.

- Activity: Regular exercise can help to control and lower high blood pressure. Patients are encouraged to enhance their engagement in daily activity or exercise.

- Nutrition: Patients are encouraged to eat a more healthy diet in line with the nutritional guidelines provided in Chapter 17. In general this means eating more fruits, vegetables, and whole grains, and eating fewer calories, saturated fats, and sugar.

- Stress reduction and relaxation techniques.

16.6 How to Stay Informed about Chronic Conditions

The more you know about a client's chronic condition(s), the better you will be able to support their health and wellness. As a working CHW, you will frequently conduct research to enhance your knowledge about a wide variety of health issues. This is particularly important because research findings, information, and practice standards are frequently updated in the fields of public health and health care. Much of this research will be conducted online.

Because so much information about health is readily available, knowing where and how to conduct research on chronic conditions and other health issues can be challenging. Remember that you have an ethical duty to stay current in your field and to provide accurate information to the client and communities you work with. You need to be able to distinguish between reliable and less reliable sources of information. If you are working directly with people with chronic health conditions, a good place to start is reviewing the information made available by your employer. Talk with your supervisor and colleagues, and study available resources including, for example, practice standards and protocols, journals, reports, and brochures.

We encourage you to become familiar with a range of reputable online sources of health information. These include your local city, county, or state health department as well as leading national sites that feature a wide range of health information including recent research findings and current guidelines for prevention and treatment, such as:

- The U.S. Centers for Disease Control and Prevention *www.cdc.gov*
- National Institutes of Health *www.nih.gov/*
- The National Institute of Mental Health *www.nimh.hih.gov*
- The National Cancer Institute *www.cancer.gov*
- The National Library of Medicine (Medline) *www.medlineplus.gov*

Other recommended sites include national nonprofit professional organizations such as those focused on specific types of chronic health conditions including:

- The American Heart Association *www.heart.org*
- The American Cancer Society *www.cancer.org*
- Foundation for Women's Cancer *www.wcn.org*
- The American Diabetes Association *www.diabetes.org*

You can also find reliable information at leading educational and health care institutions such as:

- The Mayo Clinic *www.Mayoclinic.org*
- The Harvard Medical School *www.hms.harvard.edu* and School of Public Health *www.hsph.harvard.edu*
- The World Health Organization *www.who.org*

Please note that many of these sites provide different types of information designed for either health care professionals or patients/consumers. We encourage you to review information designed for both audiences. Information designed for patients may be something that you can share with the clients and communities you work with. And while some of the language used in the resources designed for health care professionals can be hard to understand at first, the more you read these resources the more comfortable you will be with the language and concepts used by the health care providers you work with.

16.7 New Health Care Models for Chronic Conditions Management

The way that primary health care services are provided in the United States is changing. These changes are perhaps most apparent in clinics or hospitals that provide services to many low-income patients living with multiple chronic conditions. To better treat these patients, health care organizations have increasingly developed multidisciplinary and patient-centered primary care teams, promoted patient self-management of chronic disease, incorporated panel management, and the use of CHWs, and shifted their practice towards what some are labeling "upstream medicine."

THE LIMITATIONS OF TRADITIONAL MEDICAL MODELS

Traditional medical models are not always effective in managing chronic conditions.

Medicine is concerned with the proximate or most immediate causes of illness in the patient. For example, chronic conditions are generally understood to be caused by physical and biological factors, including genetics and the individual patient's knowledge and behaviors. The medical treatment of chronic conditions generally emphasizes the prescription of available medical treatments, including medications, and changes in individual behavior such as tobacco and alcohol use, diet, and exercise. This level of focus is vitally important to patients. Many CHWs work in medical settings, and their work will also focus on engaging individual patients to take medications properly and to change risk-associated behaviors.

However, when health care providers focus only at the individual level, they fail to consider the social determinants that influence a patient's health. They may fail to diagnose or address issues such as homelessness, poverty,

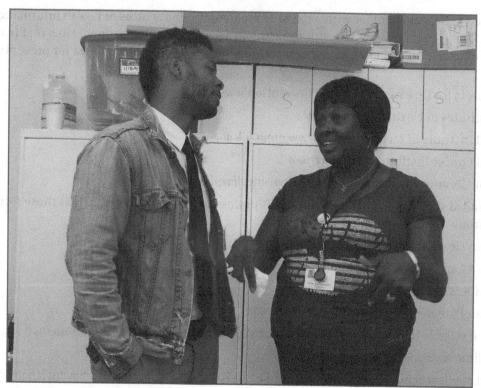

A CHW follows up with a client.

food insecurity (lack of adequate food), and a wide range of other factors addressed elsewhere in this textbook. Medicine's narrow focus on individual factors sometimes conveys a message that the patient is mostly or even completely responsible for their illness. While this may be intended as an empowering message—*"your behaviors contributed to your illness and changing them can make you better"*—it sometimes has the opposite effect, blaming or shaming patients—*"You wouldn't be so sick if you just followed our directions, took your medications, and changed your behaviors!"* This message sometimes has a negative impact on the patient's motivation for change and desire to seek out medical assistance in the future.

At its worse, licensed health care providers and patients end up in a kind of impasse or stand-off, in which each party grows increasingly frustrated with the other. The physician may be thinking:

"Why can't they get it that if they don't make big changes to their lifestyle now, they are going to end up in the hospital or worse? They shake their heads to say "Yes, doctor," but here we are again and they aren't doing anything different!"

At the same time, the patient may be thinking:

"I'd like to see this doctor walk a mile in my shoes! Where is she going to find these healthy foods in my neighborhood, and how would she afford them if she did find them? And I'd like to see her go exercise after a day juggling two jobs, a disabled husband and two grandkids! I'm too exhausted to exercise, but that doctor probably thinks I'm lazy."

16.8 Integrating Medicine and Public Health Models

Increasingly, health care providers are establishing new models that integrate medicine and public health. These models look beyond a patient's current symptoms and risk behaviors to consider how the broader social environment affects their health. They seek to intervene further "upstream" to prevent the development or progression of illness, to support patients to live healthier lives in a more comprehensive way and, in some instances, to partner with organizations, activists, and policy makers to create social change (Manchanda, 2014).

To effectively shift the focus further upstream, providers need to study and learn about the social conditions affecting the lives of patients. For example, health care professionals can study local data on public health and social issues that impacts the health of the communities they serve, such as rates of illness and death—and inequalities in these rates among populations—and data on housing, employment, food insecurity, involvement with the criminal justice system, and education (and, again, inequalities in rates of access or achievement). Zip codes are increasingly being used as a reliable predictor of health and health inequalities, and local media stories—including those provided by neighborhood and community-based media—often highlight public health and social issues. The more that health care providers come to understand these issues, the better they will understand the challenges faced by individual patients and the families who they are dedicated to serving.

When you are working as a CHW in the community, pay close attention to the environment around you. If you live in the same community in which you work, try to view it with a fresh set of eyes.

- What do you observe? What types of key resources exist?
- What types of organizations, programs and services are available?
- What is missing?
- What health risks do you notice?
- What types of social change are most necessary for promoting the health of local communities (and particularly for the most vulnerable among them)?
- What priority concerns are community members talking about?

As you provide services, apply an ecological model and the client-centered concepts addressed in other chapters of this textbook. For example, when you conduct an assessment to learn about the health status of a new patient, ask open-ended questions that invite them to share more information about their lives, including both the risks they face and the resources they have. Remember to use a strength-based approach to assess not only the factors that may be contributing to the patient's illness, but also the factors that contribute to their health. By inquiring about and acknowledging a client's strengths, you are identifying resources that may help to enhance their health. Provide case management and advocacy to support patients in addressing issues that lie beyond the individual level of the ecological model. Health is promoted when you assist clients to access new or improved resources such as stable housing and a regular source of healthy food, or when you support a new patient coming home from prison to reconnect with their family.

Yes We Can: An Example of Upstream Medicine

The Yes We Can Program developed and implemented new models for the management of childhood asthma at two sites in San Francisco, a public hospital and a community clinic. Both clinics hired CHWs to work closely with the families of children with asthma. The CHWs provided health education and case management services to support families to better understand the causes and triggers of asthma, and how to properly use prescribed medications to control symptoms. Key goals were to avoid serious asthma attacks that frequently sent children and their families to local emergency departments and often resulted in hospitalization. The CHWs conducted home visits to support families in identifying possible environmental triggers of asthma (such as secondhand smoke, dust, mold, diesel emissions and other pollutants, and pet dander) and ways to reduce these risks. Many of the families lived in local public housing developments. By conducting home visits, CHWs learned that several of these housing developments had serious mold infestations. In some apartments, the walls were covered with black mold. The CHWs partnered with the families they worked with and local community-based organizations to highlight the problem and advocate for action. This in turn contributed to the formation of a Task Force that is still working to ensure safe living environments for residents of public housing. (CDC, 2009; Legion & Madden, personal communication, 2014.)

Many people living with chronic conditions experience social isolation and benefit from opportunities to connect with others who face similar challenges. By coming together, people can share tips for effective self-management and offer emotional support and motivation for self care. In addition, connection to others and a sense of belonging are key aspects of emotional, mental, and physical health. There is a strong history in the United States, and around the world, of people living with chronic health conditions coming together to provide social support and, as we address below, to take collective social action. Building social support has been essential for some people living with mental health conditions, for survivors of trauma, for people struggling with substance use, and for people living with disabilities and chronic conditions such as cancer, HIV disease, and Hepatitis C. We encourage you to learn about the types of social or support groups that exist in the communities where you live and work. Who participates in these groups? What types of health or social issues do they address?

Because epidemics in chronic conditions, and the inequalities that characterize these epidemics, are caused in large part by social determinants, there is an urgent need to take action to address these factors. By working to create social change—such as changes to policies that limit or deny access to key resources and rights—we can also change patterns of chronic conditions within our society. For some patients, joining with others to create social change is also a prescription for their wellness. Addressing social issues that we care deeply about, such as issues of inequality and justice, can not only help to prevent greater illness and premature death in our communities, it can also be good for our own spirits, minds, and bodies (Spero, 2006).

Movements for Social Change

Social movements have changed public policies that influence American life and the health of diverse communities. These movements may take decades or centuries to achieve change, and not every effort is successful. Even when victories have been won (such as with the civil rights movement), new policies may achieve only partial change, may not be enforced or are eroded, and often require continued organizing and advocacy. Yet, social movements have resulted in meaningful changes. They have changed labor laws related to working hours and conditions, and to the exploitation of children. The civil rights movement resulted in laws to ban discrimination on the basis of sex, ethnicity, and nationality and in areas such as employment, education, and housing. The mental health recovery movement has resulted in changes in the way that people with mental conditions are viewed and treated. Activists changed policies governing research, health care, and benefits for people living with HIV disease, and helped lead the movement to find ways to prevent the spread of HIV. Movements across the United States are challenging criminal justice policies that lead to mass incarceration and impose lifelong penalties and barriers for formerly incarcerated people as they try to access employment, housing, education, food stamps, and other key resources.

For the communities that you belong to and work with:

- What types of movements have resulted in meaningful social change?
- What movements exist today that are advocating for social change?

16.9 Team-Based Approaches to Chronic Conditions Management

Increasingly, primary health care clinics rely upon a team-based approach to support the health of patients living with chronic disease. The topic of team-based practice is addressed in greater detail in Chapter 8 of *Foundations*. We will build upon that information here, emphasizing concepts related to chronic conditions management.

The members of a primary care team will vary across clinical settings. The team always includes the patient (the most important member of the team) and a licensed provider, like a physician or nurse practitioner. Teams may also include key family members (such as a parent, guardian, or a partner if they are available and willing), other licensed health care and mental health providers such as a nurse, social worker, or psychologist, panel managers (see below) and front-line providers such as medical assistants and CHWs. Some teams may integrate other specialists such as a respiratory therapist or pharmacist.

When CHWs are included as members of the primary care team, they may work with clients in a variety of ways and settings. For example, CHWs may meet clients in the clinic and in the community, and accompany clients to key medical and social services appointments. CHWs may visit clients in their homes or in other settings if clients are homeless, hospitalized, in residential programs, or incarcerated. CHWs may conduct an initial interview or intake with the client, provide health education, and support the development and implementation of an action plan over time. For these reasons, CHWs may have more time than other members of the health care team to build a relationship with the client, and to talk in greater depth about the factors that affect their health and welfare. As a result, the CHW is often the critical link between the patient and rest of the clinical team.

> **Juanita Alvarado:** At the Transitions Clinic [A clinic specializing in providing primary health care to patients coming home from prison—see Chapter 15] the community health workers meet and greet every new client first, then we set up an appointment with the doctor. Because many of the patients didn't have good experiences with health care when they were inside [in prison], the CHW usually participates in the first few visits, either before or after the doctor meets with the patient. This helps the new patients to build a connection to both the CHW and the doctor, and to feel more comfortable during their medical appointments. Then the whole clinical team meets every week, the CHWs and the doctor, nurse practitioner, therapist, and panel manager, everyone. We talk about how we can work together to support the patients, including any new patients or any patients that are having big challenges right then.

16.10 Panel Management

Panel management is a system for coordinating health care for a large group or panel of patients. The primary goal is to efficiently identify patients with the greatest health risks in order to provide timely care and prevent the progression of health conditions.

Key health information about a panel of patients is analyzed and coordinated by a designated staff member who is sometimes called a panel manager. The role of panel manager may be assigned to a medical assistant, CHW, health educator, nurse, or other staff member. By regularly reviewing electronic health data, the panel manager is able to identify "at-risk" patients such as those who have missed one or more clinical appointments, who have not returned calls or other communications from the clinic, patients with symptoms or test results that are out of range of "normal" (such as very high or uncontrolled blood pressure readings), or other signs of health risks (such as recent hospitalizations or Emergency Department visits). These patients are most at risk for disease progression, disability, and health crises such as infections, heart attacks, or stroke. The goal of panel management is to contact and connect with these "at-risk" patients and to arrange for intensive services that will result in improved health status and/or immediate care such as a clinic appointment or home visit (Willard & Bodenheimer, 2012).

For example, a Panel Manager may identify a diabetic patient who has blood glucose or Hemoglobin A1c blood tests significantly above the standard or acceptable range. This patient will be contacted and asked to come in for a medical appointment to further assess their health status, and talk about treatment options (including changes in medication, diet or exercise and access to additional services and resources). The goal is to bring the patient's blood glucose levels down to a normal or acceptable range, and to prevent further progression of diabetes and related health problems (such as infection or a loss of vision).

Because of their close relationships with patients and the community, CHWs often work closely with Panel Managers to ensure that at-risk patients are contacted and provided with an opportunity to return to care. CHWs may reach out to patients by placing calls, sending texts, or, if necessary, conducting home visits to talk with patients about their health and to ask if they would like to schedule an appointment with a provider.

While the size of patient panels and the duties of panel managers may vary from clinic to clinic, in general, panel management is:

- **Organized and coordinated**: Clinical teams meet regularly to discuss patient issues and challenges, and to ensure the coordination of care among providers and services.

- **Population based**: Panel management is designed to manage the health of a population or large group of patients who receive care from the same health care clinic or organization.

- **Data driven**: Patient data, such as blood pressure, blood glucose levels and HIV viral load, or lapses in fulfilling prescriptions for medication, are used to identify patients with immediate health risks and needs.

- **Evidence based**: Research and evaluation data has shown that panel management improved health outcomes for patients with diabetes and cardiovascular disease.

- **Provided by multidisciplinary teams**: In addition to the physician, these teams may include nurses, medical assistants, enrollment workers, clerical staff, dieticians, pharmacists, social workers, mental health professionals, case managers, CHWs, and/or health coaches. Each team generally has one person who is designated as the Panel Manager (who monitors patient data and identifies the need for immediate outreach and follow-up).

- **Focused on improving patient health outcomes**: All members of the primary-care team work collaboratively to improve health outcomes for that patient. While a doctor may spend only 10–15 minutes with a patient, the other members of the care team can provide follow-up care, ensure understanding of instructions, and assist the patient in creating their own action plan for managing their condition(s). This supports the patient to enhance their knowledge, skills, and confidence for the effective self-management of chronic disease and other health conditions.

- **Committed to preventative care**: Timely interventions and services are provided to prevent the further development of chronic disease and related complications and disabilities. Preventive care also reduces health care costs.

CASE STUDY — Keisha Mitchell (*continued*)

The panel manager at the health center informs you that Keisha Mitchell missed her last appointment with the doctor, and is two months late in refilling her high blood pressure medications. The panel manager left several phone messages for Ms. Mitchell, with no response. They ask you to try to contact Keisha, and to conduct a home visit if necessary.

After leaving a phone message and sending several texts (without receiving a response from Keisha), you decide to go to her apartment. The doctor provides you with a refill of Keisha's blood pressure medications, and you bring another pill organizer with you.

Keisha answers the door in a nightgown. When she recognizes you, she welcomes you inside and gives you a hug. She apologizes for not answering your calls and texts, and invites you to sit down. Keisha tells you that her father, Reverend Mitchell, had a stroke about two months ago, and that she took a leave from work to help with his recovery.

"We were so scared that we were going to lose him, and I've just been so busy going back and forth to the hospital and to rehab appointments with him. He was paralyzed on the right side, so he's having trouble walking and talking, but he's a strong man, and he's making progress. But his stroke has taken a toll on all of us. I try to be strong for him and for my mom (Keisha cries) . . . but it's been overwhelming. I took a leave from work and asked my daughter's father to take her in for a time, because I've just been so focused on helping my dad, and staying with my mom, and . . . I've just had to take a step back from everything else."

Eventually, you ask Keisha about her own health, and if she has been taking her medications and monitoring her blood pressure. She admits that she stopped refilling and taking her medication *"I haven't been doing any of that. I just kind of let that all go."*

Keisha gets her blood pressure cuff and takes two readings. The lowest reading is still too high at 155/100. Together you review her blood pressure medications, she takes her daily medications and fills the new pill organizer.

How would you answer the following questions?

- How did the Panel Manager identify Keisha's potential health risk?
- How did the Panel Manager and the CHW work together to take action to assess Keisha's health?
- What health risks is Keisha facing now?
- What next steps would you recommend for the CHW and the primary care team?

16.11 Patient Self-Management

Self-management of chronic conditions is rapidly becoming the new standard of care. It is a *client-centered* approach that supports patients to manage chronic health conditions over time, and make decisions about the types of treatments and services they do and don't want to participate in, and what else they will do to promote their own health (Ory et al., 2013).

Self-management represents a significant shift in the approach to chronic conditions management, and to the relationship between health care providers and patients. Traditional models of health care view the physician (or other licensed provider) as *the* health expert. The role of the physician is to share their knowledge and give informed advice to the patient. The role of the patient is to follow the directions of the physician. While this type of traditional relationship may work well for some providers and patients, ultimately, *it ignores the fact that the day-to-day management of chronic disease does not happen within the clinic or hospital*. Management happens in the context of the patient's life at home, at work, and in the community. If patients don't learn information and skills for the day-to-day management of their illness, including the confidence to make decisions, they may face increased health risks.

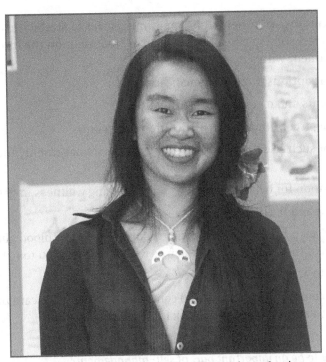

CHWs support clients to gain skills and confidence for the self-management of chronic health conditions.

Self-management places the patient at the center of a collaborative relationship with her or his health care team. While it draws on the knowledge and skills that the patient already has, it also builds and enhances skills, motivation, and confidence for the day-to-day management of their conditions. We call this "client-centered care." This approach fits very well with the concepts of cultural humility and client-centered practice that will guide your own work. As Thomas Bodenheimer, a physician and researcher and a leading expert in patient-centered primary care and the management of chronic conditions, writes:

> Sometimes called "patient empowerment," this concept holds that patients accept responsibility to manage their own conditions and are encouraged to solve their own problems with information, but not orders, from professionals. (Bodenheimer et al., 2002)

Self-management encourages patients to seek out assistance from their primary-care teams. Often, health care providers—including CHWs—teach or reinforce essential knowledge and skills for self-management, including health information about the specific illness or condition, medications or other forms of treatment. Health care providers can also help patients to enhance their ability to monitor symptoms (such as monitoring blood pressure and blood glucose levels at home), and to make informed decisions about treatments, when to seek out health care services, how to develop healthier diets and patterns of regular exercise, and more. Research evidence has demonstrated that patient self-management is indeed effective in promoting better health outcomes for patients with chronic conditions (Gordon & Galloway, 2008).

Self-management commonly includes the following strategies and actions for patients:

Develop health goals and a realistic action plan to reach those goals.

- Working effectively with their health care team
- Managing health crises or emergencies
- Finding and using community resources

Talk with family, friends and care-takers about their illness and self-management plan, and asking for help when needed.

- Some people find it difficult to ask for help. It is sometimes easier to start with a more limited and specific request such as help researching a health condition or treatment on the Internet, or to accompany the patient during an appointment with a new provider.

Evaluate available treatment options, including medications.

- Taking and using treatments and medications effectively

Manage symptoms of fatigue, frustration, sleep difficulties, and pain.

Change patterns of behavior such as diet, physical activity, stress management, and the use of tobacco, alcohol, and drugs.

- Find and maintain motivation for behavior change and promoting wellness in general

Monitor action plan progress and health symptoms.

- Patients learn to take and keep track of their blood pressure, to monitor blood glucose levels with a home meter, or to keep a record of their level of pain (such as with a scale from 0 to 10).

Make decisions about when to access health care services.

- This includes learning to communicate clearly and confidently with health care providers and family to establish a treatment plan, and to ask for help when needed.

- *What else do you consider to be an important part of self-management?*

David Spero highlights the following keys to self-management success: self-confidence, hope, motivation, and social support (Spero, 2006). While the motivation for self-management and related behavior change must come from within the patients themselves; hope, motivation, and support are often reinforced by family, friends, health workers, and community.

Please watch the following video interview [▶] with David Spero who shares his approach to supporting clients with self management.

What Do YOU Think?

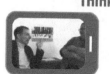

SELF-MANAGEMENT: FINDING REASONS TO LIVE, INTERVIEW

⊕ *http://youtu.be/ nRChT9oHOMM*

16.12 Chronic Conditions and the CHW Scope of Practice

CHWs are key members of primary health care teams focused on the treatment of chronic conditions, yet the role of CHWs within such teams is not always well defined. As a result, you may need help to clarify your role and the range of services that you provide. In some settings, you may find that colleagues don't understand that you can contribute more to the team. In other settings, you may be asked to provide services that lie outside of your prior training and knowledge.

The range of services that CHWs perform varies tremendously across clinical sites, based on the specific needs of the clinic or hospital, and the patients they serve. In general, the tasks and services *may* include the following:

- Outreach to local agencies, other clinics, and hospitals to make them aware of the services you provide
- Outreach to patients (for recruitment, follow-up and case management)
- Home visits, which may be because your patient is too sick to travel to the clinic
- Assistance with panel management
- Health education about chronic conditions and related health topics
- Support for client changes to health-related behaviors, utilizing client-centered counseling
- Development of client action plans for the self-management of chronic conditions, including health goals and actions to reach those goals
- Case management services and providing appropriate referrals to other agencies, programs, and services
- Accompaniment or, at the patients request, attending certain appointments with them. These might include appointments with specialists such as an oncologist (or cancer specialist), nutritionist, or with social services agencies in the community (such as a transitional housing agency or residential drug recovery program)
- Medication reconciliation and adherence counseling
- Measuring and reporting blood pressure; conducting foot exams for patients with diabetes; other health status checks as appropriate
- Health education on topics such as dietary and exercise guidelines, smoking cessation, and other health topics
- Facilitating or co-facilitating an educational or support group of patients living with a particular chronic disease
- Providing clients with information about living with a chronic condition
- Referrals to social services (as related above)
- Health system navigation

Ask your employer to clarify your role and scope of practice within the clinical team. If you are not confident about providing a particular service, tell your supervisor and ask for additional training and guidance.

Francis Julian Montgomery: I work with clients who have chronic health conditions and my work is 100 percent client-facing. It is part of how we do client-centered work and is in direct consideration of the client's needs—we literally meet people where they are at. What this means is that I travel to whatever location a patient is in, whether that be treatment, a single-room occupancy hotel room (SRO), an inpatient facility, a community-based organization, a hospital, or the street area where they hang out. We know it could be a barrier to require someone to come to our location. A health condition may prevent a patient from coming to me. For example, if someone has peripheral neuropathy and can't walk, I wouldn't see them if I couldn't go to them.

> **Richard Medina:** I had a client who was released from prison. He had HIV disease, a low T-cell count, and chronic Hepatitis C. We focused on the areas he needed help with the most. He had only one day of medication left, so first we got him the medication he needed. It turned out he had difficulty complying with his medication regimen. So we set it up that one time per week he would come in and talk to a counselor, and twice a week he would come into the clinic. He needed someplace to stay, and I was able to get him into transitional housing, but he knew some of the guys there from prison and he didn't want them knowing his HIV status. So I got him housed somewhere else. With patients with multiple chronic conditions, it's never just a one-step process.
>
> Now his T-cells are going up, and he is working on substance-abuse treatment in order to curb the urge of using drugs. He has gained some needed weight, because I got him connected to a food pantry right next door to where he is living now. It's important to provide services in the best way for the client. This allows them to make the choices they need for their health, and is the stepping-stone to life skills that will help them in the future.

16.13 Applying Client-Centered Concepts and Skills

The overarching role of the CHW is to support clients to effectively manage their chronic disease, reduce symptoms, and prevent the progression of the disease and adverse health events such as hospitalization and premature death. *This work should be consistently guided by client-centered concepts and skills designed to promote and support the client's independence and autonomy.* These concepts are addressed in detail in Chapters 6–11 of the *Foundations* textbook and include the following.

CULTURAL HUMILITY

Work to shift or transfer power away from yourself (and other providers), providing opportunities for patients or clients to claim greater control and authority for the self-management of their chronic health conditions. Strive to be aware of your own cultural identity, values and assumptions, and to avoid any tendencies to impose these standards as you work with clients. Use client-centered skills to ask clients to share their own cultural values and beliefs.

- For example, in working with Keisha, you don't want to impose cultural standards for a healthy diet. Instead, support Keisha to figure out how to change her diet in a way that fits with and honors her cultural and family traditions.

ECOLOGICAL MODEL

Remember that chronic conditions and a patient's overall health are shaped and influenced by broader social, economic, and political contexts. Try to learn about the context in which patients live, and apply this knowledge as you work together to enhance the patients' health status and autonomy.

- As you work with Keisha Mitchell, learn about social, economic and political factors that influence her health. Some of these factors pose risks to her health, and others promote her well-being.

BIG EYES, BIG EARS, AND A SMALL MOUTH

Listen deeply and carefully to what clients tell you. Observe their body language, their behavior, relationships and surroundings. Don't speak too much. Limit the use of your voice in order to provide opportunities for patients to tell and reflect upon the stories of their own lives.

HARM REDUCTION

Support clients to reduce any potential harms to their health or welfare (and harms to others). Anything that they do to reduce harms and risks to their health is a positive accomplishment. Don't impose an abstinence standard, or expectations that patients will completely stop certain behaviors (such as smoking or eating fast food) or avoid all health risks in the future. Those are not realistic goals for most people, regardless of their health.

- For example, Keisha Mitchell is not ready to change her diet radically. By applying a harm reduction model, however, Keisha may decide to cut back on certain types of food and drinks that pose risks for her high blood pressure, and to gradually increase those that promote her health.

MOTIVATIONAL INTERVIEWING (MI)

Apply MI skills including the use of OARS. When appropriate, consider using a readiness or motivation scale or ruler to support clients in assessing their readiness for change, their level of motivation and confidence.

With time and practice you will become more skilled and confident in using Motivational Interviewing. In working with Keisha Mitchell, for example, you may

- **O** = Ask Open-ended questions: "Keisha, how might you able to apply some of the skills that you have learned from your recovery from addiction to managing your high blood pressure?"

- **A** = Provide authentic Affirmations such as: "Being in recovery from drug and alcohol addiction is a big accomplishment—it must have taken a lot of strength and determination."

- **R** = Use Reflective listening to support Keisha to think about the factors that influence her health, such as her relationship with her family, her career as a counselor, and her recovery from addiction.

- **S** = Summarize key information and decisions that Keisha shares with you, such as her goal to manage her high blood pressure and her decision to increase physical activity by going to a Zumba class with her daughter.

HONOR A CLIENT'S RIGHT TO SELF-DETERMINATION

Respect a patient's right to make their own decisions about their own life, whether you agree with these decisions or not. Strive to let go of your tendencies to control a patient's attitudes, beliefs, behaviors, and choices.

- In the case of Keisha, you want to work in a way that honors her autonomy and builds upon her knowledge, skills, and values.

- *What other aspects of client-centered practice will guide your work in the area of chronic conditions management?*

16.14 Action Planning for Chronic Conditions Management

Chapters 10 and 11 provide guidance for how to work with a client or patient to develop an action plan to promote their health. Your role is to support the patient to develop an action plan that is relevant and realistic. This includes determining one or more achievable health goals for the not-too-distant future (such as within two to six months), and the actions that the patient will take to reach these goals. The actions should be ones that the patient has a good chance of successfully implementing, and should include specific details. For example, rather than "exercise regularly," or "Climb Mount Massive," actions might include something like "Walk my dog back and forth to Pine Hill Park. Start walking on Saturdays, and gradually increase to 3 times per week."

Generally, patients have a good idea of what they can do to better manage their chronic condition, but sometimes they may desire support to identify or refine the actions they will take to meet health goals. In these situations, you can provide *suggestions* for the patient to consider, reject, or accept, while keeping in mind that successful behavior change depends upon the extent to which the client can claim ownership of their plan. We also recommend normalizing the challenge of behavior change. Talk with the patient about how difficult behavior change can be, and the common cycles that people experience, including setbacks or relapse, and rethinking or revising their plans. Your ability to support a client without judgment, regardless of the challenges they may face as they implement their plan and create positive change, can play a role in their success.

Please watch the following video interview 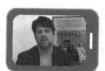 about action planning.

ACTION PLANNING: FACULTY INTERVIEW

http://youtu. be/51J58BJeQak

The Patient's Health Isn't Always Their Top Priority

Sometimes the goals that are most important to clients don't seem to directly address their chronic health condition. Clients may be more concerned about other issues, such as finding employment or stabilized housing or access to mental health services for their children. Keep in mind that the action plan belongs to the client and should reflect their authentic priorities and concerns. Remember that by supporting clients to take action to meet any significant goal, you can build trust and rapport, and lay the groundwork for future work to address new goals.

ESTABLISHING HEALTH GOALS

Developing an action plan often begins by asking clients to articulate their most important health goals. Health goals will vary among the clients you work with. Keep an open mind about the type of goals that may be most important to clients.

Goals typically represent the client's desire to change or transform some aspect of their health or wellness in order to improve the quality of their life. For clients living with chronic conditions, health goals may include:

Reduce Key Symptoms or Indicators

Most chronic conditions have symptoms such as fatigue, pain, dizziness, or loss of functions such as walking or vision. Other symptoms or indicators are specific to the disease in question and include high numbers for blood pressure, blood glucose, or HIV viral load. With good management, some symptoms can be so well controlled that they no longer have a negative impact on a patient's life.

Slow the Progression of Disease

For some patients, the focus is on slowing down the progression of a disease that may result in further disability and premature death. These patients seek to maximize the time they have to live a quality life.

Sustainable Self-Management

For some clients, their goals will include finding a way to manage illness day-to-day in a way they can maintain over time.

Increased Ability to Engage in Daily Activities

Some clients most want to re-engage in activities that are meaningful for them, such as going on vacation, attending church, caring for grandchildren, walking to the park, returning to work, and so forth.

Enhanced Autonomy

For some clients, the primary goal is not to be dependent upon others for help with the tasks of daily living, the management of medications or diet. They want to be able to live independently.

Improved Economic and Social Circumstances

For some clients, the most pressing goal may be related to finding stable housing or employment, supporting their children to stay in school or access necessary support services, reuniting with family, or other significant steps related to ensuring their basic needs (both mental and physical) are met.

Stress Reduction

Some clients may wish to enhance their ability to manage chronic sources of stress in their life. Stress management can help to stabilize or improve chronic conditions and improve quality of life overall.

Mental and/or Spiritual Health

For some clients, spiritual or religious faith plays a significant role in their lives, and in the way they view their health status.

Medication Management

For some clients, especially those living with multiple health conditions and taking many different medications, learning to and maintaining their ability to take all of their medication as directed is a major challenge.

Family Acceptance and Support

Some clients will seek to enhance understanding, acceptance, or support among their family. This might include acceptance for their diagnosis with schizophrenia, diabetes, or muscular dystrophy. Or it might mean support for changing the family diet to better promote the client's health.

Belonging

Some clients, including those with stigmatized health conditions, may seek to reduce a sense of isolation and to build a sense of connection with others. They hope to gain a sense of belonging to a group or community of people with common experiences, values, or goals.

Social Change/Social Justice

For some clients, taking part in movements to create social change or to advocate for social justice is a primary goal, and one that also enhances their own well-being.

- *What other health goals may people with chronic conditions strive to achieve?*

- *What are your health goals?*

CASE STUDY   ## Keisha Mitchell (*continued*)

CHW: So Keisha, what are your main health goals?

Keisha: Well, I guess the main one is to get the high blood pressure down. I don't want things to get worse.

CHW: Great. How would you like to begin to better manage the high blood pressure?

Keisha: Well, you know, that's been kind of the problem, I guess. The doctor told me a bunch of things I should do, but. . . . It just seemed like I had to change my whole life, so I just kind of stalled out.

CHW: There are a lot of things that help to manage high blood pressure, and you don't need to start doing all of them at once. I see how that could be overwhelming. (Keisha nods. CHW brings out Bubble Chart.) Keisha, this is a chart that shows some options that you can take to better manage your high blood pressure. Let's review this together and maybe you can select one of these options—or something else—that you want to start doing for your health, okay?

Keisha: Okay, I can do that.

(continues)

CASE STUDY   Keisha Mitchell (*continued*)

CHW: This list includes options that you already talked about with the doctor. It includes, for example: improving your diet, increasing physical activity, improving medications management, and enhancing stress reduction skills. And you can see that it includes some blank spaces for other types of actions that you might want to consider. Do any of these seem like a good place to begin?

Keisha: So I can just pick one? (CHW nods to indicate yes.) Okay, if I do that, maybe it won't be so over-whelming. I guess I'll start with exercise, because, like I told you before, changing what we eat is just a whole can of worms.

CHW: Okay, so what type of physical activities would you like to do? Is there something that you are already doing that maybe you could build up?

Keisha: Well, I'm running after my daughter and my clients all day long and that's got to count for some-thing! (Keisha laughs)

CHW: That definitely counts! What do you think about adding something to increase your physical activity a bit more? Maybe it would help to think about this as not running around after anyone else, but doing some-thing just for you? Was there a time when you were active in a way that you enjoyed?

Keisha: I played volleyball all through school. That seems so long ago now, but I really did enjoy it.

CHW: What did you enjoy the most about playing volleyball?

Keisha: Well, I liked the sense of bonding, you know, with the other girls, not the competition part so much, but just, you know, doing something together, and doing it well. It felt good (Keisha smiles).

CHW: Can you think of doing some kind of physical activity now that would feel good? Maybe something that could give you some of those great feelings you had when you played volleyball?

Keisha: Well, I guess what I do now, every once in a while, is I go out dancing with my girlfriends.

CHWs: So you enjoy dancing, and that can be great exercise. Is there a way that you might build on that to do it more regularly?

Keisha: Well, I heard there is a Zumba class over at the Community Center and I've been thinking about checking it out.

CHW: What might help you to take that step and go to Zumba?

Keisha: Well, I was thinking, you know, that my daughter Marina, she loves to dance, that maybe we could go together? I think they have a Saturday class.

CHW: So, maybe a good first step would be to go to a Zumba class with Marina?

Keisha: (smiles and nods)

CHW: Wonderful. Is this something you think you can do in the next two weeks?

Keisha: Yeah, I'll give it my best, and I'll let you know, okay?

CHW: Great, so Keisha, on a scale of 0-10, how confident are you that you and Marina will go to the Zumba class?

Keisha: Well, let me talk to Marina but if she wants to go with me, and I think she will, then that's a 9 for me. We'll definitely check it out

CHW: Great! Can you text me once you go, and then we can set up another appointment and talk about it?

Keisha: All right, I'll text you _____ (CHW's name), and thanks. Wish me luck.

Please watch the following video, 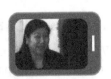 which shows a CHW who is working to support a client who has diabetes.

- What does the CHW do well in supporting the client to develop an action plan?
- What else could the CHW have done to support this client?

ACTION PLANNING, DIABETES AND EXERCISE: ROLE PLAY, DEMO

∞ *http://youtu.be/ XCOQyvhX91A*

USING A MOTIVATION OR CONFIDENCE SCALE

The Motivation Scale (as described in greater detail in Chapter 9) is a resource to share with clients as they developing or working to implement an action plan. The scale from 0 to 10 is a quick and easy way for the client to evaluate their motivation or readiness or confidence in their own plan.

For example, in the Keisha Mitchell Case Study the CHW uses a Confidence Scale to assess how ready Keisha is to start going to the Zumba dance class. There may be various opportunities in future meetings for Keisha and the CHW to assess her motivation, readiness, or confidence to make other changes.

The scale isn't a precise measurement, but it useful in highlighting goals or actions that a client is or is not highly motivated by or confident in achieving. If the client rates their readiness (or confidence or motivation) at a 7 or higher, this is an indication that their action plan is relevant or practical, and they have a good chance of moving forward (MacGregor et al., 2006). If the client rates their readiness or confidence below 7, ask them why, and what might increase it to a 9 or a 10.

- "Can you tell me why you rated your confidence at a 5?"
- "What would help you to increase your readiness to a 9 or a 10?"

These questions may help the client to refine their plan, address key challenges or doubts, scale back expectations, or add in more detail that will increase the likelihood of their success. For example, if Keisha isn't confident that she will be able to implement her action plan, she can take a step back and consider more realistic options. While Keisha may not want to make a drastic change to her diet, she may be more confident about eating more fresh vegetables and fruit at home with her daughter, or about cutting back on drinks with a lot of sugar or high fructose corn syrup.

CASE STUDY   **Keisha Mitchell** (*continued*)

Keisha: Yeah, that nutrition plan that the doctor gave me, I can't do that. I'm not going to family functions and turn my nose up at the food. I'm going to eat it, and believe me, I'm going to enjoy it! But I think Marina and I can do better at home, you know, eating more vegetables and cutting back on some of the other things. I really like that cookbook that we found that takes a healthier approach to the foods I grew up with. We are going shopping this weekend so we can try out a couple of the recipes. With this new plan, I am much more confident—like at least an 8—that we can kick it off and make some progress.

You want to support a client to develop a plan that will lead to success. If a client can't actually implement their plan, they may feel as though they failed, and this could damage any confidence the client has in their ability to actually make behavior changes that improve their health. Encourage clients to start with smaller steps and to gradually build on their successes. Behavior change is deeply challenging and typically doesn't happen all at once. Realistically, walking around the block once a week is better than not walking at all. We want clients to feel good about what they are doing to promote their own health, whatever that is, and not feel judged by us or themselves for what they were not able to accomplish.

16.15 Medication Management

CHWs working in primary health care settings often support patients with **medication management**. The goal is to ensure that the patient is taking the right prescribed medications in the proper way in order to best treat their chronic conditions.

Juanita Alvarado: At the Transitions Clinic the Community Health Workers spend a lot of time helping with medications management. Because our patients just got out of prison, where everything was done for them, many of them don't have an experience of reading a prescription or a label on a bottle of medications, and haven't had to make their own schedule for taking their meds. We spend a lot of time building trust—that is number one, and helping the client to get more comfortable managing their own health, and their medications, as well as just figuring out what is next in their lives. It is a lot.

All of our patients have chronic conditions, and most are taking more than one medication. So we meet with them a lot at the beginning and go step by step. What is this medication for? When do you take it, and how? We help them with a pill organizer if they need it. We talk about things like not skipping their medications or splitting their pills to make 'em last. We check in to make sure they are taking the medications correctly, and talking to the doctor about any problems they have. And if we do this part well, then the patients are able to take over and do it for themselves, and we move on to focus on other topics that they may want help with.

The primary health care team needs to know what medications the patient is taking and how they are taking them; and the patient needs to clearly understand what medications have been prescribed to them, why the medications were prescribed, and when and how to take the medications. There are three related components to medication management:

- Medication reconciliation
- Medication concordance
- Medication adherence

MEDICATION RECONCILIATION

Medication reconciliation compares the list of medicines that have been prescribed to the patient with the list of medications that the patient is actually taking. This is an opportunity to learn whether or not the patient and their clinical team are on the same page regarding medications.

Unfortunately, in many busy medical practices and clinics, medication reconciliation *is never done at all.* But understanding which medications the patient is taking is important in terms of managing chronic conditions, preventing potentially harmful or dangerous medication interactions (interactions between two or more different types of medications), and managing side effects.

While any member of the primary care team can do medication reconciliation, it is often done by a CHW, who may have more time to spend with the patient. Ideally, medication reconciliation is done before the patient's visit with a physician or other clinical provider. To do medication reconciliation, a CHW should:

1. Ask the patient to bring in all of the medicines they are currently taking, from all prescribing clinicians (including both those within and outside of your clinical team), and any prescriptions they may have (even if unfilled).

2. Print out a list of medications prescribed by the licensed medical providers on the patient's primary health care team.

3. Review each medication with the patient. For each medication discussed, ask the patient:
   - What do you take this medication for?
   - How often are you supposed to take this medication?
   - Are you taking the medication (and taking it according to the guidelines)? If the patient isn't taking the medication, ask them why not.

As always, document what you learn (the list of all medications prescribed, which the patient is taking, and how often).

How to Read the Label on Medications

When you ask patients to bring in their medications, ask them to do so in the pill bottles they received from the pharmacist. Review the information on the label of the medication bottle with the patient, supporting them to learn how to read and understand this information in the future.

The link below provides information about reading medication labels from the US Department of Health and Human Services Office of Women's Health. It is available online at: *http://womenshealth.gov/minority-health/taking-care-health/reading-drug-labels.html*.

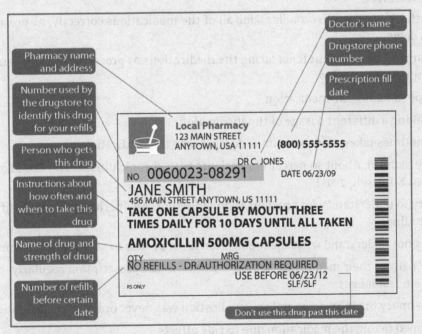

Figure 16.1 Drug Label

The labels include essential information, including:

- Instructions for how to take the medication, how often and when to take it
- The name and strength of the medication
- Possible side effects, indications of these side effects, and guidance for when to contact their doctor
- The number of refills before a certain date
- If the medication should be kept out of the reach of children
- The medication's expiration date

MEDICATION CONCORDANCE

Medication concordance means checking with the patient to see if their *understanding* about how to take a medication is the same as directed by the prescribing physician (or other provider). It is about what the patient *understands*. When you meet with patients, ask them how they take their medications. Check their answer against their prescription.

- *Concordance* means that the patient and the clinician have the same understanding of how a medication should be taken.

- *Discordance* means that the patient and the clinician have a different understanding.

Checking for medication concordance is important because research shows that approximately 50 percent of patients don't understand how to take their medications (Bodenheimer, 2008). Taking medications incorrectly can mean that they won't be effective in treating the health condition, or that the patient might experience preventable side effects or health risks.

If you find a discordance (the patient and the clinician have different understandings), be sure to talk with the patient and carefully review the directions for how to take their medications as provided on the prescription. *Make sure that the patient understands the correct way to take their medications before they leave. Ask them to write down the information clearly in their primary language.* Document the discordance you identified and be sure to inform the physician.

MEDICATION ADHERENCE

Adherence means that the patient *is actually taking* all of the medications correctly, as prescribed. It is about what the patient is *doing.*

Nonadherence means that the patient *is not taking* the medications as prescribed. There can be many different reasons for nonadherence, including:

- The patient stopped taking the medication

- The patient is taking a different dosage of the medication

- The patient sometimes takes, and sometimes doesn't take the medication

Nonadherence is very common. About 50 percent of patients with chronic illnesses do not take their medications as prescribed (Brown & Bussell, 2011).

It is important to try to understand *why* a patient is nonadherent. Again, there are many different reasons why this may be so, including:

- The patient does not understand what the medication is for or how to take it (discordance).

- The patient can't afford their medication so they don't refill the prescription regularly, or may split or skip pills to make them last longer.

- The clinic or pharmacy made an error and the medication was never ordered for the patient.

- The patient stopped taking the medication due to side effects.

- The patient is feeling better and thinks that they no longer have to take the medication (this could be an indication that the medication is actually working to help control symptoms of the disease, and should therefore be continued).

- The patient doesn't believe that the medication will help them, or does not feel that the medication helped them to feel any better, so does not see the point to continuing.

- The patient has decided to treat their chronic condition in another way, and is not taking the medication. For example, the patient may be going to a different type of health care provider for alternative treatments.

- The patient doesn't want to start a medication that they may have to take for a long time, or even the rest of their life.

- The patient is taking many different medications and it is difficult/confusing to manage it all. As a consequence, sometimes the patient forgets to take their medication, or forgets and takes a double dose of the medication.

As a CHW, your role is to use client-centered practice to talk about medications with the patient and, if they are not taking medications as prescribed, to try to find out why. Once you have learned what may be getting in the way of adherence, you and the patient can develop a plan of action. A plan of action is likely to include a follow-up appointment with the physician or other prescribing health care provider. This will provide the patient with an opportunity to raise concerns and ask additional questions about their medications, and give the physician an opportunity to explain why the medications are prescribed, discuss the pros and cons of taking or not taking the medications and, as always, to explore alternatives.

Please watch the following short videos ▶️ which show a CHW, Juanita Alvarado, working to support a patient with medications management.

- What challenges was this patient facing in terms of taking his medications?
- What did the CHW do well to support the patient with medications management?
- What else might you do to support this patient with medications management?

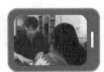

MEDICATIONS MANAGEMENT, PART 1: ROLE PLAY, DEMO

🔗 *http://youtu.be/ gleMEwoN72k*

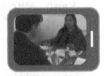

MEDICATIONS MANAGEMENT, PART 2: ROLE PLAY, DEMO

🔗 *http://youtu.be/ eLRe6wVkLuw*

16.16 Responding to Ambivalence, Resistance, and Relapse

People living with chronic conditions sometimes feel ambivalent (have mixed feelings or thoughts) about changing behavior to promote their health. At times, they may resist taking action to meet their own health goals, such as trying to change their diet. Some patients will relapse or resume older patterns of behavior that increase health risks—such as using tobacco, alcohol, or drugs, not exercising, or eating a less healthy diet.

As discussed in Chapter 9, ambivalence, resistance, and relapse are common, and we encourage you to anticipate and accept them as a natural part of life and the behavior change process. Be prepared to respond in a way that honors the autonomy of clients. Your respect may help them to get back on track. As always, let your work be guided by client-centered concepts and skills. For example:

MEDICATIONS MANAGEMENT, PART 3: ROLE PLAY, DEMO

🔗 *http://youtu.be/ F2Mndwvfu-c*

- Listen without judgment to patients' experiences, feelings, and thoughts
- Demonstrate unconditional positive regard.
  - Some clients may worry that resistance or relapse will change or harm their working relationship with you and the clinical team. They may fear your disappointment or judgment.

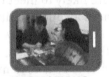

MEDICATIONS MANAGEMENT, PART 4: ROLE PLAY, DEMO

🔗 *http://youtu.be/ SVWbGyEKblk*

- Use your client-centered skills, including motivational interviewing, to support the client in reflecting more deeply about what they are thinking and feeling and what they want to do next.

- Roll with resistance (see Chapter 9). Don't try to argue or lecture a client out of their resistance to change. Share reflective statements that provide clients with a chance to further explore and understand their doubts and concerns. Honor the complex challenge of making meaningful change in our lives. Support the client's autonomy and decisions, even if you don't *fully understand or agree with them.* Remember that this work is about *the client's* life, their health, their values, beliefs, and decisions.

- If you find yourself getting stuck, wanting to give advice or rescue, note these instincts and put them aside while you are working with the client. Come back to them when you have a chance to reflect on your own or with another (such as a supervisor or other colleague). Strive to understand what was going on for *you* during the session, and where the instinct or urge to rescue or direct is coming from. Self-awareness is a critical resource for refining your client-centered approach and ensuring that your own issues don't unduly influence or undermine the health of the client.

What else might you do—or do differently—when faced with these situations?

> **CASE STUDY** | **Keisha Mitchell (*continued*)**
>
> **Please watch the following videos** that show a CHW working with Keisha Mitchell. Keisha wants to better manage her high blood pressure and develops a plan to start going to a local Zumba class with her daughter to increase physical activity. However, her plan doesn't go as expected. In the first counter role play, the CHW struggles to respond effectively. In the demo role play, the CHW displays a much more client-centered approach to supporting Keisha.
>
> - What got in the way of Keisha Mitchell's action plan? What factors made it difficult for her to be successful?
> - What did the CHW do well, and not so well, in these two role plays, and how may the CHW's approach have affected Keisha Mitchell?
>
>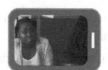
> ACTION PLANNING, REVISING AN ACTION PLAN: ROLE PLAY, COUNTER
>
> 🔗 *http://youtu.be/ g6I5omhDSHU*
>
>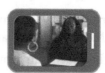
> ACTION PLANNING, REVISING AN ACTION PLAN: ROLE PLAY, DEMO
>
> 🔗 *http://youtu.be/ Clr5pcdzo74*
>
>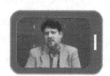
> ACTION PLANNING, REVISING AN ACTION PLAN: FACULTY INTERVIEW
>
> 🔗 *http://youtu.be/ JUtog9cd29Q*
>
> - What else would you want to do or say if you were the CHW working to support Keisha Mitchell in this role play scenario?
>
> **Finally, watch the video interview** about the role plays featuring Keisha Mitchell and the challenge of revising an action plan more generally.

16.17 Follow-up Services

You are likely to meet with most clients more than once. Each additional contact—by phone or in person—provides an opportunity to review a client's issues, questions and plans. Effective follow-up supports clients to learn and apply new knowledge and skills, and to gain confidence in their ability to manage their chronic conditions. Hopefully, these will lead to improved health outcomes. Remember that the long-term goal is for patients to be able to manage their own chronic conditions and health without frequent assistance from their primary care team.

Some follow-up services will be routine check-ins about the client's current health status and how they are doing with their action plans. Patients whose chronic conditions are not yet well managed—who may still be experiencing uncontrolled high blood pressure or blood glucose levels, for example—are likely to be scheduled for more frequent follow-up appointments. In addition to routine appointments, follow-up visits may be scheduled when:

- A client misses one or more appointments or is no longer in contact with the clinic (these clients are considered to be "lost to follow up")
- A client calls to say that their health status is worsening or that they are facing a challenge that will impact their health (such as the loss of housing)
- A client is no longer refilling prescriptions for medications, equipment, or other health resources
- The clinic learns that a client visited a local emergency department to seek treatment for their chronic condition, such as seeking treatment for an asthma attack, chest pain, or other urgent health symptoms
- A client is discharged from the hospital or another institution (drug treatment facility, the local jail, hospice, etc.)
- *Can you think of other circumstances that might prompt the clinical team to ask a client to schedule a follow-up visit?*

CHWs play a critical role in identifying and reaching out to clients in need of follow-up services. The CHW may reach out to contact the patient by phone (or text or email) to see how they are doing. They may schedule a follow-up appointment in the clinic or another setting. When the client cannot be reached in other ways, CHWs may conduct a home visit or seek out the client in other places where they may work or live. These may include a local shelter, other places where people who are homeless sleep, in residential recovery programs, hospice, hospitals, local jails, and other institutional settings.

In these cases, the goal is to provide the client with an opportunity to re-engage in services or treatment. They may ask for assistance to better control their chronic condition. They may be interested in preventing, if possible, the further progress of their disease. Or they may have other problems to address. Some clients may not want to continue services or treatment, and that must be respected too.

For those who are willing, follow-up services may include:

- Re-establishing and building (or rebuilding) a positive rapport or connection
  - Each new contact provides an opportunity to strengthen your professional relationship with patients.
- Making time for the client to discuss current priorities and concerns
  - No matter what the priorities of the primary care team are, be sure that the client's leading concerns are fully addressed during the follow-up session
- Assessing current health indicators (such as blood pressure or lung function tests)
- Reviewing and discussing information about specific health conditions such as diabetes or depression
- Reviewing existing action plan goals and steps for meeting these goals
  - One option is to use a motivation scale for the client to assess their current level of readiness or motivation
- Reviewing guidelines for taking prescribed medications correctly
- Checking in about previous referrals. Did the client attempt to access these services and, if so, what was the outcome? Are they still interested in the referral?
  - Over the course of your work with clients, life circumstances will evolve and change. Clients will face new challenges and opportunities with their families, housing, employment, education, parole, and other circumstances.
- What else do you hope to achieve during a follow-up meeting with a client?

16.18 Ending Services (Discharge or Termination)

Over time, CHWs will initiate professional relationships with new clients, while ending services to others. You may meet with (or talk to) a client just once, or communicate with them dozens or even hundreds of times. You may work with a client for a week or two, or for months or years, depending upon their interest and needs and the guidelines of your agency or program.

Ending services may be mutual, meaning that both the client and the provider or agency agree with the decision. Services may also be terminated by the client alone and, in some circumstances, by the clinic/provider alone.

Ideally, services come to end because the client's chronic condition is well managed and they no longer require ongoing and intensive support from a primary care team. But services may end (or be terminated) for many different reasons including:

- The client moves away from the area
- The client switches to a new medical provider or clinic
- The client is no longer be eligible to receive medical services at your clinic/hospital
- The client is incarcerated
- The client is upset or displeased with some aspect of the services that you and your team have provided and no longer wishes to work with you

- The clinic decides to discharge the client and no longer provide services due to behaviors such as threats or violence
- The need for specialized medical care at another clinic, hospital, or hospice
- Death

In some situations, you won't have an opportunity to work with the patient to plan for the termination of services or to say goodbye. When you anticipate that services will be ending, you and the patient can manage this process together, along with the rest of the clinical team. For example, consider the case of a long-standing client living with chronic conditions who informs you that she will be moving to another state in three months and will no longer be a patient at your clinic. Suggestions for how to manage the end of the professional relationship with the client include:

- Thank them for the opportunity to work together
- Ask the client about their plans to seek out another medical provider in their new city and state. If the client is interested, and if you are able, provide referrals for services for their new location
- Review the client's plan for the self-management of their chronic condition(s) including medications management, behavior change goals, and other actions
  - Check to make sure that the client has sufficient medications with them during their transition (this may depend upon clinic and pharmacy policies)
- Review what the client will do if their health worsens, and what signs and symptoms to watch for
- Discuss relapse prevention and what the client plans to do if they relapse to previous behaviors that may place their health at risk
- Ask the client to summarize their key accomplishments so far, including what they have learned that helps them to better manage their health
- Affirm the knowledge, skills, and confidence that the client have gained
- Ask them if they would like to provide any feedback about your own work and the quality of services received by their clinical team

CHALLENGES WITH ENDING SERVICES

Some terminations are more difficult than others. Sometimes the patient is initiating the termination of services. Perhaps they are unhappy, frustrated, or angry about the level or quality of care they received. In these cases, it is important to manage the termination process with generosity, patience, and professionalism. Some patients will cycle in and out of services at the clinic where you work. They may terminate services and re-engage with you six months or two years later. For CHWs, these situations are often awkward, particularly if you live in the same neighborhood or belong to the same community as the client and their family. You may continue to run into the client in community settings, so you want to end this professional relationship as respectfully and peacefully as possible. In these types of situations, our suggestions include:

- Listen without judgment or defensiveness
- Honor and accept the patient's decision
- Stop and reflect on the feedback that the patient provides. What could you and the team have done differently?
- If you can do so authentically, apologize for any mistakes or missed opportunities that you or your colleagues may have made
- Wish the client well
- If appropriate, keep the door open for their return to service. You might say something like "I know that right now you don't want to continue coming here for services. But, if that ever changes, please don't hesitate to contact me—we will be here for you."
- As above, review current treatment protocols, including medications
- *What else do you want to do or keep in mind as services come to an end with a client?*

Chapter Review

After studying the information presented in this chapter, practice answering some of the following questions. Think about how you would explain the concept to a professional colleague or a community member.

- How would you define and explain what chronic conditions are?
- How common are chronic conditions?
- What are some of the most common chronic conditions?
- Are chronic health conditions equally common among all communities or populations? Why or why not?
- What are some of the causes of chronic conditions (remember to apply the ecological framework!)?
- What are some of the consequences of chronic conditions—for people living with them, for their families, and for their communities?
- What are some of the available treatments for chronic conditions?
- What are some of the key ways that medical practice is changing in terms of chronic conditions management?
- What does "patient self-management" mean, and why is it important?
- What are some common goals for patient self-management? What types of behaviors may patients wish to change in order to better self-manage their chronic condition(s)?
- What is panel management, and how does it benefit patients?
- What are the key roles and tasks of CHWs who work with patients who are living with chronic health conditions?
- How can CHWs apply client-centered concepts and skills to the task of supporting patients with the self-management of chronic health conditions?
- What are the three components of medications management, and how can they promote a patient's health?
- What are some of the reasons that a client may wish to end services?

Please review the case study about Keisha Mitchell presented at the beginning of the chapter. If you were the CHW working with Keisha, how would you answer the following questions?

- What factors may contribute to Ms. Mitchell's health risks?
- What factors promote or contribute to Ms. Mitchell's health and well-being?
- What would you do or say in working with Keisha to help her to develop an action plan to manage her high blood pressure?
- How might you use OARS in working with Keisha?
    - What is an example of an Open-ended question that you would ask Keisha, and why would you ask it?
    - What is an example of an Affirmation that you would share with Keisha, and why?
    - What is an example of a Reflective listening statement that you would share with Keisha, and why?
    - What would you Summarize in working with Keisha, and why?
- Keisha takes two medications to control her hypertension, but sometimes forgets to take them. How might you help Ms. Mitchell with medications management?
- How would you help Keisha to prevent relapse or a return to prior health risks?
- How will you respond if Keisha tells you that her action plan isn't working for her and she wants to change it?
- Under what circumstances—either positive or negative—might you end your intensive working relationship with Keisha?

References

Bodenheimer, T., Wagner, E. H., & Grumbach, K. (2002). Improving primary care for patients with chronic illness: The chronic care model, part 2. *Journal of the American Medical Association, 288*(15), 1909–1914.

Bodenheimer, T. (2008). Coordinating care: A perilous journey through the health care system. *New England Journal of Medicine, 358*(10), 1064–1071.

Brown, M., & Bussell, J. (2011, April). Medication adherence: WHO cares? *Mayo Clinic Proceedings, 86*(4), 304–314.

The Centers for Disease Control and Prevention. (2009). *Yes We Can children's asthma program.* Retrieved from *www.cdc.gov/asthma/interventions/yes_we_can.htm*

The Centers for Disease Control and Prevention. (2012). Vital signs: Awareness and treatment of uncontrolled hypertension among adults—United States, 2003–2010. *MMWR,61*(35), 703–709.

The Centers for Disease Control and Prevention. (2014). *How the Centers for Disease Control and Prevention (CDC) Supports Community Health Workers in Chronic Disease Prevention and Health Promotion.* Retrieved from *www.cdc.gov/dhdsp/programs/spha/docs/chw_summary.pdf*

The Centers for Disease Control and Prevention. (n.d.-a.). *The adverse childhood events study (ACE).* Retrieved from *www.cdc.gov/ace/index.htm*

The Centers for Disease Control and Prevention. (n.d.-b.). *Chronic disease prevention and health promotion.* Retrieved from *www.cdc.gov/chronicdisease/*

The Centers for Disease Control and Prevention. (n.d.-c.). *Chronic disease overview.* Retrieved from *www.cdc.gov/chronicdisease/overview/*

Gordon, C., & Galloway, T. (2008). *Review of findings on chronic disease self-management program (CDSMP) outcomes: Physical, emotional, & health-related quality of life, healthcare utilization and costs.* Evidence-Based Healthy Aging Program and Centers for Disease Control and Prevention. Retrieved from *http://patienteducation.stanford.edu/research/Review_Findings_CDSMP_Outcomes1%208%2008.pdf*

Jones, L. (2011). *A dam brings a flood of diabetes to three tribes.* Retrieved from *http://indiancountrytodaymedianetwork.com/2011/07/05/dam-brings-flood-diabetes-three-tribes-38482*

Legion, V. and Madden, N. Personal communication, July 2014.

Lorig, K. R., Ritter, P., Stewart, A. L., Sobel, D. A., Brown, B. W., Bandura, A., . . . Holman, H. R. (2001). Chronic disease self-management program 2-year health status and health care utilization outcomes. *Medical Care, 39*(11), 1317–1323. Retrieved from *www.uky.edu/~eushe2/Bandura/Bandura2001MC.pdf*

MacGregor, K., Handley, M., Wong, S., Sharifi, C., Gjeltema, K., Schillinger, D., & Bodenheimer, T. (2006). Behavior-change action plans in primary care: A feasibility study of clinicians. *Journal of the American Board of Family Medicine, 19*(3), 215–223. Retrieved from *www.jabfm.org/content/19/3/215.full*

Manchanda, R. (2014). *The upstream doctors: Medical innovators track sickness to its source.* (Kindle ed.). Retrieved from *www.amazon.ca/The-Upstream-Doctors-Innovators-Sickness-ebook/dp/B00D5WNXPE?*

The Mayo Clinic. (2014a). Heart disease in women: Understand symptoms and risk factors. Retrieved from *www.mayoclinic.org/diseases-conditions/heart-disease/in-depth/heart-disease/art-20046167.*

The Mayo Clinic. (2014b). Retrieved from High blood pressure (hypertension). *www.mayoclinic.org/diseases-conditions/high-blood-pressure/in-depth/high-blood-pressure/art-20045868?pg=2*

Moss, M. (2013). *Salt, sugar, fat: How the food giants hooked us.* New York, NY: Random House.

National Health Statistics Reports. (2011). *Asthma prevalence, health care use, and mortality: United States, 2005–2009.* Retrieved from *www.cdc.gov/nchs/data/nhsr/nhsr032.pdf*

Ory, M. G., Ahn, S., Jiang, L. M., Smith, M. L., Ritter, P. L., Whitelaw, N., & Lorig, K. (2013). Successes of a national study of the chronic disease self-management program: meeting the triple aim of health care reform. *Medical Care, 51*(11), 992–998.

Spero, D. (2006). *Diabetes: Sugar-coated crisis: Who gets is, who profits and how to stop it.* Gabriola Island, BC, Canada: New Society Publishers.

Willard, R., & Bodenheimer, T. (2012). *The building blocks of high-performing primary care: Lessons from the field.* California HealthCare Foundation. Retrieved from *www.chcf.org/publications/2012/04/ building-blocks-primary-care*

The World Health Organization (WHO). (n.d.). *Chronic diseases and health promotion.* Retrieved from *www.who .int/chp/en/index.html*

The World Health Organization. (2009). *Global health risks: Mortality and burden of disease attributable to selected major risks.* Retrieved from *www.who.int/healthinfo/global_burden_disease/GlobalHealthRisks_report_full.pdf*

The World Health Organization. (2010). *Global status report on noncommunicable disease 2010,* Executive Summary and Chapters 1 and 2. Retrieved from *www.who.int/nmh/publications/ncd_report2010/en/index.html*

Additional Resources

California Healthcare Foundation. (n.d.). *Self-management support training materials.* Retrieved from *www.chcf .org/publications/2009/09/selfmanagement-support-training-materials*

The Centers for Disease Control and Prevention. (2009). *The power of prevention: Chronic disease . . . the public health challenge of the 21st century.* Retrieved from *www.cdc.gov/chronicdisease/pdf/2009-Power-of-Prevention.pdf*

The Centers for Disease Control and Prevention. (2013). *Summary health statistics for the U.S. population: National health interview survey.* Retrieved from *www.cdc.gov/nchs/data/series/sr_10/sr10_259.pdf*

The Centers for Disease Control and Prevention. (n.d.). Chronic disease prevention and health promotion. Retrieved from *www.cdc.gov/chronicdisease/*

Coughlin, S. (2011, July). Post-traumatic stress disorder and cardiovascular disease. *Open Cardiovascular Medicine Journal, 5,* 164–170. Retrieved from *www.ncbi.nlm.nih.gov/pmc/articles/PMC3141329/*

County of Los Angeles Public Health. (2013). *How social and economic factors affect health.* Retrieved from *http:// publichealth.lacounty.gov/epi/docs/SocialD_Final_Web.pdf*

Kaiser Family Foundation. (2014). *Fact sheet: The HIV/AIDS epidemic in the United States.* Retrieved from *www.kff .org/hivaids/upload/3029-16.pdf*

Lorig, K., Holman, H., Sobel, D., & Laurent, D. (2006). *Living a healthy life with chronic conditions: Self-management of heart disease, arthritis, diabetes, asthma, bronchitis, emphysema and others.* Boulder, CO: Bull Publishing.

National Center for Chronic Disease Prevention and Health Promotion. (2015). *Addressing chronic disease through Community Health Workers: A policy and systems-level approach.* Retrieved from *www.cdc.gov/dhdsp/docs/chw_ brief.pdf*

National Center for Chronic Disease Prevention and Health Promotion. (n.d.). *Chronic disease indicators.* Retrieved from www.cdc.gov/cdi/

National Council on Aging. (n.d.). Chronic disease self-management fact sheet. Retrieved from *www.ncoa.org/ press-room/fact-sheets/chronic-disease.html*

The Patient-Centered Primary Care Collaborative. (n.d.). Retrieved from *www.pcpcc.org*

Sledjeski, E., Speisman, B., & Dierker, L. C. (2008, August). Does number of lifetime traumas explain the relationship between PTSD and chronic medical conditions? Answers from the National Comorbidity Survey— Replication (NCS-R). *Journal of Behavioral Medicine, 31*(4), pp. 341–349.

Spero, D. (n.d.) Empowerment as Medicine. Retrieved from *www.davidsperorn.com*

Stanford School of Medicine. (n.d.). *Patient education: Chronic Disease Self-Management Program.* Retrieved from *http://patienteducation.stanford.edu/programs/cdsmp.html*

Stellefson, M., Dipnarine, K., & Stopka, C. (2013). The chronic care model and diabetes management in U.S. primary care settings: A systematic review. *Preventing Chronic Disease, 10,* 120180. doi:*10.5888/pcd10.120180*

The World Health Organization. (n.d.). Genomic Resource Centre. *WHO's Human Genetics areas of work.* Retrieved from *www.who.int/genomics/about/commondiseases/en/index.html*

The World Health Organization. *World Health Report, 2010.* Retrieved from *www.who.int/whr/2010/en/index.html*

Promoting Healthy Eating and Active Living

Tim Berthold and Jill Tregor

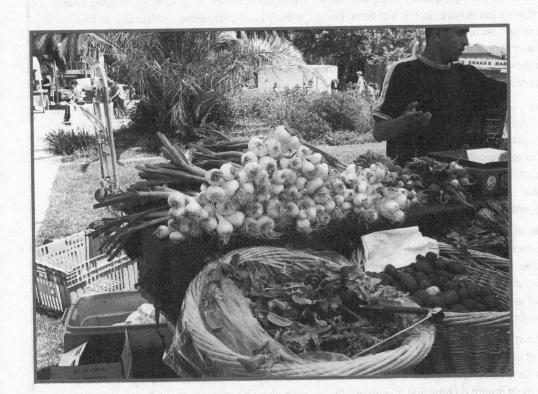

CASE STUDY   Carla Moretti

You are a CHW and work for a small health clinic that serves rural communities. Today you meet with Carla Moretti, who has uncontrolled high blood pressure. She was referred by a nurse practitioner to talk with you about improving her diet and level of physical activity.

Carla is 38 years old and the mother of a nine-year-old daughter, Roberta or "Robbie." Carla lives with her partner, Alma Lopez, and Alma's son, Mikey, age 11. Alma had a bad accident at work last year, and has been out on disability and unable to work. Carla works two part-time jobs to support her family and does most of the shopping and cooking.

When you ask Carla what the family typically eats, she says: *"Well, I don't have a lot of time for cooking, with the kids to look after and Alma being hurt. So, I'm just being honest, mostly I just microwave stuff for dinner like mac-and-cheese or those nugget things so I don't get any complaints from the kids. And the nurse told me that soda isn't so good but I don't know if the kids will drink anything else. If Alma has a good day then maybe there is some beans and rice on the stove, and I cook up some meat or chicken breasts and we have it with tortillas and my sister-in-law's homemade salsa."*

Carla continues, telling you: *"Both of us have gained a lot of weight since we met, especially since Alma's accident. Mikey, too. Robbie, my daughter, she's okay because of all the sports she does. I guess weight has been a problem for me since . . . gosh, since I was really little. All my family are on the bigger side. We used to say we were all "curvy girls"! I used to get teased pretty bad when I was in school, and when I got older I tried all kind of crazy diets. I got skinny once but (laughs), you can see it all came back! I don't need to be all bony like my sister Nancy, but I wish that I weighed what I did when I first met Alma. I met her at a bar where there used to be line dancing and (laughs) well, we both loved to dance."*

When you ask Carla about her level of physical activity now, she says: *"Not much of anything except running to the car to get to work and running back to take Robbie to her practices or games. Sometimes I take Mikey along to Robbie's practice and we walk around the field together. But Mikey isn't so into sports. He likes to stay on the couch with Alma to play their video games, though. That's their mother/son time. But really, I am just so tired all the time. If I come home from work I give Alma a kiss and say I'm gonna lie down for a minute, and next thing you know Robbie is shaking me awake and asking for dinner."*

When you ask Carla about her health goals, she says, *"Both me and Alma want to get healthier for the kids. This is the best family either of us ever had. But that nurse said I got to completely change what we eat and start doing exercise, or my blood pressure could get worse and affect my heart, or I could have a stroke just like my dad. But I need some tips on how to do it with no time and no money, because we don't have any to spare."*

If you were the CHW who is working with Carla, how would you answer the following questions?

Challenges and Strengths

- What are some of Carla's key resources and strengths?
- What are some of the key challenges and health risks that Carla is facing?

Physical Activity

- What is Carla's current level of physical activity?
- How may her current level of physical activity affect her health?
- How could Carla begin to increase her level of physical activity?
- What types of exercise or physical activity may improve Carla's blood pressure and heart health?

Healthy Eating

- What aspects of Carla's diet may promote her health?

- In what ways may her current diet contribute to her health risks?

- How might Carla improve the quality of her diet on a limited budget?

Weight

- How may the issue of weight affect Carla's health?

- What guidance would you have for Carla about her weight?

Client-Centered Practice

- How could you use client-centered practice to support Carla and her family to address issues of healthy eating and physical activity?

Introduction

This chapter provides an introduction to the health topics of nutrition, weight and physical activity. What we eat and drink, and how much physical activity we engage in, are key determinants of health and wellness. Low levels of physical activity and less healthy diets are highly associated with increased risks for chronic health conditions, including heart disease, diabetes, some cancers, and premature death.

Many CHWs who work in clinical and community settings are engaged in supporting people to increase their level of physical activity and to develop and maintain healthier diets. CHWs who work in the area of chronic disease management will spend considerable time addressing these issues as patients frequently seek to make changes to their diets and level of physical activity.

This chapter also provides an overview of the controversial connection between weight and health, and guidelines for working with clients of all sizes, including those who have been labeled as "overweight" or obese. We challenge traditional health care approaches that promote weight loss and introduce the weight-inclusive approach, an emerging model grounded in research evidence that encourages providers to stop advising weight loss and to focus on other key health issues and outcomes.

This chapter is designed to be used together with Chapter 16. It also draws upon concepts and skills presented in the other chapters on Practicing Cultural Humility, Guiding Principles, Client-Centered Counseling for Behavior Change, and Care Management.

WHAT YOU WILL LEARN

By studying the information in this chapter, you will be able to:

- Identify key challenges to changing diets and levels of physical activity

- Explain general guidelines for healthier eating and drinking

- Explain general guidelines for healthy levels of regular activity or exercise

- Analyze why a focus on health rather than weight may be most effective in supporting a client's well-being and in fostering positive relationships between CHWs and their clients

- Explain a five-step approach to providing health education about nutrition, physical activity, or other health topics

- Describe how to apply client-centered concepts and skills for supporting clients to establish healthier patterns of eating and activity

WORDS TO KNOW

Body Mass Index	Food Insecurity
Food Security	Saturated Fat

Trans Fats

Vegetarian

Vegan

Weight-Cycling

Weight-Inclusive

Weight-Normative

17.1 What We Eat and Drink

While the foods that Americans eat vary considerably based on factors such as culture, income, and geographic region, in general the diet has become less healthy over time. Today, Americans eat fewer fresh foods—such as fresh fruits and vegetables—than before, and more processed and packaged foods designed to last for months in the grocery store, and other foods that are high in salt, sugar, and fats. This pattern of eating is associated with increasing rates of chronic health conditions including cardiovascular disease, diabetes, and cancer (CDC, n.d.-c.).

FOOD POLICY

These changes in the American diet were caused by many factors, including the practices of corporate agricultural producers and food manufacturers, and government policies that have largely supported these corporate practices. A few very large multinational corporations now dominate farming and food manufacturing. The primary interest of these corporations is profit, and this has resulted in strategies for large-scale production, at low cost, of products that can be easily shipped and stored for many months on the shelves of supermarkets and in our homes.

Manufacturers have also invested heavily in the development of food products that consumers will literally *crave*. They have applied science to the development of food and drink products with just the right balance of salt, sugar, and added fats to keep us coming back for more (Moss, 2013). Visit the middle aisles in almost any supermarket or grocery store in the United States, and you will find thousands of products on the shelves that contain dramatically high amounts of sodium or salt, sugar (including high-fructose corn syrup and cane sugar) and added fats. Unfortunately, for most of the twentieth century, government policies, including agricultural policies and nutritional guidelines, supported the interests of those large corporations at the expense of our health. These practices and policies have played a large contributing role in the increased rates of chronic disease across the United States.

> ## Politics Influence Latest U.S. Nutritional Guidelines
>
> As this chapter is being written, the U.S. government is in the process of updating national nutritional guidelines. However, large corporate interests are challenging the draft recommendations of the 2015 Dietary Guidelines Advisory Committee, an expert panel of independent scientists. The advisory committee has recommended that eating less meat is not only better for human health, but better for the environment as well. American meat producers and their lobbyists are fighting hard to influence Congress to strike these recommendations from the amended 2015 guidelines (Ferdman, 2015).

HUNGER

While many Americans are consuming too much of the types of food and drink that increase risks for chronic disease, tens of millions of people do not have enough food to eat. Note that the terms **food security** (having enough food to eat) and **food insecurity** (not having enough food to eat) are increasingly used to discuss issues of hunger in America. If you are working with low-income clients, it is likely that some of these clients—and their children—regularly experience times when do they do not have enough to eat.

In 2010, approximately 17.5 percent of American household were food insecure, including about 9.8 percent of households with children (Coleman-Jensen, 2011). In 2012, the United States Department of Agriculture (USDA) reported that 8.8 percent of families had "low food security" and 5.7 percent had "very low security" (USDA, 2015). In 2014, there were 33.3 million adults and 15.8 million children who did not regularly have enough to eat (Feeding America, n.d.). Some families rely upon school lunch programs to provide at least one hot meal a day for their children. Other families are increasingly relying upon food pantries and organizations that provide free meals in the community in order to eat. Food insecurity and hunger can result in chronic undernutrition that may result in a variety of health problems including, for example, greater risks for low-birth weight, infectious diseases, and premature death.

If you work with low-income clients, you are likely to work with people for whom food insecurity or hunger is their greatest nutritional challenge. In these cases, your role may be to help them to access reliable sources of food—any food—for themselves and their families.

- *Have you or your family ever experienced food insecurity (times when you did not have enough food to eat)?*

- *How may food insecurity or hunger impact your clients' health and well-being?*

- *What local resources are available in your community that provide groceries or meals to people in need?*

17.2 Common Barriers to Changing Our Diets

Eating a healthy diet is an important part of promoting overall health and managing chronic illness. Yet, making lasting changes to our diets is often very challenging. As always, we want to encourage you to apply an ecological model to your work. Consider the wide range of factors that can make it difficult for people to successfully change what they regularly eat and drink. These factors may include the following:

FAMILY AND CULTURE

Food has an important meaning for most cultures and families. People come together to prepare and eat food, and food is often a central focus of family and cultural celebrations. The traditions established in families can be difficult to change. Family members who try to eat differently may be questioned, criticized, or pressured to conform to the traditions.

PLEASURE

We take pleasure in eating specific types of food. However, some of the foods that we may enjoy the most—such as salty French fries and chips, bacon and hamburgers, sugary cookies, or ice cream—can be harmful to our health when eaten too often.

TIME AND MONEY

Unfortunately, it often takes far less time and costs less money to eat the least healthy foods. This includes the food we purchase from fast-food chains, and the processed foods that we buy in grocery stores. Fresh vegetables and fruits are sometimes more difficult to find, depending upon your neighborhood, and more expensive than prepackaged meals.

LACK OF CONFIDENCE

Some clients doubt their ability to successfully change their diet. Keep in mind that mixed feelings or ambivalence is a natural part of the behavior change process, and that many people have tried to change their diet in the past without lasting success. This history of attempts to change their diet (and/or to lose weight) may cause people to doubt their ability to achieve changes in the future.

As with any attempted behavior change, lack of confidence can undermine success. This is why it is important to start out by seeking moderate changes in behavior that can be achieved in the short term (within several days or weeks, rather than months or years). Using the Motivation Scale (Chapter 9 of *Foundations*) can be helpful in talking about a client's level of confidence in making change. These tools help clients to select a course of behavior change action that they feel confident in taking.

PREJUDICE, STIGMA, LOW SELF-ESTEEM, AND DEPRESSION

Many people face stigma, prejudice, and discrimination based on perceptions about their weight and size. Children who are larger than average size are often teased and bullied. The stress and resulting depression may harm their health and make it more difficult to change or modify what they eat and drink, and may result in an endless cycle of weight loss and gain (Tomiyama, 2014). Clients who are facing these types of challenges require our unconditional positive regard and support.

- *What other factors may get in the way of changing what we eat?*

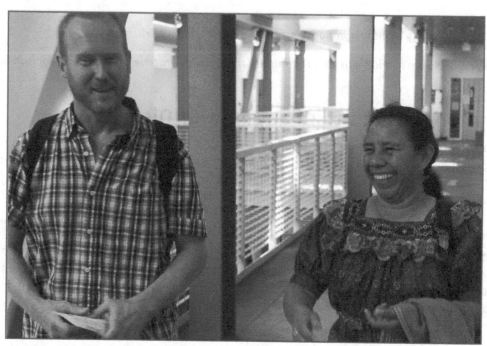

A client shares good news with a CHW.

17.3 Weight and Health

This section of the chapter addresses the connection between body weight and health promotion. Emerging research is highlighted that questions traditional health care approaches that promote dieting and weight loss. Studies show that rather than improving the health of patients perceived as overweight, the promotion of weight loss actually increases risks for physical and mental health. Emerging weight-inclusive approaches recommend that health providers focus on health and fitness issues rather than weight, and have been shown to improve health outcomes (Clifford et al., 2015; Tylka et al., 2014).

THE TRADITIONAL FOCUS ON WEIGHT LOSS

Most health care providers are trained to focus on weight as a key indicator of health. Often, one of the first steps during a health care visit is for the patient to be weighed, and their height recorded. These two indicators (and sometimes the patient's age and sex) are used to calculate **body mass index** (BMI), which is divided into four categories that range from under-weight, to normal, to overweight, to obese (CDC, n.d.-b.). In health care settings, the BMI is used to identity patients in the higher two categories (overweight and obese) and to counsel them to lose weight in order to best protect their health. Patients may be encouraged to lose weight in a variety of ways including a combination of changes to diet and exercise, participating in dieting programs and, in some cases, surgical procedures.

The focus on weight and dieting in health care is reinforced throughout our society. Children and adults who are perceived as overweight often face ongoing prejudice, bullying and discrimination. The dieting industry in the United States generated an estimated $60.5 billion in revenues in 2014 (Marketdata Enterprises, 2014) by marketing a wide range of products (pills and supplements, books, videos, diet plans and programs) that promise weight loss. Some products promise rapid weight loss and use dramatic before and after photographs and inspiring testimonials. Yet, as a result of these false promises, many people begin dieting in childhood and continue throughout their adult years, caught in a dangerous pattern of **weight-cycling** (or a repeated pattern of dieting and initial weight loss, followed by weight gain).

A Note on the Language of Size and Weight

Please carefully consider the words you use to talk about body weight and size. Our society tends to label people who are perceived to be overweight with a long list of negative and demeaning words. When health care providers echo this prejudice, and label patients as fat or obese, they reinforce the stigma of weight and related feelings of shame. While health care providers may use the term "obese" as a clinical description, it may be experienced by clients as a judgment and/or an insult.

Speak with the clients and communities you serve without using negative or judgmental language. In most cases, there is no need to assign clients with any label to describe their body shape and size. At the same time, listen carefully to the language that clients may be comfortable using to describe their own bodies. For example, in the Case Study presented in this chapter, Carla Moretti and her sisters refer to themselves as "curvy." You may wish to let these cues from clients guide you in determining which words to use to talk about weight.

THE HEALTH RISKS OF DIETING AND WEIGHT-CYCLING

Dieting to lose weight is not a sound strategy for promoting health. To begin with, dieting is not effective in promoting sustained weight loss. Research shows that the vast majority of dieters regain the weight they lost, and many gain back more weight than they lost (Jeffery et al., 2000; Mann et al., 2007; Sumithran & Proietto, 2013; Tomiyama, 2014).

Because of the combined forces of prejudice and stigma, the promises of the dieting industry and the prescriptions of medical practitioners, millions of Americans spend many years of their life caught up in the harmful dynamic of weight-cycling. Research links weight-cycling to a wide range of health risks including hypertension, cancer and other chronic conditions, bone fractures, gallstone attacks, and higher risks of mortality or premature death (Brownell & Rodin, 1994; Field, Manson, Taylor, Willett, & Colditz, 2004; Rzehak et al., 2007). In addition to the physical health risks, weight-cycling is also harmful to mental health, including lower self-esteem and higher rates of depression (Tylka et al., 2014).

Your Experience

Part of being a CHW is a commitment to self-reflection and cultural humility. This means reflecting upon your own experience with issues of body size and weight. As you read this chapter, please take time to reflect and to consider the following questions

- How comfortable are you with your body shape and size?
- Have you (or members of your family) ever tried to diet to lose weight?

(continues)

Your Experience
(continued)

- What was the experience of dieting like? What was the outcome?
- Have you (or family members) ever been judged or teased based on your body size?
- Have you ever been told by a health care provider to lose weight?
- To what extent is your own self-esteem (the way that you think and feel about yourself) influenced by perceptions about your body size and shape?
- What assumptions or beliefs do you have about people based on their body size?
- In what ways may your own experiences, values, and beliefs about weight influence your work with clients in the role of CHW?

TOWARD A WEIGHT-INCLUSIVE APPROACH TO PROMOTING HEALTH

Research evidence not only demonstrates that traditional approaches of promoting dieting and weight-loss is harmful to health, it also points the way towards strategies and approaches that are effective for promoting the health of clients while demonstrating respect for their bodies and their identities. These new models (including Health at Every Size, Health in Every Respect, and other models) have been classified as weight-inclusive approaches to health (Tylka et al., 2014).

A **weight-inclusive** approach implies respect for people of all body sizes and weight, and is compared to a **weight-normative** approach, that identifies certain people as having normal weight and others as overweight or obese. While weight-normative approaches counsel patients to lose weight, weight-inclusive approaches shift the focus from weight to focus on specific health issues, behaviors and outcomes. By taking the focus away from body weight and dieting, providers are able to support patients to develop their own culturally relevant plans to enhance health and wellness, including self-esteem. These client-centered plans are determined by the patients themselves and may include, for example, enhancing their level of physical activity by engaging in activities that are practical, enjoyable and sustainable (discussed at greater length later on in this chapter). Clients may make changes not only to what they eat and drink, but how they think and feel about food (for more information about this please refer to the resources provided at the end of this chapter). Weight-inclusive approaches also support clients to seek out support and build connection with others who are facing similar challenges, including others who are working to accept and love their bodies as they are.

Weight-inclusive approaches are based in research evidence about what actually works to promote the health of people who have been classified as "overweight" or obese. One often-cited research study was conducted with women who had been labeled overweight or obese (Bacon, Stern, Van Loan, & Keim, 2005). The women were assigned to two groups. One group was encouraged to diet and lose weight. The other group participated in a Health at Every Size (HAES) program that did not promote dieting or weight loss and focused instead on size acceptance and health goals such as healthy eating and enhanced physical activity. The group that was encouraged to diet initially lost weight, but later regained it, and experienced worse self-esteem. The group assigned to HAES achieved and sustained meaningful health outcomes including improvements to depression, self-esteem, blood pressure, and cholesterol levels and other indicators (Ibid). To read more about Health at Every Size, please see the resources listed at the end of this chapter.

A study published in the *Journal of Obesity* provides a clear description and justification for the emerging weight-inclusive approach to health (Tylka et al., 2014). This study analyzes existing research evidence to show that weight-normative approaches have failed to promote patient health, and how weight-inclusive approaches, including HAES, offer much greater promise for promoting the health of people who are perceived as overweight. Tylka and her colleagues explicitly frame the question of how providers address issues of weight as *an ethical concern.* The article questions why health care providers continue to advise dieting and weight loss when they have been shown to be so harmful to both physical and mental health. They remind us that health care providers have an obligation to avoid harming the patients they serve, and to promote optimal health.

Principles of the Weight-Inclusive Approach to Health

The weight-inclusive approach to health, is guided by seven key principles, presented here (adapted from Tylka et al., 2014).

1. **Do no harm.**

2. **Appreciate that bodies naturally come in a variety of shapes and sizes, and ensure optimal health and well-being is supported for everyone, regardless of their weight.**

3. **Given that health is multidimensional, maintain a holistic focus.**
   - In other words, look beyond weight to consider a wide range of other health-related factors and behaviors as you work with clients.

4. **Encourage a process focus (rather than end-goals) for day-to-day quality of life.**
   - In other words, meet clients were they are, and help them to engage in realistic steps to improve their life and incorporate into their daily lives

5. **Critically evaluate the evidence for weight loss treatment and incorporate sustainable, empirically supported practices in prevention and treatment efforts.**
   - In other words, think critically about what the research evidence shows us about the effectiveness of advising clients to lose weight. Draw upon existing research evidence about what works to promote the health of clients of all body sizes and shapes.

6. **Create healthful, individualized practices and environments that are sustainable (e.g., regular pleasurable exercise, regular intake of foods high in nutrients, adequate sleep and rest, adequate hydration).**
   - Build upon your client-centered CHW skills to support clients to develop and implement realistic plans to enhance their health they can maintain over time. When possible, work at the family and community-levels as well to reinforce policies and practices that support healthy living.

7. **Where possible, work to increase health access, autonomy, and social justice for all individuals along the entire weight spectrum. Trust that people move towards greater health when given access to stigma-free health care and opportunities.**

This weight-inclusive approach is consistent with the concepts and skills promoted through the *Foundations* textbook including cultural humility, client-centered counseling and case management, and support for patient self-management. To read more about weight-inclusive approaches, including Health at Every Size, please refer to the list of resources presented at the end of this chapter.

What Do YOU Think?

- *What do you think of the key principles for a weight-inclusive approach to health?*
- *How well do your health care providers put these principles into practice?*
- *How might you put these principles into action to guide your direct work with clients and communities?*

Key Arguments in Favor of the Weight-Inclusive Approach

By focusing on weight, dieting, and weight-loss, CHWs and other providers may

- Influence clients to invest time and energy in losing weight without long-term success
- Set patients up for years or decades of weight-cycling that is harmful to physical and mental health
- Unnecessarily shift attention away from more achievable health outcomes such as enhanced physical activity and improved blood pressure and glucose measures
- Stigmatize and shame people, resulting in lower self-esteem and risks for depression
- Undermine or damage a client's trust in the professional relationship

(continues)

Key Arguments in Favor of the Weight-Inclusive Approach
(continued)

By shifting the focus from weight to health, CHWs and other health care providers can

- Uphold CHW ethics
- Avoid further stigmatizing or shaming clients based on their body shapes and size
- Apply client-centered concepts and skills to support the autonomy of clients and the development of realistic and sustainable action plans to promote their health and well-being
- Support patients of all sizes to focus on key health goals and indictors such as increasing physical activity and controlling blood pressure and blood glucose levels
- Support patients to significantly improve their physical and mental health
- Develop and maintain professional relationships that enable trust and mutual respect

Please watch the following videos [▶], which show a CHW talking with a client who has diabetes and has been diagnosed as "obese" by her physician and directed to lose weight. In the counter video, the CHW demonstrates a traditional approach to the issue, and also directs the client to diet and lose weight. In the demonstration video, the CHW demonstrates a weight-inclusive approach.

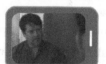

TALKING ABOUT WEIGHT AND HEALTH: ROLE PLAY, COUNTER

⚭ *http://youtu.be/ FLpx7QHjMRY*

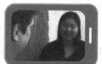

TALKING ABOUT WEIGHT AND HEALTH: ROLE PLAY, DEMO

⚭ *http://youtu. be/83EeBQuXOXo*

- What does the CHW do well in supporting the client's health and well-being?
- What could the CHW do differently to better support this client's health and well-being?
- What else would you do if you working with this client, and why?

Talking with Your Clinical Team about Weight and Health

As a CHW, you may work for a health care organization that follows traditional medical models for diagnosing and treating obesity. These traditional approaches may contradict the information we provide here, your own values, and the experience of the clients you work with. *In such a workplace setting, how can you challenge your colleagues to consider different perspectives about weight and wellness?*

If you decide to raise the issue of weight and health, do so with patience and respect for different perspectives. Anticipate that your efforts may be met with defensiveness, and the concept of a weight-inclusive approach may be dismissed by your colleagues. One way to begin is to ask your coworkers or clinical teammates to read and discuss the emerging research that challenges conventional thinking about weight and health. For example, you may ask your team to read and discuss the article by Tykla et al. on *The Weight-Inclusive versus the Weight-Normative Approach to Health*, or *Body Respect* by Bacon and Aphramor (see the References and Additional Resources at the end of this chapter). You could ask colleagues to meet together to discuss questions such as

- How may labeling patients as "obese" affect their ability to improve their health?
- Is there evidence to support encouraging patients who have tried dieting many times before—without enduring success—to start another weight-loss diet?
- What approaches are most likely to help patients of all sizes to feel respected and engaged in health care services?
- What type of approach is most likely to support patients to make and sustain meaningful improvements to their health status?

17.4 Understanding Information about Nutrition

It can be difficult to find reputable and easy-to-understand sources of information about nutrition for several reasons:

- **There are so many sources of information:** The sheer volume of information about nutrition and diet, including scientific, governmental, popular, and commercial sources complicates the task of identifying good sources of information. If you read magazines, browse the Internet, or watch television, you are constantly exposed to advertisements for weight-loss programs and products. Every year, dozens of new books rise to the top of the best-seller lists that promote new ways to achieve dramatic weight loss and improved health.

- **Distinguishing reputable information**: It can be difficult to determine the most reputable sources of information about nutrition. Agricultural and food corporations and other companies often present misleading information about the nutritional value of their products in order to promote sales. These same corporations have also invested considerable resources to influence government agricultural policies and nutritional guidelines (Moss, 2013; Nestle, 2013). At times, federal food policy has supported the interests of corporate interests over those of public health.

- **Highly specific scientific information**: Research studies, reports and guidelines about nutrition often include details that are difficult for general audiences to understand. For example, many resources on nutrition and diet include detailed information and calculations about calories, fat grams, glycemic index, vitamins, minerals, and micronutrients.

NUTRITIONAL INFORMATION INFORMED BY RESEARCH

Seek out reputable sources of information from leading health organizations that provide information about nutrition that is informed by research and presented in a manner that the communities you work with can understand. While research will continue to refine our understanding of the association between nutrition, chronic disease, and overall health, findings from tens of thousands of reputable studies indicate that *diets that feature plant-based foods (vegetables, fruits, beans, and whole grains) are better for our health and life-expectancy than diets that feature red meat, dairy, and refined and processed foods with added sugars and trans fats.*

SCOPE OF PRACTICE CONCERNS

As a CHW, you will not be expected to know or share detailed information about nutrition and health. You may provide general information about nutrition, and support clients to develop a healthier diet, often with clear guidelines provided by licensed or certified colleagues. But providing detailed information about nutrition is outside of your scope of practice, and should be left to licensed colleagues, including physicians and registered dieticians

If your duties as a CHW include supporting clients to develop healthier diets in order to promote their health, ask your employer to provide you with nutritional guidelines. If you working for a health care organization, it is important for the clinical team to be on the same page in terms of the nutritional information provided to clients.

17.5 Guidelines for Healthy Nutrition

For the purposes of this introductory chapter, we will rely on information provided by *The Nutrition Source*, a website from the Harvard University Schools of Medicine and Public Health that provides evidence-based and easy-to-understand information about nutrition. Please visit the Nutrition Source (*www.hsph.harvard.edu/nutritionsource/*) and spend a few minutes browsing the site.

The Nutrition Source provides information in a well-organized and clearly written format. For example, the first paragraph of a resource titled "What Should I Eat" reads:

> *The answer to the question "What should I eat?" is actually pretty simple. But you wouldn't know that from news reports on diet and nutrition studies, whose sole purpose seems to be to confuse people on a daily basis. When it comes down to it, though—when all the evidence is looked at together—the best nutrition advice on what to eat is relatively straightforward: Eat a plant-based diet rich in fruits, vegetables, and whole grains; choose foods with*

healthy fats, like olive and canola oil, nuts and fatty fish; limit red meat and foods that are high in saturated fat; and avoid foods that contain trans fats. Drink water and other healthy beverages, and limit sugary drinks and salt. Most important of all is keeping calories in check, so you can avoid weight gain, which makes exercise a key partner to a healthy diet. (Harvard University, 2004)

This is a harm-reduction approach. *The Nutrition Source* doesn't tell people not to drink soda, eat french fries, or enjoy an ice cream cone. Rather, they recommend that we reduce our consumption of foods and drinks that research shows increase risks for chronic diseases, and to eat and drink more of what promotes health.

Please review the Healthy Eating Plate presented on the home page of The Nutrition Source: *www.hsph.harvard. edu/nutritionsource/healthy-eating-plate/*

The Healthy Nutrition Plate highlights and provides guidance related to six key dietary categories:

Vegetables

- Eat lots of different types and colors of vegetables.
- This guidance does not apply to potatoes, including potato chips and French fries. The carbohydrates in potatoes are quickly digested and broken down into sugars that raise blood glucose levels and are associated with increased risks for diabetes, cardiovascular disease, and other chronic conditions.

Fruits

- Eat lots of different types and colors of fruit.

Whole Grains

- Eat more grains that haven't been processed, such as brown rice and whole wheat, including whole wheat bread and pasta.
- Limit refined carbohydrates like white bread and white rice. These grains have been stripped of much of their nutritional value, and are quickly digested and broken down into sugar, increasing blood glucose levels.
  - Always keep the big picture and culture in mind. Many people around the world eat white rice as a staple or a common part of a healthy diet. What often matters is what is eaten along with the rice. We provide more information about this later on.

Healthy Protein

- Remember that protein is found in many foods, including vegetables and beans, not just in meat products.
- Try to get most of your protein from beans, nuts, whole grains, and vegetables.
- If you eat animal sources of protein, focus on fish or poultry, but make this a relatively small part of your diet.
- Limit red meat and cured or processed meats (such as bacon, salami, and sausage).

Water

- Drink more water. Or tea or coffee (with little or no added sugar, if possible).
- Limit soda, juice, or other sugary drinks, as well as dairy (milk). Note that fruit juices are also a source of high amounts of sugar, although many people associate fruit juice with "healthy" eating.

Healthy Oils

- Use plant-based oils like olive and canola oils as much as possible. Fish oils are also full of vitamins that our bodies need.
  - These are the types of fats that your body needs (monosaturated and polyunsaturated fats). They help to reduce our risks for chronic disease.

- Limit the use of saturated and trans fats. **Saturated fats** include butter, lard, and other animal fats. **Trans fats** are created in the food manufacturing process by adding hydrogen to vegetable fats so that they will become solids and last a long time on the shelf. They are common ingredients in fried foods and in baked goods such as cookies, crackers, pastries, and some margarines or shortenings. Saturated fats and trans fats are associated with higher risks for chronic disease.

For more detailed information about any of these topics, please visit The Nutrition Source.

What Did You Eat Yesterday?

Helping professionals are often quick to judge what others eat and drink, and to counsel them about what they *should* eat and drink. Please take a moment to stop and consider *your own diet*. What did you eat and drink yesterday?

Breakfast: _____

Lunch: _____

Snacks: _____

Dinner: _____

- How typical was the food you ate yesterday in terms of your usual diet?
- How healthy—on a scale from 1 to 10—would you rate what you ate yesterday?
- What did you eat and drink yesterday that promotes your health?
- What did you eat and drink yesterday that may increase your risks for chronic disease?

The Benefits of Vegetarian and Vegan Diets

Shifting towards a plant-based diet is better for human health and the environment.

Extensive research indicates that animal products, especially red meat and dairy, play a significant role in the development of chronic conditions such as heart disease, hypertension, diabetes, and some types of cancer. Research also suggests a positive relationship between a **vegetarian** diet (no meat) or **vegan** diet (no animal products at all, including dairy) and a reduced risk for these conditions.

Meat production is also highly inefficient and destructive to the environment. It takes many more resources (land, water, grain to feed to the livestock, fuel, fertilizer, pesticides, and other resources) to produce meat than it does to grow grains or vegetables for human consumption. More than half of the world's crops are used to feed animals, not people (UNEP, 2010). Transporting feed, livestock, and animal products burns fossil fuels, emitting greenhouse gases that contribute to global warming. Animal waste also produces large amounts of greenhouse gas in the form of methane, in addition to polluting groundwater, rivers, and oceans. Vast areas of the world's rain forests have been cleared to grow corn and soy for livestock, decreasing the earth's biodiversity and its ability to absorb carbon dioxide from the atmosphere.

The diversion of land, water, fuel and other resources toward livestock production for those who can afford to buy meat contributes to higher food prices for everyone, and threatens the food security for those living in poverty. By the year 2050, 9–10 billion people will populate the Earth—a growth of 50 percent. "*A substantial reduction of [environmental] impacts would only be possible with a substantial worldwide diet change, away from animal products*" (UNEP, 2010, pp. 81–82).

To learn more about this topic, please see the Additional Resources provided at the end of this chapter.

17.6 Practical Guidelines for Healthier Eating

As you work with clients to change their diets, we recommend that you try to keep the following strategies in mind. Support clients to develop nutritional plans that are:

Affordable

- Recommendations for what to eat and drink must be affordable or they won't do any good (and may do harm). Keep the client's budget in mind when they are making plans for what they will eat and drink. Unfortunately, some of the healthiest foods—like fresh fruits and vegetables—are sometimes more expensive than unhealthier options, especially processed and packaged foods.

Accessible

- Not every neighborhood has affordable sources of healthy food. People who live in rural, suburban, and urban areas may have to travel some distance to find an affordable grocery store, and time and transportation can pose significant barriers. Sometimes the poorest communities have the least access to affordable and healthy food. In many low-income neighborhoods in cities it is difficult to find fresh produce (vegetables and fruit) and the produce that is available is sometimes much more expensive than in other neighborhoods.

Realistic

- Don't support a client to set themselves up for disappointment by deciding to make dramatic changes to their diet overnight. If a client eats at fast-food restaurants four times a week, it probably isn't realistic to decide never to eat fast food again. Keep harm reduction in mind. Encourage the client to begin by reducing the number of times they eat at fast-food restaurants, or to change what they order at fast-food restaurants (such as limiting or eliminating soda, or ordering a salad instead of french fries).
- It can be helpful to steer clients away from viewing any food as purely "good" or "bad." Every food may be enjoyed in moderation or on occasion.

With the Family in Mind

- For many clients, attempts to change their diet may be influenced or limited by their family. Changes may conflict with family cultures and traditions. This is especially true if other members of the family do most of the grocery shopping and cooking.
- Ideally, the family will support the client and make at least some adjustments to what the entire household eats and drinks.
- However, convincing other family members to adopt similar changes to their own diets may not be realistic. The client may have to make changes on their own, and to find ways to resist the challenges of having less healthy food and drink in their home.

Enjoyable

- Most people enjoy food. Unfortunately, some of the foods that we most enjoy are the least healthy. We have become conditioned by food manufacturers to crave certain foods high in sugar, salt, and fat.
- A healthier diet is unlikely to be *as* pleasurable, especially at first. Don't misrepresent the value of what people may give up when they limit or eliminate certain foods and drinks. Acknowledge this. Support clients to talk about this process, and listen patiently.
- Support clients to find healthier foods and drinks that they enjoy.

Nonjudgmental

- Judgment—and the shame it causes—isn't helpful to changing behaviors, or to our health in general. Clients are often sensitive to the judgments that health care providers and other professionals make about their behaviors and their health status. When clients feel judged, they may distance themselves from providers and the health information those providers share.

Francis Julian Montgomery: For people without a kitchen or cooking facilities, it can be difficult to manage diabetes, high cholesterol, or other health issues related to diet, because they cannot really cook for themselves. Because a lot of my clients eat at fast-food restaurants, I bring menus from those places and we go over the choices and things like sodium, carbohydrates, and sugar content of different items. We look for the healthiest items. That way I don't end up in the unwanted position of reprimanding a person due to the choices they make because of their income. They can go to an inexpensive fast-food restaurant and still make healthier choices. Also some congregant meal sites [places that provide free meals such as soup kitchens] are healthier than others. By learning to think about how healthy different foods are, my clients have the tools to navigate those meals.

CASE STUDY   Carla (continued)

CHW: So you want to figure out a way for you and your family to eat more healthy foods.

Carla: Yes, but we have a long way to go and, it's just harder, you know, than it sounds.

CHW: Can you tell me more about some of what makes it hard?

Carla: Well I'm just about tapped out already with everything I am trying to manage with Alma being hurt and out of work. So I don't have a lot time or energy or money to start cooking meals like those crazy cooks on TV. (Carla laughs and the CHW joins her)

CHW: I get you. You need these changes to be something that you can pull off with the time, money, and energy you already have, not adding something more to your plate?

Carla: Yeah. I just can't make this into something too crazy. But we do need to get out of rut of frozen nuggets and mac and cheese.

CHW: Okay, so . . . I am wondering if you can think of a meal that you made recently that was affordable, healthy, and not too complicated? Does anything come to mind?

Carla: Well, I don't know so well about the healthy thing, but I think maybe the rice and chicken dish we make. Alma makes the beans and she puts rice in the rice cooker, and when I get home we put some chicken breasts in the oven, with just some salt and pepper, and then we serve it up with this totally amazing salsa that Alma's sister makes.

CHW: That sounds really good to me, and I like the teamwork. So how often do you make this?

Carla: Well, not so often really. We've made it a couple of times.

CHW: So what is the biggest challenge of making your chicken and rice dish?

Carla: Well, it takes planning, and for Alma to make the beans and rice, she's got to feel up to that—you know, getting up and tending the stove. But she is starting to get stronger, so maybe we could try it again.

(continues)

CASE STUDY	Carla (*continued*)

CHW: So maybe this is something to talk with Alma about?

Carla: Yeah, this is important to both of us, and we want to work as a team to help our family.

CHW: I was wondering what you think about maybe adding some more veggies to the meal. Can you think of an easy way to do that? Do the kids eat veggies?

Carla: They do pretty good, but they each got their foods that they don't eat. But I could try salad, I think.

CHW: Salad would be great, and something else that I do sometimes is just to toss some veggies in olive oil, salt, and pepper and put 'em in a tray in the oven while you are cooking the chicken. It could be zucchini or carrots or broccoli, almost any kind of vegetable that you like.

Carla: That definitely sounds like something we could do.

CHW: So to me it sounds like you have a really good plan for making a meal that fits all your criteria: healthy, affordable, not too complicated to make, and something that the whole family likes.

Carla: Yeah, I guess so. It's good to break this down a bit, you know, to see how we can do this for at least one meal.

CHW: I am so glad to hear that. So how confident are you that this plan is something that you and the family could pull off sometime in the next week or two?

Carla: Well, as long as it isn't tonight, or every night, then it is a 10. We can do this.

CHW: This is a great start, Carla. And when you are ready, and if you want to, we can talk again and see how to keep moving forward to make other changes that fit your criteria, okay?

Carla: What we did today was really helpful, so I think it would be good to talk more about plans like this one.

CHW: Okay. Let me know when you want to meet up again, and you can always send me a text like you did this time.

Carla: Yeah, that's good for me. Thanks _____ (CHW name)

17.7 Approaches to Providing Health Education about Nutrition

CHWs often provide information about a variety of health topics to the clients and communities they work with. *How* you provide health information matters, in terms of making it relevant and useful for clients. Consider the following six-step guidelines for sharing health information about nutrition with clients:

1. DETERMINE WHAT THE CLIENT ALREADY KNOWS ABOUT NUTRITION

We recommend that you begin by asking clients to share what they already know about nutrition (or any health topic when you are providing health education). Most clients know something (and many know a lot) about the topics that impact their health. In this case, start by asking the client what they understand about the foods and drinks that are best for their health, and those that are associated with increased risks for chronic health conditions. Let the client's level of knowledge set the agenda for providing any additional health information.

2. DETERMINE THEIR INTEREST IN LEARNING MORE

Before you continue to share any information about nutrition or other health information, ask the client if they are interested in learning more. If the client isn't interested, or interested in discussing it in the moment, change the topic and move on. Respecting their wishes and priorities is essential to providing client-centered services and maintaining a strong positive connection or rapport.

3. SHARE GENERAL INFORMATION

Nutritional information and guidelines are often highly detailed and difficult to comprehend. Remember that you are not a certified nutritionist; your role is to provide more general and accurate information about healthy nutrition, and to link your clients to additional resources such as access to nutritional counseling, affordable food (including, as necessary, food pantries and hot meal programs), and other resources.

We propose the Healthy Eating Plate (discussed in the previous section) as a good place to start with general health information. Information is presented in a simple graphic, and incorporates a harm reduction approach that presents both the types of food and drinks that increase health risks, and those that promote good health.

A reasonable goal for clients is to be able to summarize:

- Foods and drinks that promote health and well-being
- Foods and drinks to limit because they increase risks for chronic disease

4. KEEP CULTURE—AND CULTURAL HUMILITY—IN MIND

When clients plan to change their diet, their decisions are often influenced by their own cultural values and practices. The role of the *CHW is never to tell clients what they should eat,* but rather to provide information and support clients to make informed decisions, keeping culture (and other factors) in mind.

For example, many people around the world have diets that feature white rice. Clients who are used to eating white rice may not wish to switch to options such as brown rice or other whole grains, even if those foods may be healthier. They may decide to cut back on the amount of white rice that they eat, and they may not. They may focus on other aspects of their diet, such as cutting back on drinking sugary sodas or eating fast or processed foods high in sugar, salt, and trans fats. Keep in mind that many people around the world eat a healthy diet that features white rice. The Japanese, for example, typically eat white rice. However, because their overall diet is balanced and healthy, people in Japan have relatively low rates of heart disease, cancer, and diabetes, and one of the highest life expectancies in the world.

5. PROVIDE MORE DETAILED NUTRITIONAL INFORMATION

In some situations, you will be asked to provide detailed nutritional information to clients about how to eat a healthier diet given their day-to-day realities, including their budget, culture, and health status. Note that nutritional guidelines may change depending upon the type of chronic condition that the client is living with. For example, there are special dietary guidelines for the self-management of diabetes, or for patients undergoing radiation or chemotherapy. As always, follow the guidance of your supervisor or your clinician here. If you have not been trained to provide this information yourself, make a referral to a certified nutritionist.

Please watch the following video ▶ role play of a CHW working with a client who is interested in changing her diet to improve their health.

CLIENT-CENTERED COUNSELING AND NUTRITION: ROLE PLAY, DEMO

🔗 *http://youtu. be/73-ebSBGQUo*

- What did the CHW do well in terms of supporting this client to make changes to her diet?
- Which client-centered concepts and skills did the CHW use?
- What would you do differently if you were the CHW who is working with this client?

6. KEEP THE INFORMATION PRACTICAL AND SPECIFIC TO THE CLIENT'S LIFE CIRCUMSTANCES

A key role of CHWs is to support clients to translate information about healthy nutrition into specific and practical guidelines for their daily lives. Don't overwhelm clients with too much information all at once. Let them control the pace of your conversation, and how much information you provide. Rather than talking about more general or abstract issues such as "What is healthy nutrition?" or "What food does your family usually eat?"—our suggestion is to keep the discussion highly focused on their specific life circumstances. For example, try asking the client:

- What did you eat for lunch today?
- What did you eat for dinner last night?

These questions are more likely to generate very detailed information about the client's diet. Follow up questions might include:

- How could you change this meal—what you ate last night—to make it healthier? Can you think of one or two things that you could do?

There are many ways to make a meal healthier, such as:

- Not eating or drinking a particular item (for example, drinking soda)
- Eating less of a particular item (a smaller order of fries)
- Eating or drinking more of an item (such as more vegetables)
- Substituting one food or drink for another (such as substituting water for soda, or a salad for a baked potato)

Another practical approach is to support clients to develop a plan for how to shop for and prepare a healthy meal for their family. This meal should be affordable and something that the client and their family is likely to find appealing. The plan could include:

- Where the client will shop
- A shopping list
- A budget
- A menu for the meal
- Recipes. Note that recipes should be easy to follow, and probably shouldn't include too many steps or ingredients or require too much time to prepare

Alma Vasquez: Especially for families who are living on lower incomes or in a shelter or an SRO [single-room occupancy hotel], I just start by asking questions and listening. I know from my work that even if people have a place to lay their head, they may not have any food. So I might ask them "Did you have something to eat yesterday?" So much information can be gotten that way.

Once you know the client's circumstances, you can start sharing information and support. For example, I might ask what they are planning to have for their next meal, and them compare that to a "Healthy Plate" to talk about healthy food. But I don't use jargon. I also keep in mind that every client is different and everyone learns at their own place. Depending on where they are at, I might help them to figure out a budget and how to buy healthier food. A lot of the time, people learn quicker by doing and observing, than by just listening. I might help a client learn to read food labels by looking together at some packaged food and cans. I might teach them how to steam vegetables in a microwave—whatever they need.

I do my own research about where produce is cheap so I can refer clients. For example, after a certain time of day, some stores cut prices. That is really valuable information. Some clients don't ever step outside of their own neighborhoods, so they may not know about resources just outside their borders. And, of course, the clients share information and tips with me, and then I pass that on to other clients as well.

CASE STUDY **Carla** (*continued*)

CHW: Carla, where does your family usually go to buy your groceries?

Carla: The SaveMore up on 6th Street.

CHW: I know that one. I've been there a couple times with my sister. What would you think about meeting up at SaveMore one day instead of meeting here at the clinic? I've done something like this a couple of times with other clients, and we had a good time. We could kind of investigate the options for food that is healthy, affordable, and not too complicated to make.

Carla: I'd like that because . . . well, I told you that I really don't like shopping, right? It would be good to get some help.

CHW: What don't you like about shopping now?

Carla: I guess I never liked it growing up and now, well, I'm just kind of in and out as quick as possible and I just grab the same old stuff.

CHW: Well, we could give this idea a try and you can let me know if it is helpful or not. The goal is really just to expand some of your options for affordable and healthy foods, and to think of quick and easy meals to make.

Carla: Okay, it sounds really helpful to me, so when could we go?

CHW: Well, let me pull out my calendar (gets her cell phone). Is there a particular day and time that might work best for you? I could meet you one day after work if that helps.

Depending upon the guidelines of your agency, other options for supporting clients to improve their regular diet may include:

- Visit the client's home (if they invite you) to talk about the foods that they have on hand and how those foods may impact their health (and the health of their family).
- Join the client on a trip to their local grocery store or supermarket to talk about healthy and not-as-healthy food choices.
- Have some sample packaged food or soups on hand at your office. Together with clients, examine the labels and recommended portion sizes of the foods, in order to enhance understanding of the levels of key ingredients and components such as sugar and trans fats.

Finally, become an expert in local resources—other agencies, programs and services—that may be of interest to the clients you work with. Conduct your own research in the community to identify possible referrals to resources such as:

- Educational and support groups related to healthy nutrition
- Food pantries
- Hot meal programs
- Programs that teach people how to prepare healthy and culturally relevant meals for their families

These kinds of resources may be found at community-based organizations, churches, adult schools, senior centers, and community colleges.

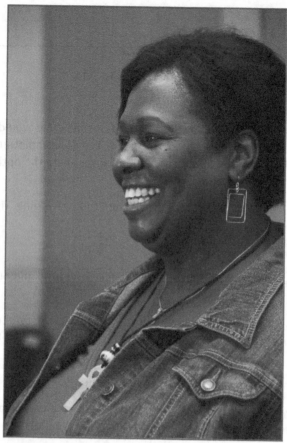

CHWs work with clients to increase physical activity and to eat healthier food.

Please watch the following three-part video series 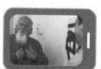, **which** shows a CHW providing nutritional information to a client who wants to better manage his high blood pressure.

HYPERTENSION AND HEALTHY EATING, PART 1: ROLE PLAY, DEMO

🔗 *http://youtu.be/ aGuViTC42G4*

HYPERTENSION AND HEALTHY EATING, PART 2: ROLE PLAY, DEMO

🔗 *http://youtu. be/271pMgUluNg*

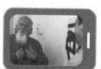

HYPERTENSION AND HEALTHY EATING, PART 3: ROLE PLAY, DEMO

🔗 *http://youtu.be/ gVlV_8iM_HA*

- What did the CHW do well in terms of supporting the client to better understand guidelines for healthy nutrition?
- What else would you do as a CHW to enhance this client's understanding of healthy nutrition?

17.8 Physical Activity

Physical activity is important to overall health and the management of most chronic conditions. Physical activity is defined as *anything* that gets the body moving. For clients with chronic conditions, who may feel out of control of their body and their illnesses, enhanced physical activity can offer a sense of control and self-mastery.

Activity or Exercise?

You may note that we use the words "physical activity" or "activity" more than "exercise" in this book. We do this because, for many people, exercise implies super-strenuous physical actions that are beyond their capacity (such as jogging for miles). When some patients hear the word "exercise" they may translate that into *"something that other people do."* Increasingly, public health and health care organizations are using the words "activity" or "physical activity" because these include a full spectrum of actions such as walking to the end of the block, around the block, or jogging. Activities include anything that gets the body moving (even if you are doing the activity while sitting down).

THE HEALTH BENEFITS OF PHYSICAL ACTIVITY

Extensive research has documented the clear health benefits of physical activity (CDC, n.d.-a.). For example, physical activity has been shown to reduce the risk of developing many chronic health conditions, including cardiovascular diseases, type 2 diabetes, some cancers, depression, arthritis, and osteoporosis. Engaging in physical activity helps to manage chronic conditions, to strengthen bones and muscles, and improve mood and mental health. Finally, engaging in regular physical activity is associated with longer life expectancy.

17.9 Guidelines for Healthy Activity

Guidelines for healthy activity levels are available from leading health organizations such as the World Health Organization, the U.S. Department of Health and Human Services, and the American Heart Association. You will find different guidelines for children and youth, active adults, seniors, and people living with illness or disability. These guidelines also vary slightly among organizations, and are refined over time to reflect new research findings.

The United States adopted the current physical activity guidelines in 2008. You can review these guidelines at the Centers for Disease Control (*www.cdc.gov/physicalactivity/everyone/guidelines/adults.html*).

The recommendations for healthy activity for adults ages 18–64 are

1. Two hours and 30 minutes (150 minutes total) of moderate-intensity aerobic activity (like brisk walking) every week, **and**
2. Muscle-strengthening activities on two or more days a week that work all major muscle groups (legs, hips, back, abdomen, chest, shoulders, and arms). This includes activities such as sit-ups and push-ups, yoga, lifting weights, or working with resistance bands.

OR

1. One hour and 15 minutes (75 minutes total) of vigorous-intensity aerobic activity (like jogging or running) every week, **and**
2. Muscle-strengthening activities on two or more days a week that work all major muscle groups (legs, hips, back, abdomen, chest, shoulders, and arms).

OR

1. An equivalent mix of moderate-and vigorous-intensity aerobic activity, **and**
2. Muscle-strengthening activities on two or more days a week that work all major muscle groups (legs, hips, back, abdomen, chest, shoulders, and arms).

These guidelines are similar to those provided by the World Health Organization and other leading organizations. It is important to highlight that benefit can be gained by engaging in these activities for just *10 minutes or more at a time. In other words, it isn't necessary to engage in activities for longer periods each time in order to benefit our health.*

A wide range of physical activities are highlighted in these guidelines, including walking and hiking, dancing, bicycle riding and swimming, aerobics, jogging, or playing sports like soccer or basketball. It isn't necessary to engage in the most strenuous forms of high-intensity activity in order to receive health benefits. Engaging in moderate activity—such as brisk walking—has the same types of health benefits, as long as it is done regularly.

Finally, while the U.S. government, the World Health Organization, and other leading health agencies recommend engaging in still higher levels of physical activity, they also acknowledge that doing any level of physical activity is better than none, and encourage people to start with a level that they can achieve and enjoy, and build from there. For example, the American Heart Association states:

> *Something is always better than nothing!*
>
> *The simplest, positive change you can make to effectively improve your heart health is to start walking. It's enjoyable, free, easy, social and great exercise. A walking program is flexible and boasts high success rates because people can stick with it. It's easy for walking to become a regular and satisfying part of life. (American Heart Association, n.d.)*

Walking and Running for Health

A study published in April 2013 showed that walking provides similar health benefits as running (Williams, 2013). In this large-scale study, walking and running were both shown to reduce risks for high blood pressure, diabetes, and other chronic conditions; though walkers do have to walk at a brisk pace for slightly longer distances than runners do to have the same benefit. This finding is significant because walking is a more realistic goal than running for many patients.

A REALISTIC AND HOLISTIC APPROACH TO MOVEMENT: THE BODY POSITIVE

The organization The Body Positive highlights the importance of exercise being joyful and authentic, rather than motivated by a desire to lose weight:

> *When exercise becomes intuitive [natural] and is more than just a means of burning calories, we find that people exercise more frequently and put an end to their stop and start (yo-yo) exercise patterns. The goal of exercising intuitively is to do it for the purposes of pleasure and release of physical and mental stress, as well as for fitness. (The Body Positive, 2013)*

When clients are new to exercise, or unsure of where to begin, consider asking the following questions:

1. What type of movement will make me feel great in my body today?
2. Are there any obstacles in my life that make it difficult for me to exercise regularly? Is so, what can I do to remove these obstacles? (The Body Positive, 2013)

17.10 Supporting Clients to Increase Activity Levels

As you work with clients to develop an action plan to increase physical activity, please keep the following concepts in mind.

INJURY PREVENTION

Ask clients to consult with a health care provider about plans to increase activity levels, and to clarify any possible risks or limitations. Physicians or other providers, including physical therapists, may provide guidelines designed to prevent injury and further harm to existing limitations or disabilities. This is particularly important if the client is recovering from an injury or serious health condition (such as treatments for cancer), has a disability, or has not been active in a long time.

GRADUAL OR INCREMENTAL CHANGE

Increasing physical activity should be done incrementally, or step-by-step. Some clients want to start out with intensive activities such as an aerobics class, jogging, or long hikes. However, they may not be prepared to be successful with such an ambitious plan, and their lack of success may become a significant obstacle to taking other more realistic actions in the future.

Talk with clients about the feasibility of their action plan. Support them to develop a plan for increased physical activity they can have immediate success with (such as within the first day or week), and to gradually build from there. An action plan to increase walking is a good starting place for many clients. Some clients may start out walking a relatively short distance and at a relatively slow pace. Over time, they may gradually increase the distance they walk, and/or the pace of their walking. Keep in mind that any level of physical activity is better than none, and that, within reason, more activity is always better for our health.

When clients are developing plans for increased activity, consider using a Motivation or Confidence Scale. Ask the client how confident or ready they are, on a scale from 0 to 10, to implement their plan. When confidence or readiness ratings are at an 8 or above, clients are more likely to have success with implementation.

Please watch the following video interview with David Spero, RN. As a nurse and chronic conditions management coach, David talks about his work to support a client to start walking. She, and her physician, doubted her ability to increase her physical activity.

- What health issues and barriers did David say his client faced?
- As a coach, what approach did David take to supporting this client to increase her level of physical activity?
- What value did engaging in physical activity have for this client?
- What did you learn that you may wish to apply to your work as a CHW?

THE VALUE OF TAKING SMALL STEPS: INTERVIEW

http://youtu. be/4ILopSTH7lk

REALISTIC AND AFFORDABLE

There are many barriers to engaging in regular physical activity: time, family responsibilities, money, past experience, mobility, pain, stress, confidence, and self-esteem. In order for most people to be successful at engaging in regular physical activity, it is important to be able to integrate the activity as an ongoing part of their life. Talk with clients about the types of activities they can do close to where they live and work, or even on their way to and from home or work. What activities can they engage in for 10 minutes or more several times a week? What activities can they do without additional expense, such as the costs of equipment or membership fees?

ACCESSIBLE

For many clients, maintaining ongoing physical activity requires that the activity be easily accessible to them. However, many people live in regions and neighborhoods where engaging in physical activity is limited by factors such as the weather, safety concerns, or the lack of sidewalks or green spaces. Support clients to brainstorm ideas for where and how they can engage in physical activities as safely and efficiently as possible.

> **Alma Vasquez:** Thinking about the client's day-to-day environment is key. We need to consider what is accessible and realistic for them. Being able to start physical activity at a low or moderate and low-impact level is really important. For example, I'll show clients some activities that we can do just sitting down together, like some stretches. Although you always need to be careful about this, it can be helpful sometimes to self-disclose a little information about your own challenges and experience. For example, I might share challenges I faced and how I started out slowly with physical activities. Sometimes it helps clients to know that you share their experience and then they are more comfortable to talk about their own challenges.

ENJOYABLE

People are more likely to be successful in meeting their action plans if they enjoy the activities. If the activities are uncomfortable, painful, or boring, they are naturally more difficult to maintain. Keep the focus on pleasurable movement and activities, and not on unattainable fitness goals. An action plan that includes dancing, or walking a child to school, may make more sense for a client than daily visits to a gym. As you think about how to approach the issue of exercise with patients, keep in mind the weight-inclusive approach. Dr. Michael Loewy, a professor and doctor in clinical psychology who is a leader in the HAES approach suggests

> *No one is too big to move around as much as feels good. I found that motivational interviewing techniques that meet a person where they are now and assesses their motivation to change, with no judgment, worked great.* (The Association for Size Diversity and Health, 2013)

Consider asking the client what kind of movement or activities they enjoyed as a child or youth. Often this question brings a smile and happy recollections of easier times, when the patient was more at home in her/his body. Those memories can often provide insight about how to move forward, in the present, to be more active.

NONJUDGMENTAL

Some clients don't feel positive about their bodies, and may feel embarrassed, frustrated, or ashamed about engaging in physical activity. They may have been teased or discriminated against in the past based on their perceived body size or shape, and these experiences and the emotions they generate can pose significant barriers to engaging in physical activity in the present. For the success of your work and the health of the clients your serve, it is vital not to impose similar judgments about body shape or size, fitness, or physical abilities. Strive to be aware of any prejudices that you may have. If you have internalized common negative perspectives and assumptions about weight, seek out opportunities to learn more about these topics, and to enhance your cultural humility.

Consider how past discrimination and emotions such as shame or embarrassment may be influencing a client. Pose open-ended questions and provide them with an opportunity to talk further about their experiences. While some clients may not want to talk about these topics (or talk about them with you), others may appreciate the opportunity. As you talk with clients about their pasts, encourage them to consider the future as well. Inquire about how they might create a different and more positive experience of being physical active. What types of resources may help them to do this?

> **Francis Julian Montgomery:** My overall goal when I am working with a client who has expressed an interest in increasing their physical activity, is to help them to do it in small, obtainable increments. The client will set their goal, and I will ask them questions to help them figure out the rest—what they are willing to do, what their capacity is, and what may be too much for them to take on. Then I help them put this into an action plan with specific steps and activities and all the other details.

WITH OTHERS, OR ON THEIR OWN?

Engaging in physical activity with others can provide motivation, companionship and safety. Some people prefer to engage in physical activity on their own. Honor the client's preferences and, if they enjoy being active with others, support them to identify opportunities to do this. This may include taking a daily walk with a friend or family member, or joining a local (and free) neighborhood or community walking, bicycling, or tai chi practice.

COMMUNITY RESOURCES

Ask the clients you work with if they know about local parks and other green spaces, organizations, or programs that support people to engage in physical activity. Do your own research to identify possible referral resources. There may be free or low-cost programs offered in the community by nonprofit or faith-based organizations, or

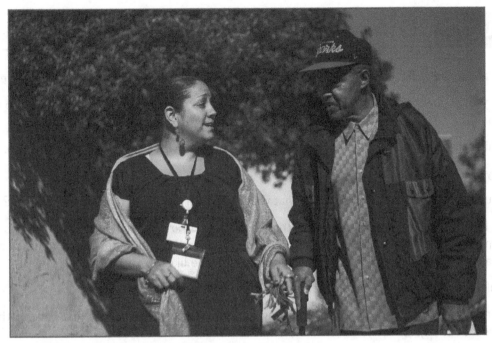

A CHW joins a client for a walk in the community.

local health departments and community colleges. Programs may include walking or swim clubs, tai chi classes, or water aerobics. There may be programs or services for people who share a specific identity such as activities for women, people with disabilities, or chronic conditions such as arthritis, cancer, or chronic pain.

CASE STUDY | **Carla Moretti (*continued*)**

CHW: So one goal that you mentioned is to increase your physical activity, right?

Carla: Yeah, but . . . (laughs). I sound like my kids with the "yeah, but" . . . it's just that I'm already so overwhelmed, so this exercise can't be too much or I'll just never do it, and then I'll feel even worse.

CHW: Okay, so let's see if we can come up with a plan that gets you moving a bit more that fits with all your other activities and responsibilities.

Carla: Okay.

CHW: So are there physical activities that you have enjoyed in the past?

Carla: Well, it's been a long time, really. But I used to do a lot more. I was on the softball team in middle school. I could run back then (laughs).

CHW: What did you like about playing softball?

Carla: Well . . . I guess a lot of things, really. I liked working as a team, doing something fun with other people, you know? We used to laugh a lot and have a good time together.

CHW: So how might you translate some of that past success into the present? What kinds of activities might you enjoy doing now?

Carla: I don't know. I can't see myself trying to play softball now (laughs).

(continues)

CASE STUDY	Carla Moretti *(continued)*

CHW: What about the walks you take around the field when Robbie is practicing or playing a game?

Carla: Well, yeah, I guess so. I mean it just doesn't seem like exercise, you know, not compared to what Robbie is doing.

CHW: Anything that gets our bodies moving counts as physical activity and is good for our health.

Carla: Really?

CHW: Uh-huh. And this walking is something that you share with someone, right, you and Mikey?

Carla: Well, I had to kind of bug Mikey to go with me at first, but now we both like it because it is kind of like a bonding time, you know? He is really into comics and those electronic games, and while we are walking he tells me all about those worlds and the characters and why he likes 'em . . .

CHW: So walking with Mikey is a good bonding time . . .

Carla: Yes and it's so great because now Mikey is my son, too. It was hard when we first got together, you know, for the kids to adjust.

CHW: So how often are you and Mikey going for walks now?

Carla: It's not regular. Maybe once every couple of weeks, during Robbie's sport season.

CHW: So are there other places that you and Mikey could go for a walk? Maybe some place right in your neighborhood, so you wouldn't have to drive there and it wouldn't take so much time?

Carla: Yeah, we are only a couple of blocks from MLK park. We could walk up there, I guess?

CHW: So is this something that you think you could try and see how it is?

Carla: Yeah, I will try to ask Mikey. Maybe Robbie and Alma could try to do the dishes—if Alma feels up to standing—and then Mikey and I could go for a short walk and that way we could each have some more one-on-one time with the kids.

CHW: That sounds like a great plan, Carla. When do you think you can make time to try this out?

Carla: I don't know, but I'll talk with Alma and find a time. . . . Maybe Friday night. Hey, we are gonna cook that chicken and rice dish, so do I get extra credit if I cook a healthy meal and do some walking on the same day? (Carla and the CHW both laugh)

CHW: Will you let me know how it goes? You can always send me a text if you want (Carla nods)

Carla: Yeah, I'll let you know, and thanks _____ (CHW's name)

CHW: Take care, Carla.

Please watch the following video 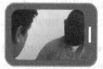, which shows a CHW supporting a client to enhance his level of physical activity and to improve his diet.

- What did the CHW do well in terms of supporting the client to make changes to his diet and level of physical activity?
- What else would you do (or do differently) if you were the CHW working with this client?

ACTION PLANNING AND EXERCISE: ROLE PLAY, DEMO

🔗 *http://youtu.be/ x9kt4EusdwA*

Chapter Review

Read the case study about Carla Moretti presented at the beginning of this chapter. Based on what you have studied and learned so far, do your best to answer the following questions:

Food and Health

- How does what we eat and drink influence our health?
- What types of factors get in the way or make it difficult for people to eat a healthier diet?
- What are the guidelines for a healthier diet?
  - What can people eat and drink less of to promote their health?
  - What can people eat and drink more of to promote their health?
- How do issues of culture and family influence what people eat and drink?
- What challenges does Carla Moretti face in terms of nutrition?
- Identify three ways that Carla might be able to change her diet to better improve her health (what changes could she make to what she eats and drinks)?
- What guidelines will you keep in mind as you work to support clients to change what they eat and drink?

Weight and Health

- What are some of the potential benefits and risks of encouraging a client to lose weight?
- How effective is dieting in terms of sustained weight loss and improvements to health?
- How does the weight-inclusive approach work to encourage providers to put the topic of weight aside and to focus on health issues when working with clients?
- What are the key principles of a weight-inclusive approach to health promotion?
- What messages would you want to share with Carla about weight and health?

Physical Activity and Health

- How does physical activity improve health?
- How much physical activity is recommended to improve health?
- What types of physical activity are beneficial to health?
- What challenges or barriers does Carla face in terms of engaging in physical activity?
- What strategies might you use in working with a client to increase their level of physical activity?
- How might you apply client-centered concepts and skills to working with Carla or another client to increase levels of physical activity?

References

The American Heart Association. (n.d.). *Recommendations for physical activity in adults.* Retrieved from *www.heart .org/HEARTORG/GettingHealthy/PhysicalActivity/FitnessBasics/American-Heart-Association-Recommendations-for-Physical-Activity-in-Adults_UCM_307976_Article.jsp?#.VlDdGHvscuc*

The Association for Size Diversity and Health, (2013). *HAES Matters: Exercise and HAES model (part 2).* [Blog]. Retrieved from *http://healthateverysizeblog.org/2013/01/15/haes-matters-exercise-and-the-haes-model-part-2/*

Bacon, L., Stern, J. S., Van Loan, M. D., & Keim, N. L. (2005). Size acceptance and intuitive eating improve health for obese, female chronic dieters. *Journal of the American Dietetic Association, 105*(6), 929–936.

The Body Positive. (2013). *Practice intuitive self-care.* Retrieved from *http://thebodypositive.org/model.html*

Brownell, K. D., & Rodin, J. (1994). The dieting maelstrom. Is it possible and advisable to lose weight? *American Psychologist, 49*(9), 781–91.

Centers for Disease Control and Prevention (CDC). (n.d.-a.). *The benefits of physical activity.* Retrieved from *www .cdc.gov/physicalactivity/everyone/health/*

Centers for Disease Control and Prevention. (n.d.-b). *About BMI for adults.* Retrieved from *www.cdc.gov/ healthyweight/assessing/bmi/adult_bmi/index.html*

The Centers for Disease Control and Prevention. (n.d.-c.). *Chronic disease overview.* Retrieved from *www.cdc.gov/ chronicdisease/overview/*

Clifford, D., Ozier, A., Bundros, J., Moore, J., Kreiser, A., & Morris, M. N. (2015). Impact of nondiet approaches on attitudes, behaviors, and health outcomes: A systematic review. *Journal of Nutrition Education and Behavior, 47*(2), 143–155. doi:10.1016/j.jneb.2014.12.002

Coleman-Jensen, A., Nord, M., Andrews, M. & Carlson, S. (2011). *Household food security in the United States in 2010.* Economic Research Report No. (ERR-125). U.S. Department of Agriculture, Economic Research Service. Retrieved from *www.ers.usda.gov/publications/err-economic-research-report/err125.aspx*

Feeding America. (n.d.). *Hunger statistics, hunger facts, & poverty facts.* Retrieved from *http://feedingamerica.org/ hunger-in-america/hunger-facts/hunger-and-poverty-statistics.aspx*

Ferdman, R. A. (2015). The meat industry's worst nightmare could soon become a reality. [Blog]. *The Washington Post.* Retrieved from *www.washingtonpost.com/blogs/wonkblog/wp/2015/01/07/why-the-governments-new-dietary-guidelines-could-be-a-nightmare-for-the-meat-industry/*

Field, A. E., Manson, J. E., Taylor, C. B., Willett, W. C., & Colditz, G. A. (2004). Association of weight change, weight control practices, and weight cycling among women in the Nurses' Health Study II. *International Journal of Obesity Related Metabolic Disorders, 28*(9), 1134–1142.

Harvard University. (2004). Exercise and the risk of stroke, heart disease. *The Harvard Medical School Family Health Guide.* Retrieved from *www.health.harvard.edu/fhg/updates/update0204d.shtml*

Jeffery, R. W., Drewnowski, A., Epstein, L. H., Stunkard, A. J., Wilson, G. T., Wing, R. R., & Hill, D. R. (2000). Long-term maintenance of weight loss: Current status. *Health Psychology, 19*(1), 5–16.

Mann, T., Tomiyama A. J., Westling E., Lew A. M., Samuels, B., & Chatman, J. (2007). Medicare's search for effective obesity treatments: Diets are not the answer. *American Psychologist, 62*(3), 220–233.

Marketdata Enterprises, Inc. (2014). *The U.S. weight loss market: 2014 status report & forecast.* Retrieved from *www .marketresearch.com/Marketdata-Enterprises-Inc-v416/Weight-Loss-Status-Forecast-8016030/*

Moss, Michael. (2013). *Salt, sugar, fat: How the food giants hooked us.* New York, NY: Random House.

Nestle, M. (2013). *Food politics: How the food industry influences nutrition and health.* Berkeley: University of California Press.

Rzehak, P., Meisinger, C., Woelke, G., Brasche, S. Strube, G., & Heinrich, J. (2007). Weight change, weight cycling, and mortality in the ERFORT Male Cohort Study. *European Journal of Epidemiology, 22*, 665–673.

Sumithran, P., & Proietto, J. (2013). The defense of body weight: A psychological basis for weight regain after weight loss. *Clinical Science, 124*(4), 231–241.

Tomiyama, A. (2014). Weight stigma is stressful: A review of evidence for the obesity/weight-based stigma model. *Appetite, 82*, 8–15.

Tylka, T. L., Annunziato, R. A., Burgard, D., Danielsdottir, S., Shuman, E., & Davis, C. (2014). The weight-inclusive versus weight-normative approach to health: Evaluating the evidence for prioritizing well-being over weight loss. *Journal of Obesity, 1.* doi:10.1155/2014/983495. Retrieved from *www.ncbi.nlm.nih.gov/pmc/ articles/PMC4132299/*

United States Department of Agriculture (USDA). (2015). *ERS-food security in the U.S.: Key statistics & graphics.* Retrieved from *www.ers.usda.gov/topics/food-nutrition-assistance/food-security-in-the-us/key-statistics-graphics.aspx#.U8iTRFaRYpE*

United Nations Environment Program (UNEP). (2010). *Assessing the environmental impacts of production and consumption.* International Panel for Sustainable Resources Management. Retrieved from *www.unep.org/ resourcepanel/Portals/24102/PDFs/PriorityProductsAndMaterials_Report.pdf*

Williams, P. T. (2013). Walking versus running for hypertension, cholesterol, and diabetes mellitus risk reduction. *Arteriosclerosis, Thrombosis, and Vascular Biology.* 2013. doi:10.116/ATVBAHA.112.300878. Retrieved from *http://atvb.ahajournals.org/content/early/2013/04/04/ATVBAHA.112.300878.abstract*

Additional Resources

Association for Size Diversity and Health. (n.d.). Retrieved from *www.sizediversityandhealth.org/*

Bacon, L. (2008). *Health at every size: The surprising truth about your weight.* Dallas, TX: Benbella Books.

Bacon, L., & Aphramor, L. (2014). *Body respect: What conventional health books get wrong, leave out, and just plan fail to understand about weight.* Dallas, TX: BenBella Books.

The Body Positive. (n.d.). Retrieved from *www.thebodypositive.org*

The Centers for Disease Control and Prevention. 2013. *Physical activity for everyone: Guidelines: Adults.* Retrieved from *www.cdc.gov/physicalactivity/everyone/guidelines/adults.html*

Health at Every Size. (n.d.). Retrieved from *www.haescommunity.org*

McMillan, T. (2014, July 16). Shift to "food insecurity" creates startling new picture of hunger in America. *National Geographic.* Retrieved from *http://news.nationalgeographic.com/ news/2014/07/140716-hunger-america-food-poverty-nutrition-diet/*

National Eating Disorders Association. (n.d.). Retrieved from *http://nationaleatingdisorders.org*

Sobczak, C. (2014). *Embody: Learning to love your unique body (and quiet that critical voice!).* Carlsbad, CA: Gurze Books.

Williams, P. T., & Thompson, P. D. (2013, April 4). Walking versus Running for Hypertension, Cholesterol, and Diabetes Mellitus Risk Reduction. *Arteriosclerosis, Thrombosis, and Vascular Biology.*

Understanding Trauma and Supporting the Recovery of Survivors

18

Tim Berthold and Janey Skinner

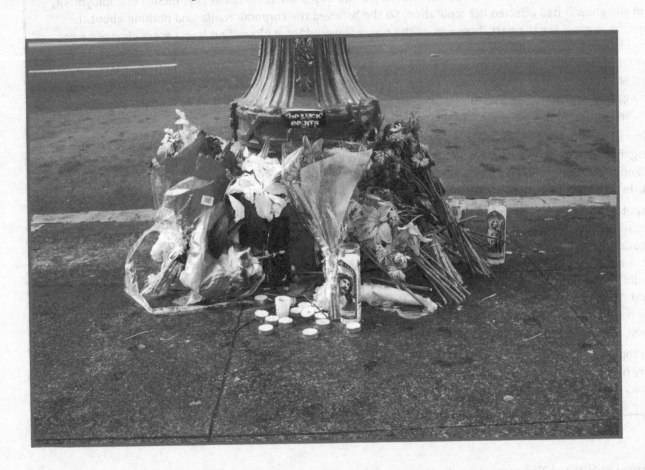

CASE STUDY Nadia Vasiliev

Nadia is a 23-year-old woman. She was born in Russia and raised in a small American city in the Midwest where her family immigrated when she was five. At 20, she enlisted in the Army and started a 12-month tour of duty in Iraq as a motor transport operator. She liked how structured the military was, each person's job made perfectly clear. She liked feeling strong and competent, and part of something larger than herself. In Iraq, Nadia learned you can never be too careful—you have to keep an eye out for explosives or other dangers, and never let your guard down. People can be laughing with you one minute, and torn to pieces the next.

Nadia might have stayed in the Army, except for one thing. About four months into her tour of duty, a corporal began to pressure her for sex. At first, it was just the usual teasing that all the women got. Then he cornered Nadia in a supply room and raped her. He told Nadia that no one would believe her if she told, and besides, everyone knew she was a whore. Nadia had dated someone in her first month of deployment, and she knew it had affected her reputation. So she believed the corporal. Nadia said nothing about the rape, to anyone. For the next three weeks, the corporal would force himself on Nadia every chance he got. She began to avoid going to eat, to the movies, or anywhere alone. She volunteered for convoys and longer transport drives, just to stay away from base. After three weeks, the corporal abruptly lost interest in her. Nadia felt relief that the assaults had stopped, but she couldn't shake the fear that they would start up again at any time. She felt angry at herself for still being scared. She told herself that she should be focused on the real enemy, the one they were sent to Iraq to fight.

After completing her tour of duty, Nadia returned home. Her parents were proud of her and her brother Sergei, who had also enlisted. Nadia told her parents only funny stories from her tour of duty, she never talked about the horrible things that happened. Nadia found work in the sales department of a regional hardware store chain and a new boyfriend, Chet, and everything was going great.

About a year after her return from Iraq, things changed. One day at a social event for veterans, Nadia refused to give her phone number to a drunken man, and he responded by calling her a whore. She began scrutinizing every man she saw, wondering if the corporal who raped her, had told them about her. At work Nadia grew more irritable. The smallest things would send her into a state of panic or anger. One day, Nadia yelled at a client who cancelled a large order, and her boss fired her. She found a new job at a fast-food restaurant, but lost that job, too. Since then, Nadia has not held down any job for long. She caught her boyfriend Chet cheating on her and broke off the relationship. She can't fall asleep, and when she does sleep, she can't stand the nightmares.

On top of this, Nadia has some uncomfortable itching and burning in her pubic area, and worries that she may have a sexually transmitted infection (STI). She decides to make an appointment at a women's health clinic. At the clinic, in addition to seeing a doctor for STI tests, Nadia meets with a CHW.

If you were a CHW and Nadia was your client, how might you answer the following questions?

- What types of traumatic events has Nadia survived?
- How may Nadia's exposure to trauma have affected her health and her life?
- If Nadia decided to tell you about her experiences in Iraq, how would you respond?
- What would your approach be to working with Nadia to heal from the trauma she survived? What concepts and skills would you draw upon?
- What is the proper role and scope of practice for a CHW who is working with a survivor of trauma?
- How may you (and other helping professionals) be affected by working closely with survivors of trauma?

- What can you do to practice self care and enhance your resilience for working with survivors of trauma over time?
- What resources exist for survivors of trauma in the communities where you live and work?

Introduction

As a CHW, you are likely to work with many clients who are survivors of traumatic events. A little over half of Americans have been exposed to one or more traumatic events, and for people living in conditions of war or civil conflict around the world, that number is even higher. The lingering effects of traumatic experiences can have a dramatic influence on the health and well-being of survivors.

CHWs and other front-line public health and social services providers are well situated to support the healing of survivors. Social support—or the lack of it—is one of the most important factors that influence how a person responds in the wake of a traumatic event. CHWs are an important part of providing social support and linking vulnerable individuals and communities to additional sources of help. However, without knowledge and skills, CHWs can also do harm.

Our goal is to better prepare you for the moment when a client discloses a trauma history to you, or asks for help in addressing their traumatic stress. How you respond in these moments can have a significant impact on the client and their process of healing or recovery. For CHWs who work with groups and communities, we provide some guidelines for how to assist the collective process of working through distress and mourning in the wake of traumatic events.

While CHWs and other nonlicensed personnel in health and human services frequently assist survivors of trauma, this work raises questions about scope of practice. It is clearly outside of a CHW's scope of practice to provide therapy, and it is clearly inside a CHW's scope of practice to apply client-centered practice to listen with compassion to a client's story and provide a relevant referral. However, between these two ends of the spectrum, there are situations that pose questions about the CHW's role. Certainly in situations of major disaster or upheaval, community health workers have been tapped to play a substantial role in psychosocial support for the affected population, both to identify cases that need the care of a licensed specialist and to foster mutual support and healing among those whose trauma symptoms are less severe (Medecins Sans Frontieres, n.d.; World Health Organization, 2001). And clients in any setting may feel more comfortable discussing their history with a CHW initially, rather than with a therapist or counselor, in part due to the stigma associated with mental health care (a stigma that CHWs can work to eliminate). Some CHWs (such as rape crisis counselors or those who work with refugees) find that speaking with clients about their trauma stories is an integral part of their job. At the same time, it is important that CHWs not work beyond their training, their agency's policies, or their personal capacity. There can be risks for the client in telling their story of trauma, as talking can exacerbate symptoms of traumatic stress, symptoms that may be best addressed in the presence of a mental health professional. We address questions of scope of practice more fully further on.

WHAT YOU WILL LEARN

By studying the information in this chapter, you will be able to:

- Define trauma and post-traumatic stress disorder (PTSD)
- Explain how common exposure to trauma is in the United States
- Identify common responses to trauma (symptoms and effects) for individuals and communities
- Identify a variety of strategies for healing from trauma for individuals and communities
- Discuss ways to promote community resiliency to trauma
- Analyze the CHW scope of practice when working with survivors of trauma, and when and how to provide referrals
- Explain and demonstrate key skills for working with survivors of trauma
- Identify strategies to support groups and communities in responding to trauma

- Discuss secondary trauma and self care strategies to enhance CHW's own resilience as service providers
- Explain secondary resilience and post-traumatic growth

WORDS TO KNOW

Cognitive-Behavioral Therapy

Historical Trauma

Post-Traumatic Stress Disorder (PTSD)

Resiliency

Secondary Resilience

Secondary Trauma

Somatic Trauma-Informed Approach

Preparing to Address the Topic of Trauma

Trauma can be a difficult topic to address. In training CHWs, we talk explicitly about traumatic events such as rape and war, and how they affect us. We do this with the intention of better preparing CHWs to work with clients who choose to talk with them about trauma.

Whenever we teach about trauma, regardless of the audience, we assume that some of the participants are survivors of trauma. We assume that others know someone close to them—a family member or a friend—who is a survivor of trauma. We assume that some of you reading this chapter are also survivors of trauma. Please know you are not alone.

Do your best to stay present as you read this chapter, just as you will need to do when listening to a client. At the same time, don't forget to take care of yourself along the way. Pay attention to the thoughts and feelings that may come up. Draw upon the skills and techniques that you already have. When something happens that stirs up strong emotions in you, what do you do to stay grounded and present? This may include deep breathing, taking a short break, drawing upon spiritual or religious practices, or thought-stopping techniques (make a conscious effort to think about something else, something less emotional that can help to calm and ground you). Over the course of this training, you will be supported to enhance your knowledge and skills related to self care (see Chapter 12).

If you are a survivor of trauma, it is possible that studying this material, and working directly with clients who are survivors, may restimulate your own trauma stories and responses. Your challenge is to develop skills for putting your own story aside when you are working with clients, so that you don't unintentionally impose your own assumptions, beliefs, or values. Clients require you to be fully present to focus on their needs. When you have the time, and are not in the midst of working with clients, it can be helpful to revisit personal memories and responses, and to continue your own path for healing or recovery. You may find time to address your experiences during meetings with a clinical supervisor. Or you may address them on your own time, by yourself or with the help of family, community or professionals.

While the topic of trauma can be difficult to study, it also brings opportunity for hope. The efforts of people who have faced and survived terrible experiences are inspiring. Witnessing the healing of survivors will bring you face to face with extraordinary people, and provides an opportunity to enhance your own resilience for facing the difficult moments that inevitably arise in every life.

18.1 Defining Trauma and Post-Traumatic Stress

Trauma is a term that is used in several different ways. It often refers to horrific events, such as child abuse and neglect, domestic violence, torture and incarceration. It can also refer to physical injuries—broken bones or burns that are treated in a "trauma unit" in a hospital. In this chapter, we are most concerned with a third meaning of trauma—the emotions, thoughts, and feelings we experience as a response to traumatic events, whether or not those events resulted in physical injuries.

According to the American Psychological Association (APA):

> *Trauma is an emotional response to a terrible event like an accident, rape or natural disaster. Immediately after the event, shock and denial are typical. Longer term reactions include unpredictable emotions, flashbacks, strained relationships and even physical symptoms like headaches or nausea. While these feelings are normal, some people have difficulty moving on with their lives. (APA, n.d.)*

Trauma affects us in many ways—physically, emotionally, spiritually, communally—when we are exposed to life's most extreme events. Trauma experiences are characterized by:

- Intense fear
- Helplessness
- Loss of control
- Bodily harm or the threat of bodily harm
- Threat or fear of annihilation (death—one's own or that of a loved one—or even of a group one belongs to, such as in the case of genocide)
- Rupture or loss of meaningful social relationships

It is worth noting that, even if the people affected by the traumatic event do not experience overwhelming fear or helplessness during the event, the severity of the event itself can still generate a post-traumatic stress reaction.

Responses to traumatic events vary considerably. In the immediate aftermath of a traumatic event, most people experience a trauma response, along with normal grieving or other reactions. For some people, that response will diminish or disappear over time, especially if they are met with support and caring relationships, and if the traumatic event is not ongoing or chronic. Yet others will experience intense symptoms of trauma that may endure for months, years, or even decades. Trauma can affect every part of a person's life—their health, welfare, work, and relationships, as well as their sense of emotional well-being.

Keep in mind that how people experience, respond to, and are affected by traumatic events is often highly subjective. In other words, people who experience the same event can be affected in quite different ways. After an earthquake, for example, one person might bounce back quickly from the initial fright and begin rebuilding with optimism, while another person might find he can't stop thinking about the disaster, and as a result feels a persistent sense of danger and instability that prevents him from moving on, months after the earthquake.

What Do YOU? Think :

- *How do you define trauma?*
- *Have you witnessed both short-term and long-term effects of trauma in your community?*

IDENTIFYING TRAUMATIC EVENTS

Many events that may be classified as traumatic, given the definition provided above. A *partial* list of events that may be classified as traumatic includes:

- Child abuse and neglect
- Sexual assault
- The death of a loved one, especially if it is sudden, unexpected, or violent
- War or armed conflict (for both military service members or combatants as well as for civilians)
- High levels of neighborhood violence, including shootings, killings, and threats
- Domestic violence, including physical, verbal, and emotional abuse
- Incarceration
- State-sponsored violence including, for example, police brutality/assault
- Torture

- Natural disasters such as earthquakes, tsunamis, and hurricanes
- Accidents such as fires and car crashes

- *What types of trauma are most common in your own communities?*

HOW COMMON IS EXPOSURE TO TRAUMA?

Unfortunately, exposure to traumatic events is very common, and much more common than many people think.

Judith Herman, a physician and the author of *Trauma and Recovery*, writes:

> *It was once believed that such events were uncommon. In 1980, when post-traumatic stress disorder was first included in the diagnostic manual, the American Psychiatric Association described traumatic events as "outside the range of usual human experience." Sadly, this definition has proved to be inaccurate. Rape, battery, and other forms of sexual and domestic violence are so common a part of women's lives that they can hardly be described as outside the range of ordinary experience. And in the view of the number of people killed in war over the past century, military trauma, too, must be considered a common part of the human experience; only the fortunate find it unusual. (Herman, 1997, p. 33)*

It is challenging to research and to document how often people are exposed to trauma. In general, rape, child abuse, and other acts of violence are underreported due to factors that include fear of retaliation or alienation (loss of family or friends), distrust of the police and/or criminal justice system, shame, self-blame, and stigma. Nations may also have a compelling self-interest to distort the reporting of war-related injuries and deaths.

The National Center for PTSD estimates that approximately 60 percent of men and 50 percent of women experience one or more traumatic events over the course of their lifetime (U.S. Department of Veterans Affairs National Center for PTSD [VA], 2014a). Some studies estimate exposure to traumatic events is even higher. In 2013, a national study in the United States showed that most people (89.7 percent) have been exposed to at least one traumatic event, and exposure to multiple traumatic events was more common than not. While post-traumatic stress disorder (PTSD) is not the only disorder that can result from a traumatic event, its prevalence serves as a rough measure of the impact of trauma (see further on for a fuller description of PTSD). About 8 percent of the population reported symptoms at some point during their lifetime that were consistent with a diagnosis of PTSD, and 5 percent reported symptoms consistent with PTSD within the previous year (Kilpatrick, Resnick, Milanak, Miller, Keyes & Friedman, 2013). While men are more likely to be exposed to traumatic events, women are more likely to develop PTSD (10 percent of women compared to 5 percent of men) (VA, 2014b). Many people also experience traumatic reactions that are distressing but do not meet the criteria for a diagnosis of PTSD, or may be diagnosed with another mental health condition. Depression, substance abuse, self-harming behaviors, aggression, isolation, and other symptoms of a reaction to trauma may appear, even without PTSD being present. To read more, please visit the website of the National Center for PTSD, *www.ptsd.va.gov/index.asp*.

Francis Julian Montgomery: Most of the clients I work with are managing multiple traumatic experiences, including being homeless in this city [San Francisco]. It's important for me to remember that trauma is invisible most of the time. A lot of people still have a misguided belief that only veterans or women who have experienced sexual assault have trauma, but the people I work with have survived all kinds of trauma.

There are strong indications that children are more likely than adults to develop symptoms of traumatic stress when exposed to abuse or disaster. Exposure to trauma at an early age can affect brain development and both physical and mental health, into adulthood. Children are frequently exposed to some form of victimization.

For example, one study showed that 71 percent of children and youth ages 2–17 were exposed to at least one incident of victimization within a year (and on average three incidents in a year)—whether a property crime (like being stolen from), a physical altercation with a peer or a sibling, or being abused physically or sexually (Fairbank, 2008). About 1 in 10 children in the United States experience maltreatment, while 1 in 4 witness domestic or community violence. About 4 percent of adolescent boys and about 6 percent of adolescent girls are estimated to experience symptoms that meet the criteria for PTSD (VA, 2014b).

Military personnel and veterans are at especially high risk of exposure to traumatic events and resulting PTSD; longer deployments and increased exposure to combat are both associated with higher rates of PTSD. Estimates of PTSD among Vietnam War veterans in the United States are as high as 31 percent for men and 27 percent for women. Estimates for veterans returning from the wars in Iraq and Afghanistan have ranged from 5 to 18 percent (Norris & Slone, 2013). These numbers, however, probably underreport the effects of trauma on veterans. A complicating factor for recent veterans is the high prevalence of traumatic brain injury (TBI), which can cause mood swings, difficulty concentrating, and behavior changes, not unlike PTSD. High suicide rates among veterans of recent conflicts (at least 22 a day, according to Kemp & Bossarte of the Department of Veterans Affairs, 2012) have drawn attention to the need for more comprehensive services and support.

Exposure to traumatic events is not evenly distributed across all populations. Communities with high rates of violence or crime, as well as refugee communities and those seeking asylum, often experience a higher exposure to traumatic events. The presence or absence of resources to overcome, escape, or transform the sources of trauma, and to support healing from their impacts, has a significant effect on whether the symptoms of traumatic stress become chronic or not.

The Legacy of Historical Trauma

Historical trauma refers to the way in which post-traumatic stress can be passed down across generations within communities that have faced extreme trauma such as slavery and genocide. Pervasive trauma can shape coping mechanisms, parenting practices and life expectations in lasting ways—especially when institutionalized discrimination continues, in new forms, into the present day. Dr. Joy Degruy Leary, for example, coined the term "post-traumatic slave syndrome" to describe "how African Americans adapted their behavior over centuries in order to survive the stifling effects of chattel slavery, effects which are evident today." DeGruy Leary considers many of the behaviors she sees in African American communities today to be "in large part related to trans-generational adaptations associated with the past traumas of slavery and ongoing oppression" (DeGruy Leary, 2005, p. 14).

Historical trauma affects many communities across the world that have experienced trauma on a mass and enduring scale. It has been documented in Native American communities (Brave Heart, 2000; Michaels, 2010), Jewish communities (Kellermann, 2013), and many others. While the nature of the historical trauma is different in each case, for those in helping professions (including CHWs) an awareness of the deep historical roots of trauma and the way that history shapes the reactions and resources of each community can be important to connecting with the client and constructing culturally sensitive pathways to healing.

- Do you belong to a community that has been hurt by historical trauma?
- How do affected communities respond to the impacts of historical trauma?

THE LANGUAGE WE USE TO TALK ABOUT TRAUMA

There are many different ways of conceptualizing and talking about trauma. We want to distinguish here between the medical language used to diagnose trauma among survivors, and the language that most people commonly use to communicate about trauma and its consequences. Our goal for this chapter is to use words and concepts that are accessible to the clients and communities you will work with as a CHW. In contrast, licensed medical and mental health providers may use the language of post-traumatic stress disorder (PTSD) to assess the effects of trauma among survivors. Those who meet the diagnostic criteria, explained in the next section, receive a diagnosis of PTSD.

Apart from PTSD, there are other diagnoses that are common among trauma survivors. They may meet the diagnostic criteria for a different stress-related disorder, such as acute stress disorder (similar to PTSD but occurring in the immediate aftermath of a traumatic event), an attachment disorder, or a dissociative disorder. Many trauma survivors experience anxiety or depression, and some develop eating disorders or substance abuse problems. And of course, some survivors do not develop any persistent symptoms at all. Because PTSD is a common and well-documented response to traumatic events—in fact, the term PTSD is often used as a synonym for trauma in popular culture—we discuss this particular diagnosis in more detail in the following section.

Debates about the Term *PTSD*

Not everyone is comfortable with the term *PTSD*. For example, some survivors of traumatic events do not want to label their reactions as a "disorder" (and point out that the events they survived, rather than their reactions to these events, are where the "disorder" lies). Others live in situations of ongoing danger where the P in PTSD might stand for "persistent" instead of "post." As we discuss later in this chapter, some have argued that PTSD is a culturally specific concept that should not be applied universally to all populations. Others may experience only some of the symptoms of PTSD, or have other manifestations of stress not included in the definition of PTSD—but still want or need support to manage these symptoms. Some people experience depression or headaches or loneliness as their primary response—not the hyperarousal or intrusive thinking associated with PTSD. And others still will describe their response to trauma in terms that are culturally or personally meaningful to them—they may not relate to the clinical language of post-traumatic stress at all. An example might be understanding nightmares as a haunting from the dead, or describing a numbing response as soul-loss.

We encourage you to talk about trauma and its consequences in way that the clients and communities you work with can relate to and understand. These are difficult concepts for some of us to talk about in any language, so using terms that are more likely to be understood is important to promoting discussion.

18.2 Post-Traumatic Stress Disorder (PTSD)

While trauma has always been a part of our history, it wasn't always acknowledged. Post-traumatic stress was formally defined as a health condition in 1982, when it was included in the *Diagnostic and Statistical Manual (DSM)* of the American Psychiatric Association. The *DSM* is the basis for diagnosis and treatment of all mental health conditions in the United States, and informs mental health practice beyond our borders as well (keep in mind that only a licensed medical or mental health care professional is qualified to provide a diagnosis).

Since 1982, research and developments in treating trauma have resulted in revised diagnostic criteria for PTSD. Today, when licensed medical and mental health professionals assess and diagnose people with PTSD they follow the clinical criteria from the fifth edition of the *DSM*, published in 2013 (*DSM-5*). There are several different diagnostic categories for PTSD including, for example, one for children six years old and younger, and one for complex PTSD. For the purposes of this chapter, we will review the most commonly used diagnostic criteria for people ages seven and older. If you are interested in reading more about PTSD and its various subcategories for diagnosis, please see the resources included at the end of this chapter.

PTSD is diagnosed in people ages seven and older if they have been exposed to one or more traumatic events characterized by death or death threats; bodily harm or threats of bodily harm; sexual assault or threats of sexual assault. This includes people who were directly exposed to a traumatic event, such as an assault, and those who witnessed the trauma. To be diagnosed with PTSD, the survivor *must show symptoms in each of four different categories, and the symptoms must have lasted for at least one month.* The four categories or symptom clusters from the *DSM-5* are: (1) intrusion symptoms [such as persistent trauma-related thoughts or dreams]; (2) avoidance [avoiding thoughts, feelings, people, places, and situations that are associated with the trauma], (3) negative alterations in cognition [thoughts] or mood [including the inability to remember key aspects of the trauma, persistent negative emotions or beliefs, and the inability to experience positive emotions, etc.], and (4) alterations in arousal and reactivity [including hypervigilance, an exaggerated startle response, problems with concentration and sleep disturbances, irritable or aggressive behavior, or self-destructive behaviors].

As CHWs, you do not need to become fluent in speaking the language of the DSM-5 in order to work effectively with clients, local communities, and colleagues. What is most important for CHWs is to be able to talk about trauma in a way that others are most likely to understand.

18.3 A Common Language for Trauma Responses

Rather than trying to use the language of the *DSM-5*, we will do our best to use more accessible language in this chapter to talk about the effects of trauma. We will begin with information about how individuals may respond to trauma, using six broad categories of trauma responses. Please keep in mind that these are not comprehensive lists of all possible trauma responses, and that some responses may belong in more than one category. In the "Collective Impacts" section later in this chapter, we address how trauma may affect neighborhoods and communities.

Exposure to trauma can have profound and lasting impacts on survivors. *Yet, how people respond to trauma is often unique. There is no formula to predict how an individual will respond to or be affected by a certain type of trauma.* Two individuals exposed to the same traumatic event may respond in very different ways. Survivors may experience some, most, all, or none of the most common responses to trauma described below. Trauma symptoms or responses may last a few months or many years, and can range in terms of severity and the degree that that they harm the survivor and interfere with day-to-day life.

PHYSICAL RESPONSES

Trauma affects the body and physical health, and these responses *may* include:

- Startle responses (strong physical responses to stimuli such as sounds, sights, smells, sudden movements, being approached from behind, etc.).

- Hypervigilance, or constantly scanning the environment for possible risks or threats.

- Increased heart and respiratory rates and blood pressure, and the release of stress hormones such as cortisol and adrenaline. These biological responses prepare the body for "fight or flight" in the face of danger. When stress responses are repeated over time, such as when someone is exposed to ongoing trauma (child abuse or neglect, domestic violence, war or torture), these same biological responses are associated with increased risk for chronic health conditions such as heart disease (see below).

- Changes to sleep and dreaming life including, for example, difficulty sleeping, or sleeping a lot, and having dreams related to trauma experiences
  - Chronic and recurring nightmares about some element of the trauma story accompanied by strong emotions such as fear or dread
  - Night terrors are strong physical and emotional reactions such as fear or dread that may interrupt sleep or cause people to cry out

- Chronic pain such as headaches, stomach pain, or nausea
  - This pain can be extreme. For some survivors, for example, it may feel as if they have had a headache that lasts for years
- Injuries such as bruises, broken bones, burns, disabilities, loss of sight
  - Chronic disability such as the complete or partial loss of sight, balance, movement, or speech, or paralysis
- Pregnancy (such as the unintended pregnancy resulting from a sexual assault), and sexually transmitted infections (STIs) including HIV disease.

Trauma and Chronic Disease

Exposure to trauma can result in long-term harm to health, including the development of chronic conditions or disease. Some of the best evidence of the long-term health consequences of exposure to trauma comes from the Adverse Childhood Experiences (ACE) Study. ACE is a large-scale research study about the long-term health impacts of childhood exposures to "adverse" experiences such as child abuse and neglect, including childhood sexual abuse. The study has demonstrated that childhood abuse results in significant, wide-spread, and long-lasting impacts to physical and mental health, increasing rates of illness and premature death (CDC, 2014).

Of the more than 17,000 adults studied, almost two-thirds reported exposure to at least one adverse event in childhood. These childhood exposures are highly associated with increased risk for a wide range of chronic health conditions including alcoholism, drug use, smoking, depression, suicide attempts, liver disease, chronic obstructive pulmonary disease (COPD), and ischemic heart disease. Childhood exposure was also associated with higher rates of sexually transmitted infections, intimate partner violence, and unintended pregnancy.

To find out more about the ACE study, go to *acestudy.org*, or the Centers for Disease Control and Prevention website, at *www.cdc.gov/violenceprevention/acestudy/*.

EMOTIONAL RESPONSES

Common emotional responses and feelings *may* include:

- Numbing or the inability to feel
- Anger or rage
- Fear or terror
- Sadness or despair
- Self-blame and guilt (including survivor's guilt)
- Humiliation and shame

- *Can you think of other common emotional responses to trauma?*

What Do YOU Think?

Please note that because trauma encompasses the most extreme human experiences, it can provoke extreme emotions such as rage rather than anger, terror rather than fear, or despair rather than sadness. These extreme emotions can be overwhelming and difficult to manage. They may inspire survivors to seek relief, escape, or regulation, such as through the use of alcohol and drugs.

It is also important to understand that some survivors are numb or devoid of feeling. This is a highly common response. It can be very confusing, however, for family, friends, and helping professionals.

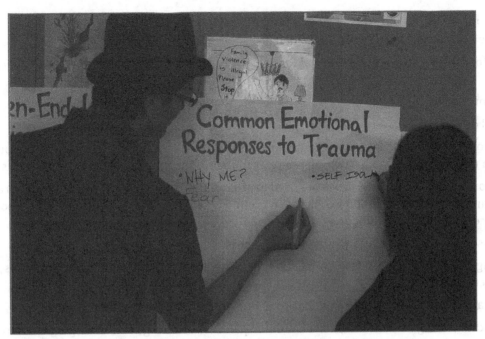

CHW students brainstorm ideas about common emotional responses to trauma.

Trauma and Numbness

Tim Berthold: I worked for a rape crisis center. I was sometimes called to the local county hospital to provide accompaniment and support to a survivor of a recent sexual assault (the survivor was always asked if they wanted someone from the rape crisis center to accompany them, and if they would accept the male counselor on call, or if they would prefer a female). The survivors were diverse in terms of ethnicity, gender, age, sexual orientation, and disability status, and experienced a wide range of different trauma responses. Numbness was common. While I had been trained to accept numbness as one of many common responses to trauma, other helping profession-als, including nurses, physicians, and the police, were sometimes confused when survivors didn't display strong emotion. They didn't understand and, in some instances, it made them doubt the survivor's experience and story. These helping professionals held assumptions about how survivors *should* respond, and numbness in the face of extreme violence was difficult for them to comprehend or believe. The lesson for me was about honoring the unique responses of individual survivors and pushing aside my own assumptions about the experience of others.

Survivor's guilt may affect those who witness or survive a traumatic event in which others were harmed or killed. Survivors are left with a feeling of guilt that they survived or escaped harm, or were not as deeply affected as others. Consider, for example, someone who survives a car crash in which other passengers were killed, or a soldier who witnesses the death of a fellow combatant.

Survivor's Guilt

Tim Berthold: I worked briefly in Guatemala with children from Mayan communities who had been orphaned during the war. One of the boys I worked with witnessed the destruction of his village, and carried with him the burden of survivor's guilt. He had been sent to the river to gather water by his mother. He was there when the helicopters arrived. He rushed back to his village and hid in some bushes as soldiers descended to torture and kill his family and neighbors. He watched as the soldiers cut the fetus from his pregnant mother before slitting her throat.

This young boy was haunted by survivor's guilt. He blamed himself for the death of his family. In his mind, "If my mother had gone to fetch water, I would have died and she would still be alive." He told me: "If I hadn't been at the river I would have heard the helicopters early and warned everyone to run and hide."

BEHAVIORAL RESPONSES

Common behavioral responses to trauma *may* include:

- Avoidance (of others, including friends and family, of work or school, or public spaces or particular types of places)

- Isolation from others

- Alcohol and drug use

  ○ The use of alcohol and drugs is common among survivors, as is addiction (to read more about the links between trauma and substance use, please refer to the resources provided at the end of this chapter).

  ○ One theory is that alcohol and drugs are used to alter, numb, or forget feelings or thoughts arising from the trauma. Indeed, early childhood pain and trauma is seen by some researchers as the root cause of substance use, abuse and addiction (Maté, 2010).

- Changes in sexual feelings, relationships, and behaviors

  ○ Including difficulty feeling safety, connection, or pleasure; avoidance of sexual experiences; or increased sexual activity

- Changes in appearance (such as the way that someone dresses or presents themselves)

- Changes in diet (eating more or less, and disordered patterns of eating such as binging or anorexia)

- Frequent arguments or conflicts

- Acting out through hurting others emotionally or physically, including through retaliation

- Hurting oneself (from self-injury, including cutting, to suicide)

- Risk-taking behaviors, such as driving too fast or engaging in unsafe sexual practices

- Returning to situations, including dangerous situations, that are similar to the original traumatic experience

- *How else can trauma impact the behavior of survivors?*

What Do YOU Think?

THE IMPACT ON RELATIONSHIPS

Trauma can touch upon all aspects of life, from performance at school and at work, to relationships with family and friends. Survivors may find it difficult to trust others or to tolerate intimacy and may push others away, including loved ones. They may stop going to work or to school, or stop performing well in these environments. They find it difficult to trust others, to feel comfortable or safe in sexual relationships, to believe that they can love others or are deserving of love themselves. They may feel betrayed by family or friends (or the church or school) and act out in anger or simply disengage or abandon these relationships altogether.

Others may develop deeper relationships or connections with others. Some may find a sense of refuge or safety at school or at work, a realm where they can exercise greater control. Some may become closer to their family or friends, or develop new friendships among others who have survived similar events or share common values.

COGNITIVE RESPONSES

Trauma can influence what people think about as well as how their mind functions. It can also affect the way that people think about themselves, and the future. Common trauma responses *may* include:

- Recurring thoughts or memories about the trauma

  ○ Such thoughts are sometimes triggered by specific factors such as physical environments, social dynamics, objects, physical sensations, sounds, or smells.

- Lack of an ability to remember the trauma or key aspects of the trauma

  ○ Dissociation is characterized by a disconnection between what's happening and one's awareness of what's happening. During a traumatic event, a person may disconnect from their thoughts and feelings, or later may seal off the memory of those events, as if they didn't happen. The continued dissociation, after the trauma has ended, can make it difficult for survivors to reclaim or integrate memories, thoughts and feelings related to the trauma experience. They may continue to experience dissociative responses in daily life when memories, flashbacks, sights, or smells restimulate some aspect of the original trauma experiences. This may manifest by zoning out or shutting down or in some way retreating from the memory and/or what is happening in the present.

Traumatic Memories

Trauma can have a dramatic affect on memory. It may cause intrusive or recurring and unwanted memories of trauma events, including flashbacks. It causes some survivors to avoid thinking about or recalling the original trauma events. For others, trauma may distort or result in the repression or inability to remember part or all of the trauma experience.

Most people have difficult remembering, in a precise or detailed way, all of life's major or minor events (*Can you remember every difficult or wonderful thing that happened in your life?*). Because of the nature of trauma and of dissociation, some survivors are unable to recall what happened to them (Brewin, 2007). For example, studies show that many people who experienced severe and documented abuse in childhood have no memory of these events (ISTSS, n.d.).

Yet it can be difficult for others—such as family, friends, and providers without specialized training—to understand how survivors can forget key aspects of the traumatic events. They may think *"If something so horrible happened to me, I'd certainly remember it!"*

As a CHW, your job is to accept that trauma can alter, suppress, or banish memories. Keep this truth in mind as you work with clients who may be trying to avoid memories, experiencing flashbacks, or struggling to remember and reconstruct what happened to them.

- Anxiety about safety and future exposure to trauma
- Thoughts of death (including more passive death thoughts or wishes, and active plans for suicide)
  - Thoughts about death are very common among survivors. These may resemble a passive desire to die or be killed in an accident. These thoughts are often related to a desire for current symptoms and suffering to end. Having death thoughts is different from being suicidal—which is defined as having a specific plan and an intention to kill oneself.
- Thoughts or fantasies about revenge
- Self-blame, shame, worthlessness
- Self-hatred
- Confusion and doubt
- Questioning why such horrible things happen, and why they happened to me, or my family. *Why did it happen to me? Why did I survive? Why did I survive when others did not?*

While we tend to focus on the negative impacts of trauma, survivors can also be affected in more positive ways. For example, survivors may, with time, gain self-confidence and self-esteem. They may identify as a strong person, as a survivor, as someone with wisdom and skills to guide their life or to share with others. They may actively seek ways to help others and strengthen community ties.

Thoughts about One's Self

Trauma can influence the way that survivors perceive or think about themselves. Some survivors develop a more negative self-image that may stem from a sense of self-blame. They may doubt their own value or worth, or see themselves as damaged, poisoned, or poisonous. They may view themselves as limited or incapable of loving or being loved. They may even experience self-hatred.

Survivors may also develop a renewed sense of their own self-worth, courage, wisdom, capability or resilience. By witnessing their own healing, and their connection with others, they may develop a deeper sense of their own strengths and values.

Concepts of the Future

Research shows that trauma can influence the way that survivors think about the future in the following types of ways:

- Loss of a sense of meaning for life
- A belief that the future will never be different from the present, that trauma symptoms will always persist and at an elevated level
- A sense of doom
- Difficulty in imagining the future or setting any future goals
- An expectation of dying early and through violence

Or, in contrast, survivors may experience:

- Acceptance of human fallibility or vulnerability
- A deeper commitment to creating a meaningful life
- A focus on the next generation (children or grandchildren) as a way to envision the future

---

The Kidnapping in Chowchilla, California

In 1976 a school bus with 26 elementary school students was stopped by armed men; the children were held captive underground for 16 hours in a buried van. They were eventually able to escape by climbing and digging their way out. Everyone was rescued; nonetheless, the experience caused trauma responses among the survivors that continue for decades.

Among other things, the children's view of the future was strikingly bleak. One boy explained that he didn't plan to have children, because "in case of an emergency there will only be time for me." An 11-year-old survivor, interviewed several years after the kidnapping, expected to die at age 12, saying "Somebody will come along and shoot me." The children lived with a fear of the future and an expectation that bad things were more likely to happen than not. (Terr, 1990, p. 164)

SPIRITUAL OR RELIGIOUS OR PHILOSOPHICAL RESPONSES

Trauma often affects a survivor's spiritual, religious, or philosophical values and beliefs. Keep in mind that not everyone is religious or identifies as being spiritual, but they may hold values and ideas that provide a sense of meaning for life. This may include, for example, a commitment to family, compassion, generosity or social justice.

Some survivors may lose their faith or sense of meaning. They may question their god or religion. They may feel betrayed or abandoned. They may stop praying or going to the temple, mosque, or church. They may feel that life has no purpose or meaning.

> **Toni Hunt Hines:** My sister used to go to church regularly, but after my son was killed, it shook her faith. She is angry with God. She can't go back. She and I, we only go to church for funerals.

Others may find that their sense of faith or meaning deepens or is strengthened. They may feel closer to their god or creator. They may establish closer relationships with their mosque, temple, church, or other religious or faith-based community. They find a renewed sense of purpose or meaning in the world.

They may dedicate their life to educating or helping others. They may join together with others who are advocating for change or social justice.

- *How else can trauma affect our sense of meaning, faith or religion?*

OTHER TRAUMA RESPONSES

We always leave space for CHWs to identify trauma responses that may not neatly fall into one of the categories provided above. It is important for you to leave the question of trauma response open as well, as you work with clients. The longer you work directly with survivors of trauma, the more you will learn about how trauma can shape and impact human lives.

- *What other categories or examples of trauma responses would you add to this list?*

18.4 Collective Impacts

When a traumatic event or series of events disrupts a community, it often rips into the social fabric of community life in addition to affecting individuals and families. Each of these three types of collective traumatic events (among others) have an impact: disasters, community-level violence over an extended period of time, and political violence or war. Each of these collective traumas has distinct characteristics—its duration, the specific needs that emerge in the wake of the trauma, the degree to which the harm was intended or accidental, and more—yet it seems worthwhile to highlight a few responses that may be found when *any* traumatic event affects or disrupts a community. The list below is influenced by researchers and providers working in the United States and internationally, in addition to the experience of the authors of this chapter and the instructors and students in the CHW program at City College.

When a community is rocked by traumatic events, the trust and interdependence of the community is altered. Some of the ways this can happen include:

- The rupture of social connections and increased distrust in the community. When a community is displaced or forced to flee or move elsewhere in the wake of a disaster or a war, many social connections are lost, sometimes permanently. In addition, the dynamics of the trauma—especially in situations of armed conflict or endemic neighborhood violence—may lead to divisions in the community. There is sometimes a tendency to blame the victim for the violence they suffered, for the risks they took, or for exposing others to collateral violence (Beristain, 2010; Lykes, Beristain, & Pérez-Armiñan, 2007; Saul, 2014).

- Inhibited communication among people, or a tendency toward silence about the trauma or anything associated with the trauma. This is especially true in cases of political violence or generalized community violence, when people may fear repercussions of talking about what is going on (Lykes, Beristain, & Pérez-Armiñan, 2007; Rich, 2009).

- Avoidance. In a context of ongoing or recent trauma, people may seek safety by avoiding participation in groups, or even going to public spaces, which can lead to increased isolation.

Human rights violations, war, and displacement often have an effect on the political voice of the community, as well. The community is denied the opportunity to participate in decisions that affect them, at many levels. And while natural disasters are not inherently political in nature, decisions about how humanitarian aid will be distributed and what will be rebuilt (or not) can be highly political. The voice of the community is constrained in important ways, including

- Transformation of community values. In the case of political violence, transforming a community's values and actions is actually one *purpose* of the violence. For example, if a community tended to support a certain ideology that was opposed by the dominant military force in the area, then the community may suppress or even reject that ideology in favor of one less likely to draw fire. Any kind of disaster can provoke a change in the sense of belonging and mutuality, when the community is disrupted for an extended period of time (Beristain, 2010; de Jong, 2011).

- Detachment from organizational processes (Beristain, 2010; Lykes, Beristain, & Pérez-Armiñan, 2007). Community connectedness has been recognized as a protective factor for many kinds of social ills. When a community is traumatized, however, people often withdraw from organizations, groups, and affiliations, weakening community organizing efforts and movements. When violence or war directly targets community organizations, there is even more reason for people to pull away from organizing. At times, the opposite response is observed, and communities are able to organize to address violence, disaster or trauma—strengthening the community's voice.

- Paralysis or inaction. The potent combination of a disruption of hope, an increase of anxiety (even panic), and a rupture of trust can lead to political paralysis. A community, or a significant portion of it, may back off from taking actions that they might have engaged in before the violence or trauma. A deep sense of hopelessness and inefficacy can take root. In cases of state torture or other forms of politically motivated violence, causing this political paralysis is sometimes not just an effect, but the purpose of the violence itself (Stevenson & Rall, 2007).

The physical insecurity of communities in the aftermath of a collective trauma is considerable. Collective traumas are never brief in duration. An earthquake might only shake the ground for a minute, but the rebuilding efforts can last for years. A war is never a single trauma, but rather a web of traumatic events that affect individuals, families, neighborhoods, communities, and even whole societies. And endemic community violence or gang warfare can last for decades. Collective traumas often generate displacement of some sort—a need to move from one place to another to seek safety—and often it is not clear at first whether this displacement is temporary or permanent. Some of the impacts of collective trauma that create physical insecurity include

- The lack of basic needs. This may include basic survival needs such as water, food, and shelter. Sources of employment, places to congregate or play, transportation, and other types of basic community services may also be lacking or unsafe to access.

- A generalized climate of fear and insecurity. It can be difficult to predict what is risky and what is safe in a climate of violence, war, or disaster. This uncertainty can contribute to decisions that are either overly cautious or overly reckless. In addition, people's freedom of movement may be significantly restricted—for example, avoiding certain corners or streets, staying away from crowds.

- Violence in response to violence. Collective traumatic events can trigger violence towards others, for example, the scapegoating of one group by another, or the cycles of retaliation that sometimes occur among groups using violence. The normalization of violence that comes about through long-term exposure can increase the likelihood of this.

One more aspect of collective traumas is the effect of the media. The media in all its forms can be an additional source of restimulation for affected communities and individuals. Through television, magazines, and social media survivors are exposed to repeating of images and other reminders of the disaster, war, or other mass trauma. This includes, for example, survivors of a major disaster like the 9/11 attacks in 2001 or Hurricane Katrina in 2005 continually seeing images of the events on television, or people who live in a community with high levels of violence seeing reports of murders and assaults on the news with great frequency. On the anniversary of major disasters or milestones in a war, images and videos of the trauma may be inescapable. These images can distort how other people perceive an affected community, leading to bias or discrimination. They can also add to feelings of overwhelm or hopelessness.

As with trauma in families or individuals, communities faced with collective trauma may also experience post-traumatic healing and growth. Groups formed to respond to the trauma may strengthen the community in new ways, or help the community find its voice. New social norms of mutual support or resistance may emerge. Often, in the immediate aftermath of a disaster, people rally to support one another. Many people step up to help others, share resources and meet basic needs. Sometimes a lively sense of solidarity and altruism can emerge in a community—even a community simply thrown together by circumstances—in the midst of a life-threatening emergency (Solnit, 2009). These community strengths should be recognized, just as much as the negative impacts of the trauma.

- *Can you think of another example of a collective trauma or disaster?*

- *Have you witnessed some of the effects described here in your community?*

- *What other effects have you observed that are the result of some type of trauma in the community?*

18.5 How Culture and Status Influence Trauma

One of the most common mistakes that helping professionals make is to assume that others share their own understanding and beliefs about trauma and recovery. Research has shown that the way that people understand and respond to traumatic experiences, and the way that they define and seek healing from trauma are influenced by culture, identity, and status (Brown, 2008; The Harvard Program in Refugee Trauma, n.d.; Mollica, 2009). Richard Mollica, a researcher at Harvard University with expertise in cross-cultural approaches to treating trauma, emphasizes the importance of paying close attention to the client's own words (in this case, regarding torture, but it could be any form of trauma). Their words say a lot about how they interpret their experience. This is aligned with the cultural humility approach that we emphasize throughout this book.

> *Critically interpreting the language a survivor uses allows a doctor to understand the meaning traumatized patients give to their experiences. Words, especially those that denote traumatic events, need to be carefully defined in the life of the patient, family, and community. While the experience of torture is a horrific event everywhere, different cultures regard its causes and consequences in different ways. In some societies torture survivors receive compassion, while in others they are blamed and punished. This understanding can aid in the healing of the survivors and, sometimes, even of society. (Mollica, 2009, pp. 18–19)*

Some research has led to questions about cultural bias in the definition and diagnostic standards for PTSD in the American Psychiatric Association's (APA, 2013) *DMS-5*. In some cultures, certain symptoms associated with PTSD may not appear at all, while others appear but are named and understood in culturally specific ways. Services that pay attention to cultural traditions and support a variety of approaches to healing are more likely to resonate with clients and communities. The following statement, again from Richard Mollica's work with Southeast Asian refugees, reflects the value of culturally sensitive services provided by a clinical team that include members of the affected community, in a role similar to a CHW.

> *. . . (T)he Harvard clinic refugee patients were the poorest members of the local communities. If they sought help in an emergency room for serious emotional distress, they ended up being committed to a mental hospital against their will, and were strongly advised to take psychotropic drugs without counseling or social rehabilitation. During the first few years of the clinic, we rescued hundreds of refugees from the mental hospital. At our clinic we provided them with all of the material (for example, housing) and emotional support (such as counseling in their own language) they needed to obtain a job, live independent lives, and care for their families. . . . (M)ost succeeded in being self-sufficient; few ever needed psychiatric hospitalization. (Mollica, 2009, p. 14)*

Refugees and asylum seekers living in the United States or Canada are also likely to have experienced multiple and severe traumatic experiences in settings with very few resources for basic survival, let alone psychological support. Their symptoms are compounded by being displaced from their country of origin and their support networks and, for some, by long stays in a refugee camp or a detention center while waiting to immigrate or receive legal status. Adjusting to life in a new country and culture also adds to their stress. CHWs should be aware of these multiple sources of stress in the lives of refugees and asylum seekers, and may find similar stresses in the lives of immigrant clients in general.

Toni Hunt Hines: Working with Latino families, especially if they are undocumented, there is such a fear of fighting back (after something traumatic has happened). They are afraid that someone will be deported if they make a complaint or do anything. It's hanging over the family's head.

Society often assigns higher status or privilege to some groups over others, and this influences trauma exposure, response, and recovery. In the United States, people of color, immigrants, members of the LGBT community, people with disabilities, and others are at greater risk of experiencing traumatic events and of encountering biased responses from the agencies charged with providing support. Among veterans of the Vietnam War, for example, ethnic minority veterans were more likely to be exposed to war-zone stressors than whites. Institutionalized forms of racism both in the Armed Services and in U.S. society as a whole added to the stressors that veterans of color experienced, prior to deployment, during their time in the war zone, and after the war (Loo, 2014). It's important for a CHW to understand this larger context when working with a client or group. As CHWs often come from a similar background as their clients, the client may feel more comfortable talking with the CHW about the role that discrimination, exclusion, or bias has played in their experience of trauma.

USING CULTURAL HUMILITY AND CLIENT-CENTERED PRACTICE

Perhaps the most significant concern is the risk of imposing culturally biased ideas and standards onto the clients and communities you work with, unintentionally causing injury or harm. *Please let client-centered concepts and skills, including cultural humility, guide your work with all clients:*

- Don't assume that you know about the experiences, beliefs, values, and emotions of others.
- Overcome biases (which are all too common in some agencies and institutions) that certain cultural groups don't want to talk about trauma, or don't experience psychological suffering in the wake of traumatic events.
- Stay curious and ask open-ended questions to learn from the only true experts in the room—the clients and community members you work with.
- Don't tell people what to do or think or believe; use your "big eyes and big ears" to give space to clients to express their own stories and wisdom.
- Don't make assumptions about how clients identify with their culture or cultures—instead, support them to explore their own choices around identity and how that impacts their well-being, especially when historical trauma is present.
- Let people chose their own route to healing (or not healing), at their own pace.
- Stay alert to the meaning that clients assign to their experiences, symptoms, and healing strategies.
- Remember that you are not responsible for rescuing, "fixing" or healing the client. You are there as a support for the client, to help the client mobilize internal and external resources to overcome the challenges they face.
- Discuss with the client (and with your coworkers, if you work as part of a team) how cultural norms may conflict with the practices of your agency. For example, mixed gender or mixed generation support groups may feel inappropriate to some clients.
- Keep learning about trauma and about the history and culture of the communities you work with. Learn about the resources within these communities that can provide culturally relevant guidance and support to survivors.

- *How else can the concept of cultural humility support the autonomy and healing of the clients and communities you work with?*

What Do
YOU?
Think ?

18.6 Healing from Trauma

Many survivors, especially those who have recently experienced trauma, question whether or not it is possible to heal or recover from trauma. The prospect may seem daunting, remote, or impossible in the moment.

It is possible to heal from trauma. But healing may be quite different than what the survivor initially hoped for. And healing is not universal; for some survivors, the effects of trauma continue to dominate significant aspects of their lives.

Finding the right language to talk about healing from trauma is challenging. While some people talk about "recovery" from trauma, others find this language confusing, especially when they compare it to the process of recovery from drug or alcohol abuse. In the mental health field, "recovery" is used to refer to "a process of change through which individuals improve their health and wellness, live self-directed lives, and strive to reach their full potential" (SAMHSA, 2014a). Another term that many people favor is "healing from trauma." Something we like about this language is that it implies a process ("I am healing") rather than a destination or outcome ("I am now healed").

What Do YOU Think?

- *What are your beliefs about healing or recovering from trauma?*

- *What language do you use for this concept?*

GOALS FOR HEALING

Trauma survivors have a broad and diverse understanding of what healing means to them. Some may hope to be restored to the person they were before they were harmed by violence or other forms of trauma. They may wish to be restored to an earlier and/or more innocent state of being. This is a common wish among survivors of childhood sexual abuse. It may be a way of grieving their loss due to trauma. However, it isn't possible to travel back in time or erase the trauma or its impacts. The trauma happened, and trauma changes us. Accepting this can be difficult, however, and often takes time, patience, and courage.

Some survivors have very specific goals for reducing or eliminating trauma responses or symptoms. These may include, for example, being able to sleep without being disturbed by night terrors, to return to work or school, to build close and trusting relationships with family and friends, to enjoy a satisfying romantic and sexual life, to be more present or comfortable with their children, or to feel joy in more aspects of their life. For trauma survivors who have acquired a disability or a physical change in their body as a result of the traumatic experience—for example, the loss of a leg or an eye—their goals may include adapting to their injury, learning to use assistive devices, and increasing their sense of independence.

Depending upon your role and scope of practice, it can be helpful to explore the survivor's goals for their health and recovery, just as you would explore a client's goals for the self-management of diabetes or depression. For example, you may ask them *"What do you hope to change or accomplish?"* or *"What are your hopes and expectations?"* And, just as you would in supporting any client to establish an action plan, assist them to establish realistic steps to take to meet goals or milestones over time. Keep in mind that gradual and incremental change is likely to be more successful than attempts to create dramatic change quickly.

MULTIPLE PATHS FOR HEALING FROM TRAUMA

Healing or recovering from trauma takes many forms. Deciding which path to follow is a highly individual matter and may be influenced by factors such as the survivor's current symptoms, their cultural and family customs, housing and financial situation, spiritual and political beliefs, and knowing other survivors who have experienced meaningful healing or recovery. Many trauma survivors choose to combine several different paths to support their healing. Just because a client is not interested in a certain path to healing at one point in time does not mean that he or she won't be open to that path at a later time. As a CHW, it may be beneficial to develop a list of referrals related to these various paths or options, including those that have a specific focus on trauma recovery, as well as some (for example, a free yoga class) that could be supportive of healing more generally.

Survivors may want to engage in one or more, or none, of the following pathways for healing.

Counseling or Therapy

There are many different types of therapy provided by mental health professionals. Therapy is often available through mental health clinics and human services agencies; some primary health care clinics also offer therapy. Many counselors also work in private practice. Therapy seeks to create a safe environment for clients to talk about and reflect upon key aspects of their trauma story, gaining new insights, knowledge, and skills. Counseling goals vary among survivors but commonly include reducing trauma responses/symptoms that are interfering with their current quality of life. Therapy may be offered as individual sessions, family sessions, or group sessions. While most counselors or therapists have *some* knowledge of trauma, there are benefits to working with a counselor or therapist who has specialized training and experience in the field of trauma. No one approach works for *all* people. A client might need to meet with more than one counselor, if that is an option, before selecting the best one to work with.

Cognitive-behavioral therapy is one of the most commonly used approaches with survivors of trauma. Over a series of sessions (over weeks or months), **cognitive-behavioral therapy** assists the client in understanding how their thought patterns and behaviors may affect them, and in learning tools to change ingrained thought patterns or behaviors that may be harmful. It often helps survivors to better understand their physical and emotional responses to trauma, manage stress, explore their trauma story (see later in this chapter), distinguish between current and past experiences, and develop new coping skills.

New approaches to counseling are always emerging, including those developed or adapted for survivors of trauma. Trauma-focused cognitive-behavioral therapy (TF-CBT), for example, was developed to meet the specific needs of children and adolescents who have experienced sexual abuse, domestic violence, the sudden death of a caregiver, or other traumatic events. TF-CBT consists of a structured short-term course of therapy for children and selected family members, both together and separately, to work with beliefs, behaviors, and family dynamics that have been affected by trauma (Child Welfare Information Gateway, 2012).

Exposure therapy is another approach used with trauma survivors and with veterans in particular. It involves asking the survivor to gradually expose themselves to images and other stimuli (situations, sounds, etc.) that are similar to key aspects of their trauma experience, with the goal of reducing anxiety and other post-traumatic symptoms. Exposure therapy using video games that simulate combat experiences has been used with military veterans. Exposure starts slowly and progresses over time *at the client's pace*.

Eye movement desensitization and reprocessing (EMDR) is another form of therapy that has been used to support survivors of trauma. EMDR is conducted by a trained professional, and asks survivors to talk about their trauma experiences while engaging in certain types of physical actions such as rapidly moving the eyes from side to side, or tapping alternating sides of the body. The theory behind EMDR is that this process allows the client to store the memory of the trauma in a different way than it was stored in the brain previously. The result for some survivors is a meaningful reduction in post-traumatic stress symptoms.

Social or Support Groups

Survivors often benefit from meeting with others who have experienced similar traumatic experiences and symptoms. This is particularly beneficial because trauma can be stigmatized and isolating. The rape crisis movement was built upon the idea that survivors benefit from meeting and forging connections with others, breaking silence, shame, stigma and isolation. Peer support and understanding can open up possibilities of healing and recovery for many groups, such as survivors of intimate partner violence, veterans, parents grieving the death of a child, and others. Some groups are facilitated by mental health professionals, while others are peer-led.

- *What type of social or support groups exist in your local communities?*

What Do YOU Think?

Educational Groups

An educational workshop, or series of workshops, about trauma often includes aspects of emotional or psychological awareness, skills, and support. These groups or workshops are sometimes called psycho-educational. They may be designed and offered specifically for people living with the effects of trauma, or other types of psychological distress (such as depression, anxiety, or compulsive behaviors). An example is the Heal the Violence group, developed by Inez Love, a CHW working in San Francisco's Department of Public Health (personal communication, October 30, 2014). Heal the Violence is designed for young people who have lost a family member to street violence. The group includes information about violence and trauma, along with opportunities for mutual support and artistic expression.

Another approach is to weave information about trauma into a more general educational group or workshop. As trauma, violence and loss are a common part of life, there is a great likelihood that any group includes people for whom trauma is a current concern. In addition, such groups may reach people who would not seek out a workshop on violence and trauma, but who would be open to a workshop on family life or wellness. An example is the groups and workshops offered by La Clinica de la Raza in Oakland, California, under their program *Cultura y Bienestar* ("Culture and Wellness"). This series includes workshops on parenting stress, grief, trauma, and other mental health topics, as well as traditional healing practices such as drumming and use of herbs (La Clinica de La Raza, 2015).

Medications

Some survivors choose to take medications that may reduce and relieve anxiety, depression, or other trauma symptoms. Clients should talk with a medical or mental health provider and carefully consider different treatment options. Clients taking medications should also meet regularly with a medical provider in order to assess the effectiveness of the medications they are taking, to monitor side effects and to revise dosages or change medications as necessary.

Acupuncture or Other Forms of Complementary Medicine

Some survivors find that acupuncture can be helpful in managing the physical and emotional effects of trauma. Acupuncture is a practice of Chinese medicine that uses needles to stimulate specific channels of energy in the body. Other survivors choose to consult with naturopaths or other practitioners of complementary and alternative medicine. As with selecting a medical doctor or therapist, it is helpful to work with reputable practitioners who have training and experience in trauma.

Somatic Therapies

Biomedical researchers have found that the effects of trauma are stored in the body and can change or rewire our neurobiology. Some survivors seek out **somatic** therapies that engage the body in ways that promote healing. Somatic therapy may include physical movements designed to help the client recognize and work with bodily sensations that arise in the present moment, as a result of the past traumatic experience or memory. Somatic therapies sometimes also use dance, theater, and yoga to engage the mind and body, to revisit memories in a new way or to create new pathways for relaxation and expression (van der Kolk, 2014).

Healing Arts

The creative and performing arts support the healing of many survivors. Music, dance, drumming, poetry, drawing/painting, theater, drama therapy, and other art forms can provide survivors an opportunity to express aspects of their trauma experience that may be more difficult to tell in conventional settings. Approaching healing through the arts is also an opportunity to incorporate cultural practices or traditions that resonate with survivors.

Social or Political Action

Some people approach healing by taking action to advocate for social change and social justice. Especially when people have been exposed to trauma at a community level, such as survivors of state-sponsored violence and armed conflicts, they may also find healing in taking collective action. Survivors of war, rape, domestic violence, and incarceration have formed organizations and movements to create social and political change. Some survivors, in fact, are not comfortable with the concept of "healing" or "recovery," as it implies an internal or individual process; they identify their journey toward wholeness with the collective pursuit of truth, justice, and peace.

- *What kinds of social action do you see in your community, in response to traumatic events?*

Spiritual or Religious Practices

Spiritual or religious beliefs and practices, including spiritual or faith-based counseling, prayer and meditation, are beneficial to many survivors. They may increase a survivor's sense of safety, provide a feeling of being accompanied and not alone, or offer hope and purpose. Healing work in a faith community can draw upon the power of tradition and ritual to help address the hard questions that inevitably arise. Survivors may create meaningful connections with others through participating in a faith community or other spiritually oriented group, including 12-step groups that may offer a way to connect (or reconnect) with a higher power.

Mindfulness

Mindfulness cultivates awareness and being present in the moment with our thoughts, feelings, physical sensations and environment. While the practice of mindfulness arose out of Buddhist meditation practices, it is now widely practiced in a secular or nonreligious way and to support those living with mental and physical health conditions. Mindfulness practices usually include breathing exercises and meditation; they can also include yoga, chanting, and prayer. Mindfulness supports survivors to notice and accept thoughts and feelings related to their trauma and healing stories. For many, it helps to create a state of awareness and clam, reducing stress symptoms. For more information about mindfulness, see the resources provided in Chapter 12 of *Foundations*.

Support from Family and Friends

The support of family and friends is often critical to a person's success and well-being. Many of us naturally turn to family and friends first to talk about intimate and difficult issues, and how those loved ones respond—whether they are supportive or not—can have a significant impact for survivors (Vogt, King, & King, 2007).

- *What are other strategies for healing or recovery from trauma are you aware of?*

What Do YOU Think?

TELLING THE TRAUMA STORY

For many survivors, telling the story or stories of their trauma experience(s) is a key aspect of healing. There are many different ways to tell these stories. Stories may be told in whole or in part, chronologically or out of time sequence. They may be told literally or metaphorically, in words or images, through art, theater, dance, or other methods. Stories may be kept private or shared with a witness or supportive other such as a friend or family member, to a group of other survivors, to a CHW, physician, or social worker.

Regardless of whom the story is shared with, and how, the most important audience for the story may be the survivors themselves. By telling their trauma stories, survivors can come to better understand their experiences including what happened, how they responded in the moment, how they have been affected since, how they live with trauma today, as well as the story of their survival and healing. In this sense, the story itself can serve as a critical resource for healing.

Please keep in mind that not every survivor will choose to tell their story, or to tell it to you. Not every survivor remembers his or her story. Consider, for example, children who were harmed at a very young age, or survivors who were sexually assaulted after losing consciousness, or survivors for whom memory has been banished and cannot be recalled.

For some survivors, telling their trauma story is an overwhelming or terrifying prospect. They may even feel that their stories will destroy them. Many people spend many years trying to escape or run away from the story of what they survived. And for others, they may begin to talk about their trauma experience and find that it is too difficult to continue. This is one reason why we never want to nudge or pressure a survivor to tell their story. Only the survivor can decide if, when, and how they want to tell their story.

My Trauma Story

Anonymous: Over time, I came to think of my trauma story like a book. At first, I buried it in the garage. I didn't want to look at it, much less read it. I didn't even want to look at the cover. It felt like, if I looked at it, I might burst into flames, like it would overwhelm or destroy me. But, at the same time, it was like a book that you can't throw away or, if you did, you would keep finding that it had been returned to your apartment.

My healing has been a slow and gradual path of learning to pick up that book—the story of what was done to me. I started by reading just a few words or pages at a time. Sometimes I waited months or years before I could read any further. What I noticed, over time, is that the more I read the book, the less afraid of it I became. Gradually, I stopped thinking of my story as this shameful secret that could destroy me, but as something that hadn't destroyed me, as something that I had been strong enough to survive. Eventually the idea of the book just kind of disappeared. It isn't a book anymore, some object outside of myself that I can pick up or hide away—it is simply another part of me. Not the most important part. Not the part that defines me, or controls me. And not just a negative part any more. Now, when I think about the trauma, I don't just see all the horrible things that happened and that I felt, I see my own strength, the part of me that survived this and that is becoming a person that is capable of love, and respect, and joy, and all the other parts of my life that are to come. Now I think of the future more than the past.

Trauma stories may be kept private or shared with others. When the trauma has affected a whole family—for example, one member of the family was killed or disappeared without a trace—it is often the case that different family members have slightly different stories, different aspects of the experience that marked them. Sometimes it is helpful for the different stories to be heard, acknowledged, and reconciled within the family—but sometimes that is not possible. At any rate, each person's story has validity, even if it contradicts the memories of other members of the family.

Telling a trauma story can also be a political act. A public accounting for and reckoning with traumatic acts, especially when those acts were carried out by the government or with the government's acquiescence—think of the Tuskegee Experiment discussed in Chapter 6, or the internment of Japanese Americans, or the campaign for reparations for slavery, or the truth commissions that have arisen in the wake of civil conflicts, from South Africa to Central America—can contribute to healing, especially if the survivors of those traumatic acts are treated with dignity and respect throughout the process.

18.7 Prevention and Resiliency

As we discussed in Chapter 3 on Public Health, the gold standard for prevention is primary prevention, meaning preventing something before it starts. When it comes to trauma, the best prevention of all is to prevent exposure to traumatic events. While it is impossible to prevent or eliminate all traumatic events, CHWs often work to reduce community violence and prevent violence in the home; to help low-income families and individuals acquire adequate housing that is less likely to burn or collapse; and to advocate with community members for safer environmental conditions (preventing certain types of disasters). All of these actions, and others like them, help to prevent trauma.

CHWs also play a role in supporting resiliency—before, during, and after traumatic events. **Resiliency**, at its most basic level, is the ability to bounce back after difficult events. Individuals and communities alike may be more or less resilient in response to a natural disaster like a flood, or an ongoing disaster such as the poverty, violence, and hopelessness that affect so many communities. CHWs can support and build resiliency within themselves, and with the clients and communities they work with. At the same time, it is very important to note that resiliency cannot erase all the effects of trauma, nor should an individual or community be blamed for lacking resiliency. Often, it is hard to know how resilient a person or community really is, until that resiliency is tested. Apart from individual or community resiliency, many other factors influence the traumatic stress response—including the severity of the incident, the duration, prior life experiences, and even our genes. Many of these cannot be easily changed.

For CHWs seeking to promote community and individual resiliency, there are significant factors that can prevent the worst effects and enhance the possibility of healing from trauma more quickly or thoroughly. Resiliency in the context of trauma could mean, for example, that a person experiences distress but not PTSD; or a person experiences short-term PTSD in the wake of a traumatic incident, but does not develop a case of PTSD that lasts for years; or that a community's social fabric resists being ruptured in the wake of a disaster, permitting the community to help its most vulnerable members and to advocate for the resources to rebuild.

The Value of Social Support

"Kids can walk around trouble if there is some place to walk to and someone to walk with." Tito, an ex-gang member (McLaughlin, Irby, & Langman, 1994, p. 219)

Some of the characteristics of resilient individuals and communities (Beristain, 2010; Mollica, 2009; Saul, 2014) include:

- Access to adequate physical and economic resources
- Adaptability and an inner sense of control or choice
- Social connectedness and mutual support

- The ability to ask for support when needed
- The ability to advocate for self and others
- A sense of purpose or meaning

  - *Can you think of ways that CHWs help communities to develop or enhance these qualities?*

  - *In what ways can you build your own resiliency as a CHW and a community member?*

In sections further on in this chapter, we discuss other ways that CHWs can support resiliency when working with individuals, groups, and communities who have experienced trauma.

COMMUNITY BUILDING

Kai Erikson defined collective trauma as "a blow to tissues of social life that damages the bonds linking people together, and impairs the prevailing sense of communality" (Erikson, 1976, p. 154). While Erikson was writing about a mining disaster, he could just as easily have been writing about New York after the September 11 attacks on the World Trade Center, New Orleans after Hurricane Katrina, or wars anywhere in the world. Because trauma is so often characterized by isolation and a kind of social wound, CHWs can help rebuild social bonds among people by working at the group and community level. CHWs may help to create mutual support groups, organize community advocacy efforts, locate and reunite families or friends who have been separated, and organize community events that give residents the opportunity to form connections. More socially connected communities have also been shown to have greater efficacy in demanding resources and attention from government agencies or others who have the power to help (Chandra et al., 2011).

Advocacy

CHWs advocate for those affected by trauma, and they support clients and communities to develop skills to advocate for themselves. Sometimes the ability to advocate develops as part of the healing process from trauma. In discussing the responses of youth in New York to the terrorist attack of September 11, Andrew Malekoff (2007) highlighted the value of working as a group to "offer opportunities for action that represents triumph over the demoralization of helplessness and despair." Some of these actions were personal—for example, writing a poem—while others were collective, such as providing advice to service providers on youth needs, or providing testimony at a public hearing. Other examples of collective advocacy in response to trauma include Take Back the Night marches (as a response to violence against women), the advocacy of refugees to return home in safe conditions, the movement in the US to reduce or abolish incarceration, and efforts (often led by torture survivors) to end the practice of torture around the world. Advocacy gives survivors the opportunity to tell their story in a larger context, propose solutions, find others who share their experience, receive affirmation, and, at least sometimes, to have the satisfaction of making a difference.

Honoring the Dead

Grieving is often an important part of healing from trauma. A violent or unexpected death may trigger traumatic stress among surviving family and friends, or those who witnessed the death. When the person who died is blamed for the death or dehumanized by labels—for example, when the victim of street shooting is labeled a "thug," or when a person in the political opposition to a repressive government is labeled a "terrorist," or when a sex worker is killed and his or her occupation is sensationalized in the media—the suffering from that trauma may be made worse as it is combined with bias, judgment, and shame. In these cases, CHWs can play a role in helping survivors to honor the dead and celebrate their memory. This can happen through working with individuals or by facilitating a group. Public events or public art can also commemorate the dead in culturally meaningful ways. For example, altars built for Day of the Dead have served this purpose in some communities. Murals, gardens, memorial statues, and public marches or ceremonies are other ways that communities have chosen to honor and remember those who died in traumatic circumstances. Such activities can assist in the grieving process; they can also assist in reclaiming public spaces, which can promote community identity, safety, and resiliency (Prevention Institute, 2013).

Client-Centered Practice

CHWs can also use their skills in health education, training, advocacy, and group facilitation to help survivors of trauma to understand what has happened to them, to normalize the trauma responses they may be experiencing, to access resources for healing and for rebuilding their lives, and to find or create meaning from the experiences they have had. Because we are social beings, it is particularly powerful to work with others to find meaning in traumatic, tragic, and unjust experiences. A strong sense of purpose or meaning has been shown to be associated with greater resiliency to trauma. CHWs can lead workshops or groups that allow survivors of trauma to share their experiences, reflect on why these experiences occurred and reframe those experiences when appropriate (for example, helping survivors of domestic violence see that the violence was not their fault), and create a sense of purpose and support for taking action in the wake of the trauma—whether those actions are individual or collective. CHWs, using client-centered and strength-based processes, can help individuals and groups suffering from trauma to tap into their own sense of choice and direction, and to adapt to changing circumstances.

It is also important for CHWs to cultivate their own resiliency. Many of the same characteristics that make someone a good CHW are associated with resiliency—such as resourcefulness, communication skills, leadership qualities, and empathy. Further on in this chapter you'll find more information about secondary trauma, secondary resiliency, and self care.

18.8 The CHW Scope of Practice

Scope of practice is a significant concern regarding the role of CHWs who provide direct services to survivors of trauma (whether they work with individuals, families, groups, or at the community level). Scope of practice is defined in Chapter 7. It provides a framework for CHWs—and all professionals—regarding the types of tasks and services that they are qualified to provide and those that they are not qualified to provide.

The most serious concern is that CHWs might exceed their SOP line by providing services that they are not qualified to offer. It is important to emphasize that CHWs do not provide therapy or act as the primary counselor for a client with trauma, and should not continue to work with a client who discloses severe trauma symptoms, behaviors of self-harm, or suicidal ideation (thoughts and a plan to kill themselves). It is vital for clients who are experiencing acute post-traumatic symptoms to work with a well-trained and licensed provider.

CHWs have an ethical duty to stay within their scope of practice and to "do no harm" to the clients and communities they serve. The risks or potential harms of working beyond your scope of practice include:

- **Harms to clients and communities**: This may include complicating, delaying, or harming their recovery or healing from trauma. It may also cause clients to feel less secure reaching out for professional support in the future.
- **Damaged relationships between clients/community and the CHW**: By exceeding your SOP you may irreversibly damage professional relationships and any trust that you have built up with a client or the community.
- **Harm to the CHW**: By exceeding your SOP, you could risk disciplinary action, reassignment, reduced scope of practice, or loss of employment. Your professional reputation as a CHW may also be damaged.
- **Harm to the agency you work for**: This could include a diminished or damaged reputation among clients and the community and possibly among other service providers and funders.

A secondary concern, at the other end of the SOP spectrum, is that CHWs will hold themselves back from providing the services they are qualified to offer to survivors of trauma. The topic of trauma has become so "medicalized" that anyone who is unlicensed is cautioned from addressing it in almost any way. Sometimes, medical and mental health professionals forget that trauma is a natural and common part of life, and that survivors and witnesses need a range of different opportunities to talk about it. Finding ways to talk openly about trauma is key not only for healing and building resilience, but also to preventing further trauma. If we caution all unlicensed providers from ever addressing trauma with the clients and communities they work with, we may unintentionally reinforce the shame and isolation that is so common among survivors. We may also give the impression that survivors of trauma should just put the trauma behind them and not talk about it, or that trauma should only be addressed by licensed professionals.

SEEKING A BALANCED AND ETHICAL SCOPE OF PRACTICE

We encourage CHWs and the agencies they work for to seek a balance between the two ends of a scope of practice spectrum. We believe that all CHWs should be prepared to use client-centered skills to listen compassionately when clients disclose a history of trauma, and to provide culturally relevant linkages to local programs and services. With the benefit of additional training, quality supervision, and close collaboration with licensed professionals, most CHWs can provide meaningful support to survivors of trauma. It is important to highlight that, in many communities, people are more likely to feel comfortable talking about a trauma experience with a trusted community member—such as a CHW—rather than going to a clinic, hospital, or therapist. Throughout the world, community members turn to CHWs in the aftermath of trauma for compassion and support. Some clients will disclose their history of trauma, and others will not. The extent to which CHWs explicitly address issues of trauma and healing with clients will depend upon the decisions of clients, and on the severity of their post-traumatic stress. In some settings, CHWs continue to address issues of trauma with their clients while receiving close supervision from a licensed practitioner. In other settings, clients with post-traumatic stress will be referred to licensed providers. Some clients will work with both a licensed provider and a CHW (as you will see in the Nadia Case Study below).

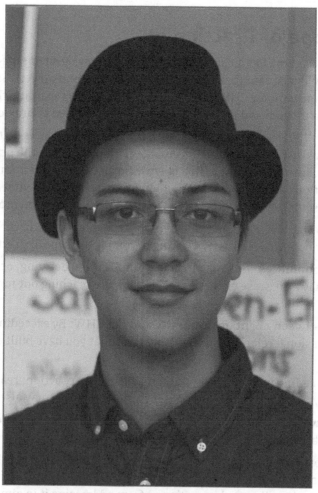

CHWs use client-centered skills to support clients to determine their own path to healing from trauma.

FACTORS THAT INFLUENCE THE CHW SCOPE OF PRACTICE

Unfortunately, there is no simple formula or hard and fast rule to tell CHWs what they can and cannot say or do in every circumstance. The truth is that the SOP of CHWs regarding trauma varies depending upon several factors such as:

- The CHW's prior training, skills, and comfort level.
  - Some CHWs have not received specific training related to trauma, while others, for example, have been trained and certified as a Sexual Assault Counselor.
- The employer's policies and protocols. For example, some agencies have adopted Trauma Informed Policies (more information is provided later on in the chapter) that provide additional training and clear guidance for considering and addressing trauma as a routine part of service delivery.
- The type of program you work for. Some CHWs work for agencies and programs that primarily address trauma (such as a domestic violence shelter) and may provide direct services to clients. Other CHWs work in settings where they rarely if ever address trauma directly with clients.
- The availability of quality services for survivors in the community.
  - When quality services are lacking in the community, or not available in the languages that clients speak, sometimes CHWs feel pressure to exceed their scope of practice. When quality services are accessible to all clients, CHWs and the agencies they work for can develop collaborative relationships and provide referrals to other providers and programs.
- The quality of the supervision you receive. If you work with communities in which trauma is common, you should receive ongoing supervision from a qualified professional who can support you to provide quality services to clients, staying within your scope of practice. Supervision also provides support for identifying and managing signs of secondary trauma and risks for burnout.
- The severity of the client's trauma response, risk behaviors, and level of distress.
  - In general, CHWs will work with survivors who have already made some progress towards establishing safety (see below) and are coping day-to-day with trauma responses. Clients who have recently experienced trauma (or recently started to face a past trauma) and who are experiencing greater distress in terms of emotional, behavioral, or cognitive responses should be referred to work with licensed colleagues and trauma-focused programs.

We encourage you, and the program or agency you work for, to carefully define the limits of your scope of practice for working with survivors of trauma. In what circumstances, and to what extent, are you permitted to address trauma? How and when should you consult with other colleagues, including licensed professionals? What types of referrals sources are you encouraged to share with clients (including those within and outside of the agency you work for)? What professional opportunities exist for you to enhance your knowledge and skills?

- *If you are working as a CHW, where do you fall along the scope of practice spectrum?*

- *To what extent do you address the topic of trauma with the clients and communities you work with?*

- *Do you receive ongoing professional development and supervision related to trauma?*

- *How well is your scope of practice defined by your employer or supervisor?*

Some CHWs Specialize in Addressing Trauma

Throughout the world, some CHWs work very closely with survivors of trauma. They may work with individuals, groups, or at the community level. For example, many rape crisis centers and domestic violence shelters train volunteers and hire nonlicensed staff who provide a wide range of direct services. These CHWs and other unlicensed providers may accompany sexual assault survivors during forensic medical exams at local hospitals, and during criminal or civil court proceedings. They may provide individual peer-counseling, by phone and in person, and cofacilitate support groups with the supervision from a licensed professional. Throughout the world, in situations of armed conflict and civil war, in refugee camps and detention centers, licensed mental health therapists are rare. Often CHWs and other lay or unlicensed leaders and providers are trained to provide support to their community.

SIGNS THAT YOU MAY BE EXCEEDING YOUR SCOPE OF PRACTICE

As we have discussed before, some of the lines between the types of services that lie within and outside of your scope of practice may be a bit fuzzy or unclear. And sometimes, despite your best intentions, you may find yourself in a situation in which you are exceeding or at risk of exceeding your scope of practice. For example, a conversation about trauma may turn into one in which you feel in over your head, or your appropriate use of client-centered concepts and skills (such as Motivational Interviewing) may prompt a client to talk about a trauma experience in depth.

Signs that you may be exceeding your SOP include:

- The client may be highly distressed and unable to contain their thoughts and strong emotions (such as fear or terror, despair, or rage).
- The client may begin to talk about issues properly addressed by well-trained professionals such as:
  - Suicide or revenge.
  - Self-harm including, for example, cutting or self-mutilation.
  - Self-destructive behaviors such as putting themselves at risk for further exposure to trauma.
  - Show signs of another mental health issue or confusing state (thoughts or behaviors that are highly confusing to you and/or the client).
  - Acting out in ways that hurt others.
  - Inability to stay or return to the present, or to shift to a safer and more neutral topic (away from their trauma story). The client may seem "stuck" in the past, in their trauma story and memories.
- You feel overwhelmed, unprepared, uncertain about what to do or say, and worried that you could cause harm to the client.
- The client is asking or pressuring you to exceed your scope of practice by asking for a diagnosis, treatment recommendations, or to talk explicitly and in-depth about trauma experiences that they have not addressed before.

Talk with your supervisor and licensed colleagues to learn more about other possible signs that you could be working beyond your scope of practice.

WHAT TO DO WHEN YOU ARE RISK OF EXCEEDING YOUR SCOPE OF PRACTICE

When in doubt about whether or not you are at risk of exceeding your scope of practice:

- **Focus on the present**: Try to support the client to shift and talk about the present and, if necessary, a different topic. Sometimes shifting physically can be helpful in shifting the client's immediate focus. For example, you may try standing up, sitting in a different location, moving to a different office, or, if possible, taking a walk with the client.
- **Demonstrate respect and kindness**: No matter what you are feeling or thinking, or what the client says or does, continue to demonstrate respect and kindness. Often, this has value in itself in terms of supporting the client's welfare and recovery from trauma.
- **Pause, stop or take a break**.
- **Comment on the process** (see Chapter 9): Speak up to draw the client's attention to the current problem or challenge that is happening in the moment between you. Sometimes naming what is happening—such as that the client's immediate distress or your own concern about scope of practice—can help to interrupt a dynamic that could do harm to the client. It can also be helpful to shift the conversation to the present.
- **Clarify your scope of practice**: Sometimes, it is helpful to clearly state your own limitations as a provider. For example, you may wish to explain that you been trained to support clients with many issues, but that when it comes to trauma experiences, your role is to help clients to connect with a professional who has further training and expertise, so that they can benefit from the best possible support. In general, clients will appreciate your compassion and honesty, and your desire for them to receive quality services.
- **Encourage the client to consider a referral**: Describe local options for therapy, counseling, or other services.

- **Seek help**: Sometimes a qualified colleague may be just a few rooms or minutes away. If necessary, step out of the room for a moment to consult with or ask for the immediate support of a well-trained colleague. With the client's permission, you may be able to bring a qualified colleague into the room or meeting to address the issues that are beyond your scope of practice.

- **End the session**: While it may be uncomfortable, sometimes you may need to interrupt the client, such as when a client is talking about issues that you aren't qualified to address. The risk of causing harm to the client by continuing the conversation may be greater than any risks from ending the session in a clear, kind, and firm manner. When your other attempts to interrupt conversations that stray beyond your scope of practice fail, consider ending the session. You might explain that you have an ethical duty to find a qualified professional to help the client with their current concerns.

> **Anonymous:** I worked as a CHW in a busy primary care clinic. One time, a client told me that she had recently been raped. She broke down sobbing. I reached for tissues and just sat with her. I wasn't sure what to do. I told her how sorry I was to hear that, and she just started to cry even harder. I didn't want to run out of the room right then, but when she was able to catch her breath and talk a bit, I told her that I wanted to bring in a colleague who had training around trauma, and would she agree to meet with someone? She agreed, so I left and returned with a social worker. We sat together and it was really amazing to watch how the social worker was able to talk with the client. I was just so relieved, and I knew that I had done the right thing because of how the client responded. She thanked us both and made an appointment to talk again with social worker later that same week.

WITHIN THE SCOPE OF PRACTICE OF ALL CHWs

We believe that every CHW who has been well-trained in client-centered concepts and skills should be able to provide the following types of services to survivors of trauma:

- Listening with patience and respect (and with Big Eyes, Big Ears, and Small Mouth as discussed in Chapter 7). Sometimes what survivors most need is an opportunity to talk about what they are going through in the company of a caring other. In this way, CHWs bear witness to the client's stories.

- Normalizing the experience of surviving trauma. Survivors often feel isolated and alone, and may believe that their experience is unusual or shameful. By acknowledging that trauma is all too common, CHWs can help to reduce the stigma that some client's face, as well as their sense of being alone.

- Reinforcing the message that help is available and that healing from trauma is possible.

- Providing linkages and referrals to local services. CHWs can support clients to connect with available quality services, including services provided by licensed mental health providers, physicians, and local programs specializing in supporting survivors of violence (including rape crisis centers and domestic violence shelters).

- Accompanying clients (and providing support) as they access new medical, mental health, legal, or other services. Sometimes, at the request of the client, a CHW will go with a client during a first meeting with a local organization such as a rape crisis center or mental health agency.

- Supporting clients to re-establish safety by focusing first on immediate physical and emotional safety, and not rushing to tell the details of their trauma story until they feel ready to do so. CHWs can help clients consider when and how they wish to address their trauma and their healing, and with whom.

- Providing a strength-based approach that highlights the survivor's key strengths and resources for health, coping, and healing.

- Keeping the focus, to the extent possible, on the present, and what the client can do now to cope, seek safety, and find a way forward in their recovery.

> **Inez Love:** I'm the first line of support. In this work, you do some counseling, but it's not the same as therapy. I would advocate and link youth to services to receive therapy, help them navigate the system. I would let them know that I can offer them what I know from my experience and my classes, and let them know that if they want more, I would recommend therapy.

OUTSIDE THE CHW SCOPE OF PRACTICE

The following types of services lie outside of the CHW scope of practice, and should be provided by other professionals with the requisite training and skills:

- Working independently (or on your own) with a trauma survivor without seeking consultation and/or supervision from a well-trained colleague.

- Crossing the line from peer counseling into therapy. Examples may include extensive exploration of the past, in-depth discussion about the details of the trauma experience, or providing interpretation of the meaning of a client's story.

- Guiding the client regarding actions or decisions that they should make in order to promote their healing. Recommending treatments or medications or paths to healing or recovery.

- Addressing issues or challenges for which you have no training and skills.

- Continuing to work with a client who discloses or demonstrates acute symptoms of trauma-related distress. If clients are highly distressed (anxious, scared, angry, etc.) and unable to maintain a calmer state, they should be referred to a qualified professional. If you aren't sure where to refer a client, refer them to a trusted colleague who can, in turn, provide an appropriate referral to a specific provider, program, or agency.

- Continuing to work with clients who indicate that they are acting out in ways that pose risks to their health (or risks to others), such as a client who has suicidal thoughts or is engaged in cutting (cutting their bodies with a razor, knife, or other sharp object), or other risk behaviors.

FACTORS THAT MAY PRESSURE YOU TO EXCEED THE CHW SCOPE OF PRACTICE

There are a range of factors that may influence the decisions you make about your scope of practice. Some of these factors may exert pressure upon you to stray beyond your properly defined scope of practice. Strive to be aware of these factors and how they may influence your practice. Some of these factors include:

- Pressure from the client. Some clients will ask, beg, or pressure you to be the one who acts as a "lead provider" or "counselor" because they have built up a positive connection or trust with you. But you will only erode or damage the quality of this relationship and any trust you have built up by offering services that are beyond your SOP.

- Desire to impress the clients or the community, your colleagues, or others.

- Ego and overconfidence in your skills and abilities.

- Desire to help/rescue/save a client in distress or crisis.

- Desire to grow your skills by experimenting or trying something new.

- Temptation to help clients by offering advice about issues and areas that are outside your scope of practice such as legal and medical questions.

- Mapping your own issues and experience onto the client. Sometimes CHWs may share questions or suggestions with a client that are influenced by the CHWs own experiences with trauma and healing. While these suggestions or advice are motivated by a desire to help, they violate guidelines for client-centered and culturally humble work, and are likely to exceed your scope of practice as well.
  - As addressed elsewhere in the *Foundations* textbook, strive to be aware of how your own experiences, values, and beliefs may unduly influence your work with clients and communities.

- A lack of services for survivors of trauma in the community where you work.
  - Your scope of practice should not be influenced by whether or not local services exist, or whether those services are culturally and linguistically accessible. You have an ethical duty to "do no harm" to the clients and communities you work with.
- Not every client will be interested in or follow up with a referral. Regardless of their decision, this does not alter your scope of practice.

Opportunities for Additional Training

We also encourage you to get as much training as possible about trauma and how to work with trauma survivors. There may be free and low-cost training opportunities in the city and county where you work provided by nonprofit organizations, departments of public health or social services, and at community colleges. For example, City College of San Francisco offers an 18-unit Trauma Recovery and Prevention Certificate. You may also wish to investigate opportunities to be trained by a local suicide prevention hotline, a rape crisis or domestic violence organization. Training generally requires a 6 to 12-month volunteer commitment from you and this, in turn, comes with additional opportunities for training and supervision. The topic of professional development is also addressed further on in this chapter.

18.9 Guidelines for Working with Survivors

In some ways, working with a client to support their recovery from trauma is similar to working with a client to support their self-management of cancer or HIV disease. In all circumstances, you have a limited scope of practice and will work in collaboration with other health care and social services providers. With all clients, you are in a facilitative role, and you will apply skills such as Motivational Interviewing to support the client to identify challenges and strengths, to establish goals and actions to meet those goals. You will support clients to identify and gain access to culturally relevant agencies, programs, and providers, and more.

What may distinguish your work around issues of trauma are your own feelings and beliefs about the issue, heightened concerns about scope of practice, and the need to consult regularly with your supervisor and other colleagues. With more experience working as a CHW, and with survivors of trauma, however, we trust that you will find that the level of knowledge and skills you have to offer are relevant and meaningful to promoting the health and healing of clients.

TO DO AND NOT TO DO

As part of the training that we facilitate at City College of San Francisco, we ask CHWs to brainstorm a list of things to *do* or say when working with a client, and a second list of things that they *don't* want to do or say. The lists are meant to fit with and build upon concepts of client-centered practice. Here is a sample of types of lists that CHWs typically create.

Not to Do

- Judge the client's experience, reactions, or current trauma responses.
- Blame the client for not responding to trauma in a different way (*Why didn't they tell their parents? Why didn't they scream? Why didn't they call the police?*).
- Take away or undermine autonomy and control, such as by directing or telling the client what they should do or think or feel. Helping professionals may do this unintentionally. Keep in mind that a central feature of trauma experiences is a loss of control, and that supporting the client to reclaim control is a key part of their recovery.

CHW

> **Anonymous:** I learned the hard way about giving back to control to clients. I was working with a young woman who had been gang-raped. She was raped and beaten and hurt so bad she was in the hospital for almost a week. Out of a desire to help and perhaps to protect, I gave her too many suggestions about what she "should" do. Finally, she just snapped at me and cussed me out. Thank goodness she did tell me off, because it gave me a chance to apologize, and for us to start a new conversation about how she did want me to support her. She gave me an opportunity to earn some trust back by going more slowly and by trusting that she could figure a lot of things out for herself. She let me know when she wanted my opinion, and I learned how important it is for people that have been hurt to be in control of their own decisions.

- Interrogate the client about their experience by asking too many questions and inquiring about details of the trauma story.

- Make physical contact with the client. Sometimes, people are conditioned to comfort others through touch (such as a touch on the arm or shoulder, or a hug). But unwanted touch may also be part of the trauma experience. Instead of touch, use words, and your client-centered skills to demonstrate and share your unconditional positive regard for the client.

- Try to "rescue" the client. Rescuing may take the form of being directive, or making decisions for the clients, and sometime threatens to violate ethical standards. This often happens when working with youth and others who are particularly vulnerable to harm. The desire to rescue is understandable—it comes from a desire to help. But it can also get in the way of client-centered practice. Be sure to slow down, as necessary, and to let the client guide their own recovery and determine how you may best support them. Reach out for consultation, supervision and assistance from your colleagues.

- Pressure a survivor to report a sexual assault or other crime, or to expect justice from the criminal or civil justice system. This is a decision that only the survivor can make. There is no way to predict how the police may respond, whether or not a District Attorney will decide to prosecute a case, or how the courts will treat the survivor, much less the ultimate outcome of a court case. Sometimes, survivors pin their recovery to the outcome of legal proceedings. Sometimes they agree to testify to please others. Decisions about reporting, filing for a protective order, or participating in a criminal trial are difficult to make, and should be carefully considered by the survivor.

- Let your own experiences and assumptions dominate. Be aware of how your own experiences—including experiences with trauma—may influence your work with clients. For example, helping professionals may guide discussions to address topics or questions that are based on their own experience and needs, rather than on the expressed desire or interest of the client. Try to notice any tendencies for your own issues to influence how you work with a client. Put these aside in the moment and return to tend to them later, on your own time (and not during the client's appointment).

- Tell the client *"I know how you feel."* You don't. You may know how *you felt*, or imagine how *you might feel*, but this is very different from knowing how the client feels. Even if you experienced a similar trauma, remember that how people respond to trauma is unique and subjective. Telling a client how they feel may engender feelings of anger and undermine rather than build trust and rapport.

- Focus on a particular aspect of a trauma event or story. For various reasons, helping professionals may sometimes want to know about a particular part of the client's experience. For example, with a survivor of sexual assault, providers may inquire about the sexual aspects of the story. This is an unintentional way of taking control away from, and may feel like a type of manipulation.

- Promise more than you can do. Promises create expectations, and when you fail to deliver or follow through, you are likely to undermine trust and rapport with the client.

To Do

- Be aware of your own tendencies for denial. We sometimes doubt trauma stories, perhaps because we don't want to believe that such horrific things truly happen, or we don't want to consider that they could also happen to us or our loved ones. If it is difficult for you to stay present and to focus on the client's story, this may be a sign that you require additional training about trauma (and/or time for your own healing).

- Listen. Listening is sometimes more difficult than it seems. It can be difficult to do well, especially if what the client has to tell you is disturbing or horrifying, or similar to something that you or a loved one has experienced. Breathe and lean in to the client's story. Don't worry about what you will say next. *Know that the act of listening and trying to really hear what a survivor is telling you can, in itself, support their healing.*

Listening Can Be Hard to Do

Tim Berthold: The first day I was in training to become a certified sexual assault counselor, I was asked to participate in a role play. Because we were being trained to do phone counseling on a rape crisis hotline, we did our role plays seated back to back (so that we couldn't see each other). My role was to play the counselor, and my fellow volunteer was given a role play script about a client who had recently been assaulted. As the role play began, I kind of blanked out. The story of the caller was so similar to something that had happened to one of my family members. I interrupted the caller to ask questions that were really about my family member's experience ("Is he still in the house?" "Can you get out of the house?" "You can call 911?").

It was a bit embarrassing, but a great training lesson. I learned how my own issues can get in the way and keep me from focusing and truly hearing the experience of a client. This topic became an area of focus for me, and for the training group that I was a part of: How can we push aside in the moment (but not forget about) our own concerns so that we can be present to witness the story of another?

- Learn to be comfortable with silence. Let the client take the time they need to reflect, to feel, and to consider what they want to say.

- Use your OARS and other Motivational Interviewing skills (see Chapter 9). Ask open-ended questions and demonstrate reflective listening to provide clients with the opportunity to reflect upon and express their experience, feelings, and values (*while keeping your scope of practice in mind!*). Provide authentic affirmations, sparingly, to support clients to recognize their own strengths and accomplishments. Summarize key messages shared by the client, and any plans or agreements that you make.

- Let the client guide the pace, focus and manner of telling their story. Be gentle in inquiring about the client's experience and responses. Let them guide the discussion and determine what they wish you talk about, when and how.

- Encourage clients to consider working with licensed professionals who have advanced training in trauma and recovery. Explain the limits of your scope of practice, and why it is important for survivors of trauma to work closely with a trained professional who has expertise in this topic.

- If you make a mistake (and all service providers make mistakes), apologize. Let the client know that you are sorry if you did or said something that was unintentionally hurtful. This may be particularly important for a survivor who was harmed by another person, perhaps someone they knew or loved who has not acknowledged or taken responsibility for what they did. Providing a sincere apology often helps to restore and enhance the professional connection or rapport between CHWs and clients.

- There may be times to share specific messages with a client, such as:
  - It is not your fault. Many survivors, including survivors of childhood abuse and neglect, and survivors and witnesses of domestic violence, believe that they are at fault. Many were told that they caused the

trauma. Depending upon the circumstances and the survivor, it may be helpful for them to hear that you don't believe that it is their fault. They may need to hear this more than once. Hearing it from others may help them to internalize this message in time.

○ I will be here for you. Some survivors have been told not to talk about the trauma events or to put it behind them. They may feel embarrassed or ashamed, and they may worry that you will be harmed if you hear what they survived, or that you may reject them. It may be helpful for you to let the client know that you are grateful that they disclosed their story to you, and that you want to do your very best to support their healing and recovery.

- Practice self care. Whether you are a survivor or not, working with survivors can be stressful, and it can lead to secondary trauma (discussed below). Enhance your skills for self care and put them into practice each day. Reach out to others—including family, friends, colleagues, and professionals—as needed, for support. If you are a survivor, watch for signs that your own trauma responses are returning or increasing, and continue to do your own healing.

THE MOMENT WHEN A CLIENT FIRST TELLS YOU ABOUT TRAUMA

Some of the clients you work with who have experienced trauma will decide to talk with you about these experiences. Stop to consider the moment when a client tells you that he or she is a survivor of trauma.

- What may be at stake for the client?
- What concerns may they have?
- What hopes may they have?
- What coping skills or strengths have they already demonstrated?
- What are your primary goals in this moment?
- Are you grounded and prepared to assist the client in this moment?
- How do you want to respond?
- How will you stay within your scope of practice?

Some clients may be accustomed to talking about their trauma experiences and responses. They may have talked about their trauma experiences many times, to many people, and have made significant progress in their healing. Other survivors, however, may have kept their trauma stories hidden. They may not have told anyone before. Or they may have told someone who did not respond in a supportive or helpful manner, and who encouraged the survivor to keep it to themselves or put it behind them.

Keep in mind that some survivors may feel nervous about telling you—or anyone—about their trauma experience, and may be fearful of how you may react (Will you believe them? Will you blame them? Will you view them or treat them differently?). Others may be terrified of confronting their own experiences in a new way, by voicing them out loud in the presence of a witness.

How others respond when survivors disclose a history of trauma can have a significant impact on their healing and welfare. Imagine, for example, a survivor who tells a family member about their trauma, and that family member doesn't believe them, or blames them in some way, or responds in a way that enhances their embarrassment or shame. In contrast, if survivors are met with patience and respect when they disclose, this can support them in taking action towards healing or recovery.

Suggestions for how to respond when a client first tells you that he or she is a survivor include:

- Respond in a calm and patient manner
- Express or demonstrate your compassion and concern for the welfare of the client
- Assess physical and emotional safety (addressed in greater detail later in this chapter)
- Follow the lead of the client. If they indicate that they don't want to talk further, or talk about a particular question or topic, accept this decision.

CASE STUDY Nadia (*continued*)

This is the second meeting between Nadia and the CHW. During the first meeting the CHW reviewed the confidentiality policy in place at the Women's Clinic.

Nadia: So, I don't know how to say this, but . . . (Nadia pauses)

CHW: (Listens and waits patiently)

Nadia: I was raped in Iraq by . . . by another soldier. It happened over and over. I was too afraid to tell. (Nadia starts to shake and puts her head down)

CHW: Oh, Nadia, I'm so sorry to know that you were raped.

Nadia: (Nadia's head is still down) I just, . . . I don't know why I'm telling you now. I don't know why I didn't tell anyone before . . . (pauses)

CHW: I'm here, Nadia, I'm listening.

Nadia: The man who raped me . . . he told me I was a whore and no one would believe me. I saw what happened to other women who reported so I . . . (starts to cry), I just kept it inside. I couldn't even tell my mother. She was so proud of me for serving our country, and my brother was still in the army, and I just couldn't tell her. I just . . . I mean, what am I supposed to do now?

CHW: Nadia, the Women's Clinic is a place to find support for what you've gone though, and for figuring out how to move forward in your life.

Nadia: (Looks up and nods her agreement. She reaches for a tissue and blows her nose.) Okay.

CHW: I imagine it might have taken a lot for you to decide to tell me about the rape today.

Nadia: I tried *so many times* to say something to somebody, but . . . I just couldn't. I didn't know how to begin. (Nadia bows her head, thinking . . .)

CHW: Well, I think you did a great job of beginning today. (Nadia smiles) What motivated you to talk about it today?

Nadia: I wasn't planning on it, but . . . I just can't get past what happened. I've been having these horrible dreams, sometimes over and over, and (pauses), I think maybe this is why I broke up with my boyfriend, and well, then I messed up at work and they fired me and . . . I guess I just tried to put everything that happened behind me but, um, it just keeps . . . I just can't get over it, and . . . I guess I need help because I don't know what I'm supposed to do. (Nadia looks up)

CHW: (nods and establishes eye contact with Nadia). You've been going through a lot, Nadia. And you have time to figure out what you want to do. We have a team of wonderful social workers here who have a lot of experience helping women who have been raped and who have survived other kinds of trauma. Would you consider meeting with one of the social workers to talk more about what you want to do and how you can heal from what was done to you?

Nadia: Yes (nods and cries and reaches for more tissues). Yes, I think it would be good to do that. I don't usually cry so much.

CHW: Well, that is why we have the tissues here (Nadia smiles). This is a good place to cry. (waits patiently)

Nadia: Thank you for listening to me . . . .

CHW: I am so glad Nina that you took a risk to reach out to me today.

Nadia (cries and nods) Thank you. I know I have some big decisions to make but I just feel like . . . I did it, you know? Finally, I said it out loud.

Topics that you *may* wish to explore with a new client (always with their consent, and in a manner that is consistent with your scope of practice within the agency where you work) include:

- Are they open to seeking support and services from a qualified professional?
- What skills and resources do they have that can help them to cope with or heal from trauma?
- How can you best support them? What are their key priorities?
- What is it like to be talking about the trauma now, in this moment?

HOW TO PROVIDE A REFERRAL

How you provide a referral is sometimes just as important as the quality of the referral. Referrals should be offered in a way that encourages the client to consider the value of the resource, while supporting their autonomy and maintaining a positive rapport or professional connection (for more information about providing referrals, see Chapter 10).

Sometimes, when a CHW provides a referral to another provider—such as a social worker or psychologist with expertise in the field of trauma—a client may feel as if you are saying (unintentionally): *"Now that you have told me _____ [about the trauma], I can't work with you anymore. Go somewhere else because I don't want to listen to these horrible things. You shouldn't have told me."* It can feed into a survivor's shame or embarrassment about their trauma story and, unintentionally, harm rapport and erode trust. It may also make the survivor more reluctant to disclose their trauma story to another.

We encourage you take extra time when providing a referral related to the topic of trauma, especially if you haven't worked with the client for very long. Explain why you are providing the referral, and how it may benefit the client. You may also wish to explain that you have a more limited scope of practice and, when it comes to the topics of trauma and counseling, you have an obligation to refer clients to opportunities to work with highly trained professionals. Finally, to the extent that you are able and willing to continue to play a role in supporting the client's health, reinforce your interest in doing so.

CASE STUDY   **Nadia** *(continued)*

CHW: Nadia, my job is to support clients to get healthier, and this means connecting you with opportunities to work with professionals who have the most training and skills for working with survivors of rape and other kinds of trauma. I have some knowledge and experience, but I am not qualified to serve as your primary support in healing from trauma.

Are you open to considering referrals to some local programs and counselors that work with survivors? If you did decide to work with one of these counselors, I could also continue to meet with you when you come to the health center. What are your thoughts about this?

Nadia: I guess so, I mean that makes sense to me. Could you continue to meet with me at least until I find someone that . . . Someone I feel good about?

CHW: Absolutely, I'd like that Nadia.

Nadia (smiles)

CHW: I will do my best to help you find a qualified counselor, someone who you feel good about working with. I have a couple of people in mind who are really great and who have a lot of experience supporting survivors of trauma.

Nadia: Okay, but I've never gone to a counselor before so, . . . I mean what is supposed to happen there?

CHW: Well, let's talk a little more about that . . .

Identifying Local Services for Survivors of Trauma

Work with your colleagues to research and develop a list of the best local services for survivors of trauma. Identify agency and practitioners that provide services in the community. What type of services do they provide? What level of training have they received? What is the cost of services, and what type of insurance may cover these costs? What languages do the providers speak? Finally, are there any eligibility requirements for clients?

ESTABLISHING SAFETY

Establishing safety is often the first step toward healing or recovery, and towards restoring a sense of control that the trauma may have stripped from the survivor (Herman, 1997; Mendelsohn et al., 2011). Safety is an inclusive concept that includes both physical and emotional safety. It may begin with gaining greater control and comfort with physical sensations and dynamics such as sleeping and eating, and coping with responses and behaviors that may put the survivor at risk. A next stage may focus on the survivor's living environment and establishing safe and stable housing and income. After these first stages of safety have been achieved, survivors can begin to address their trauma story more directly, and to focus on remembrance, integration, and mourning (Mendelsohn et al., 2011).

Not every client is ready to talk about their trauma experiences or to engage in more active forms of treatment, such as counseling. Doing so may result in increased stress, heightened symptoms (or responses) and risks. You don't want to inadvertently cause harm to a client. So, just as you would with many other clients, start by talking about more basic issues of safety and survival.

If the client demonstrates great anxiety, stress, fear or concern:

- Don't continue to engage in dialogue about their trauma story
- Provide a referral to a licensed colleague or community-based provider
- Consult with your supervisor and/or clinical team

Please note that safety is also established by assessing for the risk of suicide as described later in this chapter.

CASE STUDY   Nadia (*continued*)

It may take time for Nadia to build a foundation of safety because of her history of broken trust with the military. Talk directly with Nadia about safety and stability. Explain that it is often important for survivors to address basic issues of physical safety and stability before they begin to talk about their trauma experiences. Help Nadia to consider whether or not she is in a place in her life to begin addressing in a direct way what happened to her in Iraq. In this case study, while Nadia continues to experience common trauma symptoms including nightmares and recently lost her job, she does have a stable place to live and a growing interest in talking about what happened to her in Iraq.

The next phase is to support clients like Nadia to make informed decisions about which aspects of their trauma story they will decide to talk about, with whom, when, and how.

CHW: So Nadia, you're thinking about scheduling a time to meet with the social worker, Ms. Olivera?

Nadia: Yes, I called her and she said that we could have a first meeting, and that she could tell me about how she works with people, you know, how she does her counseling. Then I can decide if I want to work with her or not.

CHW: So, how does that sound to you?

(continues)

| CASE STUDY | Nadia *(continued)* |

Nadia: She seems really nice, and I like that I don't have to start out by telling her all about what happened. I feel kind of nervous because I just don't know what she is going to ask me, or what I am ready to . . . to talk about.

CHW: You aren't sure what you want to share with her . . .

Nadia: (nods) I don't know how I feel about talking about everything, and if I'm ready to talk about everything that happened.

CHW: Nadia, one thing I've learned about trauma is that it is really important for survivors to be in charge of their own healing, and to be the one who makes the decisions about what you talk about and when, as well as who you decide to talk with.

Sometimes, it is a good idea to back up and to consider what it would be like to start talking about trauma *before* you actually start to talk about the trauma. Does this make sense to you?

Nadia: Yes, it is helpful because, um, I was worried that someone might expect me to talk about certain things that he did to me and . . . maybe I just don't' want to talk about them.

CHW: So I think it's a great idea to consider what parts of your experience you would feel ready to talk about with Ms. Olivera, and what parts you don't want to talk about right then or ever. (Nadia nods) It might also be a good idea to figure out how you would tell her that you don't want to talk about something.

Nadia: I guess I could just say I'm not ready to talk about that part yet . . .

CHW: Good, that is really clear and helpful to the counselor too, to set your boundaries about what you do and don't talk about together. And, of course, you know that the same thing goes for me too, right? You decide what we talk about too!

Nadia: (smiles) Yes, I feel comfortable talking with you, and you haven't pressured me to talk about anything I don't want to . . .

CHW: So do you have a good idea about what you feel ready to talk about with Ms. Olivera?

Nadia: You are the only person I've told so far . . . that I was raped. I almost told the doctor when she examined me for STIs, but I didn't. And I haven't really told you a lot about what happened, right? (CHW nods) I think I need to think about this some more.

CHW: Nadia, are you someone who likes to write things down? (Nadia nods) Would writing about this be helpful to you at all in terms of figuring out some of your next steps?

Nadia: It's funny because, I wrote a letter to my mom, but I never sent it. I just kind of keep rewriting it. It is about . . . (Nadia cries) It is about what happened and I was trying to figure out how to tell her but now . . . I don't think it is really a letter anymore, it is, it is just something for me.

CHW: Do you think this letter could be helpful in figuring out what you want to say when you are meeting with Ms. Olivera?

Nadia: Well, I'm not sure. I'm going to read through the letter again. It might be different with the counselor than with my mother, but I think that writing things down, just even a little bit, could help . . .

CHW: You can also have this same kind of talk with Ms. Olivera. If it seems like a good idea, you could always start out by telling her that you are still figuring out what you want to talk about—and what you don't want to talk about—in counseling.

Nadia: That makes me feel so much less nervous. This . . . this helps me feel more ready to meet with her. I think that if I like the counselor, than I will be able to figure this out and, like you said, kind of go at my own pace.

Facilitating the End of a Meeting with a Client

Related to the topic of establishing safety, is the question of how you end a meeting or conversation about trauma with a client. You don't want to suddenly end an appointment in the middle of an important or challenging discussion, or when the client is feeling highly emotional or distressed. As discussed in Chapter 10, you have the responsibility of time management and for helping the client to anticipate the end of an appointment or meeting. For example, you might find a way to interrupt a conversation to tell the client that there are just 10 minutes left for your meeting ("I'm sorry to interrupt, but we only have about 10 minutes left and I want to make sure that we make time for . . ."). This is an opportunity to schedule a follow-up appointment and to support the client to transition from the meeting to the next agenda in their day. For example, you might ask them what they will do after the appointment. If they are facing challenges or having a difficult day, ask them to consider what they can do to take care of themselves. This is an opportunity to help clients to enhance their stress management and self care skills, and to put them into practice when they are most needed.

ACTION PLANNING

The concepts that guide you in supporting a client to establish an action plan for managing diabetes or depression are the same for working with a survivor of trauma (see Chapters 10 and 16 for more information about action plans). Assist the client to establish clear goals for their healing or recovery. With survivors of trauma, it may be helpful for them to articulate their long-term goal, and then to select a more near-term goal, something that they may be able to achieve in the next three to six months. Next, ask them to identify a series of steps or actions that they are ready to take to help them reach their goals.

Ask clients to anticipate what challenges they may face in implementing their plan, and how it may feel to achieve or not to achieve their goals. Identifying and discussing challenges may also help to normalize the complex process of recovering from trauma, which seldom happens in a clear and straightforward path.

CASE STUDY   Nadia (continued)

Since Nadia first met with the CHW, she has started working with Ms. Olivera, a social worker at the Women's Clinic, and a colleague of the CHW's. Nadia talked with Ms. Olivera about her wish to receive additional support from the CHW. Nadia, the CHW, and Ms. Olivera have all signed a release form permitting them to talk together. They agreed that the CHW would help Nadia in refining her initial action plan.

CHW: So Nadia, I'm really happy to learn that you feel good about the connection you are building with Ms. Olivera.

Nadia: Yes, I am so glad you recommended her. She really is great. But I'm glad that I can talk with you, too, because you were the first person I told, and I feel . . . I guess after being alone for so long it is good to connect with more people.

CHW: I'm happy that we can continue to work together! So, Ms. Olivera is going to be your counselor, and I am going to support you with some of the other priorities that you mentioned, like employment and housing, right?

Nadia: Yes, that will be really helpful.

(continues)

CASE STUDY | **Nadia** (*continued*)

CHW: Ms. Olivera also asked me to help you out with creating an action plan. (Nadia nods.) Did you have a chance to talk about what an action plan is?

Nadia: Yeah, I think that it is kind of like a map for where I want to go and what I want to achieve.

CHW: Yes, I like that image of the map. We encourage clients to develop maps with big goals for their life, as well as things that they can achieve more quickly. An action plan is focused on identifying a goal and practical steps or actions that you can take to reach that goal in the next three to six months. Have you started to think about what your goals are and where you want to go on your map?

Nadia: Yeah, I have been thinking more and more about this, and it's really good just to even be thinking about the future, you know, and what I really want. . . . I've talked about it some with you and with Ms. Olivera. I don't want to feel so scared anymore, and I want to start being able to trust and connect with people. And I want to be more independent. I need a job, a better job, you know, because I want to be able to afford my own place. Is that too much?

CHW: It is a really wonderful and specific list of goals (Nadia smiles). But I'm wondering what you might establish for your action plan goals. Something that you can work towards achieving in the next 3–6 months.

Nadia: Okay, that makes sense. I guess I have to start somewhere, right?

CHW: You've already started, right? You came to the clinic, you talked with me and . . .

Nadia: And now I'm working with Ms. Olivera, so, yes, I have started. (Nadia laughs.) I am already moving across my map. I'm just not sure what the . . . the destination is yet.

CHW: And your destination may change over time. For today, let's focus on one goal.

Nadia: Okay, I know that you are going to work with me on getting a job, and maybe going back to school, right?

CHW: Yes, we can continue to work toward that together.

Nadia: So maybe I could work on trying to keep building trust with people again. I'm doing that here, but I've also been thinking about the women's groups that you mentioned. Maybe I could try going to the support group thing.

CHW: Okay, that sounds like a great goal for your action plan. What are you hoping for in terms of participating in the support group?

Nadia: I want to meet some other women who have gone through similar things. And just hearing, you know, how it affected them, and . . . and trying to support each other to get . . . (pauses), stronger and just . . . better. I think it would be helpful for me right now to not be so alone with everything that happened.

CHW: I think that what you are hoping for is a good fit with what support groups are for. Have you thought about what could be challenging about participating in a support group?

Nadia: Well, I guess that, even though I want to, I still have problems trusting people. That thing that I told you about, that dinner thing that I went to for local vets—where that guy harassed me? That was so horrible. But I think a group with just women will be better. But what if I don't get along with the other women? I don't know, I guess a lot of things could happen.

CHW: Facing your trauma and finding a way forward, it does involve risks. Like we talked about before, it can also be helpful to try to anticipate these risks, and to make careful choices about them. (Nadia nods.) I am wondering if it would help you to split this goal up even further. Like, for example, what is a first step that you could take before participating in a group session?

CASE STUDY   Nadia (continued)

Nadia: Well, I guess I can find out more information about it? I mean I don't know, what they actually do or talk about, and are there other women who . . . who went through something like me?

CHW: So, for example, before you go to a support group, maybe you could find out more about it, and even meet with one of the facilitators?

Nadia: Yes, I think that would be good, kind of like how I met with Ms. Olivera before we started the counseling. And that doesn't feel as difficult, you know, in terms of a next step. I'm still moving forward on my map, but I'm taking it slow.

CHW: What questions would you want to ask the facilitator of the group? What would you want to learn?

Nadia: I don't know. . . . I guess, I want to know what actually happens in the group, like, what they talk about and, well, how does it help the women to get better. I'd also want to know if I need to talk about everything that happened to me. I know I would be going to talk about it, but I wouldn't want to feel any pressure.

CHW: Those sound like great questions to me. I think you have a really clear idea about what you want to learn about the group before you decide whether to participate or not. Would it be helpful to write these questions down?

Nadia: Yes (takes out notebook and pen), yes, I might be nervous, so . . . I don't want to forget.

(Nadia writes. The CHW waits.)

CHW: Nadia, do you have the name and phone number of the counselor who runs the group?

Nadia: Yes, I've got the card here, from before (looks for and finds the card). Yes, Ms. Sasaki, I've got it.

CHW: Okay, so I think you've made great progress already. How prepared do you feel, on a scale of 0–10 to set up a time to talk with Ms. Sasaki?

Nadia: I guess, um, I think right now it is a 9, but, I worry that it might be a 0 by the time I get ready to call . . .

CHW: It is natural that your level of confidence might change a lot when you are thinking about taking a big step. And whether you make the call or don't, or go to the group or not, I think it is great that you are considering different options for how to move forward in your healing, in taking care of yourself. Can I check in with you about this over the next week?

Nadia: Yes, next week sounds good.

CHW: Nadia, do see the progress you've already made since that day when you first talked with me?

Nadia: Yes . . . (pauses). I do see that I am moving forward. But I also see how much further I want to go.

As long as you continue to work with the client, check-in with them about their progress in implementing their action plan. Continue to normalize the challenge of recovery. Be open to the client's need or desire to question or change their plan. And remember to roll with resistance rather than digging in to lecture or try to persuade the client to stick to any aspect of their plan (see Chapter 9). Be sure to notice and reflect back the client's accomplishments—big or small—as they move forward. Remember that they may have a harder time noticing or taking credit for these accomplishments and, a growing awareness of their strengths will help them to gain confidence and a greater sense of self-determination.

How Trauma May Influence Action Planning and Behavior Change

Anyone who is attempting to change health-related behaviors may experience ambivalence and self-doubt. However, these challenges may be even more pronounced among survivors of trauma. Survivors may fluctuate back and forth among different emotions and states of readiness, and their efforts to achieve change may be complicated by trauma responses such as fear, anxiety, numbness, guilt, shame, and isolation. Remain patient, and keep in mind that neither behavior change nor recovery from trauma typically happen in a linear way from Step 1 to Step 2 and so on. As discussed in Chapters 7 and 9, the process of behavior change often includes ambivalence, doubts, relapse to prior patterns of behavior, and the need to revisit and revise action plans.

ANTICIPATING CONSEQUENCES

It can be helpful to ask clients to consider the possible consequences of their plans and decisions. It may be particularly important to do so when you are working with a survivor of trauma who is contemplating decisions that may have a significant impact on their health and relationships, such as:

- Whether to disclose or tell someone else about their trauma experience
- Whether to report an assault or other type of harm to a third party such as an employer or the police
- Whether to provide testimony in a criminal or civil court case
- Whether to "confront" someone who harmed them, such as a parent who neglected or abused them
- Whether to make a significant life change such as ending or beginning a relationship or job or moving to a new city or state

Sometimes trauma survivors rush into big decisions related to their recovery. They may be influenced by friends or families, or assumptions about what they "should do." *As a CHW, your role isn't to tell a client what to do, but to support them to carefully consider key decisions, possible consequences, and the impact on their recovery and health.*

CASE STUDY   Nadia (continued)

Nadia has been thinking about telling her parents that she was raped. She talked about this decision with Ms. Olivera, the social worker, and agreed to talk about it with the CHW as well. Ms. Olivera asked the CHW to support Nadia in thinking through her goals for talking with her parents, and the possible consequences.

CHW: Nadia, can you tell me more about the decision to tell your parents about the rape? What are you hoping will happen?

Nadia: Well, I guess I just want them to believe me, and to understand that I didn't do anything wrong. And I just don't want to hide this from them any more.

CHW: How do you think they will respond?

Nadia: Well . . . (Nadia pauses). I don't want to upset them, especially because my brother Sergei is still in Afghanistan and . . . I guess I don't think they will respond very well right away. They tend to kind of, um, get dramatic, you know? But I know that they love me, and . . . I guess I'm more worried about my dad. I think it will take him longer to accept.

CHW: So are you thinking about talking to both of your parents at the same time?

(continues)

| CASE STUDY | Nadia *(continued)* |

Nadia: Maybe I should start with my mom. She will probably tell my father, but she . . . she knows how to talk to him better than me, so maybe .... I don't have to be there when she tells him.

CHW: So your mom may be helpful in talking with your dad.

Nadia: I think so. She does this all the time, like when I decided to go into the military. He didn't want me to do it at first.

CHW: What might it be like if you don't get the response you are hoping for—right away or from both of your parents? How do you think this could impact your healing?

Nadia: Oh (cries) It would be a big disappointment, and I think . . . I would be so angry with them too—I *need* their support! But, I know that I would be okay, eventually, because, um, I've managed a lot of . . . disappointment, right? But maybe I don't need to tell them right away.

CHW: So how they respond is important to you, and you might not tell them right away.

Nadia: Yes, it is important, and I really want . . . I just want them to know that I didn't do *anything* wrong to make this happen. And I want them to know that I'm trying now, you know, to get better. But . . . I think maybe I need some more time to think about this and to figure out what to say to my mom.

CHW: If it would be helpful to you, you could practice with Ms. Olivera what you want to say to your mom . . . It might help you to figure out how you want to express yourself, and to anticipate a bit more what it might be like.

Nadia: Okay, . . . I think that could be good to figure out what I am going to say, and it will help to make it more . . . real.

18.10 Screening a Client for the Risk of Suicide

You are likely to work with clients who have thoughts or wishes about death. You may also work with clients who are suicidal and have a plan and the intention to kill themselves.

Many CHWs and other unlicensed direct service providers are trained to assess a client's potential risk for suicide, and to consult immediately with a licensed colleague and/or make a report to a third party such as the police. We will provide guidelines for assessing a client's risk for suicide (sometimes called a lethality assessment) in this section. *However, once you are working in the field, please ask your supervisor for additional training, and for your agency's policies and protocols for screening and reporting the risk of suicide.* Some employers provide training and support for CHWs to take an active role in suicide prevention and assessment, and others do not.

The risk of suicide (like the risk of child abuse or elder abuse) is not something that a CHW can keep secret. It is important for the CHW to notify all clients about the limits on confidentiality agreements, including the requirement to report any active suicidal intent on the part of the client. Confidentiality and its limits are discussed in Chapters 7 and 8 of *Foundations*, along with suggestions for how to discuss this topic with a client.

THE RISK OF SUICIDE

Suicide is not as rare as many people think. It was the 10th leading cause of death in the United States in 2010, with an estimated 38,364 suicides. Approximately 3.75 percent of adults have suicidal thoughts annually, and one million report attempting suicide. Suicide rates are higher among the elderly, youth, and young adults (suicide is the third leading cause of death among youth ages 10–24), including lesbian, gay, bisexual, and transgender youth, males (though females have more suicidal thoughts), and veterans (CDC, 2012; VA, 2014c).

Warning Signs

Some people who commit suicide do so without ever talking about it. While it can be difficult to determine if someone is suicidal, research has identified several common warning signs that may indicate an increased risk for attempting suicide. The federal Substance Abuse and Mental Health Administration (SAMHSA) provides the following information about warning signs (SAMHSA, 2014c):

> *These signs may mean that someone is at risk for suicide. Risk is greater if the behavior is new, or has increased, and if it seems related to a painful event, loss, or change:*
>
> - *Talking about wanting to die or kill oneself*
>
> - *Looking for a way to kill oneself*
>
> - *Talking about feeling hopeless or having no reason to live*
>
> - *Talking about feeling trapped or being in unbearable pain*
>
> - *Talking about being a burden to others*
>
> - *Increasing the use of alcohol or drugs*
>
> - *Acting anxious or agitated; behaving recklessly*
>
> - *Sleeping too little or too much*
>
> - *Withdrawing or feeling isolated*
>
> - *Showing rage or talking about seeking revenge*
>
> - *Displaying extreme mood swings*

To read more about suicide, please refer to the resources included at the end of this chapter, including a free online training from SAMHSA's Suicide Prevention Resource Center.

Conducting a Lethality Screening

When helping professionals suspect that a client may be at risk for suicide, they conduct what is called a lethality assessment to try to assess this risk and take appropriate action.

Keep in mind that, for many survivors, thoughts of death are very common. Trauma, after all, is characterized by a threat of death or annihilation, so thoughts and dreams (or nightmares) about death are fairly common. The challenge is to be able to distinguish between these common passive thoughts of death and an intention to kill oneself. Suicidality is not having a dream that you die, or wishing or fantasizing about death. Suicidality is defined is having a desire and a specific plan to kill yourself, including the means or method (such as poison, pills, or a gun, or a plan to drown, etc.).

SAMHSA (2014c) emphasizes that "everyone has a role in preventing suicide." They provide the following common guidelines:

What You Can Do

- If you believe someone may be thinking about suicide:
  - Ask them if they are thinking about killing themselves. (This will not put the idea into their head or make it more likely that they will attempt suicide.)
  - Listen without judging and show you care.
  - Stay with the person (or make sure the person is in a private, secure place with another caring person) until you can get further help.
  - Remove any objects that could be used in a suicide attempt.
  - Call SAMHSA's National Suicide Prevention Lifeline at 1-800-273-TALK (8255) and follow their guidance.
  - If danger for self-harm seems imminent, call 911.

The key to screening a client for the risk of suicide is to speak directly and in plain language. Ask them if they have any plans to kill themselves or commit suicide (don't use vague language like "Are you planning to hurt yourself?"). You may also explain why you are asking these questions, emphasizing your concern for the client's safety and welfare. If a client tells you that they plan to kill themselves, ask them how and when they plan to kill themselves. The risk for suicide is higher if the client has a specific plan in mind.

CASE STUDY Nadia *(continued)*

CHW: Nadia, our protocol here at the Women's Clinic, when we work with a client who tells us that they have been raped or otherwise hurt, is to ask them about suicide. Can you tell me if you have had any thoughts of hurting or killing yourself?

Nadia: Well, sometimes I have dreams, you know, that I had been killed instead of friends who died in Iraq. But, this is more kind of like wishes than anything, really.

CHW: So you haven't had thoughts of killing yourself?

Nadia: No, nothing like that.

CHW: Have you ever tried to kill yourself before?

Nadia: I thought about it before, right after I got back from my tour of duty. When I was really thinking about the rape, and feeling like . . . , like crap, and not sure that I would ever feel any different. But it was more a wish that someone or something else would kill me because I was so lost and in so much pain. I never tried to kill myself or anything like that.

CHW: The reason we ask is to try to prevent harm, and to protect your safety. And this topic of suicide is something that other providers may also ask you, like your doctor, so I want you to be prepared and to try to understand why we will bring up this topic.

Nadia: I understand. They asked in the army too, and the VA when I got out.

CHW: If you did start to feel suicidal, is there someone who you think you would talk to about this?

Nadia: I don't know. I guess what I can say is that If I started to feel that way I would do my best to call Ms. Olivera or you. I don't want to kill myself. I want to figure this out. I need to be here for my family.

If a client tells you they intend to kill herself or himself, you have a legal and ethical duty to report it immediately. **Contact your supervisor—or any available licensed colleague or supervisor—right away.** For example, if you are in the office, clinic or hospital, ask for a supervisor to join you and the client, and clearly explain that it is an urgent situation. When the supervisor arrives, let them take the lead in assessing the client and determining what further actions may be necessary. If a licensed colleague is not available, call 911 and inform the dispatcher that you are with a client who is suicidal and request immediate assistance. The 911 dispatcher will send an Emergency Responder (such as paramedics or the police) to assess the client further. If the Emergency Responder finds an immediate threat of suicide, they will transport the client to a local hospital for further assessment. The client may be held in a locked ward for several days (typically up to 72 hours) and closely monitored to prevent harm.

In these situations, a client will sometimes beg you not to call a supervisor or 911. They may be highly emotional and possibly very angry with you. Keep in mind that—regardless of what the client wants in this situation—if they have disclosed that they are suicidal, you have to make a report, and to do so right away.

Remember to document the incident as thoroughly and soon as possible. Write down the date, time, and location of your interaction with the client, what they reported to you, and the actions that you took, and the names of any other professionals or agencies involved.

Juanita Alvarado: I had a client who had recently been released from prison and he was utilizing all of the CHW services. He had a lot of mental health issues and was receiving medication from the Primary Care doctor here at Transitions. He tested dirty [a test indicated that he was using drugs] and was denied pain medications. He was very upset and was determined to jump in front of the T train. I stood by him, I calmed him down and just listened to him, I didn't care how long it was going to take. Just really listening to him, talking positive to him and what he had to look forward to instead of focusing on the pain meds and how he could get back on them. I tried to reassure him that not everyone is going to look at him like a liar and gave him a lot of positive reinforcement. After two hours he was able to calm down. I got him something to eat and I took him to Bayview Mental Health where a mental health provider evaluated him further. He didn't kill himself and I felt like I did what I could to prevent that.

18.11 Facilitating Groups with Trauma Survivors

CHWs work with groups in various ways. You may facilitate a support group for survivors of trauma, organize activities for youth affected by violence, or conduct an educational workshop in the community. Group work is especially powerful for trauma survivors, because it breaks down the isolation and the shame that is often associated with traumatic events. In a group setting, participants learn as much from one another as they do from the group leader. In this section, we offer suggestions for how to support safety and healing for trauma survivors when working with groups. You will also find more information on working with groups in Chapter 21.

Group facilitation, Scope of Practice, and Supervision

Group facilitation is a distinct skill that requires additional training and close supervision. Before cofacilitating a support group that addresses issues of trauma and recovery, seek out additional training from your employer or other local agencies or programs. Develop a detailed plan with your supervisor and cofacilitator for how to address the inevitable challenges that arise when doing group work. If possible, seek out opportunities to cofacilitate with an experienced colleague who can mentor you along the way.

As always, keep your scope of practice in mind, and seek consultation in a timely fashion. Finally, if you are facilitating or cofacilitating a group, you should receive ongoing supervision from a qualified professional. Supervision serves several key purposes. It enhances your knowledge and skills for facilitating a safe and supportive group, and assists you to develop strategies for responding to and managing specific challenges that may arise in any group. Supervision also provides a structured opportunity for you to identify and reflect upon personal issues that may arise in the course of the work, and to continue to enhance your own resiliency, self care, or healing.

It is important to be aware of the cultural traditions and beliefs of the clients or communities you serve and how they may affect participation in a group. Don't make assumptions, but do inquire, acknowledge, and allow for cultural concerns that might shape the composition or the format of the group. For example, mixed age groups or mixed gender groups might be inappropriate or create discomfort in certain communities. The purpose and subject of the group may also affect this—for example, some topics are best addressed only among men, only among women, or only among youth.

Here are some examples of groups run by CHWs related to trauma:

- **Healing circles:** The format of healing circles vary; most bring together people who have something in common such as location, culture, experiences, or kinship to support a healing goal of one or more than one person in the circle, through words, prayer, ritual, or other means; some are rooted in indigenous cultures.

- **Lifebooks or memory boxes**: A group to facilitate collecting memories for one's family or one's children when facing a terminal health condition.

- **Workshops for parents or families**: Sometimes issues of trauma and resiliency are addressed in the context of parenting or family relationship classes or general health workshops that may draw a wider audience than a trauma-specific workshop.

- **Groups as a component of other services**: Groups are often one component of a larger set of services offered in a specific setting where trauma may be common (e.g., residential housing among the homeless, support groups for veterans, assistance for transitional age youth, re-entry settings, even a homework club in a housing project)—these groups may or may not be designed around a specific goal (for example, employment or sobriety).

- **Support groups for those who have experienced a specific type of trauma**: Rape survivors, domestic violence survivors, veterans, those who experienced a common disaster.

Toni Hunt Hines: For me, the big thing was when someone said, let people help you. I'm usually someone who helps other people! But I took that in. When my son was killed, my family couldn't help me, because they lost him, too. We were all going through it. I had to let other people help me. Mostly it was ordinary everyday people who helped me, like other moms who had lost a child. I went to a Healing Circle. I have friends from that group who are like sisters now. I learned how to build up a larger network of support.

RE-ESTABLISHING SAFETY

Re-establishing safety is an important part of running a group related to trauma. Many of the suggestions provided earlier in this chapter for working with individual clients can be adapted when you are facilitating a group. You will also find more suggestions for fostering safety in a group in Chapter 21. Some practices that help with creating an atmosphere of safety in groups include:

- Creating agreements about confidentiality (while acknowledging that the CHW cannot guarantee that all group members will respect those agreements)

- Establishing and revisiting ground rules/group agreements

- Affirming people's feelings, experiences, and stories

- Allowing group members to "pass" and not speak, other than perhaps a brief check-in

- Allowing for trust to build over time, through activities that allow group members to get to know one another

Inez Love: When I developed the workshop series for transitional-age youth called Healing the Violence, I was writing something from scratch, and I learned from my mistakes. The second time around, the workshop was more uplifting and positive, because I changed the order of activities. For example, in the first round, I led the story circle, where people share their stories of losing a loved one to violence, on the first day, and that was too soon. They didn't feel as emotionally safe. The second time I introduced the story circle on the third or fourth day. Before that, I shared my story, and we had activities to get to know each other, sharing something other than their experience of violence, so they have some kind of relationship built before the story circle. In the story circle, everyone cries. It was too much to do on the first day.

Physical safety as well as emotional safety is at risk for many trauma survivors. Groups can be a powerful way to reinforce security measures and ways of maintaining personal safety, if the risk of violence is ongoing. This can take many forms, from self-defense classes (e.g., *http://modelmugging.org/*) to learning to stay safe from street violence and avoid incarceration (e.g., *http://stayaliveandfree.org/*).

SUPPORT DIVERSE MODES OF HEALING

Grieving is often an important component of healing from trauma. Groups of many kinds have helped in the grieving process, through mutual support and ceremony. Healing circles rooted in local culture and local institutions (such as a faith community, a school, a neighborhood center) have been noted as a means of healing for trauma (Prevention Institute, 2014) and working through grief is often a part of that work.

As a CHW you may be called upon to teach, share, facilitate, or practice healing techniques in which you have been trained and that fit within your scope of practice and your agency's mission, in a group setting. Examples include:

- Active listening
- Mindfulness practices
- Relaxation and stress management techniques
- Creative expression through art, music or poetry
- Creating "memory books" or "memory boxes" to tell the story of a lost loved one, or when preparing for an impending death due to terminal illness

In addition, CHWs may share basic information about trauma and traumatic stress in groups. This can help group members understand their own reactions or those of their family members and friends. It can help normalize reactions, and provide comfort to those who might be asking, "Am I losing my mind?" It can also create a space to talk about referrals or additional support services that may be available in the community.

If the group includes members who are currently in a substance abuse treatment or harm reduction program, it is advisable to communicate with the facilitators of that program and with the clients, to assess whether participating in both programs at the same time is advisable for this individual (please note that you may need to ask the client to sign a release of information form in order to talk with another service provider). Many people who use or abuse substances have a history of trauma (Maté, 2010). Discussing life traumas and grief may at times overwhelm the resources of a person also working on reducing or eliminating their substance use, and could contribute to relapse (Najavits, 2002). There are ways to address trauma and substance use in combination, but this may require additional training and supervision.

STRENGTHEN CONNECTIONS

The ability to connect and relate to others is part of healing from trauma, and part of building a group's capacity for action. Trauma often shatters or strains social connections, and groups can be an important counterbalance or response to that loss. Sometimes it is the secrecy and shame related to traumatic events (such as domestic violence, child sexual abuse, rape, or suicide) that ruptures social connections and trust. Sometimes it is the displacement of communities who must flee violence or natural disaster that leads to social disconnection. Historical trauma, also, can contribute to a sense of isolation, oppression, and invisibility.

In planning and facilitating a group, think about how connection among the group members could be fostered. For example, avoid a hub-and-spoke dynamic in the group, where every comment is directed to the leader of the group. Instead, facilitate more opportunities for mutual support and dialogue among group members. Here are some suggestions for ways to build more sense of connection in a group:

- Incorporate icebreakers and games to help people get comfortable with one another
- Sequence activities or topics, so that the group eases into more intense topics or in-depth sharing of experiences, and also eases out of those conversations
- Balance the time among different members of the group, so no single person dominates but all members have a chance to participate
- Share an everyday experience—cooking a meal, planting a garden, or fixing bicycles
- Celebrate successes and affirm strengths of all members of the group, and facilitate opportunities for them to offer appreciation to one another
- If appropriate, organize activities where group members can get together outside of the formal meetings of the group

- *What other strategies have you learned for building and strengthening the connections among group members?*

A FOCUS ON MEANING

For some survivors of trauma, making sense of what happened is central to their healing. This may involve reflecting on what happened, finding additional information about the events surrounding the trauma, and striving to better understand the factors that may have caused or contributed to the trauma. Groups may also explore the ways in which the trauma has impacted or changed the lives of individuals, families, and the community. Making meaning of past experiences is often part of a therapeutic process, processes that are clearly outside the scope of practice of CHWs. However, there are ways that a CHW can help a group understand experiences of trauma and recovery that allow for peer support and exploration.

One thing a CHW can do is share information that helps participants to understand and contextualize their experiences. For example, you can discuss with participants the legal definition of sexual assault, as it can sometimes help survivors understand that what happened was not okay and not their fault. In the wake of collective forms of violence—political violence, or disasters that are made worse by governmental actions or inactions—the CHW can support a group to gather and analyze information together, placing personal experiences in a wider context. This can also extend to a second generation or further—for example, the children of refugees may want to understand what happened to cause their family to flee, or a new generation affected by historical trauma may seek to understand that history. This process can help create a shared story of the events that took place, and can link to advocacy efforts to address the situation.

Support groups led by CHWs or other peer counselors can also challenge patterns of judgment against survivors, including self-blame. Often, behind the habit of self-blame is the desire for power over the situation—survivors want so badly to have the capacity to stop the violence or other traumatic event, that they may think, "if only I had done X, then I would not have been victimized." While it can be empowering to identify and discuss steps that clients *can* take to create greater safety in the future, or to understand what actions may have increased their risk in the past, it is never the victim's fault that they were subjected to violence, intimidation, or humiliation by a perpetrator, or by events beyond human control (in the case of natural disasters). It is important for anyone facilitating groups to develop skills in assisting participants to appreciate and honor this distinction.

- *What experiences do you have with participating in or leading support groups?*

- *Can you think of time when you gained new insight about an important life experience by sharing your story with others?*

- *What behaviors do you especially appreciate or dislike in a group leader or facilitator?*

Strengthening the Social Fabric

When the World Trade Center was attacked in September 2001, the trauma extended well beyond the attack itself. In addition to being a center of global finance, lower Manhattan is also a neighborhood, one that had to cope with tremendous wreckage and environmental contamination. Schools became a natural site for parents and teachers to meet and find ways to support the children and one another. Family support groups met every week in the first months after 9/11. Teachers and parents shared information on how the attacks had affected the children. They sought ways to support the children to feel safe again and to make sense of what happened. As parents and teachers took action to support children, they also re-established some of their own sense of agency, of power and control in the situation. These efforts were expanded to all the schools in the area, with community dinners, classroom activities, and support groups. The groups enhanced resiliency, by rebuilding social ties, sharing information, and creating a forum where the stress reactions adults and children were experiencing could be normalized and understood. This evolved into a collaborative called the Ground Zero Community Initiative. The Initiative worked toward recovery by strengthening the social connections that already existed in the community. It built on the natural ties people already had—for example, parents at a school or residents of an apartment complex—and in this way reached more people than clinical services could. The organizing experience and social ties strengthened through this process continued to serve the community even years after the 9/11 attacks. (Saul, 2014)

18.12 Guidelines for Working with Communities

In responding to trauma at the community level, CHWs often work with organizations, networks, and coalitions to organize projects or events that bring the healing process into the open and foster a public recognition of the trauma. Survivors of trauma are usually at the forefront of these efforts. You may encounter a former client in the role of community leader, advocate, or organizer.

Richard Mollica emphasizes the roles that work, giving to others, and spirituality play in the recovery of survivors of trauma. He calls these the social component of healing (Mollica, 2009). CHWs may find themselves in the role of facilitating a group or a community project focused on giving back to the community, or participating in some kind of spiritual expression or commemoration. Many times, survivors of traumatic events and situations regain a sense of autonomy and belonging by participating in their community in this way. Community action can contribute to a greater sense of social connection, which itself is associated with resiliency.

One way that healing from trauma can be shared with communities is through the arts. Any form of art may be used to promote greater understanding of trauma—painting, murals, film and video, poetry, spoken word performance, theater, dance, or music. The digital storytelling project Silence Speaks (*www.silencespeaks.org*) brings together survivors of trauma for storytelling and the creation of short personal videos. These videos are sometimes shared in community settings and used as a launch pad for deeper discussion. Jack Saul's work on collective healing has often included theater pieces drawn from the experiences of survivors. Actors collect the stories of survivors and weave them together into a performance that is then shared with and discussed by the affected community. Saul states

> By rendering individual experiences as part of a collective narrative within a performance space, the theater group creates a safe opportunity to recreate, recollect, relive, and reincorporate the memories of traumatic experience. (Saul, 2014, p. 138)

Public events that focus on healing along with a demand for change are a powerful way to engage the broader community. These can take the form of ceremonies or commemorations of a traumatic event (as discussed in the section titled Guidelines for Working with Community). Or they can be more confrontational, using mass protests or civil disobedience. They may incorporate music, street theater, or other outdoor performances. These events serve not only to bring people together in a shared experience, but also to reclaim public space and to press for concrete changes in local conditions that can help prevent further trauma. CHWs are often involved in organizing events of this type.

The pursuit of truth and justice to redress a situation of significant human rights abuses or armed conflict is often also a path toward healing, on the community level. The unresolved nature of the injury when no one has been held accountable for the harm done often leads communities to look for legal, political, or social means to document what happened and seek justice. Examples of this approach can be found at the website of the Center for Justice and Accountability (*www.cja.org*). Even if a group chooses to address a collective trauma primarily through legal or political means, opportunities for mutual support and emotional healing are often needed during that process.

Tapping into the community's own wisdom and traditions can be a powerful tool for healing. Instituto Familiar de la Raza in San Francisco, for example, offers ceremonies, community events, and drumming circles, alongside more conventional mental health counseling. They characterize their work as rooted in "a philosophy of self-determination, community empowerment, and spiritual/cultural affirmation" (Instituto Familiar de la Raza, 2015). Mentorship of younger residents by older residents is another way to promote healing and cultural sharing, including sharing of experiences of dealing with ongoing sources of trauma.

Whenever you work with community, often through a specific project or activity, be attentive to the community's interests, priorities, and direction. Voices of survivors are vital to include in any community response to trauma. Working with a community on a project related to healing from trauma and/or creating greater safety in the community can evolve into a process of community organizing or advocacy (see Chapter 23).

Envisioning Justice through a Skit about Human Rights

Janey Skinner: When I worked with Guatemalan refugee women living in camps in Mexico, we supported women's leadership in part through offering human rights workshops, together with a Guatemalan women's organization. At one workshop, the women put on a skit for others in the camp, demonstrating how to use international human rights standards to put the military generals on trial—the same generals who had led the Guatemalan Army's attack on their villages, forcing them to flee their homes and become refugees. The skit sparked a catharsis in the community, culminating with several audience members joining the actors in chasing the women who played the generals around in a big circle. There was much laughter that night, mixed with many other emotions. Over the next months, I heard people refer to the skit and the powerful image of justice it left in their minds. Also, the whole camp got to see women speaking out for once, women knowing their rights and taking leadership to tell their truths about what had happened in Guatemala. The workshops and the performances gave fuel to the long struggle the refugees still faced.

—Janey Skinner

18.13 Trauma-Informed Practice

Trauma-informed practice is growing in the fields of public health, health care, mental health, substance use and other disciplines. It encourages agencies, programs and professionals to incorporate trauma knowledge and skills into their policies and the services that they provide to clients and communities.

SAMHSA has developed a framework for a **trauma-informed approach** (also called trauma-informed care) that can be adapted and applied to any agency serving the public. SAMHSA states:

> *A program, organization, or system that is trauma-informed realizes the widespread impact of trauma and understands potential paths for recovery; recognizes the signs and symptoms of trauma in clients, families, staff, and others involved with the system; and responds by fully integrating knowledge about trauma into policies, procedures, and practices, and seeks to actively resist retraumatization. (SAMHSA, 2014b)*

SAMHSA further defines six principles that characterize a trauma-informed approach:

1. Safety
2. Trustworthiness and transparency
3. Peer support
4. Collaboration and mutuality
5. Empowerment, voice, and choice
6. Cultural, historical, and gender issues

These principles are intended to guide all aspects of an agency's operations, from what the waiting room looks like, to how plans for treatment are developed, to how staff are supervised. It requires a commitment from the highest levels of the organization; policies and procedures that support recovery and avoid retraumatizing clients; budgets for appropriate services including peer support, which could include CHWs; ongoing training and workforce development; and the engagement and involvement of trauma survivors and family members in designing and improving programs.

For CHWs and other direct service providers, trauma-informed practice means:

- Being well-trained to understanding what trauma is, how common it is, and how survivors are affected (trauma responses)
- Understanding how trauma exposure can influence current health, mental health, and addiction risks and status

- Paying attention to signs that a client may have a trauma history
- Learning to talk comfortably with clients about trauma
- The application of harm reduction principles to avoid unintentional harm to survivors who disclose a history of trauma
- Practicing client-centered skills—including cultural humility and a strength-based approach—that promote client autonomy and their unique paths for healing
- Providing referrals to appropriate community-based resources including resources for mental health and legal services.

The more you learn about trauma responses and recovery, and the more confidence you gain in listening to your client's stories, the better prepared you will be to support clients in their healing. For more information about trauma-informed practice, see the resources provided at the end of this chapter.

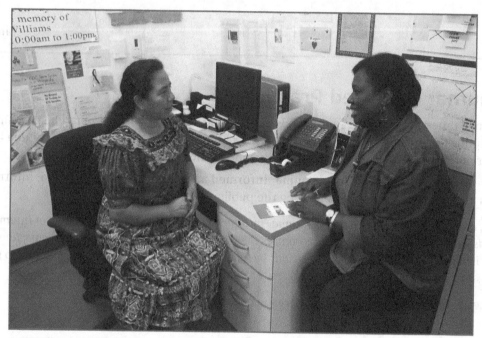

A CHW listens to a client's story.

18.14 Secondary Trauma, Secondary Resilience

Helping professionals who work closely with survivors of trauma are at risk for developing signs of **secondary trauma**. However, they can also benefit from **secondary resilience**.

SECONDARY TRAUMA

CHWs can be profoundly affected by their work with survivors of trauma. Over time, through witnessing the trauma stories of clients or community members, you may begin to develop signs and symptoms of traumatic stress reactions. These symptoms may include intrusive thoughts related to trauma stories, nightmares, and difficulty concentrating. Common emotional responses include sadness or despair, numbness, fear, anger, guilt, or shame. You may also experience fatigue, avoidance, or isolation. Your perceptions of situations may become distorted, seeing threats where there are none, or the opposite reaction, becoming insensitive to violence or danger.

In other words, even if the helping professional is not a survivor of trauma, they may develop trauma responses/symptoms through their exposure to the stories of the survivors they work with.

> **Christina:** Working with victims of sexual exploitation and trafficking, I saw directly how important it was for the organization to have safeguards and support for the staff. When that wasn't in place—not enough supervision, unclear boundaries and protocols, unreasonable workload—it made me feel overwhelmed and isolated. I was essentially the duck appearing to be calm on the surface but, underneath, desperately paddling to stay afloat. I was definitely experiencing secondary trauma, such as a sense of hopelessness and despair in the world, intrusive thoughts, and inability to be intimate with my partner. I found myself hiding away from the world, smoking marijuana and playing video games. What helped me most was the support and understanding from my friends and taking a step back from my work to focus on my education and self care.

Of course, some helping professionals are also survivors of trauma, and working with clients can restimulate or intensify their own stories and responses.

If you work closely with survivors of trauma, it is important to know that you may be at risk for developing secondary trauma, and to adapt a regular practice of self care (addressed later on in this chapter)

What Do YOU Think?

- *How are you affected by working with survivors of trauma?*

- *What can you do to monitor yourself for signs of secondary trauma?*

SECONDARY RESILIENCE

Helping professionals who work closely with survivors of trauma may also be positively affected by the extraordinary strength and resilience of clients who have faced and survived horrific trauma. Working closely with survivors provides an opportunity to witness their courage, creativity, generosity, and resilience as they seek healing. Over time, CHWs and other helping professionals may begin to internalize and benefit from these positive qualities. In this way, working with survivors can be tremendously hopeful and inspiring.

In the Presence of Perseverance

Janey Skinner: Whenever I think something is too hard or too inconvenient for me—that I just can't make it to another meeting, rally, or fundraiser—I think of Simon, a subsistence farmer in Guatemala who was active in a human rights organization I knew well. Simon always made it to the protests in the capital. He didn't miss one—he came to march, or to speak, or just to be counted among the many rallying for human rights and against the state-sponsored repression that was all too common then. To do so, Simon had to get up at three in the morning, walk four hours to the road, then take a bus another four hours to the capital. The buses were crowded—he often made the whole trip standing in the aisle. But what touched me most was his quiet seven-year-old son, always stuck to his father's side. He, too, had walked those four hours to the road, every time, and ridden the bus standing in the aisle. I think of Simon and his son, and all my excuses for not showing up just fade away. Their persistence seemed to spring from unshakable beliefs and the strength they found in taking action with others. I'm grateful if even a little bit of their resilience rubbed off on me.

While it's impossible to control the many ways that working with survivors may affect you, we believe that focusing on the client's resilience can enhance your own. Take time as you work to apply a strength-based analysis and to identify and consider aspects of a survivor's recovery that you find courageous, creative, or inspirational.

What Do YOU Think?

- *In what ways do survivors of trauma inspire you or teach you valuable lessons?*

18.15 Self Care

The work of CHWs can be both highly rewarding and highly stressful. The success and longevity of your career will be significantly enhanced by your ability to regularly practice skills for stress management and self care. Self care is even more important if you work closely with survivors of trauma, because of the risks of secondary trauma.

Please review Chapter 12 on Stress Management and Self Care. Take a few minutes to reflect about your own history of practicing self care:

● What moment of your day (today or yesterday) provided a moment of calm, relaxation, or relief from stress?

● How do you care for yourself at the end of a difficult working day?

> **Toni Hunt Hines:** I do yoga at my job every other week. And I went to a training on mindfulness. . . . I flirt with exercise—it's on my "to do" list. . . . Even learning about trauma recovery and resiliency, that's been helpful. I try a lot of different things, from different traditions. I think it is important to stay open to trying new things because everything doesn't work for everyone.

If your self care practices aren't providing enough relief from stress, research and identify new practices that might work for you. If you need help, reach out and talk with someone who may be more accomplished in their self care practice. This may be a coworker or supervisor, your own physician or therapist, or someone else in your local community. Some self care practices that may be relevant to you include:

● Ongoing counseling or therapy or other healing practices

● Mindfulness, meditation, prayer, and other stress reduction techniques

● Regular self-assessment for developing signs of secondary trauma

● Regular supervision in which you talk about how work with trauma survivors is affecting you

● Movement, yoga, stretching, exercise, or other physical activity to reduce anxiety and manage stress

● Seeking support from your own external resources such as family, friends and community-based programs and organizations

Work to develop and refine your own practical action plan for self care. Start today. Take five minutes to write down one or two ways that you can better manage stress. Then take the time—today or as soon as you can—to put one of these ideas into action. Remember that self care doesn't need to be complicated, expensive, or time consuming. A good option for many people may be some form of mindfulness practice (again, see Chapter 12). This could include 5 or 10 minutes of deep breathing. It can be as simple as:

Breathe in through your nose as you count to four, hold your breath for four counts, breath out through your mouth for six counts. Repeat. Do it two or three more times.

● *How do you feel now?*

● *Do you notice a difference?*

Swimming Laps at the End of the Day

Tim Berthold: I worked at a rape crisis center. I talked with survivors and their family members in person and over the phone. Sometimes I accompanied survivors undergoing forensic medical exams at the county hospital in the aftermath of a rape. This work was deeply meaningful. I had amazing coworkers, and the agency provided regular supervision with a therapist to help me talk about how the work affected me, and to identify challenges along the way.

(continues)

Swimming Laps at the End of the Day

(continued)

Still, it was sometimes difficult for me to separate work and my personal life. I brought the stories and the emotions home with me. I had nightmares that included details that clients told me about their own experiences. And I had nightmares about not being able to help my clients.

On my way home from work, I noticed a pool. I started to swim laps after work. I swam until I was exhausted and, as I swam, I imagined the stories that clients told me, their fear and sorrow, melting into the water. When I stepped out of the pool, I imagined leaving the stories, and their emotions, behind in the water, a safe and protected place.

This routine helped me to create a better transition back to my personal life. I started to sleep better. And this, in turn, gave me more energy for my work.

18.16 Ongoing Professional Development

We encourage you to participate in opportunities to further enhance your knowledge and skills for working with survivors of trauma. Training opportunities may exist in the city or county where you live and/or work. Many organizations offer free training in exchange for a volunteer commitment of a certain number of hours each week or month for a specified number of months. Options may include:

- Suicide prevention and crisis intervention agencies and hotlines
- Rape crisis centers
- Domestic violence shelters and hotlines
- Hospitals and departments of public health/health services
- Local colleges and universities: For example, City College of San Francisco offers several courses designed to prepare front-line providers to work in preventing violence and providing services to survivors of trauma

For more information, see the list of resources provided at the end of this chapter.

Chapter Review

To review the key concepts and skills addressed in this chapter, take time to reflect upon the following questions.

1. Test your general knowledge about trauma by answering the following questions:
   - How would you define and explain trauma if you were making a presentation at a local high school or college?
   - What kinds of events or situations are likely to cause traumatic stress?
   - How may trauma impact survivors? What are some common responses to trauma?
   - How do culture, status, and identity impact trauma?
   - What are some possible pathways or strategies for healing from trauma?
   - What are some of the similarities about working with an individual client and working with a group? What are some of the differences?
   - If you currently work as a CHW, how does trauma show up in your work? What do you currently do to support clients and communities affected by trauma, and what new ideas did you get from the chapter that might enhance your practice?

2. Research and identify resources in the communities where you live and work: What are some local resources, such as agencies, programs, or providers who offer services to survivors of trauma?

   o What activities or organizations in your community help to prevent trauma and promote resiliency?

3. Consider how you would work with a client who decides to talk with you about a trauma experience. It may be a mother whose son was shot on the street, or a client who grew up in a household characterized by domestic violence.

   o As a CHW, what is your scope of practice? If you currently work as a CHW, what policies or programs at your organization might be important when working with a trauma survivor?

   o Why are issues of autonomy and control particularly important to someone who has experienced trauma?

   o How might you use client-centered counseling in your work with this person?

   o What is something that you definitely would not want to say to this client? What is something you probably would want to say?

   o What fears or concerns come up for you when you imagine working with a client who wants to talk about a trauma experience? Where can you go to get advice, support, or information to help you address those concerns?

4. Review the Case Study information provided about Nadia throughout this chapter (including each of the conversations between Nadia and the CHW). What client-centered skills does the CHW demonstrate? For example, can you identify examples of when the CHW:

   o Demonstrated a strength-based approach?

   o Supported the client's autonomy and self-determination?

   o Used Open-ended questions?

   o Provided an Affirmation?

   o Demonstrated Reflective Listening?

   o Summarized?

   o How did the CHW work to establish safety?

   o How did the CHW support Nadia to develop an action plan?

5. Professional Development and Self Care

   o What are secondary trauma and secondary resilience? How may they affect you, personally and at work? Have you experienced either one?

   o What self care practices do you regularly practice to manage your stress and prevent burnout? What additional self care practices would you like to try?

   o What is your professional development plan for learning more about trauma? What aspects of trauma do you most want to explore? Which skills for working with survivors do you most want to enhance? Where or how can you access resources to build your knowledge and skills?

   o Identify one professional development opportunity that you can engage with in the next year that will enhance your knowledge and skills for working with survivors of trauma.

References

The American Psychiatric Association. (2013). *Posttraumatic stress disorder*. Retrieved from *www.dsm5.org/Documents/PTSD%20Fact%20Sheet.pdf*

The American Psychological Association. (n.d.). *Trauma*. Retrieved from *www.apa.org/topics/trauma/*

Beristain, C. M. (2010). *Manual sobre la perspectiva psicosocial en la investigación de los derechos humanos*. Bilbao, Spain: Hegoa.

Brave Heart, M. Y. H. (2000) Wakiksuyapi: Carrying the historical trauma of the Lakota. *Tulane Studies in Social Welfare, 21–22,* 245–266.

Brewin, C. R. (2007) Remembering and forgetting. In M. J. Friedman, T. M. Keane, T. M., & P. A. Resick (Eds.), *PTSD science and practice: A comprehensive handbook* (pp. 116–134). New York, NY: Guilford Press.

Brown, L. S. (2008). *Cultural competence in trauma therapy: Beyond the flashback.* Washington, DC: American Psychological Association.

Centers for Disease Control and Prevention (CDC). (2012). *Suicide: Facts at a glance.* Retrieved from *www.cdc.gov/violenceprevention/pdf/suicide-datasheet-a.pdf*

Centers for Disease Control and Prevention (CDC). (May 13, 2014). *Adverse Childhood Experiences (ACE) study: Major findings.* Retrieved from *www.cdc.gov/violenceprevention/acestudy/findings.html*

Chandra, A., Acosta, J., Stern, S., Uscher-Pines, L., William, M. V., Leung, D., . . . Meredith, L. S. (2011). *Building community resilience to disasters: A way forward to enhance national health security* [Technical Report]. Retrieved from *www.rand.org/content/dam/rand/pubs/technical_reports/2011/RAND_TR915.pdf*

Child Welfare Information Gateway. (2012). *Trauma-focused cognitive behavioral therapy for children affected by sexual abuse or trauma.* Washington, DC: U.S. Department of Health and Human Services, Children's Bureau.

DeGruy Leary, J. A. (2005). *Post traumatic slave syndrome: America's legacy of enduring injury and healing.* Portland, OR: Uptone Press.

de Jong, K. (2011). *Psychosocial and mental health interventions in areas of mass violence: A community-based approach* (2nd ed.). Retrieved from *www.msf.org/sites/msf.org/files/old-cms/source/mentalhealth/guidelines/MSF_mentalhealthguidelines.pdf*

Erikson, K. T. (1976). *Everything in its path: Destruction of community in the Buffalo Creek flood.* New York, NY: Simon & Schuster.

Fairbank, J. A. (2008). The epidemiology of trauma and trauma related disorders in children and youth. *PTSD Research Quarterly, 19*(1), 1–3. Retrieved from *www.ptsd.va.gov/professional/newsletters/research-quarterly/v19n1.pdf*

The Harvard Program in Refugee Trauma. (n.d.). Cultural competence. Retrieved from *http://hprt-cambridge.org/clinical/cultural-competence/*

Herman, J. L. (1997). *Trauma and recovery: The aftermath of violence—from domestic abuse to political terror.* New York, NY: Basic Books.

Instituto Familiar de la Raza. (2015). Working with our community. Retrieved from *http://ifrsf.org/mission-and-philosophy/*

International Society for Traumatic Stress Studies (ISTSS). (n.d.). Remembering childhood trauma.

Kellermann, N. P. F. (2013). Epigenetic transmission of Holocaust trauma: Can nightmares be inherited? *Israel Journal of Psychiatry and Related Sciences, 50,* 33–39.

Kemp, J., & Bossarte, R. (2012). *Suicide data report 2012: Department of Veterans Affairs* [Technical Report]. Retrieved from *www.va.gov/opa/docs/suicide-data-report-2012-final.pdf*

Kilpatrick, D. J., Resnick, H. S., Milanak, M. E., Miller, M. W., Keyes, K. M., & Friedman, M. J. (2013). National estimates of exposure to traumatic events and PTSD prevalence using *DSM-IV* and *DSM-5* criteria. *Journal of Traumatic Stress, 26,* 537–547.

La Clinica de la Raza. (2015). *Cultura y bienestar.* Retrieved from *www.laclinica.org/programs-culturaybienestar.html*

Loo, C. M. (2014, January 3). *PTSD among ethnic minority veterans.* National Center for PTSD, U.S. Department of Veterans Affairs. Retrieved from *www.ptsd.va.gov/professional/treatment/cultural/ptsd-minority-vets.asp*

Lykes, M. B., Beristain, C. M., & Pérez-Armiñan, M. C. (2007). Political violence, impunity, and emotional climate in Maya communities. *Journal of Social Issues, 63,* 369–385. doi:10.1111/j.1540-4560.2007.00514.x

Malekoff, A. (2007). Transforming the trauma of September 11, 2001, with children and adolescents through group work. In M. Bussey & J. B. Wise (Eds.), *Trauma transformed: An empowerment response* (pp. 194–214). New York, NY: Columbia University Press.

Maté, G. (2010). *In the realm of hungry ghosts: Close encounters with addiction.* Berkeley, CA: North Atlantic Books.

McLaughlin, M., Irby, M., & Langman, J. (1994). *Urban sanctuaries: Neighborhood organizations in the lives and futures of inner-city youth.* San Francisco: Jossey-Bass.

Medecins Sans Frontieres. (n.d.). *Refugee health: An approach to emergency situations.* Retrieved from *refbooks.msf. org/msf_docs/en/refugee_health/rh.pdf*

Mendelsohn, M., Herman, J. L., Schatzow, E., Coco, M., Kallivayalil, D., & Levitan, J. (2011) *The trauma recovery group: A guide for practitioners.* New York, NY: Guilford Press.

Michaels, C. (2010). Historical trauma and microaggressions: A framework for culturally-based practice. *University of Minnesota Extension Children's Mental Health eReview.* Retrieved from *www.extension.umn.edu/ family/cyfc/our-programs/ereview/docs/cmhereviewOct10.pdf*

Mollica, R. F. (2009). *Healing invisible wounds: Paths to healing and recovery in a violent world.* Nashville, TN: Vanderbilt University Press.

Najavits, L. M. (2002). *Seeking safety: A treatment manual for PTSD and substance abuse.* New York, NY: Guilford Press.

Norris, F. H., & Slone, L. B. (2013). Understanding research on the epidemiology and prevalence of PTSD. *PTSD Research Quarter, 24*(2–3), 1–5.

Prevention Institute. (2013). *Addressing and preventing trauma at the community level: A conversation with Rachel Davis and Howard Pinderhughes.* Retrieved from *www.preventioninstitute.org/component/jlibrary/article/ id-347/127.html*

Prevention Institute. (2014). *Making connections for well-being among men and boys in the U.S.* [Report]. Retrieved from *www.preventioninstitute.org/component/jlibrary/article/id-358/127.html*

Rich, J. A. (2009). *Wrong place, wrong time: Trauma and violence in the lives of young black men.* Baltimore, MD: Johns Hopkins University Press.

Saul, J. (2014). *Collective trauma, collective healing: Promoting community resilience in the aftermath of disaster.* New York, NY: Routledge.

Solnit, R. (2009). *A paradise built in hell: The extraordinary communities that arise in disaster.* New York, NY: Penguin.

Stevenson, K. M., & Rall, J. (2007). Transforming the trauma of torture, flight, and resettlement. In M. Bussey & J. B. Wise (Eds.), *Trauma transformed: An empowerment response* (pp. 236–258). New York, NY: Columbia University Press.

Substance Abuse and Mental Health Services Administration (SAMHSA). (October 9, 2014a). *Recovery and recovery support.* Retrieved from *www.samhsa.gov/recovery*

Substance Abuse and Mental Health Services Administration. (2014b). *SAMHSA's concept of trauma and guidance for a trauma-informed approach.* HHS Publication No. (SMA) 14-4884. Retrieved from *http://store.samhsa.gov/ shin/content/SMA14-4884/SMA14-4884.pdf*

Substance Abuse and Mental Health Services Administration. (October 10, 2014c). *Suicide prevention.* Retrieved from *www.samhsa.gov/suicide-prevention*

Terr, L. (1990). *Too scared to cry: Psychic trauma in childhood.* New York, NY: Basic Books.

United States Department of Veterans Affairs, National Center for PTSD (VA). (November 14, 2014a). *How common is PTSD?* Retrieved from *www.ptsd.va.gov/public/PTSD-overview/basics/how-common-is-ptsd.asp*

United States Department of Veterans Affairs, National Center for PTSD. (January 30, 2014b). *The epidemiology of PTSD.* Retrieved from *www.ptsd.va.gov/professional/PTSD-overview/epidemiological-facts-ptsd.asp*

United States Department of Veterans Affairs, National Center for PTSD. (January 3, 2014c). *The relationship between PTSD and suicide.* Retrieved from *www.ptsd.va.gov/professional/co-occurring/ptsd-suicide.asp*

van der Kolk, B. A. (2014). *The body keeps the score: Brain, mind and body in the healing of trauma.* New York, NY: Viking.

Vogt, D. S., King, D. W., & King, L. A. (2007). Risk pathways for PTSD: Making sense of the literature. In M. J. Friedman, T. M. Keane & P. A. Resick (Eds.), *PTSD science and practice: A comprehensive handbook* (pp. 99–116). New York, NY: Guilford Press.

World Health Organization. (2001). *Rapid assessment of mental health needs of refugees, displaced and other populations affected by conflict.* Retrieved from *www.who.int/hac/techguidance/pht/7405.pdf*

Additional Resources

The American Psychological Association. (n.d.). *Trauma.* Retrieved from *www.apa.org/topics/trauma/*

Armstrong, K., Best, S., & Domenici, P. (2006). *Courage after fire: Coping strategies for troops returning from Iraq and Afghanistan and their families.* Berkeley, CA: Ulysses Press.

California Attorney General's Office. (2008). *First impressions . . . Exposure to violence and a child's developing brain* [Video]. Retrieved from *www.youtube.com/watch?v=brVOYtNMmKk*

Centers for Disease Control and Prevention. (August 1, 2014). *Emergency preparedness and response: Coping with a disaster or traumatic event.* Retrieved from *http://emergency.cdc.gov/mentalhealth/*

Center for Victims of Torture. (n.d.). Healing and human rights [Blog]. *www.cvt.org/blog/healing-and-human-rights*

Cori, J. L. (2008). *Healing from trauma: A survivor's guide.* Philadelphia, PA: Da Capo Press.

Curran, L. A. (2013). *101 trauma-informed interventions: Activities, exercises and assignments to move the client and therapy forward.* Eau Claire, WI: Premier Publishing and Media.

Gutlove, P., & Thompson, G. (2003). *Psychosocial healing: A guide for practitioners.* Cambridge, MA: Institute for Resource and Security Studies. Retrieved from *https://irssusa.files.wordpress.com/2013/10/psguide_000.pdf*

The Harvard Program in Refugee Trauma. (n.d.). Retrieved from *http://hprt-cambridge.org/*

Healing Collective Trauma. (n.d.). Retrieved from *www.healingcollectivetrauma.com/*

International Society for Traumatic Stress Studies. (n.d.). Retrieved from *www.istss.org/*

Klinic Community Health Center. (2008). *The trauma-informed toolkit.* Retrieved from *www.trauma-informed.ca*

Making the Connection. (n.d.). *Veterans voices on PTSD* [Video]. Retrieved from *http://maketheconnection.net/conditions/ptsd*

Mollica, R. F. (2013). *Textbook of global mental health: Trauma and recovery, a companion guide for field and clinical care of traumatized people worldwide* [E-Book]. Cambridge, MA: Harvard Program in Refugee Trauma.

National Child Traumatic Stress Network. (n.d.). Retrieved from *www.nctsn.org/*

The Resilience Alliance. (2011). *Promoting resilience and reducing secondary trauma among child welfare staff.* Retrieved from *www.nrcpfc.org/teleconferences/2011-11-16/Resilience_Alliance_Participant_Handbook_-_September_2011.pdf*

Schiraldi, G. (2009). *The post-traumatic stress disorder source book.* San Francisco, CA: McGraw Hill.

Seeking Safety. (n.d.). Retrieved from *www.treatment-innovations.org/seeking-safety.html*

Substance Abuse and Mental Health Administration. (n.d.). *Trauma resources.* Retrieved from *www.integration.samhsa.gov/clinical-practice/trauma*

Substance Abuse and Mental Health Administration. (n.d.). *Suicide prevention resource center.* Retrieved from *http://training.sprc.org/* and *www.samhsa.gov/suicide-prevention/publications-resources*

Substance Abuse and Mental Health Administration. (2002). *Dealing with the effects of trauma: A self-help guide.* Retrieved from *http://store.samhsa.gov/product/Dealing-with-the-Effects-of-Trauma-A-Self-Help-Guide/SMA-3717*

Van Dernoot Lipsky, L. (2009). *Trauma stewardship: An everyday guide to caring for self while caring for others.* San Francisco, CA: Berrett-Koehler.

U.S. Department of Health and Human Services, Administration for Children & Families. (n.d.). *Responding to child abuse and neglect.* Retrieved from *www.childwelfare.gov/topics/responding/*

WORKING WITH GROUPS AND COMMUNITIES

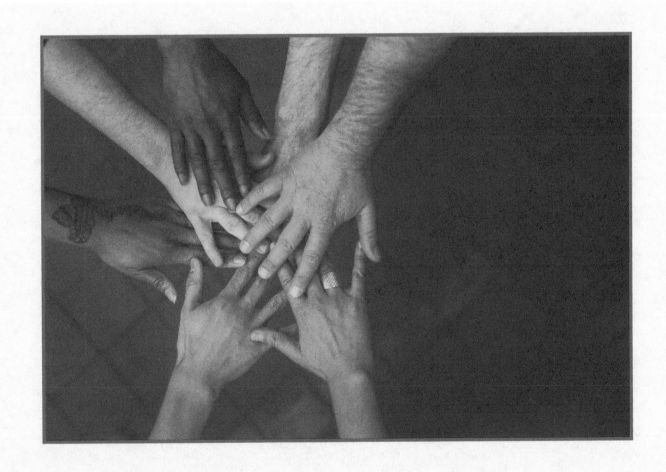

WORKING WITH GROUPS AND COMMUNITIES

Health Outreach

19

Craig Wenzl, Tim Berthold, and Emily Marinelli

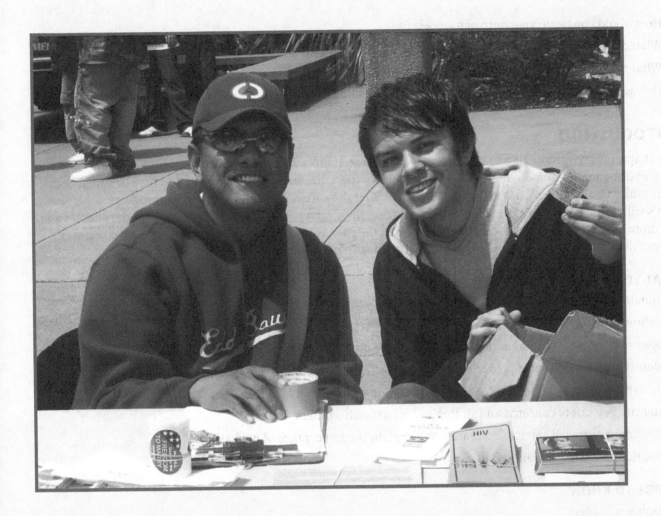

> ## CHW Scenario
>
> You have been hired as a CHW by a local health department that is concerned about the increasing rates of an infectious disease in an emerging immigrant community. Your job is to conduct outreach to the community, to provide them with information about the disease, and to support them in preventing new infections and in accessing local clinics for screening and treatment.

- How would you begin your outreach work?
- What do you want to know before you start to conduct outreach? What types of information will you gather?
- What types of resources would you rely on to guide your work?
- How would you know if your outreach program was successful?

Introduction

This chapter is an introduction to health outreach. Outreach links vulnerable communities to programs and services designed to promote their health. Some CHWs specialize in outreach services and may be called Community Health Outreach Workers or CHOWs. Even if they are not specialized outreach workers, most CHWs will participate in some level of outreach during their career. We hope that by the end of the chapter you feel more prepared to answer the questions posed in the case study above, and to bring your own experience, personality, and creativity to the task of conducting health outreach.

WHAT YOU WILL LEARN

By studying the information in this chapter, you will be able to:

- Define outreach
- Discuss the types of communities served and the health issues addressed through outreach
- Identify and provide examples of different outreach levels and methods
- Describe and apply strategies for approaching people you do not know
- Identify key safety concerns and strategies for outreach workers
- Document outreach services accurately and explain the importance of doing so
- Develop an outreach plan

WORDS TO KNOW

Key Opinion Leaders

Social Marketing

Venue

19.1 Defining Community Health Outreach

Community health outreach aims to identify, contact, and establish positive relationships with communities with increased risks for specific health conditions in order to promote better health outcomes. Additional goals for health outreach may include to:

- Increase awareness about a particular health issue (such as breast cancer)
- Promote health knowledge and changes in health behaviors (such as regular breast self-exams and mammogram screenings)
- Recruit participants for research (such as research on the effectiveness of specific breast cancer treatment options)

- Establish links to and partnerships between existing communities and existing health programs (such as between a local church and a women's health clinic)
- Increase community participation in the design, implementation, and evaluation of health programs and policies (such as development of new outreach programs to assist women of color in gaining access to breast cancer screening and treatment services)
- Mobilize community members to participate in community organizing and advocacy efforts (such as expanded access to health care)

- *Can you think of other goals for conducting health outreach?*

19.2 Qualities of Successful Community Health Outreach Workers

Outreach programs are often designed to work with communities that have experienced prejudice and discrimination, such as people with a history of incarceration, homelessness, or mental health conditions. It is sometimes difficult for an outsider to gain entry to the identified community, and to build the trust required to provide effective services. For these reasons, public health programs often recruit outreach workers from the communities to be served, with an emphasis on hiring culturally and linguistically competent CHWs. For example, when a local health department was developing an outreach program to promote breast cancer screening among Hmong women, they hired a local Hmong woman to work as a CHW.

An outreach worker named "Sheila" did HIV prevention in the predominantly African American community where she grew up.

> **"Sheila":** Everyone around here knows me as the condom lady. I drive up in my car and pop the trunk, where I keep all my supplies, and everyone crowds around asking for stuff. After they've talked with me a few times, they call me over to talk about the personal things like getting tested or how their son died of AIDS or how they just tested positive for HIV. They trust me, but even though I grew up around here, I had to bust my butt to earn that trust!

Of course, not all outreach workers come from the communities they work with. Regardless of whether or not they are already familiar with the community, successful CHWs tend to share the personal qualities outlined in Chapter 1, including self-awareness, open-mindedness, and interpersonal warmth. In addition, because all CHWs spend so much of their time building new relationships in the community, it is helpful to be:

- A "people person" who is good at talking with strangers as well as acquaintances
- Easy going and approachable
- *Extremely* patient
- Viewed as trustworthy by others; someone people feel comfortable talking to about personal issues
- Capable of earning the respect of all members of the community (and, sometimes even more important, someone who will not alienate particular subgroups within the community)
- Flexible and able to adapt to a variety of different working conditions
- Creative and willing to "think outside the box" to engage people
- Attentive to needs of communities and individual contacts
- Highly organized in maintaining outreach information, resources, and materials

- *What other qualities do you think may be especially important for outreach workers?*

One of the biggest mistakes that new outreach workers make is to imitate the style and personality of more experienced CHWs. However, the clients and communities you work with have a sixth sense for anything that is false or fake. Be your authentic self: if you pretend to be something or someone you are not, you will alienate the community and make it harder for them to trust you.

There are as many styles of outreach as there are outreach workers. There is room for all personality types in this profession. Be patient with yourself: With time and experience, you will develop your own unique approach to conducting outreach. Whether you are quiet, energetic, calm, or outgoing, your personality can inform and guide your work as a CHW.

- *What skills do you already possess that make you a "natural" outreach worker?*

- *What skills do you need to cultivate?*

What Do YOU? Think ?

19.3 Communities to Be Served through Outreach

The communities served by outreach efforts are defined by a variety of factors, including epidemiologic and other public health data that document a clear risk for a specific disease or health condition (see Chapter 3). The communities are also defined by geographical boundaries that may be statewide, or within the boundaries of a particular county, city, school district, zip code, or neighborhood. Other factors include age, ethnicity, nationality, immigration status, housing status (including homelessness), primary language, income, sexual orientation, gender, gender identity, behaviors (such as the use of injection drugs), and affiliations (such as the members of a particular labor union or religious organization).

Most communities served by outreach lack access to essential health resources and face significant barriers to health, such as poverty, lack of legal status, a history of discrimination, lack of access to educational programs or primary care services, geographic isolation, or homelessness.

> **Lee Jackson:** I do HIV outreach where it's needed most, like in areas where there's a lot of drugs and sex work. If a lot of people are injecting drugs, and people are trading sex for drugs or money, and they don't always use condoms, there's gonna be a high rate of STDs (sexually transmitted diseases), especially HIV.

19.4 Health Issues Addressed by Outreach

Outreach programs address a wide range of health issues including:

- Infectious diseases such as tuberculosis, HIV, malaria, syphilis, and hepatitis, and the need for immunizations
- Chronic diseases such as cancer, diabetes, addiction, asthma, hypertension, and heart disease
- Mental health issues (such as depression, post-traumatic stress, schizophrenia, and bipolar disorder)
- Accidents and injuries including automobile and pedestrian injuries
- Violence, including domestic violence, sexual violence, and gun violence
- Environmental and occupational health issues, including exposure to toxins and infectious agents where people live and work
- Access to key health and social services including housing, alcohol and drug treatment, and primary health care

- Enrollment in free and low-cost health insurance programs including Medicaid and linking community members to new and existing services (such as services provided through the Affordable Care Act)
- Enrollment in research studies
- Community planning efforts related to local health concerns
- Organizing and advocacy efforts related to health issues

  - *Can you think of other health-related issues to address through outreach?*

19.5 Outreach Levels and Methods

Outreach programs can operate on the level of the individual, group, institution, or population.

INDIVIDUAL LEVEL

CHWs talk one-on-one with individuals, using client-centered practice. The CHW responds to the individual's questions and concerns, and provides health information, counseling, and referrals, as appropriate. CHWs may also provide testing or screening services such as HIV antibody test counseling.

GROUP LEVEL

CHWs speak with a group from the priority population, such as clients at a homeless shelter, a youth group at a local church, or mothers at a local Supplemental Nutrition Clinic for Women, Infants, and Children (WIC). The CHW provides health education and referrals and addresses the group's questions and concerns.

INSTITUTIONAL LEVEL

CHWs work with representatives of a specific institution to reach their membership including, for example, schools, labor unions, employment sites, churches, mosques, or temples.

POPULATION LEVEL

Outreach efforts sometimes focus on a particular population within a city, county, state, or nation. This may include campaigns to reach youth, families with uninsured children, pregnant women, or smokers. Because these populations are large, the outreach methods usually include social marketing or the use of a wide range of media such as television, radio, print media, and social media to promote particular actions such as enrolling in health insurance programs, testing for HIV antibodies when pregnant, or the importance of engaging in regular exercise.

CHWs use many outreach methods, depending on the characteristics of the priority population and their preferred means of communication, the nature of the health issue to be addressed, and the type of health outcomes the program aims to promote.

STREET OUTREACH

Street outreach requires spending time in a neighborhood with the goal of locating and talking with members of a specific community, such as homeless youth. As we will discuss in the following section, what makes this approach effective (like all outreach efforts) is the ability of the CHWs to develop positive relationships with key members of the priority population. CHWs approach clients to start a conversation. While the outreach workers will have specific goals, such as promoting the services of safety net health clinics, the community often has different priorities. In order to build trust and ongoing relationships, CHWs need to listen first to the concerns and questions of prospective clients. CHWs usually carry outreach materials with them: these may include brochures, lists of referrals, first aid kits, health resources such as condoms and lubricant, and other incentives such as socks and hygiene kits (including soap, toothpaste, and toothbrushes, and so on) for people who are trying to survive on the streets.

VENUE-BASED OUTREACH

In the public health field, the term venue-based outreach refers to outreach strategies that target partic-ular places (a **venue** is a place) where the priority population spends significant time. Venues may include schools, homeless encampments, public housing units, market places and cafes, public transportation stations, job sites, bars and clubs, sports events, parks, and churches, mosques, temples, and other places of worship.

> **Phuong An Doan Billings:** At Asian Health Services we go out and try to connect the underserved populations to our clinic because one of the most important challenges for some communities is getting access to health care. The newcomers (or new immigrants) might be eligible for Covered California (health insurance for low-income families) or Medicare, but they don't know about these programs, and they are scared that they will have to pay, or their sponsors will have to pay, so they just stay home. That's why we need the outreach workers to be from the community. We go to English as Second Language (ESL) classes and nail salons and other places where the community is. For the Korean community, we go to small stores, like dry-cleaning stores, markets, or churches. To reach the Vietnamese, we also go to the churches. And to temples, pagodas. We go to senior centers, too.

● *Can you think of other venues or places to conduct outreach?*

CREATING A VENUE

Sometimes CHWs need to *create* a venue at which to conduct outreach. For example, the Mpowerment Project (http://mpowerment.org/) developed by the Center for AIDS Prevention Studies at the University of California, San Francisco (UCSF), seeks to reach young (ages 18–24) men who have sex with men (MSM) to reduce risks for HIV disease (UCSF, n.d.). In many of the cities or regions where Mpowerment projects were developed, there were no well-established venues where young MSM congregated. Mpowerment groups created the venues where the target population could spend time together: drop-in centers, BBQs, dance parties, and movie nights. At these venues and events, CHWs conduct outreach, and provide group and individual HIV prevention information, education, counseling, and referrals.

RECRUITMENT OF VOLUNTEER PEER EDUCATORS

Sometimes the best way to connect with a particularly hard-to-reach community is to recruit volunteer peer educators. CHWs identify **key opinion leaders** (people whom the community respects and looks to for guidance), build relationships and ask the leaders to participate in the outreach effort on a volunteer basis. These volunteers may receive formal training in a workshop or informal training via conversations with CHWs. Depending on the nature of the outreach program, volunteers may pass out information or other health resources, provide basic education, and make referrals to local services. Volunteers can assist an outreach program to reach more members of the priority population. While recruiting volunteers from the community can expand the reach of an outreach program, it is also time consuming and requires thoughtful recruitment, training, and supervision of volunteers. Sometimes these volunteer positions can become paid positions. Agencies may be able to award stipends to volunteers or to hire them on a part-time or full-time basis. Check with your agency to see if there is funding to support the contribution of volunteer peer educators.

● *Who are some key opinion leaders in your communities?*

Working with Key Opinion Leaders

CHWs working in a Bay Area county had a goal to increase condom use among local sex workers. They reached out to recruit key opinion leaders from the community, who in turn promoted the negotiation of safer sex and disseminated condoms, lubes, and referrals for additional services, including HIV test counseling, syringe exchange, and free and low-cost health care.

In Oakland, California, the Asian Health Center has organized Patient Leadership Councils to assist in reaching new immigrants.

> **Phuong An Doan Billings:** We do outreach to recruit people to be part of the Patient Leadership Council. We try to recruit people from each community that we serve—people who we think have potential, and we train them. We train them in leadership skills and basic knowledge about the clinic and health issues that are big in the community, and they go out and do more outreach to spread the word about the clinic. They talk to their neighbors: "Hey, I just came back from Asian Health Services today, and there is something so good about this place." They share this news and answer questions and encourage people to get health care if they need it. And they advise us about how we can do a better job serving their community.

INSTITUTIONAL OUTREACH

Many communities belong to or are represented by institutions that they trust and respect. Outreach programs can establish partnerships with these institutions to reach a specific community more efficiently. These institutions may include schools, ESL classes, churches, labor unions, clinics, or health plans, or artistic, professional, political, or community membership groups.

Partnering with Faith-Based Organizations

Community Health Workers in Monterey County, California, established partnerships with Black churches to develop and implement outreach strategies to provide HIV prevention education to their congregations. With the support of religious leaders, CHWs were able to conduct outreach to the African American community about a heavily stigmatized health issue. At several churches, ministers agreed to talk about HIV/AIDS as a part of their sermons, and CHWs facilitated workshops and discussion groups after the services.

Partnering with Public Housing

Outreach workers at the Mission Housing Development Corporation in San Francisco conduct outreach to predominantly non-English-speaking families living in public housing. Several times a year, health fairs are organized that provide residents of public housing with information and resources about a variety of health-related topics such as nutrition, cardiovascular disease, diabetes, and accident prevention. CHWs also provide weekly food distribution; and culturally appropriate, multilingual peer counseling and mentoring (Mission Housing Development Corporation, n.d.).

INTERNET AND MOBILE WEB OUTREACH

As access to computers, the Internet, and the mobile web continues to expand, CHWs have developed outreach strategies to take advantage of technology. Outreach technology continues to change and expand and can take many forms, such as:

- Create a website that appeals to the priority population, includes graphics and features to hold the interest of the audience, and is culturally appropriate. Include a blog (web log or journal) to share updates about what has been happening with your program, events that you've held, volunteer opportunities, social marketing campaigns, and so on.

- Add a web page to your agency's existing website that focuses on your program and includes information that you want the audience to discover. Update it regularly.

- Send mass text messages (i.e., messages that are sent to all group members in a mobile network or social networking app) to inform community members of events that are happening and services that are being provided, especially if they are one-time or infrequent/special events.

- Create an electronic mailing list that can serve as an Internet forum. People can join the list on their own, or you can add them to it, and they can communicate by email. Examples include Yahoo Groups, Google Groups, and so on.

- Develop a list of community members who are able and willing to be contacted by email. Send out news of interest, information, event announcements, and your outreach schedule so that they can visit your site. (This is different from an electronic mailing list because you are the only one who sends information out and participants can respond only to you and not to the entire list.)

- Create a social networking community page or group that people can view, join, and participate in and receive updates from (such as Facebook, Pinterest, Twitter, Instagram, or any current and popular technology resource).

- Make use of existing mobile apps to send out community-wide messages to priority populations.

- Add your program to the links section of related websites, resource listings, and so forth. Make sure the word gets out about the services you're providing and how to reach you.

- Use video-conferencing to connect a community of people at the same time, providing information and facilitating dialogue and support.

- Schedule and host a web seminar (webinar) when you want to reach a large number of people at a planned and scheduled time.

- Consider adding scanable graphics (such QR codes) to existing printed materials to provide a direct link to information online.

- *Can you think of other technology that you could use to conduct outreach?*

One example of social media outreach is the Community Initiative in San Francisco, a nonprofit organization working to build community and raise health awareness among gay, bisexual, and transgender men. Whenever an event is scheduled, an email is sent to the community informing them of location, time and other details. Various social media outlets are also used to distribute this information such as Facebook. (The Community Initiative, n.d.)

Another example of a social media health outreach campaign is the website developed by the U.S. Department of Health and Human Services for influenza information (USHHS, n.d.). *www.Flu.gov* provides free educational web and podcasts, Twitter, Facebook and email updates, widgets and badges, and short YouTube videos. Information is provided for all communities including pregnant women, infants, and children and older adults. Specific communities can find out their nearest vaccination location and access treatment.

Benefits to using the Internet to conduct outreach include:

1. **Privacy:** Much of your information can be provided on a website without the consumer being asked to provide any personal information.

2. **Cost-effectiveness:** You can reach a large number of people via the Internet for a small amount of money. You may be able to add a page to your agency's existing website, or you may be able to create a free Web page or other Internet resource (see Internet Resources at the end of this section).

3. **Reach:** Your Internet presence can be accessed by almost anyone at any time in any country all around the world.

Limitations to using the Internet or mobile web to conduct outreach include:

1. **Access:** Many people still do not have access to a computer, smart phone, or other mobile device because of the cost of equipment and Internet or data access.

2. **Cultural appropriateness:** For web-based outreach to be successful over time, the information accessed through the technology should be aligned with the cultural identities and values of the priority populations.

Many communities may not want to engage with you via the Internet and may prefer in-person opportunities for education, counseling, and relationship building.

3. **Privacy**: Clients may be concerned about the privacy of their communication and information online.

Priority populations with whom Internet and mobile outreach can be very effective may include:

- Youth and young adults
- Communities with greater access to the Internet
- Participants in social media sites
- People using the web to make romantic or sexual connections with others

- *Can you think of a way that you could use the Internet or mobile web to provide outreach to your community?*

SOCIAL MARKETING

Social marketing applies the same methods that businesses use to sell products (such as soft drinks or cell phones) to promote specific health outcomes. Social marketing campaigns may seek to promote immunizations or screening for breast cancer, or to prevent smoking, domestic violence, or driving under the influence of alcohol. Social marketing techniques include the use of posters, billboards, pamphlets, brochures, and social media as well as public service announcements (PSAs) on television, radio, the Internet, or cell phones. To be successful, social marketing campaigns need to analyze and understand their "target market" (the community), select a medium (such as radio or social media) that is popular with the target market, and develop a persuasive and culturally relevant message. CHWs sometimes participate in the development of social marketing campaigns, and they often work in accompaniment with social marketing to reach specific audiences.

For example, the Food and Drug Administration has launched a national campaign focused on young people under 17 to stop smoking or prevent them from starting. "The Real Cost" campaign consists of online, radio, TV, and digital game interventions. While this campaign is relatively new and still in a long-term evaluation process, the goal of the social marketing campaign is to "reduce the number of youth cigarette smokers by at least 300,000 within three years" (www.therealcost.gov). Evaluating the effective of your social marketing campaign is a key component to ensuring effective outreach.

Another example of a more targeted kind of social marketing is the American Heart Association use of various media in their Power to End Stroke campaign (www.powertoendstroke.org), including celebrity endorsements and testimonials, contests, online games and assessment tools, social media networking, and community-building events. These efforts are culturally appropriate, highlighting the needs of African American communities at increased risk for high blood pressure and stroke (American Heart Association & American Stroke Association, n.d.).

- *Have you recently seen or heard a social marketing campaign?*
- *Where did you encounter the campaign (TV, radio, the Internet, social media, a poster, billboard, or pamphlet)?*
- *What health outcome did the campaign attempt to promote?*
- *Are you a member of the "target" audience?*
- *What do you think of the social marketing message?*
- *Is it effective for you?*

- Have you ever conducted health outreach to a particular community as a CHW or a volunteer?
- Have you ever been approached by an outreach worker?
- What have your experiences been like?

- How do you like to be approached by an outreach worker?
- How do you not want to be approached?
- What are your thoughts and feelings about conducting outreach yourself as a CHW?

19.6 Planning Health Outreach

Careful planning and preparation will enhance the quality of a health outreach program. At the end of this chapter, we will ask you to develop a preliminary health outreach plan for a community that you are already familiar with. Remember, a plan is not static: it should change as you analyze your work and learn from the community you are serving.

Outreach workers are often hired to work for a program that has already been designed, hopefully with extensive planning. In these circumstances, the priority population has already been determined, along with the health issue to be addressed, goals and objectives, and outreach methods. In other circumstances, CHWs will play an important role in developing the core elements of a health outreach plan.

Regardless of whether you are developing a new outreach program or working for an established one, it may be helpful to use some of the community diagnosis methods presented in Chapter 22 to inform your work. Your research should include reviewing existing documents (such as reports by a local health department) and conducting qualitative interviews with community members. It is particularly important to learn the history of the agency you work for and its reputation in the community, as well as the reputation of other projects that may have tried to use similar outreach methods or address similar health topics in the community. Identifying past successes and mistakes can allow you to avoid errors and can assist you to build and sustain positive relationships.

DEFINE THE COMMUNITY TO BE SERVED BY OUTREACH

To learn about the community you will be working with and its health status, review available literature and reports, including reports generated by state and local health departments. Seek out available epidemiological data that will provide you with an understanding of the prevalence of the health condition you are addressing. How many people are affected by the health issue? Which parts of the community are at greatest risk? Read local papers and Internet sources (web pages, online newsletters, newsfeeds, etc.) to find out what is currently happening in the community. The most important research you will do, however, is in and with the community. Take your time getting to know members of the community and talking with them about the work you plan to do. If possible:

Identify Key Opinion Leaders

These are the natural leaders found in all communities. They do not necessarily hold positions of formal authority, but have earned the respect and confidence of the community (for more information, see the following section on Conducting Health Outreach).

Identify Potential Outreach Sites

Identify sites where the people you hope to reach spend time. If you will conduct outreach in the community (rather than via social marketing or the Internet), conduct research and talk with community members to determine the locations where you will focus your first outreach efforts (these may include parks, schools, bars, churches, hair and nail salons and barber shops, homeless encampments, syringe exchanges, drug treatment programs, or soup kitchens, depending on the population you wish to reach). If you conduct research using technology, investigate possible websites or social media sites used by the community.

Visit Local Agencies and/or Agency Websites

Visit agencies and websites to find out about the services they provide: for example, health clinics, counseling programs, educational institutions, food pantries and soup kitchens, and shelters. Some benefits of face-to-face visits include initial relationship building, fostering coalitions, and maintaining contacts for future referrals.

- *Be sure you research an agency before your first visit so that you can maximize your time while you are at the site. Be prepared!*

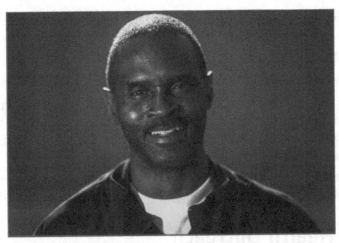

CHWs often conduct outreach in the community to link people with key resources and services.

Ramona Benson: I do street outreach and we have a flyer that talks about our services at the Black Infant Health Program. I also go out and visit local businesses and organizations like nail and beauty salons and churches. I tell them who I am and, if they have time, I tell them about our program. I ask if I can post my flyer or if they may want to pass it out. I always get some ladies that come to our program saying that they saw the flyer in their church or at a nail shop, so I know that it works to get the word out about our services.

IDENTIFY THE HEALTH ISSUE AND THE HEALTH OUTCOMES YOU WILL PROMOTE

Most outreach programs are funded to address one or more health issues such as breast cancer, hepatitis C, depression, re-entry after incarceration, or gun violence. Remember that the issues you are paid to focus on may not always be the greatest priority for the community you work with (we will address this later on in greater detail).

Your outreach efforts will be most effective if you are clear about the health outcomes you are trying to achieve. Is your goal to prevent further hepatitis C infections among injection drug users? Is it to promote testing for hepatitis C? To link people living with hepatitis C to treatment resources? All of the above? By defining your goals, and researching the health issue and the community, you can develop outreach strategies that are more likely to promote your desired outcomes. If some of your strategies aren't effective, you will be better prepared to adapt or develop new ones because you have a clear sense of what you want to accomplish.

Conduct Research about the Health Issue

A key part of your job will be to offer accurate information to community members. You need to fully understand the health issue's primary causes, consequences, available treatments, and methods for prevention. Be sure to research previous programs and outreach campaigns, if any, that addressed the same health issue in the same community. What did these programs do? What was the outcome? How did the community perceive these programs? Try to identity both the successes and the mistakes that were made by other programs, and do your best not to repeat the mistakes.

As you conduct health outreach, you will inevitably learn more about the community, and this information will guide you in revising your plan to respond to local needs, culture, and suggestions.

ORGANIZE THE OUTREACH TEAM

Take time to talk with your supervisor and colleagues in order to determine:

- The number of people you will need on the outreach team (are you going solo, or will you have a partner or two?)
- The key messages you wish to communicate to the community

- The materials you should bring to the site (written materials or pamphlets, business cards, safer health supplies, promotional materials, hygiene products, resource listings or directories, and so on)

- The referrals that you will provide

- The forms you will use to document your contacts with people and the services that you provide

- How will you dress when conducting outreach? (Casual clothing? Street clothes? Professional attire? An outreach shirt that identifies you as an outreach worker with your agency?) While this may seem like a trivial issue, how you dress often sends a message to the community. For more information about dress codes, please refer to Chapter 14.

- If you are providing outreach online or via social media, who will monitor responses and other postings, and how often? How often will you respond to the messages of others in order to build dialogue and relationships?

19.7 Conducting Health Outreach

This section discusses how to build relationships in the community, approach new clients, handle rejection, work as part of a team, manage outreach materials, and enhance your safety. While this section emphasizes outreach conducted in-person in the community, the key concepts can also be adapted and applied to conducting outreach via technology (such as social media).

BUILDING RELATIONSHIPS IN THE COMMUNITY

When you are conducting health outreach, the community will closely observe what you do and say, how you treat people, and if you remain true to your word. You need to be patient and work hard, providing the community with time to get to know and accept you. While this is particularly challenging for CHWs who work in communities that they are not a part of, even when you come from the same community you are serving, it may take time for your work to be understood and accepted.

When you are initiating a new health outreach project, begin by developing relationships with the community. Here are some suggestions for how to do this:

Contact People You Already Know

If you come from or are already familiar with the community, contact people you already know. Tell them about your new role as a CHW and the agency you are working for. Let them know what services you plan to provide and how you think these will benefit the community. Ask for their feedback and their advice about how to get your message and services out to the community. Ask for their assistance in making introductions to key opinion leaders.

Identify Key Opinion Leaders in the Community

Don't assume that you already know who they are. Key opinion leaders are not always those with formal authority (such as elected leaders), but are the people in every neighborhood and community whom others listen to, respect, and turn to for advice. If, for example, your job is to conduct outreach to homeless and runaway youth, observe and ask whom they most respect and turn to for guidance and support. Introduce yourself, explain the work you will be doing, and ask for their guidance about building relationships in the community. Take time getting to know these opinion leaders, and when the moment is right, ask them for their support and guidance regarding your outreach work: ask for their advice regarding how, when, and where to conduct health outreach in the community. Remember that relationships require constant nurturing: keep returning to visit these key opinion leaders and to continue this dialogue. Keep a confidential list of these key contacts and where to find them.

If you are conducting outreach via social media, you will also identify and build relationships with key opinion leaders, learning from the information they provide and the suggestions they may make.

Network with the Community

Network at local events and meetings and let people know what services you offer. Bring business cards and be prepared to introduce yourself clearly and quickly and explain your role as a CHW. You will need to repeat this information many times before people begin to understand who you are and what you will be doing.

Identify Community Agencies that Share Common Goals

Introduce yourself, explain what you will be doing, and explore options for strategic partnership and collaboration. For example, you may refer clients to their agency. Other agencies, in turn, may invite you to conduct outreach to community groups that they work with.

Organize a Community Forum

Work with key opinion leaders to organize a community forum to introduce yourself and your program. Invite as many people as you can. Make sure that you advertise the forum well. You can print flyers to announce the forum and carry these with you so that you can hand them out at every opportunity.

Encourage Community Involvement

Let people know that their guidance and suggestions are welcome. Let them know how they might be able to volunteer or become more involved with your program and your outreach work. Invite them to come to your agency to find out more about your services.

Listen and Observe

Your first priority should be to get to know people. Remember the diagram of the client-centered CHW with big ears and big eyes: you shouldn't be doing most of the talking. Create an actual or virtual space for community members to share information, concerns, and opinions with you. Ask them what they know about the health problem you will be addressing, the key resources in the community, and whom they think you should be talking with.

Be Patient

Don't push your agenda. Your top priority should be to listen to what the community says is important.

Keep Your Promises

If you say that you will show up at a certain location at a certain time—or post new information on a specific date—follow through with these expectations. Unfortunately, the communities you serve are likely to recall a long list of broken promises from health and social service providers—don't add to this list!

Be Respectful and Follow Through with Commitments

Send thank-you cards or emails expressing your appreciation for the community support.

- *What else have you learned about how to build effective relationships in the community?*

Alvaro Morales: For day laborers, I found out that doing outreach early in the morning wasn't a good time because this was when they were trying to find a job. The end of the day wasn't the best either, because some people were gone and those who are still there are frustrated about not finding work. So I found out the middle of the day was the best time to go. I also learned that I need to do outreach regularly so that people will get to know me and we can build trust. In the Latino community, if you find somebody who has already been working there and you can partner with them, then you will save a lot of time earning that trust. For day laborers, trust is also something that you have to maintain. Because if you stop coming, then it seems like you have to start rebuilding it all over again. That's what is so hard when you're working on a grant because the grant might end and you have to stop services. Then maybe the grant will be renewed, and you have to start up all over again.

HOW TO APPROACH NEW OUTREACH CONTACTS

When you are approaching someone for the first time, do what comes naturally—introduce yourself. At most outreach locations, you will be able to make a full introduction. Speak clearly and with a friendly, welcoming tone. Let the person know your name, which agency you represent, and why you are at the outreach location.

> Hi, I'm Janet from the Center City Health Center. I work with a breast cancer prevention project, and I'm out here tonight to let people know about the services we can provide.

Depending on the circumstances, you may or may not have a chance to share more information. Be ready to continue a conversation and to share information about health issues and your services. At the same time, be ready to back off if you need to—don't be too pushy. Be respectful of people's time and interests: they may not have the time at the moment to speak with you. If the person appears to be in a hurry, or if the outreach site is in a difficult setting, keep your message simple and brief. Distribute outreach materials if appropriate.

Every outreach setting really *is* unique. Because of this, it is important for you to learn as much as possible about the setting and the community before your first visit. If you are providing outreach in a new setting, you may feel nervous. If the location becomes a site for regular outreach, you will adapt and tailor your approach with time, gaining confidence. You will begin to recognize some of the community members and develop ongoing conversations and relationships. If you are preparing to conduct outreach online or through social media, take time to visit and explore the site and the technology before you begin. Pay attention to what people are talking about. What are their key concerns and priorities?

Depending on the outreach site and the target population, you may develop creative ways to gain access and acceptance into the community you are attempting to reach. For example, consider the following methods.

Expand your message and your outreach to *address more generalized needs* of the community. If you are providing outreach to migrant farm workers, brainstorm and network with people at the site to find out what they need. Do they need food, clothing, or school supplies for their children? You may be able to provide some things that are really needed at this location, even if these items have not been explicitly stated as part of your outreach services and goals. Network with other agencies in your city or seek donations of some of the items that are needed at the camp. By meeting some of the basic needs of the priority community, you will accomplish several goals at once. Not only will you provide important resources, but you will also build relationships with members of the community so that you can work with them more closely each time you visit their camp.

Training Outreach Workers at City College of San Francisco

At City College of San Francisco, we offered a course on conducting health outreach. During the first month, we divided students into teams of two. Each team was provided with a backpack full of HIV prevention materials, and given 10 minutes to go out on campus, introduce themselves to someone they do not know, and asked to initiate a conversation related to HIV issues.

When students are preparing to conduct outreach for the first time, they often feel nervous, embarrassed, or worried about whether or not they will be able to initiate a conversation with anyone. Once the students return to the classroom, they analyze their experience and the factors that made it easier or harder to connect with potential clients. As a final assignment, the students design and manage a three-hour campus outreach event that reaches hundreds of students. With repetition, the students gain confidence and skills in approaching potential clients. They learn to relax, have fun, and focus on their successes rather than their disappointments.

Break the ice with humor, games, or fun interactive exercises. At City College of San Francisco, outreach workers have used a variety of participatory activities such as the Spinning Wheel Game and a Talking Wall. The Spinning Wheel Game is a large colorful wheel that CHWs set up in a prominent location.

Outreach workers invite people to spin the wheel, which will land on a number that is matched to a question about a health issue (such as diabetes or nutrition). As other people gather round to see what is happening, the CHWs are able to facilitate discussions about related topics such as "What types of food and drink are best for preventing chronic conditions like high blood pressure?" or "Name two locations on campus where you can buy fresh whole fruits and vegetables." Players are provided with prizes whether they win or lose.

The Talking Wall is simply a big piece of paper—we have used paper as large as 10 feet high by 15 feet wide—with a series of provocative questions or quotes, and colorful pens also and markers available so that people can add their own comments and questions, building a dialogue through their posts. Typically, the wall focuses discussion on particular topics or themes, such as "What are health factors that contribute to diabetes in our communities?" As the wall fills up with anonymous comments and opinions, CHWs stand by to talk with participants, pass out health materials, and make referrals.

Hold an event in the community you are trying to reach. Work with your outreach team and volunteers to come up with something that will be fun. Make sure that the event allows members of the target population to participate in a way that will energize them so that they will want to get involved. Members of the Queer Youth Action Team (QYAT) in Contra Costa County, California, hosted barbeques with free food that provided lesbian, gay, bisexual, transgender, queer, questioning, and intersex youth with a safe and fun place to socialize. The CHWs were identified by colorful QYAT T-shirts, and they arranged a table with HIV prevention resources for those who were interested. They took a quiet approach to outreach and let the youth choose to initiate conversations about HIV prevention, and most did.

Don't force yourself to do things that make you uncomfortable. If you are having difficulty approaching people you don't know, be aware that this discomfort will subside in time. If you continue to have difficulty, speak with your supervisor or coworkers and listen to their suggestions.

HANDLING REJECTION

When you conduct health outreach, most people will respect your role and your contributions. But not everyone will be interested in what you have to offer, be welcoming, or act polite. Expect and prepare to handle *a lot* of rejection as an outreach worker.

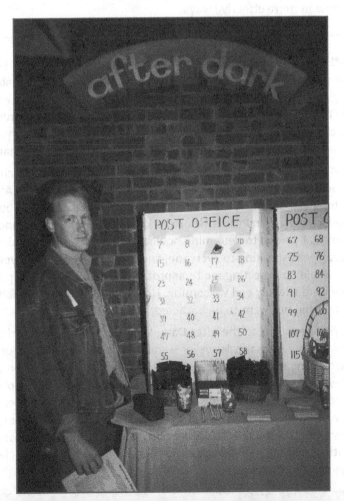

A CHW facilitates a "post-office" game at a community event to encourage people to approach his outreach table.

- *Have you ever encountered a pushy outreach worker or sales representative who didn't take no for an answer?*

- *Have you ever been followed down the street by someone who wanted to give you a flyer, ask you to sign a petition, or sell you something?*

- *What do you think of these strategies?*

- *How do they make you feel?*

Many people don't like to be approached by strangers, for a variety of reasons. If you continue to bother a prospective outreach contact after they have clearly indicated, by their words or actions, that they are not interested in speaking with you, you risk making a strong and lasting negative impression that could hurt future efforts to conduct outreach in the community. If potential outreach contacts try to ignore you or avoid you, *don't pursue them.* If they let you know that they aren't interested (by shaking their head or saying something like "I don't have time" or "I'm not interested"), consider saying something brief and polite, and move on immediately. Remember that you are likely to return to the same locations again and again, and therefore to encounter the same people in the future: leave a positive and professional impression. At a future visit to this location, you may very well have a chance to interact with the person who could not speak with you today.

Some people will be rude or disrespectful. *Try not to take it personally.* Even if a prospective contact is angry or says something vulgar or disrespectful to you (this *will* happen!), don't retaliate in kind. Keep your professionalism and your dignity. When you get a chance, debrief these encounters with a colleague, supervisor, friend, or family member. Vent your feelings in a safe place, and never with the clients and communities you work with. One angry outburst or nasty comment to a prospective client may quickly become news in the community and seriously damage your reputation.

With time, you will find that your skills as an outreach worker become more developed and fine-tuned. Encountering rejection and indifference will aid you in learning to tailor your outreach messages and interactions to reach more people in more effective ways.

Craig Wenzl: When I first began working at the Monterey County AIDS Project as a CHW doing outreach in the gay community, I thought people would be happy to hear about HIV prevention and antibody testing. But I found out right away that this wasn't always true. I was new to the community, so people didn't know me. I had to "prove" myself in order to gain their trust. At first, I was uncomfortable approaching people I didn't know at bars, events, and community gatherings. However, after doing outreach in the community a few times, I began to figure out what did and didn't work.

One method that worked well for me was to make sure that I approached and spoke with everyone at an outreach setting. For example, when providing outreach at the After Dark Bar, I started at one end of the busy bar, speaking with each patron with an introductory but nonintrusive message. I would introduce myself and ask if he or she knew about my agency and our programs. I would take the cue from that person to determine how far my interaction with him or her would go at that time. Because I was speaking to everyone, and I was aware that everyone was watching me, I knew that people would be expecting me to approach them. This gave the patrons a chance to prepare. Most people were friendly and welcoming. However, a few were unfriendly and abrupt and let me know that they did not want to be bothered.

During my first few visits to the After Dark, I was put off by the reactions of people who appeared to reject me and my message. However—and here is the key—many of those same people who initially rejected my message, later welcomed the opportunity to open up and discuss their personal interest in the topic of HIV/AIDS. I found out that many of the people who had appeared to reject me from the start were doing so because they had very close personal experience with HIV/AIDS. Either they were HIV-positive or living with AIDS, or they had a close family member, partner, or friend who was living with or had passed away from the disease. I learned the importance of being patient and not making any assumptions about prospective clients, especially those who initially rejected my approach.

RECOGNIZE AND ACKNOWLEDGE YOUR LIMITATIONS AND MISTAKES

As a CHW, you will be confronted with questions that you don't know how to answer, and situations that you are not sure how to handle. Don't be afraid to acknowledge the limits of your knowledge and skills to clients or coworkers. Rather than try to answer a question when you are not confident in your response, say that you don't know. Choose your own words and say something along the lines of: "I don't know" or "I'm not certain about that" or "I don't want to tell you anything that may not be true. Let me research this question when I get back to the office, and next time I see you, I'll let you know what I have learned." Trust us: You will need these words often!

Many of the clients you work with have suffered from prejudice, discrimination, isolation, loss, or abuse. These experiences often influence their interaction with helping professionals, and they may be watching, waiting, and expecting you to be yet another person who lets them down in some way. Inevitably, despite your best efforts and intentions, you will disappoint some potential outreach contacts and clients. For example, you might arrive late for an appointment, run out of food vouchers, forget an important detail that client told you about their life, misinterpret a statement that a client makes, make an incorrect assumption, or say or write something that triggers previous bad experiences for a client. These are natural, common, and inevitable mistakes that we all make at some point in our careers.

As a result of these types of mistakes, some clients will stop working with you and may avoid you and your agency in the future. Others may show their disappointment or anger and say something about your conduct. We encourage you to view these moments as an opportunity to repair and perhaps deepen the working relationship. A sincere apology often has remarkable power to defuse and transform anger and conflict (see Chapter 13 for more information about the power of apology). It shows that you are a fallible human being who makes mistakes, not someone who thinks that you are better than your client. An apology communicates your commitment, your desire to be supportive, and your intention to treat your clients with the respect they deserve. In many cases, it will actually result in renewed trust for the working relationship and open up dialogue that will assist you get to know your clients in a deeper way.

What words do you use when you apologize or otherwise take responsibility for doing something you wish you hadn't done? Don't apologize simply because someone suggested it to you as a professional technique: whatever you say, *it has to be authentic.*

For example:

> *I'm sorry I showed up late. I know your time is valuable, and I want you to know that I will always do my best to get here on time.*

Or:

> *I apologize. I really didn't express myself very well. I didn't mean to say that I understood what you are going through. What I want to say is that I'd like to learn about your experience and to see how I can best be supportive to you.*

We all make mistakes and do things that are hurtful to others. It is important to own your mistake and acknowledge the client's feelings that may come up as a result. Repairing a mistake can be a critical part of building a relationship with your client/contact. Respectfully saying "I'm sorry" to a client does not necessarily mean that you knowingly did something wrong. But an apology can aid in repairing a misunderstanding or conflict and provide you and the client with an opportunity to move forward in your work. Successfully managing a challenging conversation can strengthen the working relationship between client and provider.

If you haven't viewed it before, you may wish to watch the short video interview about the power of apology, included in Chapter 13.

What Do YOU Think?

- *What are your experiences with and beliefs about apologies?*

- *Are you someone who can apologize easily, or is it difficult for you?*

- *Can you think of a time when you gave or received an apology that aided in strengthening a relationship?*

- *If you have difficulty apologizing, what is it that gets in the way?*

- *What could assist you to learn how to offer a sincere apology to a client?*

YOUR REPUTATION AS AN OUTREACH WORKER

As you conduct health outreach, you will get to know and begin to feel a part of the community in which you are working. People will begin to recognize you and associate you with your work and your agency. Your reputation, both on and off the clock, will follow you wherever you go in the community, and will become one of your most important professional resources. When we asked senior CHWs how they have built and maintained positive reputations in the communities they serve, they shared ideas for what to do—and what not to do:

Table 19.1 Guidelines for Building a Positive Reputation

DON'T	DO
Don't break confidentiality in any way. This is the quickest way to end your career.	Let the client know that your discussions are confidential and be transparent about sharing information that may not be. Maintain confidential client information including notes, discussions, disclosure forms, etc.
Don't ever act like you are better than anyone else, talk down to them, or criticize anyone behind their back.	Treat everyone with equal dignity and respect.
Don't pretend to be something or someone you are not. The community will always see through your act and you will lose their respect.	Be clear about your role as a CHW, and acknowledge your own strengths and limitations. Act and speak in a way that is authentic to who you are.
Don't make things up. If you don't know about a particular topic or how to answer a question, just explain this to the community.	Be honest and do your best to get the information needed by your client and follow up as appropriate. You can say, "I'm not sure about that, but I will do research and get back to you."
Don't spend all of your time speaking with *one* outreach contact. Other people may want to speak with you, and they may feel ignored if you don't give them a chance to interact with you.	Spend your outreach time wisely and reach as many members of a community as possible without compromising the quality of your interactions.
Don't discriminate against any part of the priority population you are serving. As an outreach worker, your duty is to provide services and information to *everyone* you interact with—not just the ones you are more comfortable speaking to or the ones you would *rather* approach. Review your own reporting data to make sure that you aren't leaving anyone out—for example, are you serving women as well as men, Latinos as well as African Americans?	Be mindful of *all* people around you, and be sure not to ignore, miss, or leave anyone out!
Don't pick sides when the community you are working with is in conflict.	Stay neutral, to the extent possible, and work to maintain positive relationships with all sectors of the community.
Don't rush through engagements with people who want to speak with you.	Take the time to listen to and be kind to everyone you interact with. When you have to cut a conversation short, do so as politely as possible.
Don't make promises you can't keep. It can damage your reputation if clients feel that you do not keep your word or care enough to follow through with promises.	Know your limitations and your scope of practice. Refer clients or contacts to other professionals or relevant programs and services.
Don't flirt or have inappropriate conversations. This may be perceived as sexually charged, inappropriate, unprofessional, or unwanted.	Be friendly and professional but also mindful when a conversation is moving in a direction that it should not. Interrupt conversations that cross a line. Steer them back to an appropriate topic, or find a polite way to end the conversation.

(continues)

Table 19.1 (*Continued*)

DON'T	DO
Don't use language that is unfamiliar to the community (such as *epidemiology*): everything you want to say can be communicated using language that is accessible to your audience.	Use language that is accessible to the community. Be mindful of the words and terms that you and your colleagues use among outreach contacts. Stop to clarify any confusion or misinformation.
Don't ignore a mistake you may have made. Don't argue or try to prove that you are "right."	Apologize if you mess up or make a mistake. Owning your mistake is critical to building and strengthening your relationship with clients.
Don't push your own agenda on clients.	Listen to the immediate needs and priorities of contacts and clients. If you are talking about prostate cancer and the client is telling you he is hungry, listen to him and see if there is anything you can do to help him out. Maybe there is a soup kitchen or food pantry nearby. If you assist clients with their priorities, then they will be ready to listen to yours.
Don't forget or violate your code of ethics! For example, do not sleep with clients, do drugs with them, or give them money.	Maintain ethical and legal boundaries that support your work as a CHW.

SAFETY ISSUES

Keep in mind that some members of the community may view you with suspicion or fear, and treat you as an outsider or intruder. This is one of many reasons that it is so essential to take the time to get to know the community you will be working in, and to build respectful relationships with key opinion leaders.

Depending upon the type of outreach you are providing, safety may or may not be a major consideration. Safety issues and concerns may include:

- Losing sight of your outreach partner
- Injuring yourself in dark or dimly lit areas
- Witnessing illegal or underground activities such as selling or using drugs
- Unintentional involvement in police actions
- Witnessing arguments, threats, or violence (such as incidents of domestic violence)
- Encountering an angry, aggressive, or threatening person
- Experiencing harassment, including sexual harassment
- Theft and assault

- *Can you think of additional safety concerns?*

Your job as a CHW is to provide services to the most vulnerable and at-risk communities, such as homeless and runaway youth, injection-drug users, people returning home from prison, or people living with chronic mental illness. Often society stigmatizes these communities, and others fear them and assume they are dangerous. *Sometimes your own prejudices may influence your assessment of safety issues. Try to be aware of the tendency for this to happen and guard against discriminating against clients or communities that have already been harmed in this way. Remember that safety issues are present in any work setting and with clients of all backgrounds.*

Chapter 11 discusses safety issues in relation to home visiting and presents safety tips that apply to conducting health outreach as well. Review the safety discussion in that chapter. Here, we present additional tips and issues that are specific to doing outreach.

If you are conducting in-person outreach in the community, work with a partner or outreach team. Keep your teammates within view at all times, and check in with each other regularly. Develop a system to "signal" one another if you need some assistance, whether it be a hand signal or a code phrase ("Hey, Marcos, did you *call Dr. Standing*?") and come together immediately after the signal is given. Keep cell phones with you if possible, and keep them turned on with the sounds/notifications on for receiving text messages in case a colleague tries to reach you this way. Always allow for quick communication with other team members if you or someone else should run into a difficult situation. Listen to your instincts, which will develop over time, and pay attention to them when you feel particularly ill at ease, anxious, or unsafe.

If you find yourself in the midst of a conflict, try to de-escalate the situation using conflict resolution skills (Chapter 13). If necessary, ask your team members for assistance. Here is where a code phrase or hand signal can come in handy ("*Call Dr. Standing*"). If the situation is too intense, however, shout out for assistance. If no other team members respond and the situation is dangerous and immediate, ask for assistance from *anyone* who is nearby and might be able to assist you. If you don't see any hope for calming the situation, *leave*. Document the incident thoroughly, report it to your supervisor, and debrief it with someone you trust. *Only call the police if it is absolutely required.* Most situations will not require such a drastic measure. You want to avoid bringing the police into a community that has a history of tensions with the law (that is, injection drug or other substance users, sex workers, and so on). You could find yourself losing the trust and respect of this community.

> **Kent Rodriguez:** I always found that doing outreach with at least someone else or in a small group of no more than three people always made it easier to approach people. Safety was not an issue because someone could maintain a lookout at our surroundings while we distributed supplies. Never go out alone.
>
> Having some established "safe" words when doing outreach is a good idea. I remember my volunteers, and I had one that was as easy as "let's get coffee." If someone mentioned this at any point during outreach, we all knew that one of us was uncomfortable in the current situation and that we needed to move on.
>
> Do not be afraid to walk away from a situation that makes you feel unsafe. Make sure to take care of yourself first. This includes debriefing after outreach sessions. Talk to those you are working with about any feelings or thoughts that come up. Allow yourself time to process anything that comes up for you.

TIPS FOR SUCCESSFUL TEAMWORK

We strongly encourage CHWs to work with a partner or as a part of an outreach team for a variety reasons:

- It is safer to work in a team.
- You can reach a larger number of clients.
- You can provide more than one service at the same time (for example, some CHWs can conduct general outreach in a club, and others may provide confidential risk-reduction counseling or screening services in a more private area).
- The more diverse the outreach team, the more choice you offer potential clients. For example, a team with CHWs of various ages may provide greater comfort and access to clients who may prefer to speak with someone closer to their age.

Successful teamwork often comes down to good communication. When conducting health outreach with a partner or team, here are a few tips for working together:

- Meet with your team to clarify your goals, objectives, expectations, and the policies and protocols that will guide your work.
- Make time to review and discuss your outreach plan together, including locations, outreach materials, and referrals you will provide.

- Develop a system for responding to safety concerns, including a code that will alert you and your partners to potential danger.
- Ask for and listen to the ideas and opinions of your teammates.
- Be patient with your colleagues.
- Accept and respect the different experiences, cultural perspectives, and opinions of your partners.
- Give your teammates the benefit of the doubt: assume that they have good intentions, even when you may be upset by the consequences of their actions.
- Assert your opinions clearly, calmly, and respectfully.
- Be ready and willing to compromise.
- Learn to accept critical feedback from others without getting defensive. When you make mistakes, apologize.
- Learn to provide critical feedback to others in a way that demonstrates your respect for them. (See the section on constructive feedback in Chapter 14.)
- Make time to debrief your work together after every shift. Share your successes and your challenges. Make plans to improve aspects of your teamwork that didn't go as well as you had hoped. Look for and acknowledge the positive contributions of teammates and outcomes of your collaborative efforts.

DEVELOPING AND MANAGING OUTREACH MATERIALS

CHWs use a variety of outreach materials in the course of their work. For example, a CHW conducting street or community outreach to reduce the risks of HIV disease may carry a backpack with materials such as condoms, lubricants, safer sex guidelines, and a list of local resources for testing, counseling, and health care. Lists of resources may also be stored in a mobile phone or other digital device for ready access.

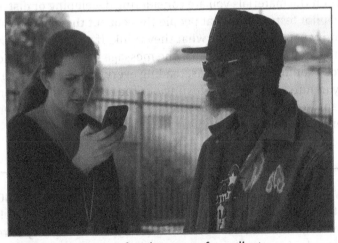

A CHW checks on a referral resource for a client.

Outreach materials may include printed brochures, pamphlets, flyers, posters, and referral cards; health promotion books, booklets, viewing, listening, or display; promotional materials such as key chains, pens, cups, toys, tote bags, and so on that have your agency logo and contact information printed on them; food, clothing, hygiene materials (toothpaste, toothbrushes, soap, and so on), or other items that are needed by members of the priority community. Of course, outreach materials may also be digital, such as the messages, graphics, videos and other resources posted online and shared via social media.

Depending on your agency and your program, you will find that some materials work better than others with your priority audience. You will want to develop a tailored mix of outreach materials that you can take to different venues or distribute in other ways.

You should plan your collection of materials carefully, based on the demographics and needs of the priority population. Trial and error will guide you as you determine what has and hasn't worked in prior visits to that site or to similar sites. Most importantly, ask the community you are serving what they think about the materials you are using. They can help tailor your outreach for optimal success.

Additionally your agency may be able to provide incentives for community members that will support your outreach efforts. These could be gift certificates, food vouchers, or stipends in exchange for community member participation in events, services, or research.

Making the Most of Outreach Materials

A CHW conducting outreach to the homeless always made a point of carrying clean socks in his backpack. Many of his clients slept on the streets and in parks and lacked clean, warm clothes, and they truly appreciated a pair of clean socks. By providing clean socks, he was able to start off a new relationship by offering something valuable to a client. This was often useful in creating an opportunity to start other conversations. For example, if a client pointed to the backpack and asked, "What else do you have in there?" the CHW was able to talk about the full range of services that he could provide.

Keep your outreach materials well organized. Be sure that they are up-to-date and undamaged. For example, make sure that none of the condoms you carry have passed their expiration date. Giving a client outdated or damaged goods is a sure way to damage their trust in you.

Often, CHWs participate in the development of new outreach materials such as flyers, brochures, or resource guides. When developing any outreach materials, or using those produced by other sources, be sure to pay close attention to the content and the messages being provided. Gather members of the priority population and ask for their input and opinions on the materials you are considering developing or distributing. Coordinate focus groups (see Chapter 23) and pilot tests to see what people think about the materials. Collaborate with other agencies who serve the priority population to see what they think. If you are purchasing or otherwise acquiring materials produced by another source, make sure that the message is culturally appropriate for your priority population(s). Make sure you examine the materials, reading every page of the brochures, reviewing websites thoroughly, watching every minute of the videos, testing out the equipment and promotional materials, and so on. The last thing you want to do is discover that you have been handing out materials that are offensive or inaccurate. Offensive materials are worse than none at all.

Craig Wenzl: When I started working as a CHW at the Monterey County AIDS Project, I once made the mistake of handing out materials that hadn't been approved or tested locally beforehand. There were some materials that had been produced by another agency to reach young African American men at risk of contracting HIV/ AIDS. I didn't read through the entire collection of materials (a series of brochures)—bad mistake!

One night when I was facilitating a small group, one of the members—an African American man—took one of the brochures out of his pocket and read it to me. He said it was offensive because it used language that he could not relate to and was clearly targeted to a more urban setting and most likely a more " East Coast " setting. As a group, we examined the materials and agreed that they weren't right for the local African American community.

This example illustrates the importance of localizing your materials if you are borrowing from another agency. Be sure to gather members of the target population together and find out what they think about the materials before you distribute them. You might be surprised at what you hear in the discussion.

19.8 Documenting Health Outreach Services

One of the most important tasks of outreach work is the documentation of the services you provide. Documentation of health outreach services has become increasingly important for a variety of reasons:

- Documentation can show what you've accomplished, and if you have met program goals and objectives.
- It provides data that can be used to find additional funding to continue or expand the program.
- It reveals the history of the program and builds a timeline of program development.
- The information gathered can assist your agency and others to develop plans to better promote the health of the community in the future.
- It enables you to be accountable to funders including, in the case of public funding, the general public (taxpayers).
- Documentation makes it possible to evaluate your program. Data are gathered in order to:
  - Determine who you have and have not reached, and highlight opportunities to reach underserved segments of the community
  - Analyze the strategies and resources, including technology, that have been most and least effective in reaching the priority community and promoting desired outcomes
  - Better understand the clients and communities served
  - Refine and improve the quality of services provided
  - Guard against discriminatory practices, such as the exclusion of certain groups from programs and services
  - Advocate for the continuation and expansion of necessary services
  - Provide evidence that can assist others to develop similar programs and services

- *Can you think of other reasons why documentation is so important?*

> **Kent Rodriquez:** When I first started doing outreach, I hated all the paperwork I had to do. I felt like all these forms just got in the way of my work, and it just took time away from building relationships in the community or talking to my clients. I didn't really understand what happened after I turned the forms in to my supervisor or how the information would be used.

Depending on the agency you work for, you may be asked to provide a weekly, monthly, quarterly, or annual report. You may have a supervisor who completes some of these reports for the program. Whatever your particular requirements, it is a good idea to keep track of *every* outreach session you complete. Use the outreach tracking forms your agency provides, or talk with your supervisor about creating such a form (increasingly these are digital forms that permit you to enter data on a computer, tablet, smart phone, or other digital device). Your agency will maintain some form of database or a calculating or totaling system to keep track of the numbers and demographics of outreach contacts. This is especially helpful if you provide outreach many times throughout the month or to a large number of different contacts. Also, you will need a simplified method of totaling the number of contacts and other services you provide in order to prepare accurate, detailed reports and to determine if you are reaching program goals.

In order for the documentation to be useful, data about the outreach services you provide are likely to include the following types of information:

- The date and time when the outreach was provided
- Outreach location(s) including physical places and addresses as well as online "locations"

- The names of the outreach worker(s)
- A count or estimate of the number of people you reached and their demographic profile:

  Often you will be asked to record demographic information about the identities of the people you serve, such as their sex, ethnicity, age, substance use, sexual orientation, homeless or marginally housed, or health status. You won't always be able to gather this information. Sometimes, you will be asked to make an educated guess about the identities of those to whom you conduct outreach, but be careful not to jump into stereotypes or assumptions. Ask for guidance about how to do this from experienced CHWs and your supervisor.

- Key services provided, if any (such as HIV antibody test counseling or health education)
- The number and type of supplies, materials, brochures, and so on that you distributed
- Key referrals provided
- Any outstanding problems or challenges encountered (such as conflicts or complaints)
- Other information that is required for your specific program

We don't recommend that you fill out outreach reports as you talk with clients, as it is likely to distract you from focusing on your interaction with them and may harm your relationship (this type of documentation is different from what you will do when you provide care management or client-centered counseling services). However, don't wait too long before you document the services that you provide. Take time during each day to stop and document your work: you won't be able to remember the details later on.

19.9 Ethics and Health Outreach

Because of the independent nature of their work, outreach workers frequently face ethical challenges, including:

- Requests for food, money, vouchers, or transportation
- Offers of gifts, sex, or drugs
- Witnessing violence, including incidents of domestic violence
- Maintaining confidentiality when working in public places
- Developing personal relationships with clients, including romantic relationships

For this reason we strongly encourage you to anticipate and prepare to respond to common ethical challenges. Review the section on ethics in Chapter 7. Talk with more experienced CHWs to learn how they handle these situations, and consult with your supervisor. Be ready to clearly explain your policies to clients—what you can and cannot do, and in some instances, why. For example, be prepared to explain the following to clients:

- Why you cannot give or loan them money
- Why you cannot accept gifts
- Why you cannot develop personal relationships with them, including romantic or sexual relationships
- Why you need to preserve confidentiality, and the exceptions to this policy (specific types of harm to the client or harm to others)
- That you don't know the answer to a relevant question, but will do your best to find out

To be successful in your career as a CHW, you will need to develop strong professional boundaries that protect both you and your clients (again, please refer to 7). Be prepared to set and maintain your limits and to stand behind them. You will often have to say "no" to clients or otherwise communicate that you cannot provide a service or type of assistance they have asked for. Some clients won't accept the boundaries you attempt to establish and may continue to push for what they want. For example, a client might say something like: "I haven't had anything to eat in two days! Can't you just give me a little cash to get something to eat this one time? I won't tell anyone about it."

Try not to let yourself get placed in a defensive position, or to spend too much time repeating your ethical obligations and professional policies to clients. Find ways to refocus the conversation on the client's issues and on the services that you *can* offer. For example, you could say: "I'm sorry, as we discussed before I can't give you money, but I can walk with you to the food kitchen which opens soon. Do you know the staff there?"

Make sure to maintain your professionalism at all times: handling these challenges with grace and compassion often results in renewed trust and the opportunity to do more substantive work with a client. If you are unable to change the focus of the conversation or the client becomes increasingly assertive or aggressive, remember that you can always walk away from the encounter. If you need to do this, however, don't do it in anger. Explain yourself clearly, calmly, and politely.

Sometimes CHWs complain that clients are trying to "manipulate" them. We encourage you to reframe the way you think about this. It may be helpful to remember that for some clients, what you perceive as manipulation is how they have learned to get the resources they need in order to survive. For some clients, these strategies may be connected to drug or alcohol use. Try not to take a client's behavior personally: it isn't about you. Respect the autonomy of your clients to make their own choices, and remember that you can only control your own words and behavior. Practice the words you will use to end an encounter with a client when you feel the need to walk away. How will you explain this in ways that asserts your own professional boundaries and preserves their dignity?

Lee Jackson: I don't lend money to my clients. Sometimes they'll ask me to lend them money and say they'll pay me back double or something like that. I explain what my job is and what my boundaries are. I tell them: "I'm not a loan shark, I'm a health worker. I'm here to get you to your appointments and make sure you're okay and get you back on your feet, and if you need housing we'll help get you housing, but I can't loan you money." Sometimes I have to break it down in a street manner and explain it to them, and they understand because then I ask them, "Do you enjoy me working with you?" If they say Yes then I'll say: "If I start breaking the laws, then I will lose my job and then there's a possibility that me and you will have to go to these agencies together because I'll be looking for a job also." So they understand. It's all in the way you explain things.

19.10 Supervision and Support

CHWs often work independently, outside of an office setting, and outreach is not always well understood or appreciated by supervisors. Depending on your agency and your program, you may or may not receive regular supervision.

While we hope that each of you has the opportunity to work with a knowledgeable and supportive supervisor, the truth is that not all supervisors have the skills necessary to provide effective guidance and support to CHWs. Despite this, you have a professional responsibility to do your best to develop and maintain a positive working relationship with your supervisor. A positive relationship with your supervisor is essential to doing effective work, preventing stress and burnout, and maximizing your job satisfaction and opportunities for advancement. Ask for regular meetings with your supervisor and take the opportunity to inform them about your accomplishments as well as the challenges that you face in the field. Remember to turn in documentation of your work in a timely fashion.

When you face an immediate challenge and do not have a supervisor (or another coworker) nearby to consult, rely on what you have learned about ethics, safety, and representing your agency. You will not always know how best to respond to problems that arise in the field. Sometimes, it is better and safer to remove yourself from a situation as soon as possible rather than to try to respond or resolve it in the moment. When this occurs, document what happened and report to your supervisor as soon as possible. (For more information about supervision, see Chapter 14).

Because CHWs do a lot of outreach work in such an independent fashion, they may feel isolated and wish for more professional support. Other CHWs will best understand the nature of the challenges that you face and are best equipped to provide meaningful support in terms of how to handle the stresses of the job and to enhance the quality of services that you provide. Try to identify someone you trust to talk with about the challenges you face on the job. Our recommendation is to seek out a mentor who has years of experience conducting health outreach. This senior CHW may work at your same agency or with another organization. In many parts of the country and around the world, CHWs have formed local support groups that provide them with an opportunity to meet regularly with peers. These groups function both as a source of support and of ongoing professional development.

Chapter Review

To review the concepts and competencies covered in this chapter, we would like you to develop a health outreach plan for a community that you belong to and know well. Please do your best to complete the following worksheet based on what you already know about your community and the information presented in this chapter.

1. Select a community that you know well. Define the community to be served (ethnicity and other demographics, location, and so on). Be as specific as possible.

2. Define the health issue to be addressed by the outreach program.

3. What is the objective of your outreach program (what do you want to accomplish as a result of the outreach services provided)?

4. Who are the key opinion leaders in the community? How will you identify others? What are three questions that you would like to ask these key opinion leaders?

5. Identify actual or virtual (online) places (such as social media sites) where you can reach and contact community members.

6. List three institutions that are respected by the community that you can work with:

7. What outreach level might you use to conduct your outreach?

8. Which types of outreach methods would you select?

9. What types of outreach messages or materials will you share with the community?

10. What types of information will you gather to document the outreach services you provide? How might this information be used to improve the quality of your program?

References

American Heart Association and the American Stroke Association. (n.d.) Retrieved from *www.powertoendstroke.org*

The Community Initiative. (n.d.). Retrieved from *http://thecommunityinitiative.org/*

Mission Housing Development Corporation. (n.d.). Retrieved from *www.missionhousing.org/03_resident-services.php*

U.S. Health and Human Services (USHHS). (n.d) FLU.gov. Retrieved from *www.flu.gov*

University of California San Francisco (UCSF). (n.d.). *Mpowerment*. Retrieved from Center for AIDS Prevention Services, *http://caps.ucsf.edu/mpowerment*

Additional Resources

Affordable Care Act. (n.d.). Retrieved from *www.healthcare.gov*

Asian Health Services. (n.d.). Retrieved from *www.asianhealthservices.org*

Bourne, A. (March 2011). Social marketing and HIV prevention. *Making It Count Briefing Sheet 6, Sigma Research*. Retrieved from *http://makingitcount.org.uk/files/MiC-briefing-6-SocialMarketing.pdf*

The Center for AIDS Prevention Studies at the University of California, San Francisco. (n.d.). Retrieved from *www.caps.ucsf.edu*

Centers for Disease Control and Prevention. (2012). *The road to better health. A guide to promoting cancer prevention in your community*. Retrieved from *www.cdc.gov/cancer/dcpc/pdf/CancerToolkit.pdf*

Community Tool Box. (n.d.). *Using outreach to increase access*. Retrieved from *http://ctb.ku.edu/en/table-of-contents/implement/access-barriers-opportunities/outreach-to-increase-access/main*

Cruz, Y., Hernandez-Lane, M. E., Cohello, J. I. & Bautista, C. T. (2013). The effectiveness of a community health program in improving diabetes knowledge in the Hispanic population: Salud y Bienestar (Health and Wellness). *Journal of Community Health, 38*, 1124–1131.

Evans, P., Aungst, T.D., Massey, C. & Bartlett, D. (2015). Expanding clinical and information services to the ambulatory older adult through community outreach programs. *The Consultant Pharmacy, 30*, 31–7.

Health Hotlines. (n.d.). Retrieved from *www.nih.gov/health-information/health-info-lines*

Lefebvre, C. R. (2013). *Social marketing and social change: Strategies and tools for improving health, well-being, and the environment.* San Francisco, CA: Jossey-Bass.

University of California, San Francisco. (2013). *The UFO model intervention replication manual: Outreach and education.* Retrieved from *www.ufomodel.com/outreach*

Facilitating Community Health Education Trainings

Jill Tregor

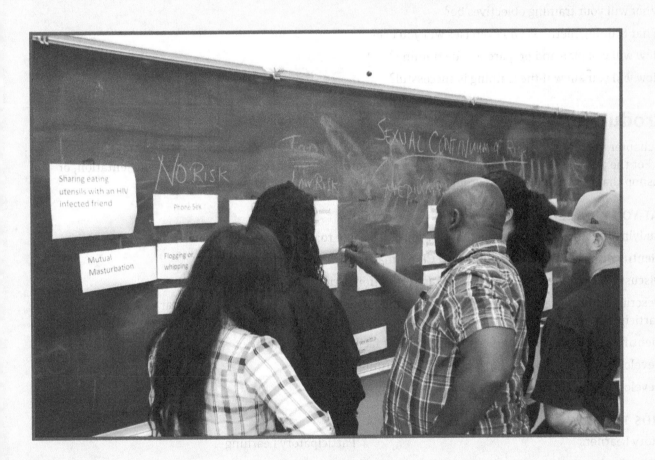

CHW Scenario

You receive a call from a staff member at a local nonprofit agency that does violence prevention work. She asks you to facilitate a two-hour training on stress management for a team of CHWs who do frontline work in the community. You are knowledgeable about the topic of stress reduction, but haven't facilitated this type of training before. What additional information would help you to plan for this training?

Please consider how you would answer the following questions:

- How will you gather this information?
- What will your training objectives be?
- What training methods and exercises will you use?
- How will you plan and prepare for the training?
- How will you know if the training is successful?

Introduction

This chapter addresses the knowledge and skills necessary for facilitating a training or educational presentation. For the purposes of this chapter, we will use the word "training" for any type of class, presentation, or workshop that CHWs facilitate for groups.

WHAT YOU WILL LEARN

By studying the information in this chapter, you will be able to:

- Identify different types of training that CHWs may facilitate
- Discuss some of the ways that people learn new information and skills
- Describe and apply approaches to training commonly used by CHWs, including popular education, participatory learning, and problem-based learning
- Identify and respond to common challenges that facilitators may face
- Develop a training plan, including goals and learning outcomes
- Develop a simple evaluation of a training

WORDS TO KNOW

Auditory Learners	Participatory Learning
Conscientization	Popular Education
Kinesthetic Learners	Problem-Based Learning
Learning Outcomes	Visual Learners

20.1 An Overview of Training

As a CHW you may be asked to facilitate or cofacilitate all or part of a training. These trainings may vary in many ways including:

FOCUS OR MAIN TOPIC

CHWs facilitate trainings that address a wide range of public health topics including:

- Chronic illness such as diabetes, high blood pressure, substance use, depression, and cancer

- Infectious diseases such as hepatitis, tuberculosis, and HIV
- Reproductive health topics, including family planning and pregnancy
- Violence, including domestic violence
- Healthy relationships, including parenting
- Environmental or occupational health
- Civil rights and human rights
- Stress management

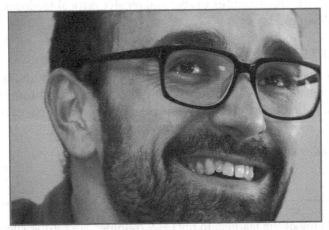

CHWs facilitate health education trainings about a wide range of topics.

- *Can you think of other topics that CHWs might address in trainings?*

Francis Julian Montgomery: It's vital for people like myself—African American and middle aged—to have a chance to learn about chronic conditions. Many trainings leave people out, such as people of color or gender minorities, by not including language and information that is geared for them. I want to make sure that a person like me can get the information they need.

PURPOSE OR GOAL
The primary purpose or goal of trainings may include:

- To share and learn new health-related information
- To promote changes in health-related behaviors
- To promote self-management of chronic conditions
- To share and learn new skills such as stress management, risk reduction, health outreach, or advocacy skills
- To build leadership skills, capacity, and autonomy
- To promote teamwork and community building
- To support a community planning or organizing process

- *Can you think of other goals for trainings?*

DURATION

Trainings may last anywhere from 30 minutes to eight hours or more, and may even take place over many days or weeks.

NUMBER OF FACILITATORS

Sometimes you will facilitate trainings on your own, and sometimes with a cofacilitator or as part of a training team. When you are starting out, it is helpful to observe other facilitators and to facilitate trainings as a part of a team. This will provide you with opportunities to give and receive critical feedback, and to learn new skills and approaches from trusted colleagues.

AUDIENCE OR PARTICIPANTS

CHWs facilitate trainings for a wide variety of audiences including youth, parents, coworkers, clients, members of a faith community or other group or organization, people diagnosed with chronic illness, and professionals such as teachers, physicians, police, and staff and volunteers of community-based organizations.

- *Can you think of other groups who might participate in trainings?*

> **Alma Vasquez:** Many of the learners in my CHW trainings are former clients. The training teaches them job readiness skills in addition to CHW skills. When they are done with the training, they can take their passion for helping and make it a career.

LOCATIONS

Trainings take place in a wide variety of locations, including:

- Schools
- Clinics or hospitals
- Churches, mosques, temples, and other religious or faith-based organizations
- Juvenile hall, jails, or prisons
- Work sites
- Housing sites, including public housing and homeless shelters
- Community-based organizations
- After-school programs
- Recreational sites
- Cultural and arts organizations

- *Where do trainings take place in your community? Where have you been when you participated in a training?*

PREPARATION

Facilitating trainings can be intimidating, especially if you feel uncomfortable speaking in front of groups. Most people who lead trainings start out feeling nervous and unsure about what to do. I have been making presentations and conducting trainings for many years, yet I still feel nervous before a training session. The good thing is that being nervous motivates me to do my homework in order to *prepare* for the training. By the end of this chapter, my hope is that you will have the building blocks to develop interesting and engaging trainings and learner-centered activities, and will feel confident that you already have the qualifications necessary to be a great facilitator. Remember, even mistakes in planning can lead to great learning opportunities, as long as you are able to think "on your feet" and adapt to changing or unexpected situations.

An Early Experience as a Trainer

Jill Tregor: My first paid job in the community was with an organization that worked to prevent and respond to hate-motivated violence (when people are threatened or attacked due to their real or perceived ethnicity, religion, sexual orientation, gender, or gender identity). We often received requests for presentations about hate violence from schools and other organizations. Occasionally, I had time to learn something in advance about the group I would present to, but more often I showed up to the training without knowing much about the participants because I really didn't understand how important it was to do so. I thought my material should be what guided the format for the training, not the audience, and not even what I hoped would be the outcome(s) for the training.

Because I knew a lot about my topic, I wanted to just *tell* people about hate violence. But quite often the people in the trainings also knew a lot about the topic, because their communities had been the targets of hate-motivated violence themselves. I didn't think about how boring it might be for them if I just stood up at the front of the room and talked for 30 minutes or more, although I knew I did not like to be a participant in trainings like this. Because I didn't always have a training plan, or the training plan I had was overly simplistic, it was also possible (or likely) that I would end a training without covering topics or concerns that the participants were most eager to learn about.

Eventually I realized that I needed help, and looked for opportunities to become a better trainer. I talked with my coworkers. I read books, went to workshops, and participated in trainings for trainers. I observed what experienced trainers did. I finally learned to prepare for *every* training I do, and to tailor each training to fit the needs of the group I am working with. Now my first step is to make sure I know who my participants are, and what it is they want to know or learn about.

20.2 Understanding How People Learn

TYPES OF LEARNERS

Many people think of the process of learning as one in which an "expert" talks about what they know, and the "learners" simply listen. The learners are assumed to have understood what they heard, even though there may be no evaluation to determine whether or not they did. Perhaps you experienced (or still experience) school in this way: the teacher lectures or gives an assignment, and then you, the student, are assumed to have understood. In reality, people learn in *many* different ways, including:

- **Visual learners** need to see the material they are learning. They might prefer films, photographs, drawings, or observation. For example, to learn how to facilitate a training, this type of learner may want to observe an experienced trainer in action.

- **Kinesthetic or tactile learners** need to interact with the material they are learning, to move around, touch, or practice doing what it is they are trying to learn. This type of learner may want to practice how to facilitate a training by conducting part of a training activity with an experienced cofacilitator.

- **Auditory learners** learn by listening. This learner might enjoy a lecture, a film, or a small or large group discussion. To learn how to facilitate a training, this type of learner may want to listen to a detailed lecture or presentation about training skills.

Of course there are other types of learners as well. I find that I am most likely to learn if I am given the opportunity to interact with the trainer/educator *and* the material. I want to ask questions, have discussions, and to understand how the ideas being presented can be applied to my own life and work experiences and the knowledge and skills I already have.

While some people may be *primarily* one type of learner, all of us learn in more than one way. In any training, you will be working with a diverse group that learns in a variety of ways. If you rely on only one teaching method, you will limit the effectiveness of trainings.

What Is Your Experience as a Learner?

Think about a training session or class that was *not* effective in facilitating your learning.

- What made it difficult for you to become actively engaged in learning?
- Did the trainer or teacher talk too much?
- Did the training value your own experience and knowledge?
- Did the training or class invite your participation?
- What could the trainer or teacher have done to improve the class?

Now think about a training or class that *was* effective in facilitating your learning.

- What did the trainer or teacher do to make you feel comfortable?
- What kind of activities most engaged you?
- What styles of teaching worked best for you?
- How did you know that this training or class was effective for you?

20.3 Approaches to Teaching and Training

There are many approaches to facilitating trainings. For the purposes of this chapter, we will emphasize three approaches that are commonly used in the field of public health to actively engage training participants in learning and teaching: popular education, participatory learning, and problem-based learning.

POPULAR EDUCATION

Paulo Freire is considered one of the world's most important thinkers about education. He is widely known in the field of public health as a key theorist and practitioner of "**popular education**." Freire lived and worked in Brazil, where it was illegal to vote unless one was literate (able to read and write), leaving the poor without a voice in elections. Freire worked to address the problem of illiteracy, teaching sugarcane workers how to read in just 45 days. He initiated a national literacy campaign, which ended when the Brazilian government was overthrown.

Freire recognized that unless a learner's own experiences were recognized and valued, truly significant learning could not occur. Education that starts *where people are* has the potential to transform lives. Freire's approach suggested that education that supported people in identifying and analyzing important problems in their lives, and in better understanding how those problems are connected to larger social issues and dynamics, could lead them to develop and implement actions to change and improve their circumstances.

Freire called this process **conscientization**, or the development of a critical consciousness about social and political realities. He also strongly believed that the true purpose of education should be liberation and the promotion of social justice.

> One cannot expect positive results from an educational or political action program which fails to respect the particular view of the world held by the people. Such a program constitutes cultural invasion, good intentions not withstanding. (Freire, 1970)

When Freire taught farmworkers how to read, the workers also talked about and analyzed their personal experiences with poverty and injustice. They came to realize that these were not individual problems, but larger problems created by social inequities and oppression. Freire believed the final step of the popular education process comes when the development of critical consciousness leads to *praxis,* when the participants use their knowledge to take collective action to promote social justice and the welfare of their community.

Have you ever taken a class in which the teacher lectured the entire time? Freire called this "banking"—a traditional teaching method that treats learners as though they are containers into which information is poured, with the expectation that the learner will be able to repeat back the information exactly as it was told to them. As a learner, it is easy to become so accustomed to this approach that we may have difficulty adjusting if we are invited to more actively participate in our education. In contrast to this approach, Freire encouraged teachers or trainers to recognize, value, and call forth the experience, the knowledge, and the wisdom of students or participants. Though it can be comfortable to be taught via the banking method instead of being an engaged participant, there is research to show that learners actually retain much more of what is being taught if they are given opportunities to apply the information/learning as soon as possible.

Popular education supports learners in "speaking their own word," rather than repeating back the language, analysis, and ideas of trainers, or anyone else. *To learn more about popular education, review the resources provided at the end of this chapter, including the Paulo Freire Institute.*

Popular education is commonly used to guide the work of CHWs and community workers. The Bayview/Hunter's Point neighborhood of San Francisco is a neighborhood with some of the highest levels of poverty in the city, where residents are hospitalized more than those from any other neighborhood, primarily for preventable conditions (HOPE SF, 2013). In 2002, a pair of residents started planting flowers and vegetables in a number of places around their block, including the median strip in the center of their street, which had been "a dumping ground for everything from engine oil and beer bottles to garbage and brake pads" (Yoffee, 2003). What began as an effort to beautify a small block has become, over time, a means to build community by bringing diverse neighbors together to focus on everything from eating and distributing healthy food to actively organizing against major sources of pollution in the neighborhood. Community members recently began to market their own products, including jams and honey made from the fruit they grew and the bees that pollinate their gardens. While the founders had basic ideas about gardening and neighborhood improvement, over time the project has spread to other blocks, and become a source of free and nutritional food. By sharing their experiences and educating each other, Quesada Street residents have become experts and outspoken leaders for San Francisco as a whole about the health concerns of Bayview/Hunters' Point, food policy and access to healthy food, and health care policy (Quesada Gardens Initiative, n.d.).

Sergio Matos: Most education in this country assumes that students know nothing. Popular education is the exact opposite. It holds that people are a fountain of wisdom and knowledge and experience, and they bring all of that life experience and history to education and training. As a CHW, you really need to validate that. We call it liberation education because it provides an opportunity for freedom and critical thinking and organizing for social justice. Liberation education is about the wisdom in the group, not of any one individual.

PARTICIPATORY LEARNING

When CHWs engage people in all aspects of the learning experience, when they presume that a learner is also a teacher, the process of **participatory learning** has begun. Other ways to describe participatory learning are interactive learning, or sharing knowledge. As with popular education, participatory learning views the learner as more than a recipient of information. A participatory learner is involved in identifying what she needs to know, how she would like to learn new information, and in all learning activities. You might say that the learners identify not only what their problems are, but the solutions to these problems as well. This approach to learning eliminates the idea of there being one expert: we are all experts when it comes to figuring out the solutions to our own life's problems and challenges. To learn more about participatory learning, please refer to the resources at the end of this chapter.

CHWs are trained to view clients as the experts about their own lives. Clients are the only ones who can properly decide about making change in their lives. We encourage you to apply these same concepts to understanding what makes for the best learning opportunities for people. You could say that participatory learning is "client-centered learning," a parallel to the client-centered counseling that CHWs use when working with individuals (see Chapter 9).

Community-Based Training Is Like Client-Centered Practice

Consider your approach to training as similar to doing client-centered work with individual clients. Let the community take the lead in determining what they want to learn, and why. Ask for their input and use the information they share to guide you in setting up the training workshop or class. During the training, stop and reflect: Whose voice is taking up most of the space in the room? If you are speaking more than the participants, you may not be doing "community-centered training." Let the voices, experiences, values, and ideas of the participants dominate the learning environment. Remember that after the training is over, it will be up to them to use the knowledge they generate to promote their own health and well-being.

PROBLEM-BASED LEARNING

Another way to engage a community in the learning experience is to organize them into teams that work together to discover solutions to real-life problems. As with the methods described above, **problem-based learning** (PBL) encourages people to think in a critical way. Instead of just memorizing somebody's idea of "the right answer" to a problem, team members talk to and challenge each other to develop their own solutions. Under this model, there are a range of possible answers that represent the experience, ideas, and values of the group. One significant benefit of this approach is that the group members get to know each other as individuals and learn how to work together as a team. This creates a sense of community, as well as building relationships across differences such as class, ethnicity, immigration status, language, and culture.

One challenge is that people can become accustomed to education or training that promotes "yes" and "no" or "right" and "wrong" ideas. It is sometimes uncomfortable, at first, for people to engage in learning that is less defined. People may look to you for guidance and judgment. In this case, problem-based learning may require additional explanation, and additional patience from you in your role as facilitator.

CHWs use participatory learning, popular education, problem-based learning, and other methods that actively involve community members in the process of learning. These methods respect the experience, knowledge, and wisdom of learners, and support them in using their knowledge to take action that will promote their health and well-being.

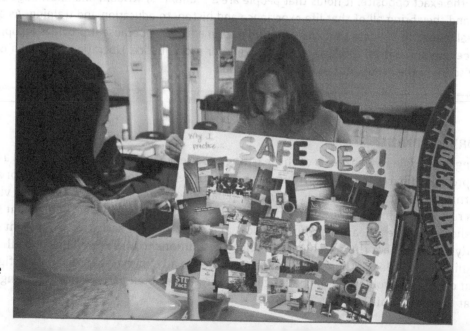

Participants create a collage to learn about the topic of safer sex.

- *How might you apply these approaches to learning as you facilitate a training on stress management for the team of CHWs?*

20.4 Deciding If Training Is the Right Strategy

Training is often suggested as the strategy to address many community health issues. But training may not always be the best way to address the challenge at hand. It may be more effective, for example, to conduct community health outreach, to facilitate a support group, to engage in community planning, or to facilitate community organizing and advocacy.

How do you figure out whether training is actually what a group needs?

The following questions are designed to guide you in deciding whether or not to conduct training:

- What does the group want to accomplish?
- What does the group want to learn to help them reach their goal?
- Are there other ways to accomplish these goals?
- What makes you think that training is the best way to accomplish it?
- Is there a better way to get the information to people?
- Is there an interest in training as the method to learn the material?

In order to answer those questions, you will need to figure out:

- Who is the audience?
- Will participation in the training be voluntary or required?
- Would learning be better in a formal or informal setting?
- Is the group highly diverse (with different backgrounds, identities, and levels of knowledge about the training issues)?
- What are the possible barriers between you and the audience? For example, how may differences in age, race, language, gender, sexual orientation, national origin, and literacy level affect your ability to facilitate an effective training?
- Will the audience be expecting an "expert" as the teacher? What qualifies you to be the one to lead the session?
- Are you hoping to teach concepts or skills?
- What will the cost of the training be? What is your budget? Is there a more cost-effective way for participants learn the material?

There is no simple formula to determine whether training is the right strategy use. Based on the answers to these questions, use your best judgment to decide whether training is the right approach for the challenge at hand. It is often helpful to talk these issues and questions through with trusted colleagues.

20.5 How to Plan and Prepare Trainings

How will you prepare for the stress management training that you have been asked to facilitate?

Your first task is to ask questions. You need to know what the agency supervisor wants the training to achieve, what the CHWs need, and what resources are available for this training.

The following list of general questions does not necessarily have to be answered in any particular order, but we recommend that you find out as much as you can about each one.

- If you have been asked to conduct this training by someone else, *what are their primary goals*? In the case study presented at the beginning of the chapter, what are the agency's goals for the stress management training? What do they expect CHWs to learn in the two-hour workshop?
- What do the participants *want to know*? What do the CHWs who will participate in the training most want to know about stress reduction? Do they want to learn specific stress-reduction techniques such as meditation? Do they want to talk about how the stress of their work is affecting them?

- What do those who will participate in the training *already know*? For example, have the CHWs participated in stress-reduction workshops before? What do they currently do to manage their stress?

CONDUCTING AN ASSESSMENT BEFORE DESIGNING A TRAINING

You will facilitate a better training if you understand what the participants already know and want to learn. If possible, conduct a *preassessment* to gather this information and prepare for the training. The assessment doesn't need to be complicated or lengthy; it just needs to provide you with some basic information. There are a number of options for how to gather the information, each with its own strengths and weaknesses. These options are described in greater detail in Chapter 22.

Interview Stakeholders or Possible Participants

Interviews with potential participants, or another professional who works with the participants, provide useful information for planning a training. Ideally, for the stress management training you have been asked to provide, it would be best to interview the CHWs who will participate in the training. You might be able to visit the agency and talk with them in person, or set up a conference call. Prepare a list of *open-ended questions*, being careful not to take too much time with the people you are interviewing (you don't want folks to think you are disrespecting the value of their time). Decide how many people you are going to interview. Once you have conducted a few interviews you can review your notes for common themes.

If you are able to speak with the CHWs who will participate in the stress management training, your questions might include:

- What is your level of interest in attending this training?
- What do you hope to get out of this training?
- What type of stress is most common in your job?
- What types of training, if any, have you already received in stress reduction?
- What do you do now to manage stress?
- What topics do you not need me to cover in detail?
- What would you most like to learn about?
- What kind of trainings do you most enjoy? How do you best learn new information or skills?

- *What other questions would you want to ask?*

What Do YOU Think ?

Administer Surveys

Your agency might use a survey to gather information about future trainings. In general, surveys ask *closed-ended questions*. You need to decide on your goals before you design the survey, and think about the type of answers that people may give to the questions you ask. You can conduct a survey by phone, via the World Wide Web, by distributing paper copies, or with an in-person interview. Survey questions can be of many types, including multiple choice, yes/no, or *interval rating* (such as a Likert Scale, which asks people to rate their feeling or opinion on a 0–5 or 0–10 scale).

Learning to develop a good survey is an art that takes practice. It includes balancing the need for information against the likelihood that for the survey taker, time and patience may be limited. For more information about using surveys, please see Chapter 22 and the resources provided at the end of this chapter from the LimeSurvey Manual and the National Association of County and City Health Officials.

Conduct a Focus Group

Chapter 22 also presents information about focus groups. Briefly, this is an opportunity to bring together six to twelve members of a common group or community to facilitate a discussion about specific topics and record their responses. It is often used as part of a community diagnosis process, to develop new public health programs or educational materials or to evaluate programs, and it may be useful in designing a training as well. Focus groups take a lot of time to prepare for and, depending on the nature of the training, it may be a bigger project than the training itself merits.

Facilitating a Training on Domestic Violence

Several years ago, I assisted in developing a domestic violence training for people who worked at a family law court. The group I was working with, which included several judges, felt that court employees did not always know what to do when someone experiencing family violence came to them for assistance. The next task was to find out what the court employees themselves thought about the issues.

To develop the training, I conducted a preassessment that included a survey of all court employees, brief telephone interviews with select individual employees, and a focus group discussion with about six of the employees. Keep in mind that this assessment was part of a well-funded and ongoing program, so we had the resources and time to conduct a fairly comprehensive assessment.

When I conducted telephone interviews with court employees, I asked the following questions:

1. Have you had previous training about domestic violence? If so, who provided the trainings, and when/where were they held?

2. What were the strengths and weaknesses of those trainings? What did you like? What didn't you like?

3. What type of information might assist you to do your job better when working with victims of domestic violence?

4. If you had the opportunity for more domestic violence training, what would you most like to learn?

The questions were designed to give me ideas about possible topics for the training. Question 2 was an opportunity to find out if certain topics or training approaches were either particularly effective or ineffective. Questions 3 and 4 might seem repetitive, but sometimes asking the same question in a slightly different way brings out new information. Even if we had not held focus groups or distributed a survey, these phone calls gave me essential information that assisted to formulate our training agenda.

You will decide how to conduct an assessment based on the amount of time and other resources you have, how easy it will be for you to contact the participants, and what you and the participants are comfortable doing.

ARE YOU THE RIGHT PERSON TO FACILITATE THE TRAINING?

Once you have determined that training is an appropriate strategy to meet the needs of the community or organization, there are still other questions to be answered. Are you the right person to deliver this training? Do you have the expertise and knowledge required? If your answer to that question is "no," you may be able to learn new information and skills that will prepare you to take the lead. Or you may want to identify someone who is more knowledgeable about the topic, and ask that person to facilitate the training in your place, or to work with you as cofacilitator. Even if you are highly knowledgeable about the topic, you should still consider whether you are the right person to facilitate the training. In general I find that having a cofacilitator improves my ability to be an effective trainer. With two of us, we are more likely to notice a participant who needs extra support, or adjust our material if we hit a bump in the road.

Perhaps the most important issues I consider before deciding to do a training, are the potential barriers that may exist between the training participants and me. I don't believe that a facilitator must resemble the people participating in the training, but I do believe that it is helpful if participants feel they can relate to the facilitator in some way. It is also true that if I share things in common with participants, I may better understand their questions and concerns. If I don't share things in common with the group, I want to consider whether our differences are going to get in the way of their learning experience. When I trained public school teachers in the Central Valley of California about the topic of hate-motivated violence, I acknowledged that I was *not* a schoolteacher and that I was not from a rural area myself. My cotrainer grew up just a few miles away from the training site, so while she, too, had never been a schoolteacher, she was able to assure people that she had some insight into who they were.

Cultural identity and issues of class, ethnicity, age, gender, and language are among the most obvious differences that may exist between you and the people you are hoping to train. Sometimes any or all of those differences might be such significant obstacles that you are not the right person to lead the training. Other times, by acknowledging the differences, by allowing for different points of view during the training, and by doing plenty of homework ahead of time, you can be an effective trainer.

ESTABLISH GOALS AND LEARNING OUTCOMES

Once you have gathered the information you need from stakeholders and potential participants, it is time to establish the goals and learning outcomes or objectives for the training. (For the purpose of this chapter, we will use the terms *learning outcomes* and *objectives* interchangeably.) The feedback you received, whether from a survey, an interview, or a focus group, will be a critical part of determining what these goals and objectives will be.

What is the difference between a goal and a learning outcome? A goal is the broad statement about where we want to go or what we want to accomplish, and is generally an abstract idea. A **learning outcome** should be as specific as possible about what participants will know and know how to do as a result of the training. A straightforward way to remember the differences between a goal and an outcome may be to think of the goal as what you (the trainer) want participants to know, and an outcome should not only be specific but measurable. In other words, you should be able to assess or evaluate whether or not you achieved a learning outcome and the participants in the training walked away with certain knowledge and/or skills. To learn more about developing goals and objectives, refer to the resources at the end of this chapter from the American Library Association and the Association of Learning and Research Libraries.

Here are the goals and two of the learning outcomes we established, after we conducted a preassessment for the training with the family law courts described above:

Training Goals

1. To increase awareness of the impact of exposure to domestic violence on victims and their children.

2. To increase the ability to understand and respond to families in crisis.

3. To increase the number of families experiencing domestic violence that are linked to appropriate resources, including legal, mental health, and housing services.

Learning Outcomes

1. For staff who work at the family court to be able to identify at least three symptoms of post-traumatic stress (PTS), and at least one example of how PTS could affect how a victim of domestic violence presents herself at the court.

2. For staff at the court to be able to list at least three new resources they could offer to survivors of domestic violence and their children.

Training goals and learning outcomes should reflect the abilities and desires of participants. What are the possible goals and learning outcomes for the training on stress reduction that you have been asked to facilitate?

Goals:

Example: To reduce stress for workers and volunteers doing violence prevention work.

Write down additional goals here:

1. _____

2. _____

Learning Outcomes:

Example: All participants will be able to demonstrate a three-minute breathing exercise designed to reduce stress responses.

Write down additional learning outcomes here:

1. _____

2. _____

CREATE A TRAINING OUTLINE

After identifying the training goals and learning outcomes, you are ready to develop a detailed outline of what you will do in the training. What information will you cover? What kinds of training methods are you going to use? Be specific about every step and topic you are going to cover. This will assist you in many ways, including allowing you to determine what you really have time to cover.

There are many ways to outline a training plan. Here is an excerpt of the outline format I used for the court training.

Table 20.1 Section 1: Introduction to the Training

OBJECTIVE/ SCOPE	KEY CONTENT	ACTIVITY	MATERIALS	WHO IS RESPONSIBLE?
A. To review the purpose and content of the training.	1. Mission, history, and primary tasks of the family court's Domestic Violence Project. 2. Review the training agenda, goals, and learning outcomes.	1. Facilitator presents information and invites questions and discussion.	1. Agency brochure; handouts with training agenda, goals, and learning outcomes.	1. Jill
B. To understand common signs of post-traumatic stress among victims of domestic violence (DV) and their children.	1. Define post-traumatic stress (PTS) and common trauma responses among victims of DV.	1. Show video about DV. Provide definition of post-traumatic stress and facilitate discussion. 2. Facilitate small-group activity to identify common trauma responses. Review the work of small groups with all participants. Highlight common trauma responses. Respond to questions and concerns about trauma responses.	1. Video: *The Impact of Domestic Violence on Families*. 2. Handout with definition of post-traumatic stress, and questions for small group participants. Flip-chart paper and pens for small-group brainstorming. One paper for each small group (of three to four participants) with a different category of trauma response, including: physical, emotional, cognitive (thoughts), spiritual/religious, and behavioral responses.	1. Tony and Jill

Now try using the same format to develop a plan for the training you are scheduled to facilitate on stress management.

(continues)

(continued)

Table 20.2 Section 1: Introduction to the Training

OBJECTIVE/ SCOPE	KEY CONTENT	ACTIVITY	MATERIALS	WHO IS RESPONSIBLE?
A. Example: To provide an overview of the goals and learning outcomes for the training session. B. Fill this in: What's next? C.	1. Goals and learning outcomes developed for the session. 2. 3.	1. Presentation and large-group discussion of the goals and learning outcomes. Ask if there are other items people want to cover. 2. 3.	1. Flip-chart paper and pens. Handouts. 2. 3.	1. Your name here! 2. You! 3. You!

20.6 Tips for Facilitating a Participatory Training

You will develop your own approaches and training methods with time and experience. In the meantime, here are some tips I've learned along the way that I hope will be useful to you.

PREPARING THE TRAINING

- **Identify a safe, comfortable place for the training** that is accessible to all participants. Will people be able to get there easily by bus, car, or on foot? Will there be seats for everyone? If there are stairs, is there also an elevator for those who are unable to use the stairs?

- **Ask about the language needs of the participants.** Do the trainers speak the same language as the participants? If you can't afford to pay for interpreters, see if there are community members who are willing to volunteer to play that role. Is there someone who requires sign-language interpretation? If so, make sure they have access to an interpreter and a comfortable place to sit where the participant can clearly see the interpreter and still be part of the group. Otherwise, you will need to let people know that the training is not accessible to all.

- **Assess child care needs.** If possible, try to arrange for child care, or have a plan for how to handle children if participants bring them. Participants will appreciate knowing their children are safely occupied so that they can focus on the training. If you can't afford child care (which is likely to be true most of the time), it may be possible to provide some toys and materials for the children to play with.

- **Pack up the training materials well ahead of time,** including extra pens and paper, plenty of copies of any handouts, newsprint and an easel, markers, tape, and anything else you will be using. Make sure you haven't left anything out. I have usually made up a box with everything I will need at least two days ahead.

- **Identify the need for technology.** If you plan to show a video or DVD, make sure that the appropriate technology (such as a laptop and LCD projector) will be available at the training site, or bring what you need with you. You definitely do not want to waste valuable time at a training discovering that your systems aren't compatible or don't work at all.

- **Get to the training location at least thirty minutes in advance** so that you have plenty of time to set up the room, and to deal with any unexpected problems related to the space.

- *What else would you want to do to prepare for the training session?*

FACILITATING THE TRAINING SESSION

Setting the Stage

- **Set up the room:** Depending on the topic and expected number of participants, I usually like either a full circle or a U-shape. I set up chairs (and tables, if appropriate) ahead of time or request them to be set up as I need. If participants will be working a lot in small groups, you might want to set up tables with seats for four to five each throughout a room. What matters here is the comfort of the participants, the ability for everyone to hear and see, and the opportunity for participants to interact with each other, and not just with the trainer(s).

- **Introduce yourself and welcome all participants:** Tell them what topics the training will address. Review the training goals and learning outcomes, and the day's agenda so that they know what to expect. Invite and respond to their questions or concerns. Make sure participants know when breaks will occur, where the restrooms are, and any other logistical information they might need.

- **Establish clear ground rules:** Suggest some ground rules to the group and ask them if they would like to add to the list. Sample ground rules include: "No interruptions—let each person finish speaking before you begin," "Turn off cell phones," "Maintain confidentiality—don't share anyone's private or personal information with people outside of the training," and "Offer respect to all of the participants, even if you disagree with them." Ask everyone for their support in following the ground rules: this will be helpful if anything happens during the session that creates an unwelcome interruption or disturbance.

- **"Step Up, Step Back":** Ask participants to monitor their own participation in the training. If they are someone who tends to speak a lot, encourage them to "step back" and allow other voices to be heard. If they are someone who tends to be quiet, encourage them to take risks and speak up so that others may benefit of their insight and experience.

- **Use icebreakers or opening activities** to assist participants to relax and build trust. This will assist people to prepare for the work at hand, and perhaps allow them to meet some or all of the people in the room. There are thousands of great ideas for icebreakers on the World Wide Web (see the resources provided at the end of this chapter). Be guided in your choices by how much time you want to spend on this activity. Take into consideration the degree to which the participants already know each other or not.

- *What else would you want to say or do at the beginning of a training?*

Organization and Logistics

- **Keep to the training schedule:** You will break trust with the participants if you start the training late or don't finish on time. If for some reason you cannot start on time, I encourage you to start within 10 minutes of when scheduled.

- **Schedule breaks during the session,** particularly if you are working for more than an hour. People need time to stretch, use the bathroom, and return phone calls. They will be more capable of giving their full attention to the training if you let them know that they will be able to take care of these needs.

- **If possible, provide healthy refreshments for participants:** Fruit, water, fresh vegetables, and dip are good things to provide, and also provide reassurance that you are concerned about the welfare of participants.

Clarity

- **Tie your points together:** Show how one idea leads to the next. Check in regularly with participants to see if they understand what you are saying and doing. Ask them if they have any questions or concerns. Watch for their body language. If you see looks of confusion on their faces, ask if you are communicating clearly enough.

- **Build on earlier lessons:** They may be lessons learned at a different time entirely, or lessons learned earlier during the same session. Clearly identify—or ask participants to identify—how one training session or topic builds upon or connects to another. This helps to reinforce learning.

- **Repeat your main points** during the course of the session as a way to emphasize your message. If you do your job well, the participants will begin to take on this role for you.

- *What else would you do to organize the training and to ensure that participants understand the information provided?*

Engaging Participants

- **Don't talk too much!** Give people many opportunities to ask questions and to express their own knowledge and expertise.

- **Ask questions:** Acknowledge that everyone in the room has knowledge and experience to share. Your role is to facilitate learning, not to be the only source of information. I like to start a training by asking people to introduce themselves and answer a few questions. I might ask, "How long have you worked here?" "What do you hope to learn today?" "What is one thing you would like to share with other people about your experience with this topic?"

- **Ask participants to work in teams:** There are many methods for getting people into smaller groups including both teams of two and larger groups of three to five. You can ask people to group themselves by twos or threes, "count off," assign people to a group as they enter the workshop (put a symbol on their name tag). When people work in small groups they are more likely to actively participate. For many, small-group work is where their best learning occurs.

- **Engage participants in problem-based learning** instead of telling them what they need to know. For the stress-reduction workshop, you might assign participants to small teams, and ask each team to develop a proposal for what they and their agency can do differently to reduce stress among frontline workers.

- **Keep people moving:** Sitting in one place throughout a training often makes it difficult for people to stay alert and to learn effectively. I often ask people to move around the room, meeting in different small groups, or writing down their ideas on large sheets of paper posted on the walls.

- **Provide games and exercises:** Once people are in small groups, they often enjoy an opportunity to compete in some way with the other groups. Teams might play a version of Jeopardy or another popular game show. Questions to be answered should reflect the material that you want the participants to learn.

- **Role-play:** This is one of the best ways for participants to practice new skills. Teams can be given a scenario to act out, which they present to the other participants in the workshop or training. Or you can ask for volunteers to participate in a role-play in order to demonstrate a situation, challenge, or skill that the group is learning about.

- **Have teams teach each other a new skill:** For example, you might give each group a handout about a different stress-reduction method. Each group is given enough time to understand and practice the method, and to make a plan for how to teach it to others. Each group will make a presentation to the other participants about a stress-reduction method.

- **Use real-world examples as case studies:** When I led trainings about hate crimes, I told stories about the cases that I had worked on as a victim advocate (maintaining the confidentiality of the parties involved). You can use these stories and case studies to ask what participants might have done differently, or even to assist them to learn what *not* to do. You can draw upon stories in the news, historical events, films, or literature.

- *What else would you do to actively engage training participants?*

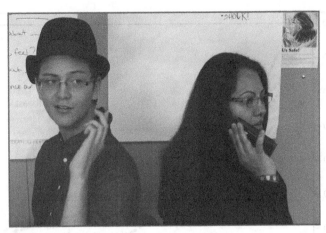

CHWs participate in a role play training.

Romelia Rodriguez: I facilitate a lot of trainings in the community, and there is a big difference between being a facilitator and being a teacher. Teachers might want to control the agenda in the workshop, but as a facilitator, someone who understands popular education, I know that the group should control the experience of the training. It's not my job always to be in control or to know the outcomes of the workshop. I need to make space for the group to speak up, to share their experiences and their knowledge. It is harder sometimes for people to give up this control. But popular education is about sharing power, about being equal with the group, about knowing that the most important knowledge comes from the group. Because the learning that happens is for them, and we hope that it leads to action, and these actions must be carried out by the community.

ENDING A TRAINING

- **Make sure you end on time:** Even if you have not been able to cover all material, you must respect people's time and end when you said that you would.
- **Acknowledge that people may still have questions** and let them know where and how they can continue to learn about the topics addressed in the training. Give people a way to contact you if they don't already have that information.
- **Thank everyone for their participation.**
- **Ask for feedback:** You may want this in writing, as answers to a questionnaire, for instance, or you may ask students to discuss the "plusses and deltas" for a training. There is more information later in this chapter about some evaluation methods for a training.
- **Make sure that you leave the training space as you found it:** This is particularly important if you are using space that was donated. Make sure the hosts want to invite you back.

PRESENTING STATISTICS IN A TRAINING

In general, we advise you to use statistics and numbers sparingly in the trainings you facilitate. Unless statistics are presented very well, they can be boring and difficult to understand. However, if you have a really punchy, simple statement, like "More women have died this year in St. Louis due to domestic violence than due to cancer," then use it. See Chapter 22 for more discussion about this.

Please refer to Figure 20.1 below.

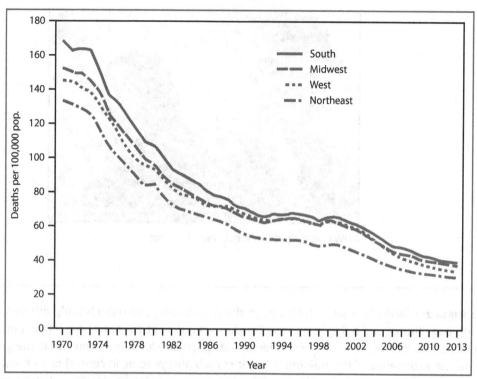

*Per 100,000 standard population.

† Stroke cases are identified using underlying cause of death with codes 430–438 (1970–1998), and I60–I69 (1999–2013) in the *International Classification of Diseases, Eighth, Ninth and Tenth Revisions*. ICD-10 replaced ICD-9 in 1999, and its new classification scheme has had a net effect of increasing counts of stroke as an underlying cause of death by about 6 percent starting that year.

§ *Northeast:* Connecticut, Maine, Massachusetts, New Hampshire, Rhode Island, New Jersey, New York, Pennsylvania, and Vermont; *Midwest:* Illinois, Indiana, Iowa, Kansas, Michigan, Minnesota, Missouri, Nebraska, North Dakota, Ohio, South Dakota, and Wisconsin; *South:* Alabama, Arkansas, Delaware, Florida, Georgia, Kentucky, Louisiana, Mississippi, Maryland, North Carolina, Oklahoma, South Carolina, Virginia, Tennessee, Texas, West Virginia, and District of Columbia; *West:* Alaska, Arizona, California, Colorado, Hawaii, Idaho, Montana, Nevada, New Mexico, Oregon, Utah, Washington, and Wyoming.

The age-adjusted death rates for stroke in all U.S. Census regions in the United States generally decreased from 1970 to 2013, although the rates in all regions were relatively stable from 1992 to 1999. From 1970 to 2013, the rate decreased an average of 3.3 percent per year in the South, 3.2 percent in the Midwest, 3.3 percent in the West, and 3.4 percent in the Northeast. Throughout the period, the rate was the highest in the South and lowest in the Northeast region.

Figure 20.1 Age-Adjusted Death Rates for Stroke, by U.S. Census Region—United States, 1970–2013
Source: Centers for Disease Control and Prevention (2015, April 10). MMWR, 64(13), 371.

- *In Figure 20.1, what is the central point that the creators are trying to make?*

- *Would you use a graphic like Figure 20.1 in the training you are facilitating?*

- *Do you think most training participants would be able to understand this table?*

What Do YOU? Think ?

Can you think of another way that the material could have been presented? Now, please review Figure 20.2, below.

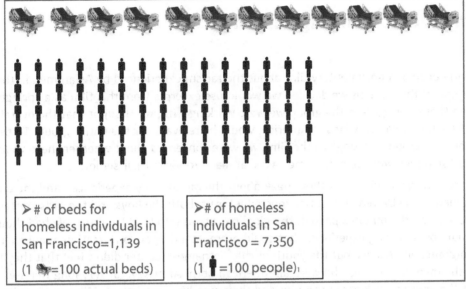

Figure 20.2 Beds for Homeless People in San Francisco, 2013
Source: San Francisco Human Services Agency, 2013.

- *What story is Figure 20.2 telling?*

- *Does Figure 20.2 make a different impact on you than Figure 20.1? In what way?*

What Do YOU Think?

20.7 Responding to Common Challenges

No matter how well I plan a training, something unexpected is certain to happen. Mostly, this is a good thing, but sometimes it makes the work more challenging. Recently, one of my cotrainers was over one hour late and I couldn't reach her by phone. I had to decide whether to adjust the agenda and hope she showed up later in the day to do her part, or whether to go ahead and facilitate a section of the training that I didn't feel confident about. I decided to gamble that my colleague would show up eventually. I rearranged the agenda slightly, hoping that if I moved her segment to a bit later in the session, she would be there. Sure enough, she showed up, her training segment went extremely well, and I didn't have to be responsible for material that I didn't know very well.

Following are several other challenges that you are likely to face when you facilitate trainings, and my suggestions for how to handle these situations.

One of My Worst Training Mistakes

Mike, a colleague, and I were asked to facilitate a series of trainings about interracial conflict for immigrant teenagers at a Vietnamese youth center. The Vietnamese youth had recently experienced a series of conflicts with some African American youth. We spent a lot of time trying to think about appropriate ways to work with the group, given that they had life experiences that were enormously different from our own. Mike is Chinese American, I'm Caucasian, and neither of us are immigrants. We did not know much about these young people, although we were advised by one of the adult staff members that many of the boys probably wouldn't want to participate in any group activities and that some were current gang members.

(continues)

One of My Worst Training Mistakes

(continued)

Mike had recently been in a documentary film about the racism experienced by Asian men in the United States, and for one of the sessions we decided we would use excerpts from this film as a springboard for discussion. Though there were girls in the group we were working with, we thought that the overall message of the film, about facing racism as Asians in America, would be relevant for the entire group. To the degree that we worried about the group "relating" to the film, we were concerned about whether these young people would relate to Asian men who were, in some cases, at least 20 years their senior.

Several of the men in the movie cry as they speak about the racism they experienced and the difficulties they faced as Asian men in the United States. Unexpectedly for us, both the boys and the girls started laughing during these scenes. As the minutes passed, the giggling turned into loud laughter. We had thought watching the film would be a moving experience that could promote a deeper conversation about their own experiences as immigrants and Asians, but the youth at the Vietnamese Center didn't feel that they had much in common with the men in the film, who were all American born. After several very long minutes during which we tried to get the youth to talk about the film and their own life experiences, Mike and I realized that we had completely missed the mark.

This was not the time for a lengthy examination of what had gone wrong. We needed to quickly change direction and find another way to open a door to communication and connection with the participants. We took a short break. I felt overwhelmed and uncertain about what to do next. Thankfully, Mike is both a quick thinker and someone not willing to give up easily. He suggested we ask the group to do a writing exercise. We reconvened, and Mike handed out paper and asked the youth to start writing about their own experiences. We made it through the difficult moment without the youth themselves seeming to be aware that there had been any problem at all. Eventually, we were able to recapture their interest and to get them talking and reflecting about their own lives, the recent conflicts with the other youth, and how they could respond in ways that were positive for both groups.

As trainers, our plan didn't initially meet the youth where they were, and the gap between our assumptions and their reality was enormous. Remember what Paulo Freire said: unless a learner's own experiences are recognized and valued, real learning cannot occur.

In retrospect, we could have turned down the request to conduct these trainings, offering referrals to other sources. Alternatively, we might have sought out a cotrainer, perhaps someone from the Vietnamese community, who could have assisted us in developing a curriculum that our participants could better connect with. We might also have asked the staff at the Community Center for the opportunity to meet with some of the youth prior to the training, to learn more from them about what they were interested in and how we might engage them. None of those ideas would be wrong. While Mike and I had spent a lot of time preparing for the trainings, we needed to spend it differently. We were talking to each other, when we needed to be talking to others.

- *What do you think happened during the training at the Vietnamese Youth Center?*

- *If you had the chance to do this training, what would you do differently?*

What Do YOU Think?

A PARTICIPANT WHO IS ARGUMENTATIVE OR DOMINATING

You are likely to encounter a training participant who is argumentative, who has something to say about every statement you make, who is disrespectful to others, or in some other way makes it difficult to proceed smoothly with the training agenda. Each of us has a different tolerance for this type of behavior. It is important to consider, however, how these behaviors may affect the other participants. As a facilitator, it is your responsibility to ensure a productive learning environment for *all* participants. Once I realize what is going on, I rely on several strategies to try to manage this type of challenge.

The ground rules established at the beginning of the training can be useful when challenges arise. If a person is openly disruptive, it is up to you to remind the individual that everyone agreed to follow the ground rules. If there is a person who is dominating the discussion, I make a point of calling on others to speak. I might even begin to call on people who have not raised their hands or spoken up on their own. I might say, "Let's make sure we hear from everyone today." I have also spoken with disruptive participants one-on-one, during a break. I might say something like: "I see you have a lot to say, and I really appreciate that, but today I need to make sure that everyone gets an opportunity to participate. If you have questions or comments you want to make to me, we can always check in after the training session is over."

If I am working with a cotrainer, one of us will take responsibility for keeping their eye on the "room temperature," making sure that disruptions are handled quietly, perhaps even by asking the person to step out into the hallway to talk for a minute, and asking them if they can agree to be present without being disruptive.

During one particularly challenging training session, a participant became so disruptive that we stopped the training. One of the cotrainers stepped out into the hallway with the person causing the disruption, and the other trainer stayed inside with the other folks in order to hear from them what they wanted and needed from the situation. Sadly, we ended up asking the disruptive person to leave the training, because she was unable to make a commitment to peaceful participation. The experience really underscored one basic truth of community health work: no matter how much you plan, the unexpected can, and will, happen. It will be how you respond to the bumps in the road that will determine your success.

Francis Julian Montgomery: One challenge I have is managing the participation of someone who is excited, even exuberant, about the training. I try to make sure I am still encouraging them even while I may have to limit their participation so that others can have a chance to speak up.

WHEN PARTICIPANTS ARE NOT INTERESTED IN THE TRAINING

As with the training mistakes that we made with the group of Vietnamese youth (described above), there are times when the agenda is simply not the right one for the situation or the participants. While there is nothing to stop you from plowing ahead and ignoring the problem, that does nothing to accomplish the training goals or those of the participants. In the situation I described, I was fortunate to have a cotrainer who was great at thinking on his feet. The experience also illustrates how valuable it is to have a Plan B along with your Plan A at all times—alternate methods of delivering your message, or even other topics that could be covered. It is all right to put aside your own agenda and to check in with participants about the training. If you learn that the training isn't working well for them, put aside the planned agenda and try using other methods to reach the learning outcomes and the needs of the group.

DOING OR SAYING SOMETHING THAT OFFENDS TRAINING PARTICIPANTS

Perhaps my biggest fear is that I am going to say or do something that offends the group I am training, undermining trust and perhaps the opportunity for future partnerships. At the same time, I know that despite my best efforts, I will make mistakes, and from time to time I will unintentionally do something that offends someone. Hopefully, when this occurs, it will be brought to my attention in some way. Ideally, participants will speak up to let me know that they are upset. If I don't learn about the problem, I won't have an opportunity to respond and to restore trust and collaboration. When participants tell me that I have done something that they experienced as offensive, hurtful, or disrespectful, I want to give them my full attention. This is the most important time to be fully present, to listen deeply, and not to respond defensively. I want to understand their experience and point of view so that I can respond in an appropriate manner and prevent similar mistakes in the future. In these moments, I have come to realize that I don't need to explain or defend my actions. What I need to do is to honor the experience of the participants. Even if I didn't intend to be hurtful, I listen, apologize, and try not to repeat the error. When I have done a good and honest job at this, often I have deepened the quality of our relationship by showing that I am a human being who makes mistakes, takes responsibility for them, and expresses my intention to build a respectful professional partnership.

Similarly, when a cotrainer and I have had some sort of strain or disagreement with each other during a training, I have found it critical to address it both directly and quickly. Training participants deserve and need your full attention. If you are distracted by some sort of discomfort between yourself and your fellow trainer, you could be distracted from the work you are there to do.

20.8 Evaluation of Trainings

How will you measure what people learn during a training? For most trainings, you will want to keep the evaluation fairly simple. Determine what you want to know. What information will allow you to do a better job next time you conduct a training? Do you want feedback about your presentation skills? Do you want to know how much people learned? What their favorite part of the session was?

An evaluation can be as simple as asking participants to respond anonymously, in writing, to four questions: What did you think of the training? What did you learn? What else did you want to learn? What would you change about the training? Or it can be a series of questions about each section of the training.

Here is a sample of a brief evaluation for the stress management training mentioned at the beginning of the chapter.

1. Name two things that you learned as a result of today's training.

2. How much has your knowledge of stress management increased as a result of this training?

   0 1 2 3 4 5 6 7 8 9 10

   Not at all   Neutral   A lot

3. Would you recommend this training to others?

4. What suggestions do you have for how to improve this training?

To learn more about evaluation, review the resources at the American Evaluation Association (*www.eval.org*).

Chapter Review

PLAN A TRAINING

You have been asked to facilitate a two-hour training on stress management for CHWs and volunteers at a local nonprofit agency (the case study presented at the beginning of this chapter). You have a month to prepare the training.

1. What steps will you take to plan this training?

2. What do you most want to know in order to prepare for the training? How might you conduct a preassessment to prepare for the training? What questions might you ask?

3. What do you want the participants to come away with at the end of the training? What might be some of the training goals and learning outcomes?

4. Explain what Paulo Freire called *conscientization*, or *critical consciousness*, and how this concept could be applied to the training you will facilitate.

5. What training methods will you use? How will you engage different types of learners?

6. Develop a specific training plan for at least two learning outcomes using the format provided in this chapter.

7. How will you evaluate this training?

References

Centers for Disease Control and Prevention. (2015). QuickStats: Age-adjusted death rates* for stroke, by U.S. census region—United States, 1970–2013. *Morbidity and Mortality Weekly Report, 64*(13), 371.

Freire, P. (1970). *Pedagogy of the oppressed.* Clearwater, FL: H & H Publishing. (Original work published 1968).

HOPE SF. (2013). *For residents: Health, 2013.* Retrieved from *http://hope-sf.org/health.php*

Quesada Gardens Initiative. (n.d.). Retrieved from *http://www.quesadagardens.org*

San Francisco Human Services Agency. (2013). 2013 homeless point-in-time count & survey. Retrieved from *http://www.sfgov3.org/modules/showdocument.aspx?documentid=4819*

Yoffee, P. (2003, September 2). Bayview block in bloom. San Francisco Chronicle. Retrieved from *http://sfgate.com/homeandgarden/article/Bayview-block-in-bloom-Two-neighbors-create-2558862.php*

Additional Resources

American Evaluation Association. (n.d.). Retrieved from *www.eval.org/*

American Library Association. (n.d.). Retrieved from *www.ala.org/*

Association of College and Research Libraries. (n.d.-a). Retrieved from *www.ala.org/acrl/*

Association of College and Research Libraries. (n.d.-b). *Writing measurable objectives.* Retrieved from *www.ala.org/acrl/aboutacrl/directoryofleadership/sections/is/iswebsite/projpubs/smartobjectives*

Center for AIDS Prevention Studies. (n.d.). University of California, San Francisco. *Good questions/better answers: A formative research handbook for California HIV prevention programs.* Retrieved from *http://caps.ucsf.edu/uploads/goodquestions/index.html*

Freire Institute. (n.d.). Retrieved from *www.freire.org*

International Institute for Environment and Development. (1995). *Participatory learning and action.* Retrieved from *www.iied.org/participatory-learning-action*

LimeSurvey Manual. (n.d.). *How to design a good survey (guide).* Retrieved from *http://manual.limesurvey.org/How_to_design_a_good_survey_(guide)*

National Association of County and City Health Officials (NACCHO). (n.d.). *Achieving healthier communities through MAPP.* Retrieved from *www.naccho.org/topics/infrastructure/mapp/upload/MAPP_Handbook_fnl.pdf*

National Education Association. (n.d.). *Research spotlight on project-based learning. www.nea.org/tools/16963.htm*

National Park Service. (2002). *Community toolbox. Facilitation tools: Icebreakers.* Retrieved from *www.nps.gov/ncrc/programs/rtca/helpfultools/Toolbox/fac_icebreakers.htm*

Northern Illinois University, Faculty Development and Instructional Design Center. (n.d.). Problem based learning. Retrieved from *www.niu.edu/facdev/resources/guide/strategies/problem_based_learning.pdf*

University of Durham. (n.d.). *Participatory action research toolkit: An introduction to using par as an approach to learning, research and action.* Retrieved from *www.dur.ac.uk/resources/beacon/PARtoolkit.pdf*

Woods, D. R. (1996). *Instructor's guide for problem-based learning: How to gain the most from PBL (3rd ed.).* Hamilton, Ontario, CAN: McMaster University, Department of Chemical Engineering. Retrieved from *http://chemeng.mcmaster.ca/pbl/chap2.pdf*

Group Facilitation

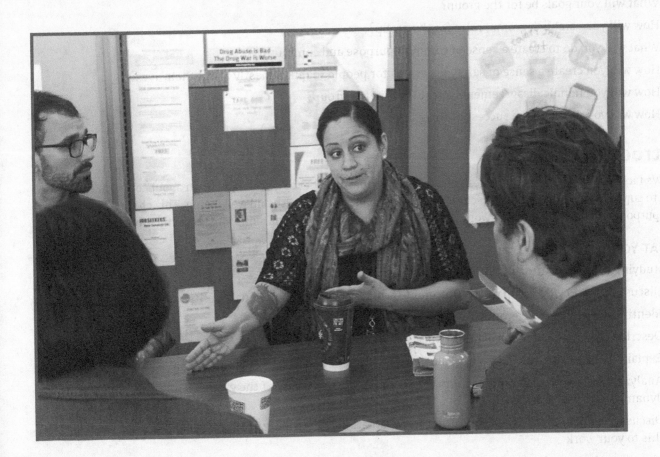

Philip Colgan, Joani Marinoff, and Tim Berthold

21

> ## CHW Scenario
>
> You have been asked to help start a group in your community for people who are newly diagnosed with a chronic illness. The purpose of the group is to support participants in better managing and living with their illness, and in preventing further complications.

- What will your goals be for the group?
- How will you establish ground rules for the group?
- What will you do to create a sense of common purpose and community?
- How will you create a sense of safety necessary for people to talk honestly about their lives?
- How will you handle disagreements or conflicts in the group?
- How will you measure the success of the group experience?

Introduction

CHWs facilitate a variety of groups designed to bring people together to discuss and learn about common concerns and to support each other in taking actions that will enhance their health and well-being. This chapter will address the purpose and benefits of group work, and it will present knowledge and skills for successful group facilitation.

WHAT YOU WILL LEARN

By studying the information in this chapter, you will be able to:

- Discuss how and why group work is different from working with individual clients
- Identify and describe different types of groups
- Describe the unique benefits of group work
- Explain four key stages of group work and analyze the roles and tasks of facilitators at each stage
- Analyze how issues of power and authority, including the authority of the group facilitator, influence group dynamics and processes
- Discuss the importance of self-reflection and evaluation to becoming a skilled group facilitator and apply this to your work
- Identify and respond to common challenges of group work
- Discuss and apply ethics to group work, including issues of cultural humility, boundaries, and confidentiality

WORDS TO KNOW

Cohesion

Contagion

Self-Disclosure

21.1 The Dynamic Nature and Purpose of Group Work

The groups that CHWs and other helping professionals facilitate create a space for people with common experiences or interests to join together and support one another in experiencing some type of change. Learning from one another in a structured environment, with a trained facilitator, can open new possibilities for people's thinking, feelings, and behaviors. Groups in their most basic form and function have the power to enhance social connections and build community: this in itself can support and increase well-being.

Group work is different from working one-on-one with individual clients because it provides the opportunity for dynamic interaction among several individuals. Group members form working relationships with other participants, and through their interactions they come to understand themselves better. Members improve their communication and other interpersonal skills and take action to make changes in their lives. *This makes group work unique: the group itself becomes the agent of change for the participants.*

As we will emphasize in this chapter, key roles for group facilitators are to create and maintain the necessary safety for members to be able to participate, and to support the leadership of the participants themselves. When members begin to take responsibility for the group process and relationships, supporting each other to make positive life changes, the facilitator has also supported their empowerment.

Facilitating groups is not easy. With training and the support of regular ongoing supervision, many CHWs find facilitating groups to be a particularly engaging and rewarding part of their work.

21.2 Key Factors among Groups

Before we describe the types of groups most commonly facilitated by CHWs, we want to identify additional key possible differences among the groups that CHWs facilitate. These include the following factors:

GROUP SIZE

Some groups are smaller, others larger, and they may range in size from three to thirty or more members. Both very small and very large groups pose challenges for participants and facilitators. You may find that groups with approximately six to twelve participants allow for dynamic interaction between members and a diversity of experience and points of view, without being so large that they are difficult to manage.

CLOSED GROUPS

Some groups include the same people who participate regularly over a specified time period. Groups with a defined membership generally select members in advance through an invitation, application, or interview process, and do not accept new members for a stipulated period of time, such as the next time that a new group forms, or when there is a need for new participants.

OPEN GROUPS

Some groups are open to anyone who fits the membership criteria. For example, Alcoholics Anonymous meetings are public and open to anyone interested in attending. Open groups, sometimes referred to as "drop-in" groups, may be ongoing, with members rotating in and out as they wish. Facilitating drop-in groups can pose particular challenges (see *The Work of the Facilitator in the Initial* Stage further in this chapter).

DURATION OF THE GROUP

Some groups, such as certain educational groups, may meet just one time. Other groups may continue to meet for several weeks, months, or even years. Some groups are highly structured, as described below, and may always meet for six or eight or ten weeks, and then start up again with new members. The duration of the groups you facilitate will depend on the agency you work for, the community you work with, the issues the group addresses, and the common purpose that brings the members together.

THE GROUP FOCUS ISSUE OR TOPIC

Check online or in the back of your city or county's free paper, if you have one, and you will find a large number of groups addressing a wide variety of topics. CHWs may facilitate groups addressing any number of health-related topics, such as parenting, recovery from drug use, living with disabilities, depression, supporting family members living with different health conditions, sexual assault, domestic violence, surviving the death of a loved one, negotiating healthy relationships, healthy pregnancy, living with disabilities, diabetes, asthma, or other chronic health conditions. The list of possible topics is almost endless.

- *What issues or topics are addressed by groups that take place in your community?*

- *What additional topics or issues would you like to see addressed?*

What Do YOU Think?

LOCATION

Groups may take place in a variety of settings, including nonprofit agencies, clinics and hospitals, schools, faith-based institutions, local departments of public health, recreational centers and facilities, correctional facilities, community centers, group homes, and housing developments.

PURPOSE OF THE GROUP

Some groups are designed to educate participants about a specific health issue such as family planning or hypertension. Other groups aim to support members in changing health-related behaviors, such as smoking, parenting practices, or patterns of drug use. The purpose of other groups is to build self-esteem, community, and a sense of belonging. Most importantly, facilitators and group members need to have a clear understanding of and a commitment to a common purpose that brings them together.

The reasons people decide to participate in a group include:

- To break isolation and build community
- To learn from others who have had similar experiences
- To talk about experiences, identities, feelings, and ideas that may not be understood or accepted in other settings, including the family
- To learn information and skills to better manage a specific illness
- To learn more about oneself
- To change behaviors and take action to enhance health and well-being
- Participation may be mandated by the court or other agency, for example, an anger management or parenting skills group.

- *Can you think of other reasons why people participate in groups?*

GROUP STRUCTURE

Some groups begin with a highly developed structure, purpose, membership criteria, and even an agenda for meetings that are established by the sponsoring program and the facilitators. In others, decisions about the structure of the group are determined by the participants. Educational groups tend to be the most structured. For example, a diabetes education group might always meet once a week for five weeks and have an established purpose and agenda that the facilitator uses to guide each meeting. At the other extreme, social groups are often much more flexible; and the purpose, length, and topics for discussion are determined collaboratively through discussion by the participants and facilitator(s). For example, see the description of a social group for Latino men presented later in this chapter.

GROUP MEMBERSHIP CRITERIA

Membership may be loosely or specifically defined. For example, a group addressing violence in the community may be open to anyone who lives in the community. In contrast, some groups may be open only to people who fit a more specific profile, such as single fathers, Native American youth under the age of eighteen, or African American men living with prostate cancer.

PRESENCE OF A FACILITATOR

Some groups don't have a facilitator. For example, a group for Latino college students might function without an outside facilitator. Other groups may have one or more facilitators.

NUMBER OF FACILITATORS

Sometimes you will facilitate groups on your own and on other occasions with a cofacilitator. Educational groups are more likely to be facilitated by just one CHW. We recommend cofacilitation as the best model for support groups. As part of your training, we hope that you will have the opportunity to work with an experienced cofacilitator. Later on in your career, you may have the opportunity to aid in training a new group facilitator.

ROLE OF FACILITATORS

In most groups, facilitators have a strongly defined leadership role. As we will discuss in this chapter, the facilitator is responsible for setting the clear intention for the group, creating a safe environment that encourages participation and dialogue through providing group agreements or guidelines, assisting to prevent and resolve conflicts, and for modeling how to provide meaningful support. In other groups, such as the social groups that we will discuss in this chapter, the leadership role of the facilitator is less pronounced. In that case, the facilitator's key role is to support the leadership and empowerment of group members, who make most or all of the key decisions about membership, purpose, ground rules, and the topics addressed during group meetings.

Regardless of the level of formality and structure of the group, and the authority of the facilitator, CHWs should always be supervised and guided by client and community-centered practices designed to enhance the capacity and leadership of group members themselves.

For the purposes of this chapter, we will emphasize three different types of groups that CHWs commonly facilitate: educational, support, and social groups.

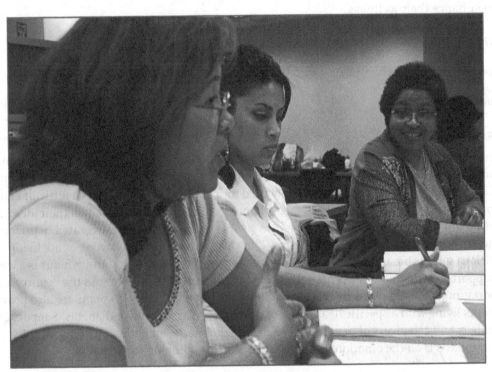

Breaking participants into small groups gives everyone the chance to participate.

21.3 Types of Groups

What Do YOU Think?

- *What type of groups have you participated in?*

- *What motivated you to participate in the group(s)?*

- *What were the benefits for you?*

- *What was your experience like overall?*

There are many different types of groups, including a wide range of therapy groups facilitated by licensed mental health providers such as social workers, counselors, psychologists, or psychiatrists. For the purposes of this textbook, we will focus on the types of groups most commonly facilitated by CHWs, and will refer to them as *educational, social, and support groups*. Different agencies and regions of the United States and the world may refer to these types of groups by different names.

EDUCATIONAL GROUPS

Educational groups bring people together who are seeking to learn new information about a specific health topic. Some examples of educational groups include an educational group that focuses on the prevention of a particular illness or health condition, a group to support behavior change with those with a desire to quit smoking cigarettes, and a group learning stress reduction practices such as meditation. Other groups provide people newly diagnosed with a health condition, such as asthma, lupus, or hepatitis C, with information about the condition, how to manage it, and how to prevent progression of the disease. The groups typically focus on enhancing health-related knowledge and skills, and provide an opportunity for people to share questions, concerns, feelings, and knowledge that they have gained through their own experience.

In general, educational groups are time limited. Once the basic health information has been covered, the group ends. Some groups might meet just once, and others might meet four or five times, depending on the nature of the health issues. Educational groups might be held in a variety of locations, including a clinic or hospital, schools, and community-based and faith-based organizations. Educational groups are commonly facilitated by one CHW, but may be cofacilitated. The emphasis is on providing health information that will assist participants to enhance their wellness.

- *Can you think of other examples of educational groups that are offered in your community?*

- *Who facilitates these groups?*

- *What issues do they address?*

SUPPORT GROUPS

Support groups may or may not have a facilitator. They provide a place for people who share a common experience, concern, or goal to meet and talk together, and to provide each other with support for improving their health or life circumstances. These groups are widely used for people who have survived difficult experiences (such as rape or the death of a family member), face stigma and discrimination based on their identity or behavior (such as for Latino immigrants, transgender women, or people who have been incarcerated in prison), share risks for a specific health condition (such as HIV, hepatitis C, or risk from smoking tobacco), or are living with a disease or health condition (such as breast cancer, alcoholism, or depression). Alcoholics Anonymous is a well-known example of a support group. Rape crisis centers and domestic violence agencies across the country also commonly facilitate support groups for survivors. Increasingly, clinics, hospitals, and health plans are also providing support groups for patients living with a specific health risk or disease such as asthma or diabetes. Support groups for the family members and caregivers of people with cancer, Alzheimer's, and other chronic conditions may also be provided. The emphasis is on the emotional support that peers can provide to each other.

- *Can you think of other examples of support groups that are offered in your community?*

- *Who facilitates these groups?*

- *What issues do they address?*

Alma Vasquez: When I first started facilitating groups I was a little nervous, but it gave me the opportunity to align myself more with the clients and gave me the opportunity to step outside a one-on-one meeting and see a client in a community setting. My first group was a Latina Support group with migrant Latina women. It was a great experience to see a group of women who shared experiences and see them interact. They got a sense of belonging, and also a sense of home. To speak their native language freely helped them to feel welcomed and embraced. They now had a safe space to share.

I also had an experience facilitating a group inside a jail. It allowed me to come in as a facilitator, but also as a human being. Some of the men had never had a healthy relationship with a woman. This was the first time for them to have a respectful interaction with a woman, a relationship with

(continues)

(continued)

appropriate boundaries, and with someone who could bring resources to them inside the jail. It was a humanizing feeling. I was culturally humbled by it. Lock-up has its own culture. There is a way things are done—a lifestyle they've become accustomed to. I was bringing a little bit of the outside to them—they are the forgotten generation.

SOCIAL GROUPS

Support groups are not familiar to or appropriate for all communities. Some people feel that support groups are a culturally specific model, that they emphasize problems or challenges, and that they are based on therapy groups. For these reasons and others, some communities prefer to form and facilitate social groups. Social groups tend to be less formal than support groups and are generally characterized by greater autonomy of the group members. For example, participants often take responsibility for determining what the group will address, membership criteria, ground rules, and when and how the group will meet. A key role of facilitators is to support the leadership of the members, to assist in fostering a sense of community, to step in when needed, and to resolve conflicts or address issues that the members themselves may not be prepared or willing or able to address. The emphasis is empowerment and community building.

A Social Group for Latino Men

A local health department, concerned about the increase of HIV infections among Latino men who have sex with men (MSM), asked a community-based agency to start support groups for this population. When the agency conducted interviews with this community, they found little interest in attending traditional support groups. However, the men did report a sense of isolation and the lack of meeting spaces in their home county. Instead, they visited urban areas outside of the county to meet other men. The men were very interested in creating meeting spaces and a stronger sense of community nearer to home.

Based on this formative research, agency staff initiated a social group that met for dinner on a weekday evening. Eventually, the men decided to cook dinner together, using the agency's large kitchen on a night when they could use it with privacy. Together, the participants determined when and where they would meet, what they would talk about, and decided to keep the group open to new members. While the CHW who facilitated the social group informed participants that his primary job was to work on HIV-prevention issues, he didn't push any particular agenda for discussion.

As the men began to build relationships with each other and to establish a basis for trust, they began to talk about a range of issues including coming out, family and community acceptance, dating, sex, healthy relationships, drug use, and HIV and other STIs (sexually transmitted infections). Over the course of a year, participants reported increased comfort with their sexual orientation, a deeper sense of belonging to a community, and increased commitment to and confidence in their ability to negotiate safer sex.

Please watch the following video interview ▶ with Alma Vasquez, a CHW working in San Francisco. Ms. Vasquez talks about her experience facilitating a support group for Latinas.

GROUP FACILITATION: CHW INTERVIEW

🔗 *http://youtu.be/36IBED_1Nvk*

21.4 The Unique Advantages of Group Work

What Do YOU Think?

- *Reflect on your experiences participating in different types of groups. What was it about the group that was most helpful to you?*

Participating in group work is different in many ways from working one-on-on with a service provider. Dr. Irvin Yalom identified several factors that make group work unique, based on his years of work as a mental health clinician. He identified twelve therapeutic (beneficial or healing) factors that people who participated in groups reported as being particularly helpful to them (Yalom, 1995). While Dr. Yalom comes from a clinical perspective, the 12 factors that he identified hold true for the types of groups facilitated by CHWs.

1. **Installation of (or building) hope:** Hope is a strong motivator and is one primary reason people give for beginning a process of change.

2. **Universality (or building a deep connection with others):** Universality refers to the human experience of finding that one is not alone. While each person's problems may be unique, connecting with others who have experienced similar events, circumstances, and emotions can be a powerful experience, particularly for people who have survived traumatic experiences or whose identity or behaviors are stigmatized by the larger society. Finding commonality with others assists to quiet self-doubts that may arise when one feels isolated and alone with a difficult experience. For example, the rape crisis movement created safe spaces for survivors of rape to meet together and provide each other with meaningful support, breaking silences and isolation.

3. **Altruism (or true generosity to others):** Altruism refers to acts of unselfish giving to others. Research has shown that in interpersonal relationships where individuals find a high degree of satisfaction, they sometimes act for the benefit of the other without expectation of return. In social or support groups, participants develop a connection that fosters generosity and unselfish giving to other members. The experience of providing meaningful support to others in need can also boost the self-esteem of those who offer support.

4. **Corrective recapitulation of the primary family group (or healing from bad family experiences, and learning new ways of building healthy relationships):** Essentially, this means that group participants may have the opportunity to replay the tape of earlier experiences with family and to learn emotional responses that are more productive and supportive of good health. For example, if one was the victim of trauma in childhood, one can now develop the skills to put a stop to abuse in adulthood.

5. **Development of socializing skills:** Group participation provides a rich opportunity to improve interpersonal skills such as listening more deeply to the experience of others, expressing feelings, handling conflict, negotiating safe and meaningful relationships, or promoting health and wellness. Participants receive feedback and support from their peers in practicing behaviors that reinforce their health and that of their families and communities.

6. **Imitative behavior (or the influence of role models):** In groups, people observe others making choices that they might like to incorporate into their own lives. By observing the behavior of others, participants learn different ways of communicating and living. This is the same process by which younger children learn from observing their older brothers and sisters. For example, participants might learn from one another new ways to manage anger, reduce stress, or cook traditional foods that are lower in calories.

7. **Interpersonal learning (or learning from interactions with others):** Interpersonal learning means that we learn more about how our own behavior affects and is perceived by others, as well as how to create meaningful connections and offer support. The advantage of the group experience, in this regard, is that participants don't have to guess at the impact of their actions. Under skilled leadership, the group can explicitly assist the members to understand themselves in an interpersonal context and can develop and enhance the skills essential to creating and maintaining healthy relationships with others. For example, participants might learn new ways to respond to differences of opinion, to receive feedback from others, and to take responsibility for actions that are harmful or hurtful to others.

8. **Group cohesiveness (or creating community and experiencing a sense of belonging):** This may be the most powerful factor of all. Group cohesiveness refers to the feeling of belonging to a group of people you admire and want to be a part of. When the group is working well, participants may experience a sense of deep connection and commitment.

9. **Catharsis (or the expression of strong emotion):** Catharsis is the experience of having expressed strong and often difficult emotions in a way that feels healthy, productive, and healing. Catharsis requires a safe environment that supports not only the expression of experiences and emotion, but also the opportunity to reflect on the meaning of these emotions. For example, survivors of sexual assault may express emotions

that are difficult for them to share anywhere else. Through expressing these emotions, survivors may begin to better understand how assault has affected their lives and their individual paths to recovery.

10. **Imparting information (or sharing information with others):** Group participants share information with each other, including information about what they do to promote their own health and well-being. Because group members share a common connection and experience, the information they share with each other is often highly relevant. Hearing information from someone you know and respect is generally much more powerful than reading about it in a book or brochure. For example, people living with HIV disease might share information about how they navigate the health care system to get the care they need or what they do to manage stress or depression.

11. **Existential factors (or life choices and meaning):** It has been said that group work recapitulates (or repeats) key aspects of life. The behavior of members in the group, including positive experiences of handling conflict and building connections with others, can motivate participants to make similar choices elsewhere in their lives.

12. **Self-understanding:** In many cases, people who participate in groups gain new insights and knowledge about themselves, the way they interact with others, and the feelings and thoughts that may unconsciously influence their behavior. This is often associated with increased acceptance of themselves and enhanced self-esteem.

These twelve factors have been identified as key opportunities and benefits from participating in groups.

- *Have you ever experienced or benefited from participating in a group in any of the twelve ways described above?*

- *As a group facilitator how would you encourage or support the development of these key factors?*

- *Can you think of other factors that contribute to the power and benefit of group participation?*

21.5 Group Functions and Processes

The group itself—through the power of its **cohesion** or togetherness—influences people to try new ways of thinking, feeling, and behaving. While every experience is unique, groups often share common processes. By understanding these common processes, you can be prepared for the sorts of things that might come up in the group you are facilitating. The following section is adapted, with some additions, from the American Group Psychotherapy Association (American Group Psychotherapy Association, 2007).

THE GROUP AS A SOCIAL SYSTEM

It is helpful to think of a group as its own culture, with its own rules, roles, boundaries, and values. As a facilitator, it is helpful to keep in mind these cultural processes are continually arising and changing within groups.

Rules: Members establish group norms with the assistance of facilitators. These rules, sometimes called guidelines or agreements, cover expectations about everything from being on time, to when and how much to talk, to respecting different experiences and opinions, to practicing nonviolence in all interpersonal interactions. They are similar to the ground rules that govern our participation in classes or trainings and at work and are essential in building trust and creating a safe environment to support inclusive participation.

Roles: Group members will likely find a role to perform within the larger circle of group work. The facilitator's role is clear: to assist the group to achieve and maintain cohesion. Finding one's role is frequently the task of early group membership. People report greater calm and less anxiety once they establish what they can expect of others. Facilitators can aid in acknowledging and appreciating the role that each participant plays in the life of the group.

Boundaries: Boundaries are enforced by rules, and they assist in making a group physically and emotionally safe to explore new challenges and new choices. Boundaries overlap with the ground rules discussed above. They include maintaining the confidentiality of participants, and professional relationships between participants and facilitators. The boundaries that will guide group work must be developed at the beginning of a new group in order for members to feel comfortable participating. For more on boundaries see the section titled Ethics and Group Facilitation at the end of this chapter.

Values: Groups universally come to value openness, honesty, and respect in interpersonal communication. They also value interpersonal safety, including confidentiality, and creating opportunities for participants to learn, grow, and change. Groups may wish to speak openly about shared values and to revisit them during times of conflict.

BENEFICIAL AND HARMFUL GROUP PROCESSES

Group processes may be beneficial or harmful (or neither).

Beneficial Processes

Beneficial processes include the following:

Conflict management and resolution: For some participants, the group offers an opportunity to experience a healthy resolution of conflicts. With skilled leadership and facilitation, group members can experience conflict as a natural and inevitable part of life. They learn strategies for managing conflict that lead to greater understanding of themselves and others.

Contagion: Contagion refers to the spread of attitudes or behaviors from one member to the group. It can be either harmful or beneficial. It may be harmful to the group process when, for example, it undermines the willingness to address difficult issues, or it reinforces discriminatory treatment of group members or other behaviors that may be harmful to participants. At its best, contagion represents the spread of positive attitudes and behaviors to others, such as an attitude and feeling of hope, or a desire to listen and support one another.

Cohesion: As identified above as a key benefit of group participation, cohesion is a sense of belonging to a community. It motivates members to achieve positive growth and change. A cohesive group often feels that "We are growing and changing in positive directions together, and we are all important members and contributors to this process!"

> **Andrew Ciscel:** I really like cofacilitating groups, because I get to witness people connecting with each other, building community, and feeling good about what they accomplish. The key aspect of groups is the sense of friendship and community that the participants create with each other. This motivates them to keep coming to the group, and it creates a kind of mutual responsibility. They support each other to get a clearer sense of their own goals—and the inspiration for what they want to achieve or change.

Harmful Processes

Harmful group processes work to defeat the primary task of the group and include the following:

Subgrouping: Subgrouping, *or w*hen part of the group splits off and forms a subgroup, may also be either beneficial or harmful. When it is harmful, subgrouping may occur when individual members' differences are not resolved and become a source of division. This can threaten the cohesion of the group as whole. At its worst, subgrouping results in discrimination against certain members based on real or perceived differences in experience, identity, values, or beliefs. The group may ignore, isolate, insult, or fail to provide support or validation to these members.

Contagion: Contagion may be harmful to the group process when, for example, it undermines the willingness to address difficult issues, or it reinforces discriminatory treatment of group members or other behaviors that may be harmful to participants.

Absence: An individual member's lack of ability to be physically and psychologically present due to any number of personal reasons. Carefully screening participants in advance about their ability to be physically, emotionally, and intellectually present can prevent this.

Avoidance: When the group is unable or unwilling to approach important topics, including issues or conflicts that arise among members, the group can become ineffective and lifeless. Avoidance can include an individual member's psychological defenses as well as the group's defenses as a whole.

It is the responsibility of the group facilitator to address and minimize the harmful factors identified above, and to maximize those factors that are beneficial. This is skilled work and takes time to master. Again, specific and ongoing clinical supervision is essential to the development of solid group facilitation skills.

21.6 The Roles and Abilities of Group Facilitators

For the group to be effective in its work, the facilitator(s) must be adequately prepared for the intellectual, emotional, and behavioral challenges that group members will bring and create.

KEY ROLES OF GROUP FACILITATORS

A comprehensive study of leadership functions identified four key roles of group facilitators (Lieberman, Yalom, & Miles, 1973):

1. **Executive Function:** Executive functions are those that manage the rules and boundaries of the group, assisting to create and preserve safety and to prevent and resolve discriminatory treatment. They include setting the clear purpose or intention for the group, assistance in the development of group guidelines or agreements, resolution of conflicts, time and space management, as well as other administrative tasks that keep the group on task. The facilitator monitors each member's participation and acts to create opportunities for those who have been silent to be able to speak, and for those who have spoken a lot to listen more.

2. **Caring:** Caring refers to the group facilitator's ability to convey to each group member individually, and to the group as a whole, that their well-being matters. This is done in many ways, including listening attentively to the contributions of each group participant, respecting the experience and perspective of each participant, asking members if they would like to speak, and acknowledging the positive contributions of each member.

3. **Support for the Expression of Emotion:** The group facilitator sets the tone for the group and supports and affirms the expression of feelings, personal value statements, and personal attitudes.

4. **Support for Expression of Meaning:** The group facilitator effectively assists the group as a whole, as well as the individual members, to understand themselves more deeply and thoroughly. The group facilitator does this by inviting individuals and the group to talk about the significance and meaning of their participation and experience. For example, a facilitator might ask questions such as: "There aren't any public places for gay and bisexual Latino men to meet here, and many of you have spoken about being hesitant to come out in your families and churches. How do you think that affects you?" "What do you think it would be like to be able to come out and to be fully accepted by your families and communities?" "What role does this group play in your life?" "Last week, we touched on some powerful topics. Did anything take place during group that had particular meaning for you?" These questions are also designed to provide opportunities to the group to talk about issues that have particular significance and meaning in their lives.

PREVENTING DISCRIMINATORY TREATMENT

A responsibility for preventing and intervening to stop discriminatory treatment is another key role for group facilitators. In societies characterized by bias, prejudice, and discrimination, group members are likely to act these out. Intentionally or unintentionally, participants may sometimes act in ways that exclude, confront, shame, or punish people who are perceived as belonging to groups that historically face discriminatory treatment. For members who are the targets of this behavior, the group experience may repeat the very traumatic experiences that negatively impact their health. For this reason, groups often define membership criteria in ways that are designed to create a safer environment for members from a common community, such as Latino men who have sex with men or Native American women.

Nothing can damage the life, value, reputation, and success of a group as powerfully as uninterrupted prejudice or discriminatory treatment of participants. As a facilitator, one of the most important roles is to carefully monitor the group and to quickly intervene to restore respect, equity, and safety if you observe discriminatory treatment. This will also be discussed later in this chapter in the section on Ethics and Group Facilitation.

KEY ABILITIES OF FACILITATORS

The success of group work is also enhanced by the ability of the facilitator to do the following:

Show Up: The effective group facilitator is personally, emotionally, and intellectually present to assist the group to create and maintain a safe environment for personal exploration. Facilitators need to learn to let go of their own agendas and emotions and to concentrate on the participation of group members.

Pay Attention: The effective group facilitator pays close attention to all the communications of the group as a whole as well as the individual members so that people feel heard and cared for.

Tell the Truth: The effective group facilitator is able to see and comment on both potentially harmful and beneficial group dynamics including, as referenced above, dynamics of subgrouping, avoidance, and conflict. The facilitator keeps the focus on telling the truth about what is taking place during the group.

Let Go of the Outcome: The effective group facilitator trusts that the individual members will do their best to learn from the group. Letting go of the outcome expresses your deep faith in the capacity of group members to be responsible for what they get out of the group.

21.7 Facilitation Techniques

The following techniques are used to fulfill the basic role and functions of group facilitators:

NAMING

Naming means to acknowledge a dynamic that is happening in the group such as prolonged silence, tension, anxiety, fear, bias, subgrouping, exclusion or conflict. These dynamics may be neutral (silence), positive (enthusiasm, support for a group member, a deep common connection, humor, silence), or negative (such as discrimination against certain group members). The idea is to name or to ask the group to name what is happening in order to provoke reflection and learning about the nature of the group dynamic or interaction or to interrupt potentially harmful behavior. The facilitator might comment on the process ("So, it seems like people aren't talking right now. What is coming up for you?"). The facilitator could ask the group to name what is happening ("What is going on in the group right now?"). This is an opportunity for the group to analyze their interactions, increasing their knowledge and communication skills.

SILENCE

Silence in a group can be uncomfortable, but often serves a beneficial purpose. Facilitators and participants should strive to become comfortable with silence, instead of rushing to say something. People often require time to reflect on what has been said or what has occurred, and to identify their feelings and thoughts, before they speak. When silence arises naturally in a group, try to sit back and just let it be for 10 to 20 seconds. See what will happen. Maybe a new idea will come up, or perhaps somebody who hasn't participated will speak up. Even if nothing new happens, that is all right.

Facilitators can also ask the group for a moment of silence. This can be useful to give people a chance to reflect on something that has just been said. Sometimes, the facilitator may need a few moments to reflect and figure out what to do next. Asking for silence in these moments is a way to take care of yourself, so that you can take care of the group.

FOCUS ON THE PRESENT TENSE

Encourage participants to stay in the here-and-now and to address recent events, especially in regard to any interactions going on within the group itself. The material of early life experience and injury or trauma is best addressed in therapy with licensed professionals. If or when issues arise from earlier experience, guide participants to reflect on how these prior experiences may influence the present—what is happening right here and now. For example a facilitator may ask "What is happening right now for you? Might there be any pattern you recognize in your decision-making that is not in your best interest right now? What kind of support would be helpful from us in the group right now?" Remember the present tense is the *only* time any of us have to learn something new, make a different choice, and create positive change.

Andrew Ciscel: I cofacilitate a recovery and wellness group. Everyone has had some type of mental health challenge—either in the past or in the present. They come to the group to support each other. Sometimes people talk about really big or hard issues. We allow space for people to talk about what is important to them, and to have an emotional release when they need it. Then we help to shift the conversation to the coping skills that people can use in the present to manage memories and emotions. The focus is on what they can do to in their daily lives that promotes their wellness. The participants get really engaged in sharing ideas and strategies with each other.

GUIDING INCLUSIVE PARTICIPATION

Not all members will speak up and actively participate in group discussions. Yet it is important for the group to hear all voices and to benefit from the input of all members. A key role of the facilitator is to support all members in talking and sharing their experiences, ideas, and feelings, and to guard against dynamics that are dominated by a minority of speakers (see Common Challenges in the section titled Challenges of Group Facilitation).

MAPPING THE CONVERSATION

A technique that can be helpful for understanding group interactions is to map the conversation. Start by drawing a representation of the group, as in Figure 21.1, that shows where each group participant sits. During the group conversation, draw in:

- Solid directional arrows to indicate when one member speaks directly to another
- Dotted lines to indicate a statement made to the entire group

It is easiest to do this when there are two facilitators, and one can focus on mapping part of the conversation. They might do this for just 5–10 minutes or so. After the group session ends, the cofacilitators can analyze the map and talk about what it indicates about patterns of communication within the group. Who is speaking most often? Who is not speaking as much or at all? How often are comments being made to the entire group? Your analysis can assist cofacilitators to shift the way that they to direct the flow of conversation in order to increase the participation of all members, and to prevent just a few members from dominating the discussion.

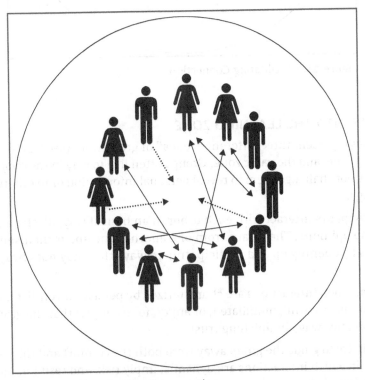

Figure 21.1 Mapping the Conversation

- *What does the map provided above tell you about participation in the group?*

FACILITATING CONNECTION

Sometimes, group interactions are dominated by prolonged conversation between one group member and the facilitator. Your role as group leader is to facilitate interaction and dialogue among *all* group members. Imagine, for example, that you ask an open-ended question to the group, and Peter answers. Instead of responding to Peter, you might ask the group as a whole, or another member, what they think about what Peter just said. (See Figure 21.2.) This technique is sometimes referred to as triangulation, and is used to foster more inclusive participation so that all members benefit equally from the unique power of group dynamics.

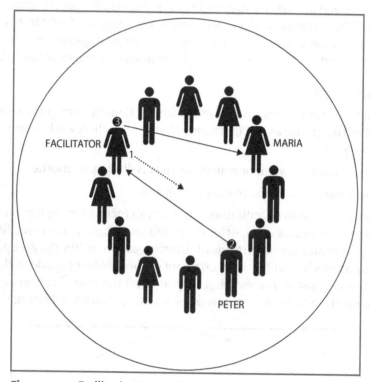

Figure 21.2 Facilitating Connection

GUIDING PARTICIPANTS INTO THE LEARNING ZONE

The three concentric circles represent three different "zones" of group work (see Figure 21.3). These are the comfort zone, the learning zone, and the panic zone. Groups often like to stay in the *comfort zone* because it is easy and familiar and does not challenge them to reveal personal information or to otherwise take risks that can inspire learning and change.

In the *learning zone,* participants interact with each other in an honest way, disclosing their own life experiences, feelings, and opinions. They learn from one another and about themselves. The learning zone implies taking risks by opening up and participating in ways that may not always be familiar or comfortable.

A group is in the *panic zone* when interactions are characterized by persistent conflict, and when one or more members become so emotional (fearful, humiliated, or angry, for example) that the group can no longer interact in a safe and productive way, diminishing trust.

A successful facilitator will try to guide the group away from both the comfort and the panic zones, and to stay close to the learning zone in which interactions are dynamic, imply risk, and result in meaningful learning and motivation for positive action.

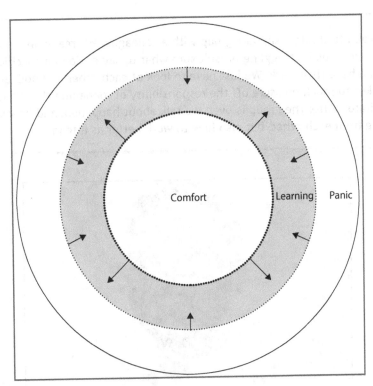

Figure 21.3 Learning Zones

COFACILITATION OF GROUPS

Sometimes CHWs will facilitate groups on their own, and sometimes with a cofacilitator. While each model poses slightly different challenges, in both circumstances you are responsible for ensuring the physical and emotional safety of participants and successful group interactions that provide members with information and support designed to promote their health.

We encourage CHWs who are facilitating groups for the first time to seek out opportunities to cofacilitate with an experienced colleague. Through working together, you will be able to observe, practice, and learn essential skills and techniques.

When working with a cofacilitator, you will want to meet in advance to plan how you will work together to create and sustain a positive group process. Take this opportunity to clarify your goals for the group, how you will establish membership criteria and ground rules, and your approach to ensuring group safety and responding to conflicts. The more that you and your cofacilitator are on the same page, the more effective the group process will be. The success of groups suffers significantly when cofacilitators are unable to work together in a collegial, respectful, and coordinated fashion. During your planning, talk about how you wish to handle differences of opinion that may arise between the two of you.

Be sure to check in with each other between each group session, to debrief what occurred in the last session, and to make plans for the next. This is the time to raise concerns about individual members, the group process, and cofacilitation. It is also an opportunity for you to talk about any personal issues or challenges that have come up as a consequence of facilitating the group. For example, you might have a strong reaction to a particular event that occurred in group that is related to your own life experience. Talking about this openly and honestly with your cofacilitator can ensure that your personal issues don't unduly influence the group process.

If you are unable to productively work through challenges or disagreements between you and your cofacilitator, make an appointment as soon as possible to talk with a supervisor and ask for guidance and support for moving forward in a productive fashion. This is your ethical obligation to the group. You must always put their interests and welfare above your own and address your own challenges, no matter how difficult, in order to keep your ethical commitment to the group and its members.

> **Andrew Ciscel:** I facilitate a support group with a colleague. We really understand each other, and know that if one of us is struggling or isn't sure what to say or do in a specific situation, that other will notice and have their back. We just have to look at each other and nod, and the other knows to step in. It takes so much pressure off the responsibility of managing the group when you have a good cofacilitator. After the group is over, we talk about happened, and how we handled it. We keep learning from each other, but also how to work better as a team.

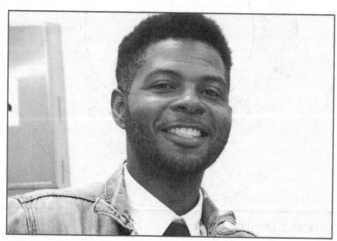

CHWs cofacilitate groups that bring people together to talk about common experiences and health issues.

21.8 Autonomy and Control

Issues of autonomy and control are essential to consider when facilitating groups, just as they are when working with individual clients, or families. Keep client-centered concepts in mind, including cultural humility, and practice in ways that transfer power from you as a service provider to the participants in the group. Always keep in mind that a key outcome for all the work that you do with clients is to support and enhance their autonomy and self-determination.

THE POWER AND AUTHORITY OF FACILITATORS

Regardless of the level of formality and structure of the group, CHWs should always be guided by client and community-centered practice designed to enhance the leadership of group members. Facilitators also need to acknowledge the power of their authority as group leaders, and to be open to constructive feedback. Skilled facilitators are also conscious of inviting all group members to share different opinions, experiences, and belief systems.

Group participants often give power to the facilitator even if the facilitator doesn't want it. For example, participants will often wait for the facilitator to set the agenda, to respond to a comment, to offer support to a member, or to intervene in the early stages of a potential conflict. A skilled facilitator works in ways that encourage participants to demonstrate their own leadership in these moments.

Because group members may defer to the authority of the group facilitator, it is particularly important that facilitators don't bring their own issues, concerns, and experiences into the group or otherwise make the group about themselves. Working with a cofacilitator can be helpful here. During your check-in meetings, try to assess whether or not your own issues may be influencing the group discussions or dynamics.

COMMUNITY AND PARTICIPANT EMPOWERMENT

Perhaps the most important measure of the success of a group is the extent to which it fosters the participation and empowerment of its members. While group facilitators must be strong leaders in order to ensure nondiscrimination and safety for all members, *the transformative power of the group process to promote life changes must come from the participants themselves.* As a facilitator, you will support group members, to the extent possible, to establish ground rules, to identify common values and goals, to develop skills in providing meaningful support to each other, and in honoring differences and resolving conflict. When this occurs, participants emerge from the group process more competent and capable of employing these same skills in other relationships and areas of their lives. A truly healthy and effective group may not require much participation, intervention, or direction for the group facilitator: members learn how to keep the group process on track and to support each member in gaining the confidence to make significant life changes.

Strong group facilitation skills are often embodied by a quiet but firm leadership style that becomes more prominent when events occur that could be harmful to members, and stays in the background when participants are engaged in dynamic and supportive discussion. As always, be aware of your tendencies to dominate the life of the group and to unconsciously undermine the autonomy and leadership of participants.

21.9 Professional Boundaries and Supervision

As a group facilitator, you are highly likely to face challenges related to establishing and maintaining healthy professional boundaries. Your ability to handle these challenges will be greatly improved by self-reflection and self-awareness, and by seeking out regular supervision and support from experienced colleagues.

SELF-AWARENESS

Our own experiences, feelings, opinions, culture, and values sometimes get in the way of providing culturally sensitive and client-centered services (you may hear this phenomenon referred to as "countertransference" by those who work in mental health settings). The most effective group facilitators are those who recognize that their own issues may be stimulated (or become active) and are prepared to take action to minimize the potential damage to the group.

Because group work is dynamic and requires the development of relationships between group members, issues related to our own relationships are likely to be restimulated. These may include unresolved issues in our family of origin, current relationships and family, or our prior experience participating in different types of groups. For example, if your role in your family of origin (the family or families you grew up with) was to be silent when conflicts developed, you may feel uncomfortable about speaking up or addressing conflicts, even if that is part of your role as group facilitator.

Signs that the facilitator's own issues may be getting in the way of the work include:

- Finding it difficult to listen to what others are saying
- Strong emotional reactions to what occurs in group
- A tendency to avoid particular topics, dynamics, or group members
- Making assumptions about the experience, values, emotions, or ideas of others
- Negative reactions, thoughts, or feelings about certain group members
- Paying less attention to some group members than others
- Strong opinions or judgments about the behaviors or beliefs of clients
- A strong desire to share personal information

- *Can you think of other signs that a CHW's own issues might be getting in the way of their ability to work effectively with clients?*

- *Can you identify personal issues (we all have them!) that might get in the way of your work?*

An effective group facilitator is *not* one who has it all together and who has worked through and resolved all personal issues that could possibly interfere with their ability to provide effective services: this isn't an attainable goal! The key is to recognize what personal issues may be restimulating for you, to do what you can ahead of time to address these issues, and to seek out supervision for support when your issues are restimulated.

All CHWs, regardless of whether or not they facilitate groups, have an ethical duty to develop self-awareness and to identify personal issues that could get in the way of their work. This challenge is also addressed in Chapters 1, 6, and 7.

To reflect on whether or not personal issues may be getting in the way of your work, think about what you say and do during group work. When you speak, are you doing so for the benefit of the group, or to fulfill a personal need? If you find that you have a thought that you are compelled to share, it may be about yourself rather than the group. If you find that the motivations are more personal than professional (the feeling that I *must* share my point of view), try not to speak until you have a chance to reflect on and to understand what is influencing you. Chances are it is you (and not the group members) who wants to hear your story.

As always, we strongly encourage you to reflect on and talk about these personal issues with others. This may be a colleague, your cofacilitator, a counselor, or a trusted friend, and your supervisor. The most important thing is not to avoid these insights, but to investigate and strive to understand them. Remember that you need to do this not only for yourself, but also out of concern for the welfare of group members and other clients. If you are facilitating a group, you should receive regular supervision. Some of the many things to explore during your supervision are personal issues that are being restimulated by group work and how you are handling them.

- *What resources do you have to reflect on personal issues that may get in the way of your work with groups and other clients?*

- *Who can you talk to about these issues?*

GUIDELINES FOR SELF-DISCLOSURE

Self-disclosure means that a CHW or other helping professional shares personal information about themselves with clients (please refer to Chapter 7 for more information about the topic of self-disclosure). As a rule, we encourage facilitators not to disclose personal information about themselves to the group. Self-disclosure can sometimes change the dynamic of the group to focus on the experiences, needs, and ideas of the facilitator rather than of those in the group. This risk is particularly significant because of the unique power and authority of group facilitators. Self-disclosure should never be used as a way to connect with a client or establish rapport. Although this may feel like an easy way to make connections, there are better ways to do this such as building trust with honesty and compassion over time.

If you consider disclosing personal information to the group, we suggest the following five guidelines, with the primary goal of minimum self-disclosure and shifting the focus back toward the client or group as soon as possible:

1. In general, don't disclose personal information to the clients you work with or the participants of a group.

2. Consult with your cofacilitator or supervisor in advance about the potential risks and benefits of self-disclosure in the group environment. What information are you considering sharing with the group, and why?

3. If you decide to self-disclose, be certain that you know how it will legitimately benefit the group. If you are motivated to disclose information for a personal reason, or to build rapport, please don't disclose. Let your client-centered and group facilitation skills do the talking for you.

4. When disclosing, be brief. You may reveal a fact about yourself, but should not share the details or take time and attention away from the group participants. For example, the facilitator of a group for people living with HIV disease may disclose that they are also living with HIV disease (we are not making a value judgment about the wisdom of disclosing such information). But they should not go on to share additional information (such as to explain how they were infected, how many T cells they have, or what kinds of medications they take, etc.). This is likely to unduly influence the focus, direction, or safety of the group.

5. Never disclose current sexual behavior or current drug use.

We strongly encourage you to talk with coworkers and your supervisor about the issue of self-disclosure before you consider doing it. Ask them to share their beliefs and practices in relation to self-disclosure.

- *What are your personal beliefs and guidelines about self-disclosure?*

- *Would you ever disclose personal information to a client?*

- *If so, what information might you share, when, and why?*

- *What do you think the risks of self-disclosure may be in your situation?*

- *What questions about self-disclosure might you discuss with your supervisor?*

SUPERVISION IS ESSENTIAL FOR GROUP FACILITATORS

Supervision is essential for CHWs who facilitate groups. Quality supervision should be provided on a regular and ongoing basis, ideally by someone with extensive experience facilitating groups. This is often a licensed professional with many years of experience.

The function of good supervision is to ensure that group members are provided with a safe, supportive, and effective environment that promotes reflection, learning, and change. It is also designed to support CHWs and other facilitators to enhance their self-awareness and their overall skills for facilitation. Supportive supervision serves to create an environment in which a CHW can talk about what is going on in the group, ask questions about techniques or courses of action, explore strategies for dealing with challenging group issues or individuals, discuss ethical and boundary issues related to their own feelings and experience in the group, and receive positively framed critical feedback and other helpful suggestions. The content of a supervision session is confidential unless there are mandated reporting issues determined by the supervisor (such as child or elder abuse, domestic violence, etc.).

21.10 The Stages of Group Work

Various authors have described a predictable sequence of stages that represent the development of emotional and physical safety necessary for a well-run, high-functioning group. Knowing about these common stages may assist you to identify how your own group is progressing and to anticipate and manage challenges that may arise. Bruce Tuckman's memorable names for these stages are Forming, Storming, Norming, Performing, and Adjourning (Tuckman, 1965). Marianne Schneider Corey and Gerald Corey (2006) build on Tuckman's work to describe the stages of group work as follows.

THE INITIAL STAGE (FORMING)

At the beginning of a new group, members may be somewhat hesitant to participate and may have concerns about whether the group facilitators are competent, whether the group offers a format that will be useful to them, if they will be accepted and come to belong, and more. Participants may be on their best behavior and be cautious about sharing their life experiences, challenges, and doubts. In the beginning stages, people are searching for structure and safety that will support them in taking risks and sharing more intimate and difficult information.

Bruce Tuckman called this the *Forming Stage*. The group forms around its tasks and boundaries. Participants decide what they want to accomplish, how to define membership, and what the ground rules are that will allow them to function well together. There is a high sense of individuality at this stage.

The membership functions in the initial stage are to begin to participate by sharing relatively safe personal information, telling stories about life experiences, cooperating to set rules for the group for attendance and confidentiality, and establishing expectations of each other and the facilitator(s).

The Work of Facilitators in the Initial Stage

In the first stages, the facilitator's task is to clarify the purpose and intention of the group, and to establish physical and emotional safety by assisting the group to identify common goals, expectations, and ground rules that will guide their participation. Overall, your goal in the initial stage of group work is to assist the group in creating an atmosphere of safety, shared purpose, and intention.

You will assist the group to anticipate differences in terms of their experiences, opinions, beliefs, and values. This is important to do at the beginning of new groups, as is framing conflict as a natural, inevitable, and often productive aspect of life and group work. You can also assist the group to establish agreements about the way they will handle disagreements and conflicts, and you should emphasize that a key part of the group's role is to ensure that conflicts don't spiral out of control in way that is harmful to individual members and the group itself. To read more about conflict resolution concepts and skills, please refer to Chapter 13.

As the facilitator, you direct the flow of communication, encouraging but not pushing all members to participate and ensuring that no individual group member dominates the discussion or pushes an agenda that does not resonate and is not supported by the group as a whole.

A strategy for assisting the group to establish safety is to assist members to recognize the similarities they share with others. In the beginning, encourage each group member to speak, and assist them to identify experiences, ideas, feelings, and values that they share in common. These opportunities for sharing in the initial stage should be relatively "low risk" sharing activities whose main purpose is to build connections and relationships among members. It is important that each person identify at least one other person in the group who appears to share some point of view, experience, or value system.

Any similarity between members, however superficial, opens the door for personal sharing. This is one reason why the membership of groups is often structured around common identities and experiences. For example, groups might be established for Cambodian women living with breast cancer, Latino parents with a child who is developmentally disabled, or men diagnosed with high blood pressure. Active participation in the group is one predictor of a positive outcome, so getting people to join with others right from the beginning is important. You can do this by asking everyone to share their name and something about themselves. Ask everyone to share one expectation that they have about participating in the group.

Be sure to reinforce any behavior that is for the good of the group. If someone arrives breathless and says, "I worked really hard to be here on time!" respond with positive affirmation about the effort and reinforce how important it is to use the full time allotted for the group. Be generous and explicit with your praise. Draw upon concepts for client-centered practice addressed in other chapters, such as Carl Rogers's concept of unconditional positive regard (Chapter 7) and the motivational interviewing technique for providing affirmations (Chapter 9). When a participant first takes a risk to share something personal, thank them for this contribution. When one participant offers support to another, point out that this is the kind of support that is important to provide in the group.

Please note that drop-in groups may have different participants from session to session and may essentially remain in this Initial Stage of group development. These groups can be a challenge to facilitate, as a few regularly attending members may be ready for deeper interaction. As long as there are new members at every meeting it is essential to keep the group focused on the guidelines and be attentive to members who may want to share more deeply with vulnerable self-disclosure. This can be risky when new members are unknown to the facilitators and to the group—so maintain attention on the safety of all participants, even gently asking members to be mindful of boundaries when sharing sensitive material.

Sample Group Agreements or Guidelines

Group guidelines or agreements can be developed with participants, although this process may take some time. Over the years we have come to recognize the essential elements of working group guidelines and present them here. They may be adjusted for your groups and settings.

Confidentiality

- Not repeating personal information shared by other participants without their permission
- A commitment not to address conflicts within the group outside of group meetings

(continues)

Sample Group Agreements or Guidelines (continued)

Communication

- Make room for different speaking styles
- Step up, and Step back (don't dominate group discussions. Make space for all members to actively participate and share their experiences and ideas)
- Value deep, uninterrupted listening
- Silence is okay, it often supports reflection
- Avoid giving unsolicited advise or suggestions to other group members
- Speak when it's your turn—one person at a time

Inclusion

- Honor different experiences, identities, cultures, values, and beliefs
- Work to build community that values the participation of all group members
- Learn to avoid and to interrupt bias or discrimination against any member. This most frequently occurs as microaggressions or subtle and often unnoticed behavioral patterns that can serve to offend or exclude others, for example rolling your eyes, making faces, or using subtle body language that can feel hurtful to others

Using the Group as Practice

- Group is an opportunity to practice new skills, such as communication skills related to listening, providing support to others, encouraging and accepting different points of view, and working to prevent and resolve conflicts.

Anticipate and Address Challenges

- Challenging moments, including differences of opinion and conflicts, occur naturally among people and are likely to occur within groups
- Disagreement is common and essential to support. Work to create a group culture where any participant is able to disagree with any other, and support them to voice these disagreements in a direct and respectful manner
- Expect that participants will make mistakes in group, and do your part to help make these opportunities for learning
- Demonstrate a willingness to forgive yourself and other group members

Qualities We Value

- Not judging the experiences, beliefs, cultures, behaviors, or identities of others
- Respect
- Timeliness
- Honesty
- Humility
- Kindness

Facilitating a Support Group for Middle-School Youth

The Initial Stage

Tim Berthold: When I was starting my career in public health, I facilitated a support group for seventh and eighth graders at a middle school. The school counselor referred students to the group whom she considered to be "at risk" (this included students struggling with academic, family, and personal issues). The group met for eight weeks in a confidential space and provided participants with a hot lunch. I was initially surprised that students were willing to participate in such a group, and was inspired by their ability to cocreate a supportive group experience that addressed genuine concerns affecting their lives.

During the first session, I asked each student to introduce themselves and to share one hope that they had for the group. At the very least, everyone introduced themselves to each other (this was a large middle school, and not everyone knew each other's name). Occasionally, someone expressed a hope ("I really hope this group can be different and everyone can really try to respect where everyone is coming from") that resonated powerfully with other members and sparked an initial discussion.

From there, we set up expectations and ground rules designed to make the group a safe and productive place to be. As facilitator, I introduced certain ground rules, such as privacy (confidentiality), and asked participants to talk about why it is important to them. Confidentiality was a big concern for the students, as many had experienced hurtful rumors, or had a friend or family member break a promise to keep something private. The group would then identify other ground rules to guide participation, such as the importance of accepting different experiences and points of view, and of respecting the participation of all members, including not using put-downs (making negative comments about other group members). Not only did this result in a set of ground rules and expectations to guide the group process, it also provided members with a first experience of working together with a common purpose.

Together the students brainstormed and prioritized a list of topics to be addressed during group. They never had difficulty identifying issues for conversation, and worked well together to prioritize the lists. When it was difficult for the group to decide which topics to select, the participants voted to select the issues they most wanted to talk about: the topics with most votes formed the agenda for the next six weeks. The agenda selected by the participants generally included topics such as family conflict and divorce, dating and sexual involvement, alcohol and drug use, peer pressure, depression and suicide, and immigration and discrimination (a significant percentage of students at the school were immigrants).

During the first session, I made a point of encouraging each member to participate. For example, I might turn to a student and say: "Julio, is there anything you would like to add to the ground rules?" I also tried to model ways of affirming their participation by making comments such as "Thanks, Julio, I agree that maintaining the privacy of what we talk about here is really important for our success," or "You did a great job of working together to express your expectations for the group."

THE TRANSITION STAGE (STORMING AND NORMING)

In the transition stage, members begin to talk more directly about the issues that motivated them to participate in the group. People work to establish trust by talking honestly about their lives. Some participants may resist hearing the truths of others, or acknowledging certain aspects of their own experience and behavior, particularly those that may imply making changes. This is a rich and productive stage in the life of the group when issues and challenges are identified.

Tuckman called this the *Storming Phase,* when conflicts may emerge and people with apparently different agendas seem to struggle for attention. The necessary group task is to develop tolerance and patience for the process of becoming a group with a common purpose.

The membership functions in the transition stage are to interact in ways that affirm participation. In many cases, this means that group members will begin to identify and name their fears out loud, including fears of revealing certain aspects of their life experience and identity, of being rejected or accepted by the group, of intimacy or getting too close to others in the group. The other main task in this stage is to learn how to listen; to accept, validate, and support other participants; and, most important, to accept and respect people with different experiences, identities, and points of view.

The leadership functions of this stage are to assist participants to resolve ambivalence about becoming a group. The ambivalence of this stage may be marked by behavior that is confusing to a beginning group facilitator. But, to the experienced group facilitator, the necessary emergence of ambivalence—"I want to change and I don't want to change"—signals that people are becoming emotionally more involved in the group, and a group identity is beginning to emerge.

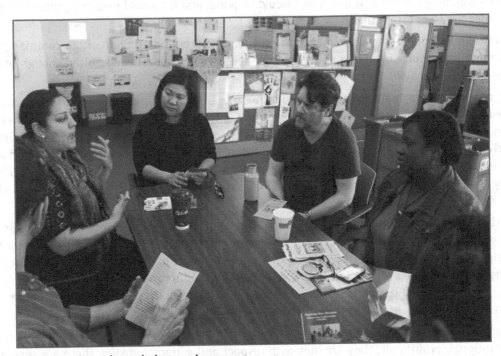

Group members share their experiences.

The Work of Facilitators in the Transition Stage

The group facilitator's job at this stage is to assist the participants to see that differences and conflicts can be resolved. As a facilitator, you will need to become comfortable witnessing and responding to ambivalence, anger, and conflict. Keep in mind that ambivalence to change is natural and common, and apply your skills for rolling with resistance as appropriate (see Chapter 9). You will need to develop skills in assisting members to reflect on their experiences and their participation in the group and to demonstrate empathy for each other's point of view. Tuckman called this the *Norming Phase,* where individuals settle down, become a group, and create new norms for emotional and social interaction. Members are committed to the group and find that they can trust each other even if they disagree.

A key role for the group facilitator is to assist each member to be viewed as valuable to the group. You do this by using your active listening skills to support participants in identifying, validating, and striving to understand different points of view. The end of this stage is marked by group members having a solid sense of safety within the group—a sense of belonging by choice and by inclusion.

Facilitating a Support Group for Middle-School Youth (continued)

The Transition Stage

Tim Berthold: Middle school (seventh, eighth, and sometimes ninth grade) is often a difficult time for students. Not only are the students going through adolescence, but the school environment is often characterized by popular and unpopular groups, bullying, teasing, and discrimination. It is only natural that participants bring some of these dynamics to group. A key part of my job was to watch for and to quickly respond to early expressions of conflict. For example, one group member might roll their eyes as another was talking, and turn to another participant or make a disrespectful comment (such as "That's nothing new coming from *you*" or "Yeah, but *you're* always depressed anyway."). While the form of put-down always varied, I made sure to respond right away. I also kept in mind that, while I was watching for conflict to emerge, group members were watching me to see if and how I would respond, and if I would keep my promise to enforce the ground rules they had established.

In general, I would first direct my comments to the entire group, reminding them of our common purpose and ground rules, and emphasizing that every member deserved respect. This was often enough to interrupt and stop the negative behavior.

If, however, an individual or individuals continued to tease or otherwise disrespect other members of the group, I would address them directly by saying something like: "K., remember our commitment to follow the group ground rules." I would also make time to address my concerns to K. privately, after group, explicitly describing the behavior that I had observed and why I found it harmful. I always tried to do this in a respectful and supportive way, encouraging the participant to rejoin the group and to make positive contributions. Occasionally, I would ask the student to apologize to the target of their behavior and let them decide when and how to do so.

If I judged the behavior to be more harmful, I would have immediately interrupted the group and removed the participant who had put down another member. Depending on the nature of what they did, they might not be invited to return. Acting in a prompt and effective method to remove a serious threat to the welfare of the group is important to preserving its integrity and your leadership (I facilitated five or six groups at the middle school, and never reached a point where a member had to be asked to leave).

In these moments, I want to ensure that when a group member shares something that seems highly personal, emotional, or difficult, they are met with respect and support. Ideally, there are several participants in the group who do this naturally and well. As group facilitator, I also tried to model this. For example, during a discussion about depression, a student said that his older brother had killed himself three years before. While he was clearly emotional, he also continued to talk about what had happened. We listened and, when he stopped, I acknowledged what a significant loss the death of a family member is, and asked him if he wanted to talk about how the death of his brother had affected him. Generally, other group members will follow this lead and rise to the occasion, offering condolences and listening to whatever else the participant cares to say. If something occurred that might be harmful in the moment, I would intervene and say something like: "H. just shared something really important with us. That isn't easy to do. The purpose of this group is to be able to talk about the real things that happen in our lives, to listen to each other, and to provide support." If I were concerned about the individual participant who took a risk to share something personal, I would check in with them as soon as the group ended, in a private space.

In general, the young people were naturally good at providing support to each other in these moments. I would make sure to acknowledge and reinforce this. For example, I might say something like: "I was impressed today with how supportive you were when S. was talking about his brother. That is what this group is all about."

THE WORK STAGE (PERFORMING)

The most in-depth work takes place at this stage. The individual members and the group as a whole commit themselves to the deeper work of understanding the issues that trouble or challenge them, and identifying what they can do to address these problems. For example, this is the stage when the Latino men's group talked about the people they had lost to the HIV epidemic; about not being accepted by their families; about their desire for community, healthy relationships, and love; and what they can do to create healthier and more satisfying lives.

Tuckman called this the *Performing Phase,* when the group is functioning best, offering members opportunities for self-expression and personal growth within the functioning of the group as a whole.

In some groups, this is the stage in which members examine behaviors that are harmful to their own health or that of others. They move beyond health information to consider making changes in behavior. The deep work comes with understanding the full impact of thoughts, feelings, and behaviors in one's own life as well as on others. It is through sharing these experiences and insights in the group and creating connections with other members that participants gain the motivation and commitment to changing and growing in other relationships and areas of their lives. Group members provide support to each other in making changes, and report on their progress in future sessions.

The Work of Facilitators in the Work Stage

The facilitator's function at this stage is to assist members to access and express their emotions and thoughts in the here and now, and to reflect on the meaning of their experiences. As always, the group facilitator works to maintain the emotional cohesion of the group by addressing any behavior that may be harmful and is not adequately addressed by the members themselves. Facilitators also ask the group to focus on actions that they can take, including changes in behavior that will promote their health and well-being and that of others.

Essentially you will work to assist the group members to understand and respond to each other in supportive and positive ways. You continue to resolve problems created by misunderstandings, and to assist group members to see each other's points of view. You steer the conversation toward topics that are beneficial for the participants' growth and away from conversations that reinforce unhelpful behavior. The effective group facilitator continues to assist individual group members to understand how their behavior in group affects other people. The facilitator assists individuals in understanding how they can try out new knowledge and skills with people they trust—the other group members.

In this stage of the group process, the facilitator does not need to speak or step into discussions unless there is a good reason. Good facilitation includes being able to trust group members to stay on track with their discussions, interactions, and values, and understanding that the leadership of group members is critical to the ultimate success of the process. Be aware of your tendencies to impose your own agenda on the group. If you are working with a cofacilitator, discuss these issues to ensure, to the best of your ability, that the work of the group is guided by the interests, experiences, emotions, and values of the members rather than the facilitators. Any actions that members decide to take to promote their health must be their own, in order to maximize the chance that they will follow through in making those changes.

Facilitating a Support Group for Middle-School Youth (*continued*)

The Work Stage

Tim Berthold: During this stage, I monitored participation and provided opportunities for all members to talk. For example, I might turn to a member who has mostly been silent and say: "Esther, what are your thoughts about this topic?"

(continues)

Facilitating a Support Group for Middle-School Youth (continued)

An important part of my role as facilitator was to guide members to reflect on the meaning of their experiences. The members of the youth group did this naturally, as talking about what matters is a common part of adolescence. For example, when the youth group was talking about the issue of depression, which was a common experience, I might ask something like: "So how does being depressed influence your life?" (or "How does depression affect your life at home or your performance at school?" or "Does being depressed change the way you think or feel about yourself?"). If we had done our work well up to this point, the group would have created an environment in which the participants wanted to share their experiences, feelings, and ideas.

By this stage, group members were generally skilled at supporting each other in identifying possible actions to improve their lives. Occasionally, as a facilitator, I might ask something like: "What do you think would be helpful for you to do about this situation?" In addition, I watched for members who, out of an effort to be supportive, might try to give advice or otherwise tell another participant what to do. In such a circumstance, I might say something like: "That sounds like a great suggestion, but we need to keep in mind that everyone is unique. Is this something that you might be interested in?"

While in some ways working with youth can be more challenging than working with adults, in other ways the very nature of adolescence supported the middle-school students in talking about real issues in a real way. A guiding principle for every group I facilitated was some version of "keeping it real." This meant that group members could drop the false front they sometimes showed to parents, teachers, and each other, and talk about common challenges, like depression, in a very direct way. They were also able to identify realistic steps that might encourage them to make positive changes rather than suggestions that were out of reach for most people.

THE FINAL STAGE (ADJOURNING)

The final stage of group work consolidates what people have done and allows them to say "good-bye" in a healthy fashion. Tuckman calls this the *Adjourning Phase*. Participants confront the realization that the group—like other aspects of life—may end before they are ready. Simultaneously, members report that they incorporate what they have learned in group into their lives.

Membership issues at this stage include expressing feelings about any missed opportunities and other losses, as well as risks taken in group and positive changes made. Ambivalence returns as people are both ready and not ready for the experience to end. For those who have had a satisfying experience, saying good-bye provides yet another opportunity to be in the here and now with emotions, thoughts, and new behaviors. For those who wish for more, the experience of closure provides a way to acknowledge the limitations of self, others, and relationships. Most people experience a little of each.

The Work of Facilitators in the Final Stage

Leadership functions at the final stage are, as before, to guide members to experience and express their thoughts and feelings as they confront the ending of the group. It is also time to revisit and reinforce the commitments that participants have made to enacting changes that will enhance their health and wellness.

Facilitating a Support Group for Middle-School Youth (continued)

The Final Stage

Tim Berthold: Each time I facilitated the support group at the middle school, I was struck by how difficult it was for participants to say good-bye.

(continues)

Facilitating a Support Group for Middle-School Youth *(continued)*

One activity that I have used to end a class or group takes just a few minutes. It requires an eight- to ten-foot length of colored ribbon, one for each participant. The group stands in a circle, and one participant begins the activity by sharing something that they appreciate about the contributions that another participant made to the group, handing them the other end of their colored ribbon. This member in turn selects another, acknowledges something positive about their participation in the group, and hands them the other end of a second piece of colored ribbon. At the end of this brief activity, all group members have been acknowledged and appreciated by others, and a web of ribbon has been created that visually represents the interconnections among all group members.

With the middle-school students, I also asked each member to share something meaningful that they learned from the group, something they plan to do to promote their own health, and one resource they can realistically turn to when they face life challenges.

It was typical for group members to stay late after the last group, talking further with each other, with the facilitator, and with the school counselor (who was invited, with permission from members, to attend the last session).

It is not unusual for people to have a tough time saying good-bye to an experience that has become valuable. A key role is to support members in saying good-bye to the group and affirming the connections they have made, the knowledge and skills they have gained, and the changes they intend to make.

What Do YOU Think?

- *What do you do to say good-bye to a group when it ends?*

- *What sorts of activities would you choose to facilitate?*

Ramona Benson: I facilitate a couple of different groups for women at the Black Infant Health Program. One way I measure my success is when women who were in a group before come back to speak to a new group. They might share what they went through and what they learned, because they want to give back and help other women. And they might tell me: "I'm in school now. I'm working for my GED or my Associate's Degree." One lady said, "Can I get a referral to a therapist?" And that's success to me because they are still working to change their life, and not ashamed to reach out and ask for help.

21.11 Challenges of Group Facilitation

The "client" in group work is both the individual participant and the group itself. The group is the agent of change, and maintaining an environment that *supports group learning* is the responsibility of the facilitator.

COMMON CHALLENGES

Some of the common challenges to facilitating a successful group include the following.

The Culture of Individuality

The United States places great emphasis on the individual, often at the expense of the group or community. The society often celebrates the right of individuals to go their own way, and to oppose the will of the group. These cultural values and messages sometimes make it difficult for people to work collaboratively in a group setting. They may feel restricted by the group process and start to rebel by asserting their unique needs.

Unclear Intentions of the Group

Group members are often unclear, and sometimes suspicious, about the intentions of the group. What is it trying to accomplish? What are its values? Is it right for me? Will the group accept me? These doubts can undermine safety and participation.

Unconscious Issues

Group work is affected by unconscious and unspoken issues that group members bring with them, such as unresolved experiences with their families or other groups. These issues may be acted out in any number of ways including blaming, criticizing, denial, trying to please others, or attempting to control the dynamic and focus of the group.

OTHER COMMON CHALLENGES

- Members who do not actively participate.
- Members who dominate discussions.
- Put-downs, insults, threats, or attacks on any member of the group.
- Prejudice, cultural bias, or discriminatory treatment targeting any group member related to their identity or perceived identity.
- Development of subgroups or cliques.
- Persistent negativity from individuals or the group: Sometimes groups get stuck focusing on what isn't working well in their lives. It is important for members to be able to talk honestly about the challenges they face. But it is also important for them to talk about and to support each other in taking positive actions that will improve the quality of their lives.
- Members bringing private issues between themselves into the group: Sometimes group members have pre-existing relationships as friends, family, or coworkers, and sometimes new personal relationships are established by members outside of the group. Sometimes conflicts within these relationships are brought into the group. The group is not the proper place to raise or resolve these issues, and this situation may place other participants in the very awkward or harmful position of being asked to take sides, to provide critical feedback, or to aid in resolving the conflict. None of this is appropriate, and group facilitators must be prepared to set a firm boundary.
- A participant who is under the influence of drugs or alcohol: Ground rules for many groups include not coming to group after drinking alcohol or using drugs. This can change the behavior of a group member and may contribute to many of the other challenges identified here. If you suspect that someone has been using, pull them aside and privately address your concerns in a way that does not scapegoat or shame them. Focus on any conduct that may not be in line with your ground rules. You may need to ask this group member not to participate in the current group session. If the behavior continues in future sessions, you may need to ask the member to leave the group permanently.
- Breaking confidentiality: This is one of the most powerful ways of harming or destroying safety and trust in a group. Facilitators can prevent this by strongly reinforcing the ground rules that require members to maintain the privacy of all members. If confidentiality is broken, it must be addressed immediately and decisively. In some circumstances, it may result in expelling any member who has broken the confidentiality of any other member.

- *Have you experienced these challenges as either a group participant or facilitator?*
- *Can you think of other common challenges that you might face as a group facilitator?*

- Lack of support for group members in moments of vulnerability: People sometimes participate in group to talk about intimate and challenging issues that they are not comfortable discussing elsewhere. Participants understandably have a strong expectation that if they share personal information in the group (such as mental health challenges, HIV status, or gender identity), it will be received with respect. If this does not occur, it may also harm the ability of the group to establish or maintain trust and safety and to continue working productively together. Group facilitators should model how to provide respect and support to participants who share intimate information, and intervene to restore respect if it is not provided in these moments.

- Other situations of conflict: Please refer to Chapter 13 for more information about handling conflict. We encourage you to anticipate conflict as an inevitable part of the group process and to discuss it with the group up front, developing mutual ground rules to guide the way you will respond in the moment of conflict. We encourage you to share some of the information addressed in Chapter 13, including concepts such as shifting from certainty to curiosity, from blame to contribution, and disentangling intentions from impact.

- Crisis situations: These may include reports or threats of violence or other physical harm to self or others, including the disclosure of suicidal thoughts or plans. When such situations arise, they immediately become your number-one priority. You may have to interrupt the group (or ask a cofacilitator to continue) as you meet with the individual or individuals involved, and you may be required to report this information to legal authorities. When a group member experiences crisis, it also affects the group and should be addressed with all participants. The focus here should be on the impact on the group, and personal information about the member undergoing a crisis must be kept confidential. Whenever a crisis emerges, be sure to report it to your supervisor and to debrief it with your cofacilitator.

- Resistance to "keeping it real": Sometimes group members will try to keep conversations on a more superficial level, avoiding the issues that brought them to the group in the first place.

Expect to face some of these challenges, and more, when you facilitate groups. Briefly, we wish to highlight classic mistakes that facilitators sometimes make, and share a few tips designed to enhance the quality and effectiveness of your work with groups.

CLASSIC MISTAKES THAT FACILITATORS MAY MAKE

Because facilitating groups is such challenging (and rewarding) work, it is inevitable that we will make mistakes along the way. Some of these common mistakes include the following:

Avoidance (or doing nothing)

For a variety of reasons, including a lack of comfort with anger or conflict, facilitators sometimes fail to act when events take place that may be harmful to group members. Members must be able to trust that facilitators will take action swiftly and effectively to stop harmful dynamics such as insults or discriminatory treatment. If facilitators fail to do this, they are modeling avoidance, and may send the message that the problematic behavior is acceptable. Avoidance can quickly undermine the integrity and effectiveness of the group process. While handling conflict is difficult, it is an ethical obligation. When facilitators don't step in to resolve a conflict that members themselves are unable to prevent, they are putting their own self-interest and needs above those of the group members.

Dominating the group process

Facilitators sometimes forget that the group exists for the benefit of the members, not themselves. When facilitators dominate the group process, they undermine opportunities for participants to express themselves and to claim their own leadership potential.

Imposing personal values or opinions on the group

It is common for the personal issues of helping professionals to unconsciously influence our work with clients and groups. Unfortunately, when we impose our own values or opinions (about faith, relationships, love, sex, treatment options, behavior change, politics, and so forth), we undermine the autonomy of participants. Effective group facilitation requires being able to get out of our own way; to leave our own experiences, feelings, and ideas outside of the meeting space; and to listen, encourage, and support group members in expressing their own values, doubts, emotions, and opinions.

Failing to demonstrate and model empathy and support

Participants need to know that facilitators care about them, want to learn about their life experiences, and will support them in taking positive steps to promote their health. Responding with empathy and compassion when members share something personal and difficult about their lives also provides participants with a model for how to do this.

Disagreements or conflicts between cofacilitators

Cofacilitators may disagree about a range of issues. This is natural. However, when these disagreements are shared with the group, or result in a conflict that influences the ability of facilitators to work cooperatively together, it undermines the integrity, quality, and effectiveness of the group process.

- *Have you faced or witnessed other challenges to effective group work?*

- *Which of these challenges do you think will be most difficult for you to address?*

SUGGESTIONS FOR GROUP FACILITATORS

Interview and screen potential group members

We recommend, if appropriate, conducting brief interviews to screen potential group participants. This is an opportunity for you to explain the focus of the group to potential members. It is also an opportunity for the prospective member to determine whether or not they are interested in participating in the group. During the interview, try to assess whether the prospective member is ready to make positive contributions to the group process. When people are unable to make use of the group as a learning environment, it is unethical to include them in the group, where their behavior may be a threat to the integrity of the work of others.

Regular meetings for cofacilitators

As described above, meet with your cofacilitator to plan the group, and check in after every group meeting to debrief what happened, to identify potential challenges and areas of disagreement, and to come up with a coordinated plan of action for the next group meeting.

Regular meetings with supervisors

CHWs who facilitate groups should have regular meetings with a supervisor who can provide guidance regarding the work and support for personal issues or challenges that may arise as a consequence of facilitating group work.

Participate in professional development opportunities

Seek out opportunities to enhance your skills. Identify skills that you would like to enhance, such as resolving conflict, cofacilitation, or self care. Talk with your supervisor to see if there are opportunities to attend local workshops or trainings. Consider enrolling in a class at your local college or university.

Self care

Facilitating groups is deeply rewarding work. As you have learned in this chapter, it is also often challenging. Make time to do the things that assist you to relieve stress and prevent burnout. Refer to Chapter 12.

- *What other suggestions would you share with a colleague who was preparing to facilitate their first group?*

21.12 Ethics and Group Facilitation

The foundation of ethical practice for facilitating groups is the same as for individual practice as outlined in Chapter 7. Everything that CHWs do should be designed to put the best interests of the client first (in this case, the group and its members). The difference between group work and individual work is that the client is, for ethical decision making, both the group and the individual.

CONFIDENTIALITY

Some ethical issues are relatively easy to understand, such as preventing discrimination, physical violence, or threats of violence. Other ethical issues are more complex, such as the boundaries of confidentiality. The ethical duty of the CHW is clear: clients' rights to confidentiality are the same as with any individual counseling relationship. What is said to the CHW is held in the strictest confidence with only a few exceptions (see Chapter 7). But what about the boundaries of confidentiality within an agency? Should you, as a group facilitator, be allowed to share client information with other agency workers? Are you obligated to divulge information you think would benefit the client in work with another agency professional? The answers become complex when agencies don't have explicit guidelines about intra-agency policies and when those policies aren't made explicit to clients.

What about confidentiality between group members? What can a group member expect from the group with respect to privacy? In fact, the group member can only expect what one would expect from any human interaction. There is no law to prevent other group members—nonprofessionals, that is—from talking to people who are not in the group, or talking to other group members outside of group time. The best that can be hoped for is that group members pledge to each other that what is said in group stays in group. This is a mutual promise made by group members, but it does not carry the weight of law.

The group facilitator should make the limits of confidentiality clear to group members as they join the group. This is best done by facilitating a discussion among group members about privacy. The group facilitator can guide the group toward the mutual promise of confidentiality and be ready to intervene should the promise be broken. It is best to get the group to come to a consensus about their pledge to each other, with the understanding that everyone in the group will work to enforce that rule.

CULTURAL HUMILITY

An integral part of ethical practice as a group facilitator is the ability to demonstrate cultural humility (see Chapter 6). Group facilitators need to understand the dynamic of power in their role in groups and demonstrate cultural humility in the following ways.

- Develop a deep understanding of one's own culture, biases, stereotypes, and prejudices in order to be aware of how they may inform your perspectives and strategies in groups.
- Inquire about and listen to the opinions and concerns of the group as you make decisions together about issues such as group guidelines, goals, topics, and activities.
- Work to transfer power (see Chapter 6) away from the facilitator and to the group members themselves. This is their group and it should, to the extent possible, reflect their priorities, knowledge, experience, and values.
- Pay attention to who is participating in the group, and how. Make space for different styles of participation. Invite—but don't pressure—all members to speak up and share their experiences, feelings, and opinions.
- Introduce group guidelines, techniques, and activities in a way that invites all members to express their questions, concerns, and ideas.
- Don't continue with a particular technique or activity if it isn't working for the group.
- Stay open to feedback from group members and your cofacilitator. Pay special attention to any indication that you may be imposing your own cultural biases and values.
- Be ready to demonstrate to the group that you can take responsibility for your own mistakes and know how to offer an authentic and warm apology when necessary (see Chapter 13 on Conflict Resolution Skills).

CONSULTATION AND SUPERVISION

Finally, every group facilitator and cofacilitator should meet regularly with a supervisor. This is your opportunity to raise ethical concerns and other challenges and to receive direction and support from a trained professional in how best to respond to these issues. If you are ever confused about how to handle a potential problem in a group, seek guidance as soon as possible from your supervisor.

Chapter Review

DESIGN YOUR OWN GROUP

Develop your own model for a social or support group that you would facilitate. Please develop a realistic model based on the information in this chapter. Choose a community to serve, and health issues to address, that you are already familiar with.

1. Describe the community that will participate in the group.
2. What health issue or concern does the group have in common?
3. What are the membership criteria for the group?
4. Describe the structure for the group:
   - Where will you meet and how often?
   - How many times will the group meet?
   - Will the group be open or closed?
   - How will you start and end each group session?
   - What ground rules will guide the work of the group? How will these be established?
5. What will some of the primary goals for the group be?
6. What will you do to promote participation of all group members?
7. How will you work to promote the leadership of group members?
8. How will you know if you have been successful in facilitating this group? What outcomes will group members achieve?

References

American Group Psychotherapy Association. (2007). *Practice guidelines for group psychotherapy: A transtheoretical guide to developing and leading psychotherapy groups.* Retrieved from *www.agpa.org/home/practice-resources/practice-guidelines-for-group-psychotherapy*

Lieberman, M. A., Yalom, I. D., & Miles, M. B. (1973). *Encounter groups: First facts.* New York, NY: Basic Books.

Schneider Corey, M., & Corey, G. (2006). *Groups: Process and practice* (7th ed.). Belmont, CA: Brooks/Cole.

Tuckman, B. (1965). Developmental sequences in small groups. *Psychological Bulletin, 63,* 384–399.

Yalom, I. (1995). *Theory and practice of group psychotherapy.* New York, NY: Basic Books.

Additional Resources

Agazarian, Y. (2004). *Systems-Centered Therapy for Groups.* New York, NY: The Guilford Press.

Community Tool Box (n.d.) Retrieved from *http://ctb.ku.edu/en/table-of-contents/leadership/group-facilitation/facilitation-skills/main*

Community Toolbox offers extensive online resources for community building curriculum. See Chapter 16: Group Facilitation & Problem Solving—Section 2. Developing Facilitation Skills provides general discussion, checklist, and Power Point slides.

Corey, G. (2015). *Theory & practice of group counseling.* Boston, MA: Cengage Learning.

Kaner, S. (2014). *Facilitators guide to participatory decision making.* San Francisco, CA: Jossey-Bass.

Rosenberg, P. R. (1984). Support groups: A special therapeutic entity. *Small Group Research 15*(2), 173–186.

Systems-Centered Training. *www.systemscentered.com/*

Community Diagnosis

22

Susana Hennessey Lavery, Mele Lau-Smith, Alma Avila,
Janey Skinner, Jill Tregor, and Tim Berthold

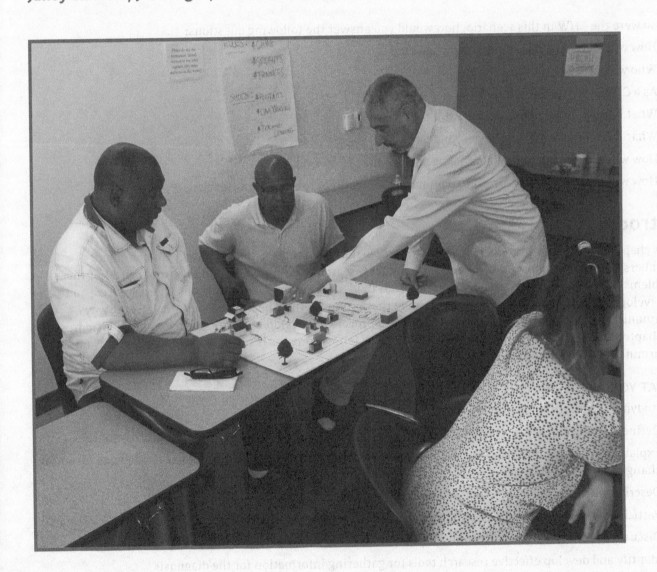

CHW Scenario

You work for a coalition of nonprofit agencies in a county with a large and diverse Native American population. Native communities are concerned about the high rates of low birth weight and infant mortality that their families experience. You've been asked to work with Native American communities to conduct a community diagnosis. Together, you will gather information to guide the development of an action plan to advocate for policies that will reduce the rates of low birth weight and infant mortality.

If you were the CHW in this scenario, how would you answer the following questions:

- How will you begin this community diagnosis?
- Who will participate in this diagnosis?
- As a CHW, what will your role be?
- What types of information do you want to gather?
- What types of research might you conduct?
- How will the information you gather be analyzed?
- How will this information be used to promote the health of the communities at risk?

Introduction

This chapter provides an introduction to community diagnosis, a process and a strategy for community members to identify important concerns and conduct research to better understand the root causes of these problems. The diagnosis also supports communities in identifying their own strengths and resources, and in developing a plan to advocate for social change that promotes their health and welfare. In some ways, community diagnosis resembles the client-centered process of developing a care management plan addressed in Chapter 10. As a CHW, your role in the community diagnosis process is to facilitate the leadership and self-determination of the communities you work with.

WHAT YOU WILL LEARN

By studying the information provided in this chapter, you will be able to:

- Define community diagnosis and discuss key concepts and methods related to community diagnosis
- Explain how community diagnosis is used to guide public health programs and efforts to advocate for social change
- Describe and apply seven key steps in a community diagnosis process
- Participate in the design and execution of a community-centered and strength-based community diagnosis
- Discuss the role of the CHW in community diagnosis
- Identify and develop effective research tools for gathering information for the diagnosis
- Summarize and analyze research findings
- Explain how research findings are used to develop an action plan

WORDS TO KNOW

Assessment of Community Strengths and Assets

Content Analysis

Institutional Review Boards

Leading Questions

Needs Assessment

Qualitative Data

Quantitative Data

Root Causes

Sample

22.1 Defining Community Diagnosis

Community diagnosis is the process of identifying community concerns or problems, uncovering their root causes, and developing a clear plan to overcome them. Many communities have experienced people coming in from the outside to conduct research that does not lead to any meaningful benefit or positive change. In contrast, a community diagnosis involves community members in all phases of research and planning, and supports them in making all key decisions along the way.

Community Diagnosis is Participatory

Community diagnosis uses methods and frameworks of the larger field of participatory research, often called community-based participatory research (CBPR) or participatory action research (PAR). One distinction is that while community diagnosis is specifically focused on identifying assets and problems in a community, CBPR and PAR can be used either in the diagnosis phase, or later to evaluate the implementation and impact of community projects or changes. You may find inspiration for your own community diagnosis project by looking at examples of any form of participatory research.

What these research methods have in common is that they are designed and conducted by the community rather than by outside experts, although outsiders may be involved in the research or even sometimes initiate it. These methods are also explicitly tied to a process of community organizing, advocacy, or action to transform or improve community conditions.

COMMUNITY DIAGNOSIS IS STRENGTH-BASED

Traditionally, public health workers have done **needs assessments** on behalf of the community. These needs assessments can provide a false view of what's happening in the community because they frequently focus on the negative—the risks, problems, and lack of resources and skills. While all communities have problems, they also have strengths. When a CHW works with an individual client, the CHW supports the client in identifying the client's own strengths and resources. Working at the community level should be the same. For this reason, community diagnosis incorporates an **assessment of community strengths and assets**. The strengths of any community are numerous, and may include their shared experience, culture, wisdom, skills, and history, including histories of resistance and past accomplishments. Resources may also include the ability and desire to work together; a vision for the future; commitment to justice and peace; formal and informal leaders; parks; faith-based, educational, health, and social services agencies; community groups and associations; and existing employers with safe working conditions that pay a living wage. The positive elements evident in all communities should always be highlighted in a community diagnosis and used in planning for solutions (Kretzmann and McKnight, 1993; NACCHO, 2013).

- *What are some of the many strengths and resources in the community or communities that you belong to?*

- *Identify at least five resources that promote the health of your community.*

A FOCUS ON ROOT CAUSES

A community diagnosis must go beyond the surface, to conduct an in-depth analysis of the **root causes** of the issues and concerns a community identifies. Research that does not identify root causes is likely to result in a simplistic or superficial understanding of a problem or concern. This can lead to solutions that "blame the victim" or place responsibility for fixing the problem on the very people who have already been most harmed.

For example, consider the high rates of infant mortality within the Native American communities mentioned at the beginning of this chapter. An analysis of the causes of this problem that stays on the surface might identify factors such as low rates of participation in prenatal care and breastfeeding. An analysis that goes deeper—beneath the surface of the problem to consider its root causes—might identity factors such as institutionalized racism; unequal access to basic resources including quality housing, education, employment, health insurance, food, and safety; hazardous working conditions; living in poverty in neighborhoods characterized by high levels of crime and lack of safety; and the chronic stress that these inequalities produce (see Chapter 4). This type of analysis will guide the community in determining what actions they wish to take in order to reduce infant mortality rates.

An analysis of root causes assists the community to view their work as part of a larger movement. For example, in tobacco control, many of the smoke-free policies that exist today at the state level started at the local level in cities and towns. In San Francisco in the 1990s, a local youth agency diagnosed and compared tobacco advertising targeting different neighborhoods alongside the history of targeting communities of color and low-income folks by the transnational tobacco industry. The results of their community diagnosis influenced statewide and national efforts to restrict tobacco advertising. We now see restrictions on tobacco advertising as one of the key pillars of the international Framework Convention on Tobacco Control (*www.who.int/fctc/en/*). These local policies shaped the need for statewide, national, and global policies and treaties to control the actions of transnational tobacco companies.

Root Causes

The ideal way to prevent any health problem is to transform the root cause or the place where the problem starts. The root causes of many health issues lie in how systems (political, economic, health, educational systems) are structured to perpetuate power imbalances that result in health inequalities between populations. For example, growing inequality in income and wealth in the United States, along with the lack of a national "living wage," leads to working-class people being unable to acquire the goods and services necessary for a healthy life. On a global level, the way that the corporate-led global economy is structured often results in the same outcome.

WHEN TO CONDUCT A COMMUNITY DIAGNOSIS

Community diagnosis serves many purposes and may be conducted at different times in the life cycle of a community program, project, or movement. Sometimes the community diagnosis will be initiated by the community itself, and sometimes by others such as the city council, mayor's office, or local department of public health.

Some groups come together to improve the general health of their community, but have not yet decided which particular issue or problem they want to tackle first. These groups might conduct a broad community diagnosis to clarify what issues the community is most concerned about and what types of change they want to prioritize.

Other groups have already identified the issue or problem they want to work on, such as infant mortality. These groups might conduct a community diagnosis because they need to gather data and information to guide and support the actions they will take to address the problem. Often, the diagnosis assists the community to further define the problem and their proposed solution or action.

Finally, many groups do both. They start with the broader diagnosis to prioritize an issue or concern, and then they conduct a more targeted diagnosis to further define potential solutions and actions to create change.

THE ROLE OF THE CHW

Regardless of the community or communities you belong to and the organization you work for, as a CHW, your role in a community diagnosis is to support and facilitate diverse leadership from the community. Your role is not to make key decisions about the diagnosis: the community must identify their own issues of concern, design and do the research, analyze the research data gathered, and develop their own action plan. As a CHW, you may assist in facilitating meetings and support the community in deciding what types of research tools to use and how to develop and implement them. Equally important is the CHW role in connecting the community to key resources. If the community wants to do a survey, a literature search, or a GIS map, and has never done this before, you may be able to connect them with an expert who can provide technical assistance. You may also arrange for additional training to build new skills within the community.

When you provide client-centered services to individual clients, one of your key roles is to ask simple open-ended questions designed to aid them in clarifying their strengths, risks, needs, and goals, and the steps to reach those goals. Similarly, when you assist in facilitating a community diagnosis, you ask open-ended questions that will support the community in sharing experience, knowledge, and proposed solutions. These questions might include, for example: "What do you want to know about the problem you have identified? Who else would you like to invite to participate in this community diagnosis? What does this information tell you about the problem of infant mortality? What factors seem to contribute to this problem? What are some of the most important strengths and resources in your community? What other strategies might assist you to promote greater equality and to reduce low birth weight and infant mortality?"

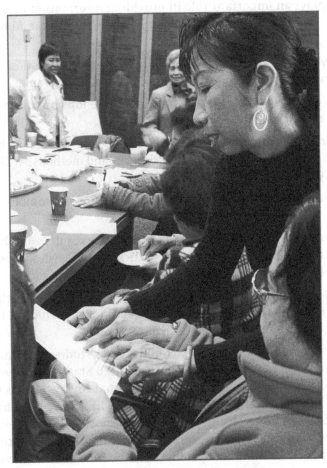

A CHW facilitates a community planning process.

If you participate in a community diagnosis, ask yourself the following questions along the way to reflect on whether or not you are doing community-centered work:

- Who identified the issues, concerns, or problems that are the focus of the community diagnosis?
- Were all segments of the community invited to participate in the community diagnosis?
- Have you treated all community members with courtesy and respect?
- Did the community determine what type of research they wanted to conduct? Who developed the questions that were used in the surveys, focus groups, or other research tools?

- Who analyzed the research findings? How active was the community in this process?

- Were any key sectors of the community left out of the process? If so, why?

- Did the community develop their own action plan? Who participated in these decisions?

- Have you or your professional colleagues attempted to influence the outcome of any part of the community diagnosis? In what ways?

- Were you able to comfortably accept decisions made by the community, especially when they were different from the decisions that you would have made?

WHEN RESEARCH IS NOT COMMUNITY-DRIVEN

Most research is quite different from a community diagnosis; it does not invite community members to participate in a meaningful way in its design, implementation, analysis, or dissemination (sharing of results). CHWs are often hired to work on public health research studies. As we discuss in Chapters 3 and 4, research plays an important role in providing information to guide efforts to promote community health and eliminate health inequalities. However, not all research studies are equally valuable.

If you are considering a job with a research study, we encourage you to ask questions to determine how the research will benefit the community. These questions might include, for example:

- What issues or questions are the focus of this research? Are these topics and questions important to the community in which the research will be undertaken?

- To what extent will researchers involve local community members in the research process and project? Have community members been consulted about the research focus and methods? Will community members be hired to work on the study?

- How might the information gathered by research ultimately be used to promote the health and well-being of the community?

- How will the results of the study—including positive and negative results—be shared with the community and with the subjects of the research (the people who participate in surveys, questionnaires, and focus groups or who donate blood or other biological samples)?

- What is the past record of the lead researchers (sometimes called principal investigators)? Have they made efforts in the past to share research findings with the communities they studied? Has their research been used to promote the welfare of the communities they studied?

Increasingly, researchers are changing the way they conduct their studies to be more responsive to community needs. For example, all research studies in the United States that involve gathering information from people must be approved by human subjects or **institutional review boards** (IRBs) to ensure that the research is ethical and does not harm participants. Historically, IRBs have been based in institutions—such as universities—that conduct research and have been composed of fellow researchers. Recently, community-based IRBs have been developed to evaluate the ethics of proposed research in communities. For example, the Native Hawaiian Health Care System (NHHCS) Institutional Review Board (IRB) was established to:

> . . . maximize the benefits and minimize the risks of research in Native Hawaiian individuals and communities but additionally to educate researchers to build capacity within communities so that communities can participate in and partner with research that addresses existing community health concerns. (Shore et al., 2014, p. 10)

KEY CONCEPTS OF COMMUNITY DIAGNOSIS

Community diagnosis is based on concepts of popular education and models from Africa, Latin America, and other parts of the Global South. It is greatly influenced by the work of Paulo Freire and Orlando Fals-Borda in Latin America, and Miles Horton of the Highlander Institute and Kurt Lewin in the United States (Minkler &

Wallerstein, 2008). Popular education is discussed in more detail in Chapter 20. Community diagnosis does the following:

- Educates and raises the consciousness of all participants, including community members and CHWs assisting with the research (Tsark, 2001)
- Values knowledge generated from the life experiences of the community (Tsark, 2001)
- Actively involves the language and cultural values of community members in both the design and implementation (Arble & Moberg, 2006)
- Prioritizes issues of gender, race, class, and culture in the design and analysis of the research (Minkler & Wallerstein, 2008)
- Values collaboration, ensures that all partners are involved equally in the research process, and recognizes the strengths that they bring to the process (Israel, Schulz, Parker, & Becker, 1998; Minkler, 2006)
- Begins with an issue of concern to the community with the aim of combining knowledge and action for social change to improve community health and eliminate health inequalities (Israel, Schulz, Parker, & Becker, 1998; Minkler, 2006)
- Seeks the participation of all members in development of the research questions, as well as the design, data collection, analysis, and dissemination of the results (Tsark, 2001)
- Exposes and examines issues of power and power relations, and works to promote individual and community empowerment (Tsark, 2001)
- Seeks political action, social change, or both (Tsark, 2001)

22.2 Key Steps in Conducting a Community Diagnosis

A community diagnosis generally consists of at least seven steps:

1. Define the community and bring them together
2. Choose a focus for the community diagnosis
   - For example, infant mortality, gun violence, homelessness, or heart disease
3. Select research tools
   - These may include, for example, conducting research at the library or on the Internet, researching existing policies, conducting qualitative interviews with or administering a survey to community members, facilitating a focus group, counting physical objects, mapping community resources and risks, or developing other visual documentation such as Photovoice.
4. Conduct research
5. Summarize the research findings
   - Often the information and data that you gather will be large or technical (or both), and it must be summarized in a way that makes it understandable to the community.
6. Analyze the research findings
   - Community members analyze the information that has been gathered to learn more about the root causes of their concerns and the community's strengths and risks, to guide them in taking action.
7. Develop an action plan
   - Community members determine—guided by the research findings—what they can do to create social change and promote their health and well-being, such as advocating for culturally competent services, transitional housing programs, closure of the incinerator, or stricter controls on emissions.

Chapter 23 will introduce you to the community action model, which incorporates many of the steps in this chapter. The community action model builds on community diagnosis to implement an action plan and advocate for policy changes that promote social justice.

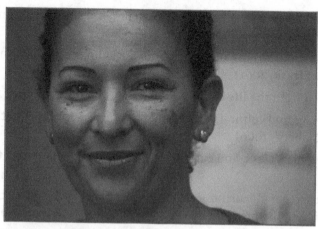

CHWs may help to facilitate a community diagnosis process, working to promote the leadership and decisions of community members.

STEP 1: IDENTIFYING AND BRINGING THE COMMUNITY TOGETHER

A community may be defined and brought together to conduct a community diagnosis in different ways. As discussed in other chapters, the community or population may be defined by factors such as geography (neighborhood, city, county, and so on) or by other common characteristics, including ethnicity, nationality, language, risk factors, interests, gender, or sexual orientation. Remember, however, that all communities are diverse in some way. A truly meaningful community diagnosis will actively reach out and invite all members of the community to participate. The process will ensure that all voices can be heard, including those that are sometimes marginalized in the community, such as the voices of youth, seniors, immigrants, or people with disabilities.

The community diagnosis process may begin with a series of meetings at accessible locations such as a community center, school, or social services agency. These meetings, as well as the community diagnosis process itself, should be advertised and promoted throughout the community. Enlisting the participation of formal and informal leaders or key stakeholders will aid in ensuring that the entire community learns about what is going on. This may include asking local media, schools, faith-based organizations, service organizations, businesses, unions, and activists to assist in getting the word out. For more information about how to identify and build relationships with formal and informal leaders in a community, see Chapter 19.

- *How would let your community know about a community diagnosis that was about to begin?*

- *Who are some of the key stakeholders in your community?*

- *What parts of the community are sometimes left out of efforts like this?*

- *How would you reach out to invite them to participate?*

What Do **YOU?** Think **!**

STEP 2: CHOOSING A FOCUS

The next step in the process is for the community to select a specific problem or concern that will be the central focus for the community diagnosis. Sometimes the focus has already been selected, and this is the reason that people have come together to conduct a community diagnosis. At other times, community diagnosis will lead the group to identify issues that the community wants to change. You play a critical role in this process. As you sit in on discussions, listen carefully for themes and issues that the community feels passionate about. Reflect these ideas back to the group, to assist them in defining and clarifying the focus for their common work.

We recommend that the community apply some or all of the following criteria to choose the issues or problem they will work on. Ideally, the focus of the community diagnosis will meet the following criteria:

- **Meaningful:** Addressing this issue will make a real difference. It will result in a significant improvement in people's lives.

- **Reach:** Addressing this issue will impact many people.
- **High need:** There is an underserved population or geographic area that has a high need related to the issue.
- **Public support:** It will be easy to get support from the public and community leaders to address the issue.
- **Political will:** There is political will within the community to address the issue.
- **Practical:** The expertise, time, and resources are available to address the issue.
- **Clear target:** There is a clearly defined policy-making body (such as a city council or health commission, county board of supervisors, or state legislature) that can influence the identified issue or concern.

The next step will be for community members to create a list of the questions to guide them in learning more about the issue they identified. The following questions can aid the community in coming up with their own list:

- What don't you know about the issue?
- How is the community hurt by the issue?
- What factors and forces are creating the issue or making it worse?
- Is there a law or policy that deals with your issue?
- Do other communities experience the same issue? What have they done to address this problem?
- What does the research say?

Example: Reducing Tobacco Advertising and Sponsorship

Questions to answer:

- How many people smoke in my community?
- What are the health hazards of tobacco use?
- How does tobacco use hurt our community?
- How do the tobacco companies target our community?
- How much money do the tobacco companies make on selling their product and how much do they give away?
- What local organizations and events take tobacco money?
- How do the tobacco companies benefit from giving money to these events?
- Who can decide not to take the tobacco money? What is the decision-making process?
- Which local organization or events (if any) have refused to take tobacco money?
- What can groups do rather than take tobacco money? What are some alternative sources of funding?

STEP 3: SELECTING RESEARCH TOOLS

Once the list of questions has been developed, the community will decide which research tools are best to use to find answers. A research tool or method is what you use to gather information about the identified issue or priority concern. Your community diagnosis may use one or many research tools depending on the type of information you want to gather. As a CHW, you play an important role in bringing resources to communities. You may have the opportunity to invite a consultant who is familiar with evaluation, epidemiology, or research to meet with your group and work with them to design the diagnosis. This person can give you advice about which types of research to conduct and how to do it.

You may use some or all of the following types of research (we'll talk about each one in the next section):

- Research at the library
- Research on the Internet
- Research at city hall, city departments, state and federal government
- Research to count physical objects
- Focus groups, community groups, community forums

- Surveys
- Community maps and diagrams
- Visual documentation such as Photovoice or video

Different Types of Information

Research tools will assist you to gather quantitative or qualitative data. Both are useful in better understanding the problem that the community has identified.

Quantitative data: This type of information lets you know how many times something is happening, how many people share the same experience or opinion, or anything else that can be measured numerically or by counting. Surveys, mapping, counting, and public health data records are all good ways to get quantitative data. When you hear "quantitative," think of numbers.

Qualitative data: This type of information gives you an in-depth or deeper understanding of how people feel about or experience an issue. Interviews, focus groups, and community forums are all good ways to get qualitative data about your issue. When you hear "qualitative," think of words and pictures.

An Example of Quantitative and Qualitative Data

The Question: How does smoking hurt our community?

Quantitative data: The number of people who report that their health has been harmed by smoking, the number of tobacco billboards or ads in a community, or data from the local health department on the number of people in the community who smoke and the number of people with chronic diseases that are caused by smoking such as emphysema, lung cancer, and heart disease.

Qualitative data: Real-life stories of how smoking hurts the community; the story of someone who died too young because they smoked; how a group of parents feels about tobacco advertising that targets their community; or how people feel about limiting smoking in public housing.

When to Use Different Types of Research

Table 22.1 provides information to aid you in deciding when to use a specific research tool.

Table 22.1 Uses of Specific Research Tools

TYPE OF DIAGNOSIS	DESCRIPTION	WHEN TO USE IT	WHEN NOT TO USE IT
Library	Visit a local library and work with librarian and library computers to research your topic.	For access to local statistics, resources, and history that might not be available elsewhere.	If the information or data is available on the Internet.
Internet	Use search engines like Google or reputable health sites like www.cdc.gov to get data or to network.	To do a quick initial search; a broad search; to access records/data unavailable locally.	If the information does not come from a reliable source.
Existing Policies, Regulations	Research at local, state, and federal level whether there are existing policies relevant to your topic and whether they are being enforced.	This should be a standard part of your diagnosis!	This is always relevant!

(continues)

TYPE OF DIAGNOSIS	DESCRIPTION	WHEN TO USE IT	WHEN NOT TO USE IT
Count Physical Objects	Visit sites and count actual items to assess their prevalence in the community (like # of alcohol ads, condom dispensers, etc.).	Useful when you want to demonstrate how much something is occurring in your community. This quantitative data always is more powerful if coupled with qualitative findings.	If the subject you're researching isn't connected to a physical object that can be counted.
Community Forums	Organize evening or weekend community meetings to gather community input, feedback, perceptions, and experiences.	When you want information from the community at large and want to raise awareness that an issue is being addressed.	If you do not have the resources available, as Community Forums are labor intensive.
Focus Groups	Strategically choose 6–12 people representing a variety of views on your issue. Facilitate a discussion to get their perceptions and experiences.	When you want to get deep and in-depth qualitative information about your issue. This information complements information from community surveys.	If you want to be able to talk about what the community as a whole thinks about an issue—you may need to survey at least 300 people to get that broader view.
Survey Individuals	Decide on the number of people you will survey. Come up with a survey or questionnaire to use to ask those people what their opinions are on the health issue you are concerned about. Then come up with a survey design (decide how many to survey, where, etc.) and conduct the survey.	When you want a representative sample of the community's responses in an organized way. This information goes well with focus group information. Survey information can be counted, such as the number and percentage of those surveyed who share similar experiences, risks, or opinions.	May not provide you with the qualitative "stories" you are looking for. Complements information from qualitative research.
Qualitative Interviews	Set up individual interviews to find out more about what people think, or why people feel the way they do.	When you want deep information such as explanations, quotes, stories, and detailed descriptions of people's experience, behavior, attitudes, feelings, and opinions.	When you want statistics—since interviews will not get you statistics or other quantitative data.
Community Map	Take a large piece of paper and "map" a place such as a neighborhood, inside a store, etc. Plot important items you are looking for. Can also use Google Maps or other online mapping tools. Some cities and counties have websites with specific mapping tools (like GIS) for that community.	When you want a visual representation of a place. For example, to show how many liquor stores or parks are in your neighborhood. Also when you want to compare the locations of two things—for example, traffic lights and car crashes.	When it is difficult to define the community geographically.
Photovoice (traditionally done with still photographs, can also be done with video)	Use cameras to document or take pictures of the issue you are working on. Usually, these pictures or videos are shared and discussed first among residents in a focus group, and then may be used later to tell the public or a policy-maker about the problem.	When you want a rich discussion with community members about how they see the problem. When you want to show the media or policymakers what's happening in your community.	When you don't have the resources.

Participating in research is where community members really begin to feel as though they are working toward change. Be sure to provide training or skill-building sessions as necessary so that community members have the skills they need to do the job. This phase of a community diagnosis can be exciting!

STEP 4: CONDUCTING RESEARCH

This step requires a lot of organization! It may mean making trips to the library or calling up agencies to ask them for information. You may need to design survey tools and train community members in how to use them to collect information. If you conduct focus groups or community forums, you will need to work with the community members to identify the questions you want to ask, and recruit people to participate in the groups or forums. Depending on how complicated the research plan is, you may want to connect the community with specialists for assistance—for example, a librarian might advise the group on library or Internet research, or your local public health department may be helpful in developing or reviewing a community survey.

A Word about Bias

It is possible to conduct a community diagnosis so that you learn only what you want to hear. If you think that the community should start a campaign to close a nearby waste incinerator, you can set up the community diagnosis to increase the chances that this will be the final outcome or recommendation. But this type of manipulation contradicts the true purpose of a community diagnosis: to gather information without prejudice and to let the community express their own concerns and their own ideas for change.

Common ways that bias can undermine a community diagnosis include:

- Determining who participates in the community diagnosis—such as including only people who already agree with a certain position.

- Asking **leading questions** or questions that lead people to the answers you want them to provide. An example of a leading question is: "Do you think that racism is one of the most important factors contributing to high rates of infant mortality in the community?" An open-ended and unbiased question would be: "What do you think are some of the most important factors that contribute to high rates of infant mortality in the community?"

- While you should avoid leading questions, it can be helpful to ask questions with a list of answers to choose among. These "multiple choice" questions may help people to think about the topic from different angles. They also make it easier to count the responses. An example would be, "Which of the following do you think contributes to infant mortality in this community? (a) lack of clinics (b) poor transportation (c) racism (d) other. When you include the option of "other" you also decrease bias, since it allows the community members to add their own ideas. (Make sure you give them the opportunity to state what they mean by "other.") If all of the options you list for a question are very similar, then that introduces bias, because it guides people to think only one way.

- Summarizing data to highlight information that supports your position, withholding data that does not, or presenting it in a confusing way.

- Guiding the analysis or trying to do the analysis for the community, and telling them what the data says.

- Guiding the development of the action plan, by calling on and supporting the voices of people who agree with you, or by asking questions that lead people to the type of action that you think is best.

As a CHW, allowing your own bias or that of your agency to influence the results of a community diagnosis is likely to undermine the community's trust in you. It may also weaken and damage, rather than strengthen, the community's own capacity. It is a violation of your ethical commitment to respect the right of communities to choose their own course of action.

Library Research

Library research can provide access to local data, history, and other resources that might not be available elsewhere. We recommend that you start by finding a librarian and asking for a general orientation and guidance in researching your topic. Librarians are experts in conducting research and are there to provide training, guidance, and support. You can also use library computers to find local, statewide, national, or international information and resources. Librarians can even help you research current laws and policies related to your topic. Ask the librarian for assistance with the computers and how to enter keywords to find your information. Keywords are those you enter into a computer or Internet search program that tell it what to look for.

For example, a group of youth advocates in San Francisco was concerned about peers who smoked *bidis* (cigarettes hand-rolled in South Asia, without filters). This became the focus of their diagnosis and their project. Neither the city health workers nor the youth advocates knew much about bidis, so they decided to go to the city library to research whether bidis contain tobacco or other harmful substances, and whether smoking bidis is harmful. Their search at the library revealed that bidis do contain tobacco and other unknown substances. They found out that smoking bidis can cause cancer, just like smoking other types of cigarettes. They also found out that bidis are often rolled by women and young children who work 12 to 16 hours a day for little pay.

Library privileges are easy to get, usually requiring some proof of where you live (such as a driver's license, utility bill, or anything that shows where you live). Colleges and universities also have libraries and often allow community members to use them. If it is difficult to go to the library in person, remember that some libraries offer many resources online.

Internet Research

To research information on the Internet, go to a search engine such as "Google," "Google Scholar," "Bing," or others, and type in keywords, such as "bidis" or "bidi cigarettes" or "bidis and health." Be sure to try different keyword combinations to do a broad enough search. Research on the Internet allows you to get the most updated research findings on your topic. It also assists you to connect with other organizations working on similar issues (so you can see what other groups are doing, what materials they are using, and what research they've done).

Be sure to look at sources of data from local governments, such as the local health department, and private organizations, including universities and foundations. Information that you may find on the Internet includes health statistics that can assist people to better understand the scope of the problem, its causes, and the consequences.

Note: It is important to verify sources when searching the Internet. Health information on the Internet varies in quality . . . *anyone can post health information on the web!* For some tips on assessing the reliability of a website, visit *www.nlm.nih.gov/medlineplus/healthywebsurfing.html*.

Here are examples of reputable public health websites:

- The Centers for Disease Control and Prevention: *www.cdc.gov*
- Office of the Surgeon General, Reports and Publications: *www.surgeongeneral.gov/library/reports.htm*
- Healthy People 2020: *www.healthypeople.gov*
- Partners in Information Access for the Public Health Workforce: *www.phpartners.org*
- MedlinePlus: *www.nlm.nih.gov/medlineplus/*

- *What is the website for your local city, county, or regional health department?*
- *What kind of health data or information can you find there?*

Research Existing Laws and Policies

A key component of many diagnoses is to research existing laws. There are many laws, regulations, and policies that already exist at the city, state, or federal level that may influence the issue your group is working on.

Within city government various city departments also have policies that may be relevant to your work. For example, many cities have laws that limit the amount of advertising in corner stores. A group of community advocates concerned about tobacco and alcohol advertising in neighborhood stores might find that their city limits outdoor advertising to no more than 10 percent of window space. They could identify stores that exceed this amount and work with city enforcement agencies to get unhealthy advertising reduced in their community.

You can begin the process by going to city hall or onto the city website to search for the city agency with jurisdiction over your issue. For example, if you want to find out about local laws regulating signs and advertising, you could start by getting on your city's website and searching using the key words "sign laws." You might be directed to the city planning department or the city municipal codes that include these laws. This type of research requires patience and persistence. Every system is organized differently, but the more you familiarize yourself with city, state, and federal systems, the easier it becomes. Sometimes the best you can do is find a phone number and start by calling and asking for assistance. Your local public library may also be able to help you with this. Try a variety of methods to find the person or city agency responsible for addressing your issue. Don't give up!

Counting Physical Objects

Counting physical objects can show how aspects of the physical environment positively or negatively affect the community. For example, if you wanted to show how often tobacco companies promote their products to children, you could come up with a checklist, visit all the stores in your neighborhood, and count how many times each store has tobacco ads located below three feet in height or near candy.

Things you might count:

- The number of grocery stores selling fresh produce (vegetables and fruit)
- The number of fast-food restaurants in the community
- The number of liquor stores and bars in the community
- The number of after-school recreation facilities or programs for school-aged children
- The number of clinics or physicians accepting Medicaid
- The number of colleges, adult schools, or employment training programs in the community

- *What else might you count as part of your community diagnosis?*

What Do YOU Think?

To conduct this type of research:

- Work with community members to design a standardized tool or checklist to document how often something (such as alcohol or tobacco advertising) occurs, where it occurs, and any other important information they want to gather.

- Work with community representatives to develop a research plan. Do they want to count objects in all stores in your neighborhood, or do they want to visit a **sample** (a representative selection) of all stores citywide? What are the geographic boundaries of the neighborhood?

A youth group at the Vietnamese Youth Development Center in the Tenderloin neighborhood of San Francisco were concerned by the high concentration of corner stores and their influence in the community. They felt that the strengths in their community were overlooked, and the neighborhood got a bad rap in the media. They developed a one-page tool and visited 35 corner stores and rated them based on: presence of healthy, fresh food; quantity of alcohol/tobacco ads; compliance with signage, permit posting, and other laws; and other issues. They applied a point system to the responses and plotted them on a spreadsheet that they used to create a map of the stores (see Figure 22.1) that got either a "rotten," "half," or "whole" apple based on the points assigned to each store, to highlight strengths and problems in the neighborhood. They then presented the map to a number of community groups, which resulted in the creation of the Tenderloin Healthy Corner Store Coalition (www.healthytl.org). The map is updated annually, and stores that improve their healthy offerings get recognition for their efforts.

Surveys

You can also find out what the community thinks by surveying a sample of individuals. You might survey youth, parents, teachers, agency leaders, or members of any group. Surveys can be completed in apartment buildings, on the street, at community events, and in waiting rooms. Sometimes surveys are done in two neighborhoods with different characteristics to compare and contrast. The important thing is to take the time to prepare your survey questions and set up a good survey design that will represent the community you are working with.

Developing an Effective Survey

Start by working with community members to identify the type of information they want to gather and how that information will enhance their understanding of the focus issue or concern. Next, create a list of questions to include in the survey that are designed to gather this information. Narrow the questions down to no more than two pages. Use straightforward language and don't use abbreviations. Finally, put your questions in a logical order, from the general to the more specific.

Start the survey with the questions that are the most interesting and least threatening. Save the more difficult questions for the end, and avoid leading questions (for example, a question starting with "Don't you think . . . ?").

As much as possible, use closed-ended questions for surveys rather than open-ended ones. This will allow you to collect data and analyze your findings more easily. When including questions that ask people to compare or rate items, be sure that the scale includes options from both extremes. Keep this simple (for example, *poor, okay, great*). If you want to give respondents a list of answers or categories to choose from, try to keep it fairly short (no more than five choices). Questions that ask people to remember things from the past should focus on the near past in order to document accurate information (for example, "How many times in the past month have you . . ."). Many groups bring in someone with evaluation experience to review their survey tool and make suggestions.

Once you have your survey in draft form, pretest it with a few people representing the group you want to survey to ensure that all the questions are clear and invite responses that are useful to the community diagnosis. Finally, come up with a brief memo to attach to the survey describing who you are, why you are doing the survey, and how you will use the information gathered. You will want to hand this out to everyone whom you ask to participate in the survey.

The survey in Figure 22.1 was developed and used by Literacy for Environmental Justice to assess community attitudes and feelings about tobacco advertising in the Bayview Hunters Point neighborhood of San Francisco.

Facilitate Discussions with Community Members

Other strategies to find out what the community is thinking include:

- Inviting the community to attend local forums or meetings
- Visiting community agencies and groups
- Facilitating focus groups

Community Forums

Invite community members to a large meeting or community forum to talk about the issue or concern you are investigating and to share their experiences, feelings, and opinions. A community member may introduce the forum or meeting and explain the community diagnosis process, what you are doing, the type of information you hope to gather, and how you intend to use it. Let the audience know that their knowledge and information will be used to guide efforts to promote the community's health. You may identify specific questions and facilitate a structured conversation in one large or several small groups. Or you may decide to use an open microphone and let community members speak up as they choose about the issue that you are addressing, such as low birth weights and high rates of infant mortality. Appoint two or more people to take notes in order to document the information shared during the meeting. Community forums can be effective ways to discover various perspectives on an issue and to generate a range of ideas about how to approach it. Other techniques used in forums involve putting questions or maps on easel paper and asking community members to "vote" or "comment" with sticky dots or notes.

Figure 22.1 Tobacco Advertising Survey (Literacy for Environmental Justice)

With the following survey, we would like to find out from you how you feel about tobacco advertisements in your community at your community corner/liquor stores here in Bayview Hunters Point. We would appreciate your spending a few minutes to complete this survey. The results from this survey will be used to fight the placement of tobacco ads in our community.

First, we would love to learn more about you.

Age: ☐

Gender: Male ☐   Female ☐   Transgender/Gender Variant ☐

Zip Code: ☐

What is the primary language you speak at home? ☐

What's your ethnicity? ☐

Do you or any family members smoke cigarettes? Yes ☐   No ☐

On average how many cigarettes do you/they smoke? _____

What brands do you/they smoke? _____

Where do you or your family members buy your cigarettes?

_____ In the BVHP   _____ Elsewhere: where? _____

Did you know that the tobacco industry provides incentives to stores
to advertise and promote tobacco?   Yes ○ No ○

Where do you see advertisements for tobacco?

_____ Outside of stores _____ Inside stores _____ Magazines _____ Movies _____ Other

What brands of cigarettes do you see advertised the most? _____

Are you aware that there are tobacco advertisements in your community liquor stores?

Yes ☐ No ☐

Name one way that you think tobacco companies advertise tobacco: _____

Do you think that tobacco ads influence young people to smoke? Yes ☐ No ☐

What about tobacco ads do you think is influential: _____ Pictures _____ Messages _____ Slogans _____ Other

Do you think that the tobacco companies should compensate the city/public for the
harm caused by tobacco advertising and use?   Yes ○ No ○

Would you support efforts to reduce advertising in the community?   Yes ☐ No ☐

If yes, what are some ways we might try to do this? Would you support:
- Trying to get the tobacco companies to pay for city efforts (GN) to reduce exposure to tobacco promotion for youth
  and others   Yes ☐ No ☐
- Amending the Lee Law (that restricts ads in store windows) to reduce advertising?   Yes ☐ No ☐
- Getting programs to replace tobacco and alcohol ads with ads about healthy eating and healthy and sustainable
  communities?   Yes ☐ No ☐

Visits to Community Agencies, Associations, or Groups

Compile a comprehensive list of the agencies, associations, or groups in your community. Come up with a standardized survey or interview guide that outlines the questions you want to be sure to cover in your visits. Try to put the questions in order so that they flow from easier to more difficult and prepare them so you can sort and group responses (make clusters of similar responses). Determine whom you will talk to at the agency. Visiting local agencies is an opportunity to build relationships and identify potential allies who will support the community diagnosis and advocacy for social change.

Facilitate Focus Groups

A focus group is essentially an interview conducted with a group of 6 to 12 people. Focus groups generally last one to two hours, address one main topic or issue, and ask five or six questions to guide a discussion. Here, we devote more space to describing focus groups, because they are often a great research tool to learn more about commonly held experiences, ideas, and feelings. However, not every community diagnosis will use focus groups, and not every kind of information you want to learn is best gathered by focus groups. Focus groups are a great tool to use when you want in-depth information about a specific topic.

Resource for Conducting Focus Groups

We can only provide the briefest introduction to the focus-group process here. Learning the skills required to facilitate a productive focus group takes time and experience. The best possible beginning would be to observe a focus group, or even to take part in one as a participant. There are many resources, in books and on the Internet, that can provide more information, such as the Free Management Library, an online resource for nonprofits (*www.managementhelp.org/evaluatn/focusgrp.htm*) and The Community Tool Box, a community health resource (*http://ctb.ku.edu/en/table-of-contents/assessment/assessing-community-needs-and-resources/conduct-focus-groups/main*).

Why Use a Focus Group

Like a community forum and qualitative interviews (see following sections), a focus group provides an opportunity to gather more in-depth and potentially surprising information. Focus groups also give people the opportunity to interact *with each other*, in addition to responding directly to a question. The conversation that participants have with each other is the richest part of any focus-group process.

How to Facilitate a Focus Group

Focus groups should not be facilitated by one person. You should always work with others to determine your focus group goal(s) and questions. And in addition to the participants whom you invite to take part in the focus group, you will need someone to act as the moderator or facilitator, as well as someone to act as the recorder and to document what participants say.

1. **Identify your goal:** A clearly stated goal will better serve to keep you on track throughout the focus group. What is it that you want to learn? How will that information be helpful to the community diagnosis?

2. **Formulate your questions:** Your questions must be open-ended but inspire conversation. A question that is too open could leave participants confused or overwhelmed. It's smart to start simply, with questions that are easier for people to understand and answer, and build to more complex questions.

   A sample set of questions might look like this:

   A. What do you like about living in the neighborhood?

   B. What are your concerns with safety in your neighborhood?

   C. How do these safety concerns affect the community?

   D. What needs to change to promote safety in the neighborhood?

   E. _____?

   F. _____?

3. **Recruit participants:** Generally, you want to make sure there are enough people in the room to keep a good conversation going, but not so many that some participants won't have a chance to speak. Eight to 10 people in the focus group is ideal. In planning the number of participants, anticipate that one or more individuals may not show up. Generally, if 12 people have confirmed that they will participate, 10 will show up. If everyone shows up, it would still be a manageable size for a focus group, and if fewer than 12 show up, you will still have enough people to keep the conversation flowing.

- *Diversity of perspective:* Often, having people who are similar in some way is useful—for example, having all the participants come from the same neighborhood, all be single parents, or all be of the same gender, age, or ethnicity. Other times, it's helpful to have more diversity. You might hold several focus groups on the same topic. Talk with your colleagues about what you think the right mix will be for the information you wish to learn.

- *Incentives for participation:* If you have a budget for this, small gift cards or other incentives will be appreciated by the participants and encourage them to show up for the focus group.

Conducting a Focus Group with High School Students

In a focus group with ninth-grade students to identify the after-school activities they most enjoyed, and the factors that encouraged or discouraged participation in these activities, the facilitator was aware that students could lose interest very quickly. The facilitator worked with several youth to develop the questions for the focus group. The facilitator also had the students draw a picture that showed the after-school activity they would offer if they were in charge, and if resources were not a problem. The students were asked to stand up and present their idea to the group. The facilitator could assess the enthusiasm that peers had for the idea as well as ask questions about any details that might be of interest. Asking them to write their name, age, gender, languages spoken at home, and languages spoken with friends also helped to increase participation and dialogue.

---

4. **Create the right environment:** Build rapport and trust: Participants need reassurance that you and the other group members are trustworthy. Let people know what you are doing and why, and follow through on any commitments you make to the group.

- *Power dynamics:* Will everyone in the room feel equally empowered to speak up? If a person's supervisor is present, they might not be comfortable talking about certain job-related concerns. In certain cultures, women are expected to defer to men, and are therefore less likely to speak up if men are present. Some power dynamics can be handled through good facilitation, however. If some people are more dominant participants than others, the facilitator can say, "I'd like to hear from some of the people who haven't spoken yet."

- *Consider the interests and strengths of the group you'll be convening:* Different groups of people may require different strategies in your facilitation.

- *Facilitation:* Don't try to control the conversation too much, but make sure that you get answers to your most important questions. Understand that people build ideas by talking to each other and asking each other questions. Let that happen!

- *Child care:* Depending on the group you are bringing together, it is a good idea to have a plan for child care. Offering child care might enable some people to participate who would otherwise decline.

- *Refreshments:* Providing healthy snacks and drinks is an important way to thank your participants, and to make sure they get the brain fuel they need to participate fully.

- *Languages spoken:* Know the language needs of your participants, and arrange for interpretation, if necessary. You might consider holding more than one focus group if you have enough participants to hold, for example, an all-Russian language group as well as an all-Spanish language group.

- o *Documentation*: Documenting the focus group accurately is very important. Use a tape or digital recorder, and test all your equipment ahead of time. Bring plenty of extra batteries and blank tapes. Also plan to take your own notes. You want to keep track not just of what people say, but of how they say it. For example, people's body language is important to notice. Ideally, one member of your team will act only as the recorder and not do anything else. Be sure to inform participants that they are being recorded.

5. **Making it work:** How you facilitate the group will shape what you learn, and also how the community members will feel about participating in future activities. Please keep the following suggestions in mind:

- o *Ground rules*: Setting basic ground rules allows everyone to know what to expect. You might suggest some, and then ask those in the group if they have any they want to add. Post them on flip-chart paper so everyone can keep them in mind.

- o *Confidentiality* is important to discuss. You need to assure participants that what they say will be treated confidentially by you, and they in turn need to agree to keep what they hear and say confidential.

- o *Agenda*: Plan to spend between 60 and 90 minutes, and not more. You should have a clear agenda that you share with participants at the beginning of the session.

- o *Facilitation suggestions*: Make sure that everyone has the chance to speak. Let people know what you are going to do with the information they have provided.

6. **Analysis:** As soon after the session as possible, write down your thoughts and review your notes. Spend some time with your fellow facilitators and share your reflections. Identify strongly held views, major areas of agreement among participants, and surprising information. Generally, you will do a content analysis similar to what is explained in the next section related to qualitative interviews. Content analysis is a way of identifying common themes that are shared by focus-group participants (and is explained in greater detail below).

Qualitative Interviews

Sometimes you want to gather in-depth information about people's experiences, feelings, and opinions expressed in their own words. You may be looking for insights into sensitive or controversial issues, or want to learn more about the history of the community. This kind of data is gained by qualitative interviews, or structured conversations with people. The insights of the CHWs quoted in this textbook were obtained from qualitative interviews.

Like focus groups, qualitative interviews can strengthen or provide a context for other data and statistics that you gather and may show *why* people feel the way they do. Qualitative interviews can provide quotes from community members that serve to attach meaning to the numbers or statistics you have gathered. Qualitative results also help community advocates evaluate how well projects were implemented and provide feedback from community members on the process involved in implementing social change efforts. Finally, qualitative interviews reveal unexpected positive or negative outcomes of your efforts.

Conducting Qualitative Interviews

Ideally, qualitative interviews should feel like a conversation. Ask people about themselves in relation to the issue at hand. ("When did you first become aware of the high infant mortality rate in your community?" "How does this problem affect you and the community?" "What do you think causes or contributes to this problem?" "What do you think should be done to reduce the problem of infant mortality?") In general, people like to be asked to share their opinions. Similar to surveys, start with nonthreatening questions. People may not want to answer very personal or difficult questions until they get comfortable with you and the process. Open-ended questions are best. As people begin to answer questions, use probing follow-up questions to get more information such as, "Can you tell me more about that?" or "Is there anything else you wanted to say about this issue?" Sometimes it is useful to stay silent and give the person you are interviewing time to reflect and respond. Use your client-centered counseling and motivational interviewing skills (see Chapter 9).

You can encourage the person being interviewed (the respondent) with positive feedback and by paying attention to nonverbal cues and body language. Don't share your views on the subject in case this may influence what the respondent says. Finally, let the respondent know that you are taking notes to be sure to remember key points. If you are looking for material you can quote, use a recorder to make sure that you get it right. Let the person you are interviewing know you are recording the interview. They will be reassured that you will not distort what they say. It is unethical to record anyone without that person's knowledge and consent. If you think there is any reason to believe the person you are interviewing might get upset with your using the interview, clarify the situation by asking them to sign a release form giving you permission to use the interview for the specific purposes that you tell them. This can also reassure people that the interview will not be used for any other purposes.

Release of Information

I, _____, give _____ [name of interviewer] permission to use material from this interview only in material created by the Tobacco Free Project.

Signed and dated:

_____

Note: If the person you are interviewing is younger than 18 years old, a parent or guardian must give permission.

The Most Important Question

After you have finished the interview, but before you turn off the recorder, always ask if there is anything else the person wants to tell you. Don't suggest what that might be. Wait for as long as it takes for the person to decide that they are done. Some of the most interesting insights come when people answer the question you didn't think to ask.

Content Analysis of Responses

There are different ways to analyze qualitative interviews. Transcribing the interview—writing it down word for word from a recording—often helps with this. To identify key themes from one interview or common themes from more than one interview, do a **content analysis** of what was said. A content analysis is a way of summarizing what people said by grouping, comparing, and counting their responses. You can do a content analysis of interviews by looking for common themes or categories in what people said, identifying issues that come up again and again, or that the respondent gave particular importance to. A theme might be something like: appreciation for neighbors; lack of education or good schools; the closing of a big employer in the community; conflict between certain segments of the community; or racism. In your summary and analysis of the interviews, look not only for opinions and themes that were shared among the respondents, but also for particularly strong or powerful opinions. Write down insightful quotes to include as part of your analysis. To find out how common particular themes are, you can create a simple table (see Table 22.2) to identity the themes mentioned and to count how many people mentioned them.

Table 22.2 Sample Summary of Qualitative Interviews

MAJOR THEMES	OUT OF 20 INTERVIEWS, NO. OF PEOPLE WHO MENTIONED THE THEME:
Close relationships with neighbors	8
Closing of shipyard	12
Poor quality of local schools	6
Racism	15

Community Mapping

Mapping can be a powerful research strategy. Maps are used to provide a visual image of the risks and negative influences that impact a community, such as sources of environmental pollution, dangerous crosswalks or intersections, or very-poor-quality housing. Maps can show the distribution of illness and death in a community or region such as homicides, infant mortality, or other conditions. Maps can also show the strengths and resources in a community that promote well-being and health, such as quality housing, parks, schools, public transportation, health centers, and grocery stores.

A classic early example of a map that was used to guide public health work is the map that Dr. John Snow drew of cholera deaths in London in 1854 (see Figure 22.2). As you can see, the map revealed that a large number of deaths had occurred near the location of the Broad Street Water Pump. The map assisted Dr. Snow to convince policymakers to turn off the pump, which resulted in a dramatic decline in cholera cases and deaths. The map also led to a new understanding of how cholera was transmitted from person to person, eventually resulting in new strategies for prevention (UCLA, n.d.; Kukaswadia, 2013).

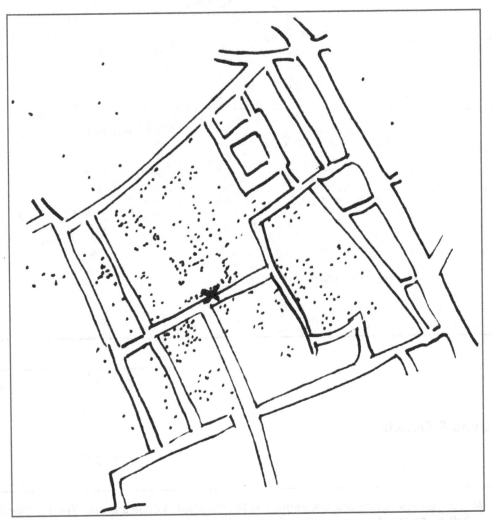

Figure 22.2 Map of Cholera Deaths in London, 1854 (The X marks the location of the Broad Street water pump)

Mapping is increasingly used by local, national, and international health agencies to identify populations with the highest health risks, and to better understand the factors that contribute to those risks. Mapping is often done using Geographic Information Systems (GIS) that rely on information gathered from satellites and other sources to create detailed electronic images. For example, the Youth Leadership Institute worked with the San Francisco Department of Public Health to map the distribution of tobacco permits across the city. This map (Figure 22.3) shows that permits are concentrated in districts with high numbers of youth, people of color, and low-income people. Pay attention to the section labeled "Soma/Tloin D6." In fact, the low-income Tenderloin neighborhood is located in a district with 270 permits while the high-income Marina (D2) only has 50, a glaring health equality issue.

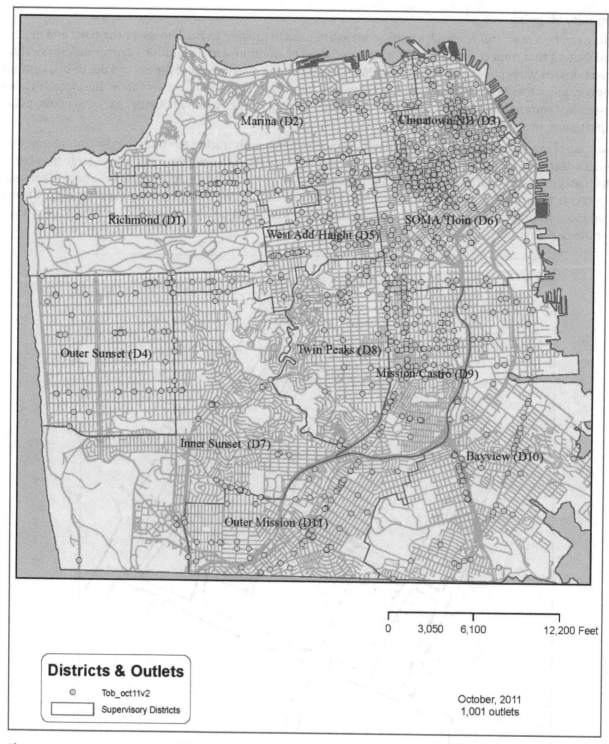

Figure 22.3 Map of Tobacco Outlets and Sale Permits in San Francisco: A Comparison of Two Neighborhoods (Approximately half of the city of San Francisco is shown in this map)

Mapping doesn't require advanced technology, however; it can be done by hand, with graph paper, on top of paper maps of your neighborhood or city, or through using web resources such as Google Maps or Google Earth (*maps.google.com* or *earth.google.com*). Taking a walk or a drive through the neighborhood is also a good way for the people involved in the community diagnosis to get ideas for what they want to show in a map. To read more about mapping and GIS technologies, please see the resources at the end of this chapter.

Photovoice

Another resource for conducting a community diagnosis involves using cameras to document what is happening in a community. This powerful tool is known as Photovoice (Wang & Burris, 1997). For example, a project conducted by Legal Services for Prisoners with Children, "Invisible Punishment: Photovoice Challenges the Prison System," gave cameras to formerly incarcerated women and family members of prisoners to record the impact of high rates of incarceration on communities. As with other tools of community diagnosis, a key aspect of the Photovoice process is bringing community residents *together* to analyze the photos that they themselves took. The photos served multiple purposes: they sparked conversation and analysis among the family members who took the photos, they demonstrated in compelling ways the impacts of incarceration through a traveling exhibit of the photographs, and they strengthened the bonds and activism of the community involved. Through Photovoice, the participants could analyze the effects of their social environment as shown in the photos, to identify problems and possible solutions (D. Willmott, personal communication, April 9, 2009).

Community mapping and Photovoice produce compelling visual representations of what is happening in the community. Many CHWs and community advocates use photos, maps, and diagrams when presenting public testimony to local policymakers or when discussing their issue with the press.

Literacy for Environmental Justice

A project supported by the Tobacco Free Project was carried out by Literacy for Environmental Justice (LEJ), a nonprofit agency, and a group of youth advocates. They were concerned about the lack of fresh and healthy foods in the corner stores in their community. They visited the 11 stores in their neighborhood and drew maps of the inside of the stores. They created simple maps for each store. The following diagram (Figure 22.4) recreates a map produced by the youth advocates for one of the 11 stores: Jimmy's Market. The map shows that 35 percent of all products sold at Jimmy's Market were nonfood items, 27 percent were alcohol and cigarettes, 24 percent packaged food, 10 percent all other beverages, and just 4 percent were meat and fresh produce.

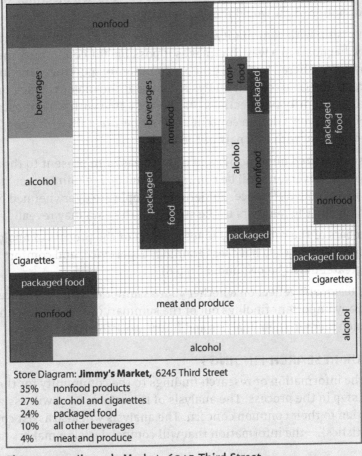

Store Diagram: **Jimmy's Market,** 6245 Third Street

35%	nonfood products
27%	alcohol and cigarettes
24%	packaged food
10%	all other beverages
4%	meat and produce

Figure 22.4 Jimmy's Market, 6245 Third Street

The Focus Project

Since 2005, the Tobacco Free Project (TFP), a program of the San Francisco Department of Public Health, has funded the FOCUS Project. FOCUS is a collaboration of the Chinese Progressive Association (CPA) and People Organizing to Demand Environmental and Economic Rights (PODER). The collaboration grew out of a desire to support the empowerment of working-class immigrant communities in Southeast San Francisco and to improve the dire environmental health conditions in those neighborhoods.

CPA/PODER conducted a community diagnosis to understand how the local environment influences tobacco use and resulting health problems, and what role the transnational tobacco industry plays within these working-class communities of color. They created a map to show the results of their community diagnosis. The resulting map of San Francisco showed that the greatest numbers and concentrations of tobacco outlets were located in communities with the highest levels of poverty and the greatest number of immigrants and people of color. These communities also had the highest rates of smoking. The maps were used to show that the number of tobacco retail outlets put the community at greater risk of tobacco-related health inequalities—greater rates of illness and death.

Ultimately, this research influenced decisions about local policy and how to prevent exposure to environmental health risks, including tobacco. To give just one example of a policy changed through the community diagnosis and advocacy of CPA and PODER, the San Francisco Board of Supervisors passed an ordinance in 2010 to restrict smoking in public areas such as farmer's markets, homeless shelters, and outdoor dining areas at restaurants (San Francisco Tobacco Free Project, 2010).

STEP 5: SUMMARIZING YOUR RESEARCH FINDINGS

If you collected three hundred surveys, and want community members to analyze them, would it be helpful to hand out all three hundred copies of the two-to-three-page surveys at a meeting? What would community members do with this information? How would they analyze it?

CHWs often work in partnership with community representatives to assist in summarizing the information gathered for a community diagnosis in a way that makes it possible for community members to understand. Qualitative data—information gathered by focus groups, community meetings, and interviews—is often hard to summarize. You can perform a content analysis to look at the major themes that emerged. You may also want to highlight strong minority perspectives that do not agree with what most people tell you for the community to consider. If you haven't done a content analysis before, talk with your supervisor or ask an experienced colleague to assist you with this part of the work.

Quantitative data can be summarized numerically and is much easier to present to the community, using charts and graphs. However, not everyone will be comfortable analyzing numbers or statistics, so the way that you present this data can make a big difference. Sometimes, people are overwhelmed by data and statistics, and have difficulty seeing beyond the numbers to the story that the data may reveal.

You don't want some members of the community to feel left out of the process of analyzing the findings of the community diagnosis simply because they have less training, experience, and comfort talking about statistics (we address this point in greater detail below, under Step 6).

Most important, work as a team, and reflect on whether your assumptions and prejudices are influencing the outcomes. Are you leaving any important findings out of the summary? Are you presenting the community with accurate information to guide them in their analysis and future work together?

STEP 6: ANALYZING YOUR RESEARCH FINDINGS

Now it is time to present the information or research findings to the community for them to analyze and interpret. This is a crucial step in the process. The analysis of the information will assist community members to identify a possible solution to their common concern. The analysis will also assist community members to identify the "startling statistics"—the information that will compel decision makers to do something about the issue.

As the community is reviewing the information gathered, you may use the following types of questions to guide their analysis:

- What does the information tell them about the issue they investigated?
- Who in the community is most affected by the problem?
- What percentage of people who participated in the research seem highly concerned about the problem?
- What does the community think about the causes and consequences of the problem?
- What are their proposed solutions?
- Do different parts of the community have different experiences or opinions—for example, do women express different opinions from men, do youth express different opinions from elders? Are there any differences in opinion based on where people live in the community?

Important Things to Keep in Mind

Don't take the data at face value

There are different ways to interpret the same data. For example, your data may show that there has been a decrease in the number of reported illegal tobacco and alcohol sales to minors. This could mean that: (1) fewer merchants are selling tobacco and alcohol to minors, or (2) less enforcement is taking place due to a lack of funding or some other reason. It is important to look deeper to discover the whole story.

Information or data gathered cannot always tell the whole story

For example, data that has been collected at the neighborhood level cannot be used to say what is happening in different neighborhoods or in all neighborhoods. Focus groups and interviews give you information only about the people you interviewed. When describing this type of data, always notes such as, "Of those people surveyed, 80 percent reported . . . " or "Survey respondents reported that . . . " or "Focus group participants felt. . . . "

Allow the community residents time to absorb the information and react, before jumping to action ideas

The results of the community diagnosis may well be surprising or distressing to those who live in the community. On the other hand, there may be important community strengths or aspects of community history that were not captured in the diagnosis—discussing the results with the community may provide an opportunity to add more detail to the picture.

Phuong An Doan-Billings: As someone who works as a CHW, you get trained to look at information in a certain way. But when you bring the information to the community, sometimes they close the door, they don't want to hear it. You have to figure out how they feel when you share bad news—for example, that nail salon chemicals can cause cancer. They don't think that's something they want to know. They'll think, you mean I harm myself, my customers, everyone who works here? And they will feel very, very sad. You assume that it's good information for people to know, but they don't feel that way. Someone might think, "It's not personal—it's a community issue," but that's an American way of thinking. The Vietnamese way is more indirect. You can't talk right into their face. What we do is, we find out what they don't like to hear, and then present that in a delicate way. It's a cultural difference—and that's why we are here as CHWs.

Preparing Your Findings in a Visually Compelling Format

Once the community has analyzed and interpreted the data, we recommend that you develop a clear way to present it to others. You will want to share your key findings with allies who will assist you to advocate for changes in the community and to policymakers who have the power to make certain changes. How you present the data often can make all the difference in terms of whether or not people will understand it or want to act on it (also see Chapter 23).

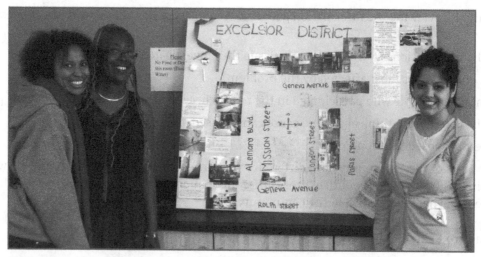

City College students share a map of health risks and resources in their community.

The community group analyzing the data should try to identity the five top findings that will become their "startling statistics." What information is most compelling to the community? What information supports their final analysis? What information will be useful in engaging policymakers to take action on the community's behalf?

Tip: You are looking for startling statistics that:

- Show how your community is adversely affected by the issue compared with other communities
- Show that your community is concerned about the issue and wants something done about it
- Show that your community understands the issue and has done their homework around it
- Show that policies already exist that address the issue
- Show that local solutions exist to address the issue

There are many ways to present your data, including:

- Tables
- Pie charts
- Bar or line graphs
- Photos
- Maps
- Pictures
- Case studies and quotes

Literacy for Environmental Justice:

How One Group Presented Their Findings in a Visually Compelling Format

As described above, youth advocates working with Literacy for Environmental Justice (LEJ) were concerned about the lack of healthy food sold in their community, which had very high rates of diabetes and other chronic diseases. They were also concerned about the health problems caused by smoking and alcohol.

(continues)

Literacy for Environmental Justice:
(continued)

The youth drew a map of 11 local stores showing the products that they sold. From this information, they created a pie chart showing the types of products sold at the stores in their community. The pie chart shows, for example, that 26 percent of the items for sale in neighborhood stores were alcohol and cigarettes, and only 2 percent of the items for sale were produce (vegetables and fruit).

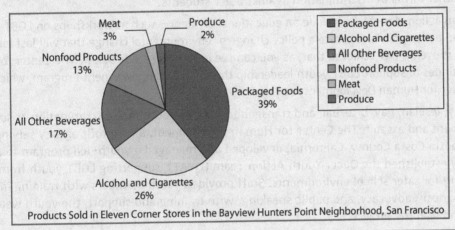

Products Sold in Eleven Corner Stores in the Bayview Hunters Point Neighborhood, San Francisco

- *What do you think of the way that Literacy for Environmental Justice presented information using a pie chart?*

- *Is the information easy to understand?*

- *Can you think of other ways that you could present this information?*

STEP 7: DEVELOPING AN ACTION PLAN

Based on the analysis of research findings, community members work together to develop an action plan to address the concerns they identified and to create changes to promote health. An action plan lays out the steps the community may take to make or advocate for change. This process should be as inclusive as possible, providing an opportunity for all members of the community to participate if they choose. Getting this process right is more important than doing it quickly. If you rush and forget to include certain members of the community, you risk losing support for your action plan or creating a new conflict and problem in the community. Be as transparent or open and honest as possible about this process: let everyone know how and when they can participate.

- *What are some possible actions that the Native communities mentioned at the beginning of this chapter could take to reduce high rates of low birth weight and infant mortality?*

The work you have done in the community diagnosis to map out potential allies and opponents will be especially helpful as you create an action plan. You will need allies at all levels—from the grassroots to City Hall. It's often helpful to identify a specific policymaker who might be sympathetic to your ideas and who has influence with other policymakers. This person could become a champion who helps you attain your policy goals. Yet even champions sometimes need to be convinced or persuaded to achieve the results you want.

You will learn how to develop an action plan in detail in Chapter 23.

Queer Youth Action Team

The Queer Youth Action Team (QYAT), a project of the Center for Human Development in Contra Costa County, California, was a group of lesbian, gay, bisexual, and transgender (LGBT) high-school-aged youth who came together in 2000 to address health concerns related to HIV, harassment, and discrimination. With support from CHWs and other staff, the youth conducted a community diagnosis to guide them in developing an action plan. This plan involved advocating for new policies at local school districts to prohibit harassment and other forms of discrimination against LGBT students.

In general, while an action plan might include an educational element—such as workshops on LGBT health—the primary focus of an action plan is to create a policy change or environmental change that will last long after the specific campaign is over. QYAT achieved that, as you can see in the case study below. The Center for Human Development continues to support LGBT youth leadership through the Empowerment Program, which grew out of the QYAT (Center for Human Development, 2001).

Across the country, lesbian, gay, bisexual, and transgender (LGBT) youth face discrimination at school, including harassment and assault. The Center for Human Development, a nonprofit agency serving youth and families in Contra Costa County, California, developed and managed a youth-led program to address these issues. They established the Queer Youth Action Team (QYAT), supporting LGBT youth from local high schools to advocate for safer school environments. Staff provided youth members with training in skills such as community diagnosis, advocacy, and public speaking. With training and support, the youth were able to take ownership and lead the project.

The QYAT members decided to advocate for local school districts to adopt and implement antidiscrimination policies to protect the rights and well-being of LGBT students. Their first campaign would focus on the West Contra Costa Unified School District (WCCUSD). The youth developed and submitted a resolution to the local school board; conducted outreach to garner support for the resolution; developed and sent out press releases; conducted interviews with print, radio, and television news agencies; and spoke at a school board meeting in February of 2001. At the same time, statewide advocacy achieved a change in state law (AB 537) that set standards for how schools should ensure safety and freedom from discrimination for LGBT students. The QYAT's advocacy helped shape how AB 537 would be enforced in Contra Costa County.

A description of their work can be found in the manual, "Make It Real: AB 537" published by the Gay-Straight Alliance Network (GSA), the Friends of Project 10, & American Civil Liberties Union of Southern California (2001). The manual explains the QYAT's planning process:

> We developed a strategy chart outlining our long-term and short-term goals, and identifying our allies. . . . We also asked ourselves more personal questions such as what were our strengths and weaknesses as a group as well as what type of tactics we were going to use. (GSA et al., 2001, p. 36)

The QYAT members also organized a forum for LGBT and straight students to talk about their experiences in high school and the need for stronger antidiscrimination policies.

> On March 8, 2000, QYAT organized a youth forum called "Give Us the 411" at the Richmond Unity Church in West Contra Costa County, specifically for students in the district. The event was a major success, with youth both queer and straight showing up from all over the district to tell us what they thought about homophobia in their schools. With some animated discussion, everyone came to the conclusion that there were some major problems that needed to be addressed in the district regarding homophobia. . . .

> Yet undoubtedly, the most unforgettable part of the forum was [were] the school climate surveys and personal stories the youth left. As we read each story, I felt something inside of me begin to stir. Why are we treated differently because we are queer? It seemed so unfair to me. . . . That was the moment we all became emotionally invested in this fight. (GSA et al., 2001, p. 36)

(continues)

The QYAT developed a draft resolution and antidiscrimination policy for the school district to consider. After a lengthy struggle to get the resolution on the school board's agenda, QYAT members started to advocate on behalf of the policy:

> *We went out into the community and collected over 200 signatures of WCCUSD constituents. We created QYAT postcards of support, hundreds of which were sent to different board members. Finally, we collected 40 letters of support from parents, teachers, PFLAG members, various religious organizations, PTA groups, as well as the teacher's union, all of which urged the board to pass our original version of the resolution.*

> *On February 7, 2001, a year after our efforts had first begun, came the day of the WCCUSD Board meeting where the fate of our resolution would be decided. . . . A few days prior to the event, QYAT sent out media advisories to local news agencies, and in response KQED, KPFA, KGO [radio stations], the San Francisco Chronicle, the Contra Costa Times, and Contra Costa Television showed up to witness this historic event. With the community out in full force and wearing hot pink stickers in support of QYAT, we began our presentation with legal information, statistics, and personal testimonies of students. Many students felt uncomfortable being seen at the meeting, so their stories were told by other youth, who pointed out the author's reluctance to be identified. There were more than 30 speakers in favor of QYAT's resolution. (GSA et al., 2001, p. 37)*

As a result of their organizing and advocacy efforts, the WCCUSD became the first school district in Contra Costa County to pass a new policy prohibiting harassment and other forms of discrimination against LGBT youth.

> *With a unanimous vote, the board passed the amendment, and the crowd simultaneously broke out in a roar of cheers. At that moment my eyes flooded with tears as I hugged my fellow QYAT members in celebration of our victory. It was the greatest feeling ever to watch the crowd of students and adults light up with hope and enthusiasm where once only fear and hopelessness existed. (GSA et al., 2001, p. 38)*

Not only did this project result in new policies to protect students from discrimination, it also empowered youth leaders who learned how to successfully do their research, explain their diagnosis in compelling terms, and use that information to organize and advocate for policy change and social justice.

Chapter Review

YOUR COMMUNITY DIAGNOSIS

Think about a community you belong to or know well. Apply the information presented in this chapter to answer the following questions:

1. Define and describe the community that will undertake the diagnosis.
2. What is the focus of the community diagnosis? What issue will the community address?
3. What are you trying to find out about your focus or issue? What questions are you asking about your issue? List at least five questions here.
4. What research tools will you use to you find this out? How will you do your research?
5. How will you work with community members to analyze your findings and come up with "startling statistics"? List three to five "startling statistics" here!
6. How will you prepare your findings for the community and policymakers (in charts, graphs, written form, with pictures, or in packets)?
7. What type of actions might the community take to address their priority concern and create positive changes?

References

Arble, B., & Moberg, D. P. (2006). Participatory research in development of public health interventions. *Translating Research into Policy and Practice, 1*(6), 1–4.

Center for Human Development. (2001). *Empowerment program.* Retrieved from *http://chdprevent.server283.com/our-work/supporting-active-youth-leaders/empowerment-program/*

Gay-Straight Alliance Network, Friends of Project 10 & American Civil Liberties Union of Southern California. (2001). *Make it real: AB 537 activism.* Retrieved from *http://66.160.205.104/ab537/pdf/manual.pdf*

Israel, B. A., Schulz, A. J., Parker, E. A., & Becker, A. B. (1998). Review of community-based research: Assessing partnership approaches to improve public health. *Annual Review of Public Health, 19*, 173–202.

Kretzmann, J. P., & McKnight, J. (1993). *Building communities from the inside out.* Chicago, IL: ACTA.

Kukaswadia, A. (2013, March 11). John Snow—the first epidemiologist [blog]. *PLOSblogs, Public Health Perspectives.* Retrieved from *http://blogs.plos.org/publichealth/2013/03/11/john-snow-the-first-epidemiologist/*

Minkler, M. (2006). Community-based research partnerships: Challenges and opportunities. *Journal of Urban Health, 82*, ii3–ii12. doi:10.1093/jurban/jti034

Minkler, M., & Wallerstein, N. (2008). *Community-based participatory research for health* (2nd ed.). San Francisco, CA: Jossey-Bass.

National Association of County and City Health Officials (NACCHO). (2013). *Recommendations on characteristics for high-quality community health assessments and community health improvement plans.* Retrieved from *www.naccho.org/topics/infrastructure/CHAIP/*

San Francisco Tobacco Free Project. (2010). *Comprehensive smoke-free policies in dining, entryways and hallways.* Chinese Progressive Action. Retrieved from *http://sanfranciscotobaccofreeproject.org/case-studies/shs-laws/*

Shore, N., Park, A., Castro, P., Wat, E., Sablan-Santos, L., Isaacs, M., . . . Seifer, S. D. (2014). *Redefining research ethics review: Case studies of five community-led models.* Seattle, WA: Community-Campus Partnerships for Health. Retrieved from *https://ccph.memberclicks.net/assets/Documents/PapersReports/crp-chapter2.pdf*

Tsark, J. A. (2001). A participatory research approach to address data needs in tobacco use among Native Hawaiians. *Asian American Pacific Island Journal of Health, 9*, 40–48.

University of California, Los Angeles (UCLA), School of Public Health, Department of Epidemiology. (n.d.). *John Snow.* Retrieved from *www.ph.ucla.edu/epi/snow.html*

Wang, C., & Burris, M. (1997). Photovoice: Concept, methodology, and use for participatory needs assessment. *Health Education & Behavior, 24*, 369–387.

Additional Resources

Advancement Project/Healthy City. (2013). *Try this: Participatory asset-mapping with Wikimaps.* Retrieved from *http://v5.healthycity.org/en/blog/try-participatory-asset-mapping-wikimaps*

Association of Asian Pacific Community Health Organizations. (n.d.). *CBPR toolkit.* Retrieved from *www.aapcho.org/resources_db/cbpr-toolkit/*

Centers for Disease Control and Prevention, Division of Heart Disease and Stroke Prevention. (2015, March 3). *Maps.* Retrieved from *www.cdc.gov/dhdsp/maps/*

Checkaway, B., & Richards-Schuster, K. (2008). Participatory evaluation with young people. East Battle Creek, MI: W.K. Kellogg Foundation. Retrieved from *www.wkkf.org/resource-directory*

Collective Impact Forum. (n.d.). Retrieved from *www.collectiveimpactforum.org/*

Community Tool Box. (2014). *Chapter 3: Assessing community needs and resources.* Retrieved from *http://ctb.ku.edu/en/table-of-contents/assessment/assessing-community-needs-and-resources*

The Examining Community-Institutional Partnerships for Prevention Research Group. (2006). *Developing and sustaining community-based participatory research partnerships: A skill-building curriculum.* Retrieved from *www.cbprcurriculum.info*

Legal Services for Prisoners with Children. (n.d.). Retrieved from *www.prisonerswithchildren.org*

Pain, R., Whitman, G., Milledge, D., & Lune Rivers Trust. (n.d.) *Participatory action research toolkit: An introduction to using PAR as an approach to learning, research, and action.* Retrieved from *www.dur.ac.uk/ resources/beacon/PARtoolkit.pdf*

Papa Ola Lokahi. (n.d.). Retrieved from *www.papaolalokahi.org*

PhotoVoice: (n.d.). Reframing the World. Retrieved from *www.PhotoVoice.org*

San Francisco Health Improvement Partnership. (n.d.). Retrieved from *www.sfhip.org/*

San Francisco Tobacco Free Project. (n.d.). *Community capacity building and community action model.* Retrieved from *http://sanfranciscotobaccofreeproject.org/actions/*

Shimeles, H. (n.d.) *Community-based participatory research kit for Artreach Toronto G.O.A.L. youth workshops.* Retrieved from *http://avnu.ca/avnu/uploads/2014/04/GOAL_CommunityBasedParticipatoryResearch.pdf*

Treuhaft, S. (2009). *Community mapping for health equity advocacy.* Oakland, CA: PolicyLink. Retrieved from *http://opportunityagenda.org/files/field_file/Community%20Mapping%20for%20Health%20Equity% 20-%20Treuhaft.pdf*

Community Organizing and Advocacy

23

Alma Avila and Janey Skinner

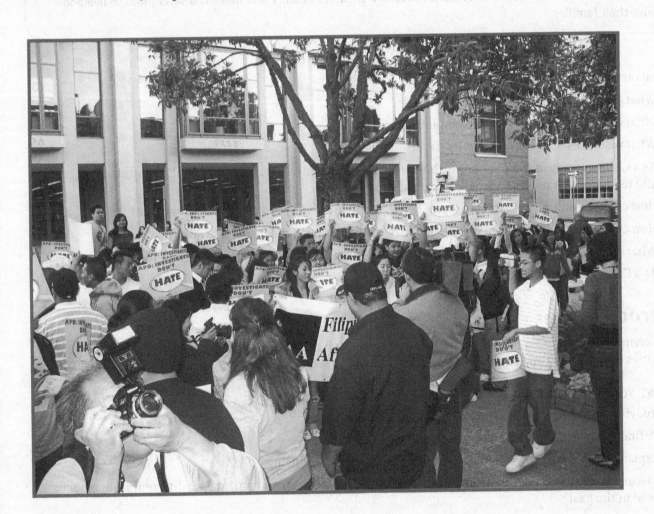

CHW Scenario

A local community is deeply concerned about increasing gun violence. This predominantly low-income Latino and African American community includes a large number of public housing units, along with single-family homes and small apartment buildings. The community faces a wide range of other health concerns, including high rates of asthma and diabetes. The neighborhood has a city-funded health center, schools, a park, and several churches, temples, and nonprofit agencies that provide social services. Many community members have a long history of participating in social movements, including civil rights movements.

Recently, a young mother and her infant were killed by stray bullets during a drive-by shooting. Over 400 community members attended the memorial service. The community wants to find a way to prevent further shootings and deaths. They want to reclaim their community and make it a safer place to live and raise their families.

Based on the situation described above:

- What are the community's primary concerns?
- What other challenges does the community face?
- What resources does the community have?
- As a CHW working in the community, how would you bring members together to talk about their concerns and to identify strategies to promote social change?
- How could community organizing promote the health and safety of the community?
- How could technology be used to help mobilize the community and increase awareness?
- What possible actions might the community take? What solutions might they work toward?
- As a CHW, what are your roles and responsibilities in the community organizing process?

Introduction

This chapter provides an introduction to the basic knowledge and skills that CHWs use when supporting communities in organizing and advocating for social change and social justice.

WHAT YOU WILL LEARN

By studying the information in this chapter, you will be able to:

- Define and discuss community organizing
- Explain the difference between advocacy and community organizing
- Discuss at least two ways that contemporary models of community organizing are different from models used in the past
- Explain the five steps of the Community Action Model (CAM)
- Discuss the CHW's roles and responsibilities in the community organizing process, and put them into practice
- Apply the Community Action Model to issues facing the communities you work with
- Explain the importance of integrating news media and social media into community organizing efforts

WORDS TO KNOW

Community Organizing

Media Advocacy

Policy

Power Analysis

Social Media

23.1 Why Organize?

We all want to live in healthy communities. Yet many communities lack access to the basic resources necessary for health such as clean water and air, safety, housing, food, education, employment, health care, and civil rights. They face a wide range of other public health problems such as high rates of infant mortality, heart disease, HIV/AIDS, drug use, incarceration, or homelessness. They may live close to an oil refinery or waste incinerator.

It is to face these challenges that communities come together and organize for social change. They want a better life for themselves and their children.

Because CHWs have a special relationship with communities, they are often ideally situated to facilitate community organizing efforts. CHWs are also skilled at connecting community members to information and resources that can assist them to find solutions to their identified problems or concerns.

A LITTLE HISTORY

The concept of community organizing is not new. Throughout history, people excluded from power and decision making have come together and organized to assert their needs. Organizing campaigns have achieved significant improvements in people's lives, and the gains of one campaign (such as a new law recognizing community rights) can serve as a platform to pursue further goals. Consider the following examples:

- Labor movements organized to demand safe working conditions, the right to organize, limits to working hours, and a living wage.
- The feminist movement organized to demand the right to vote and other civil rights protections for women and girls.
- The civil rights movement allowed communities of color to gain new rights and access to essential resources.
- Disabled communities organized for civil rights protections to pass the Americans with Disabilities Act.
- Cesar Chavez and the United Farm Workers (UFW) won rights for better working conditions and treatment for California farmworkers.
- The Queer Youth Action Team (QYAT)—as described in Chapter 22—gained protections against discrimination in local high schools.
- In Bolivia, communities organized and fought off the efforts of Bechtel, a large transnational corporation, to regain control over regional water resources.

- *Can you think of other examples of successful community organizing campaigns and movements from the United States or elsewhere in the world?*

- *What about the history of communities that you belong to?*

- *Have these communities organized to advocate for social change in the past?*

- *Are they currently organizing?*

- *Have you or your family and close friends participated in any of these efforts?*

The term *community organizing* was first used in the late 1800s by U.S. social workers to describe their efforts to coordinate services for newly arrived immigrants and the poor (Garvin & Cox, 1995). While community organizing has contributed to national movements and resulted in major changes in policy and social conditions (the right to vote, the 1964 Civil Rights Act), it often begins at the local level when a group of people come together to talk about a common problem or vision. The history of community organizing shows that communities do have the power to challenge and change social and political situations that have a negative impact on their health.

23.2 Defining the Community

Which communities participate in community organizing efforts? There are many ways to define communities. Early leaders in the field of community organizing defined "community" as "a group of people living in the same defined area, sharing the same basic values, organization, and interests" (Rifkin, Muller, & Bichmann, 1988). More recently, public health researchers examining how diverse communities affected by HIV define themselves arrived at this definition: "A group of people with diverse characteristics who are linked by social ties, share common perspectives, and engage in joint action in geographical locations or settings" (MacQueen et al., 2001).

Communities share something important in common. Members of a community may live in the same neighborhood or region. They may share a common gender, gender identity, sexual orientation, ethnicity, religion, cultural identity, nationality, immigration status, disability, health condition, profession, political affiliation, values, or other identity or interest. Communities can even exist virtually, linking people with an affinity through the Internet and with social media. Communities may organize locally or within a region, county, nation, or even internationally. For example, the campaign to win the vote for women in the early 20th century was a national campaign; the Montgomery bus boycott, the first major campaign of the Civil Rights Movement in 1954, was a local campaign, with national implications. Other campaigns are too localized to ever draw national attention, such as a high school protest over dress codes, a neighborhood mobilization to get speed bumps installed, or a rent strike to change a landlord's behavior.

What is most important is that the members of the community identify for themselves what they share in common, rather than having their identity defined by anyone else.

- *How do you define community?*

- *What communities do you belong to?*

- *What communities have you worked with?*

What Do YOU Think?

23.3 What Is Community Organizing?

Community organizing is a process by which people, usually a group of people who have been denied resources and participation in the decision-making process, work together to create social change that results in meaningful improvements in their lives. These meaningful improvements may be a policy change—such as access to new resources and rights—or a change in the social or physical environment, such as improved health and living conditions. Community organizing identifies and supports leadership from within the community, and increases their capacity to work together and take effective action for social change. In this way, the balance of power and resources shifts toward the community.

Community organizing often involves advocacy, but not all advocacy is linked to community organizing. They both work with and for people to reach a common goal. Advocacy is a broad term; it can be used in the sense of advocating for the needs of a client when working with an individual or family, but in this chapter we are focused on advocacy for policy changes that affect a broader population. The following list presents some of the similarities and differences between community organizing and advocacy.

Advocacy:

- Is defined as working on behalf of people, including those who may not be able to speak for themselves, to help them gain access to specific resources

- Is the act or process of supporting a cause or a proposal

- Usually means working to get a policy passed or implemented by those who have the power to make policy (e.g., a board, council, legislative body, or executive authority)

- Can be either "grass roots" or "professional" in leadership

- Often uses the testimony (or voices) of experts alongside community members directly affected by the policy in question

- May or may not involve community organizing

> **Phuong An Doan Billings:** Every year there is an Immigrant Day in Sacramento [the state capitol of California]. Many different immigrant groups and communities go. My agency, Asian Health Services, participates. We rent some buses and take those who want to go up to Sacramento. We go to express our opinion, and there is always a big demonstration. This is advocacy. Immigrant communities still face so much prejudice. We need more respect for our histories and cultures and contributions to California and the United States.

Community Organizing

- Mobilizes the community to do for themselves, to advocate on their own behalf.
- It is usually led by "grassroots" leaders, sometimes with the support of professionals.
- Helps to shift power into the hands of the people.
- Develops skills of community residents.

Please note that within the field of public health, community organizing often takes a more collaborative focus to build bridges among allies and to persuade policymakers.

WHY IS COMMUNITY ORGANIZING SO IMPORTANT?

Community organizing is important for many reasons. It is one of most effective strategies for creating lasting social changes that will improve the lives and health status of large groups of people. For example, community organizing efforts significantly expanded the rights of disabled people for access to basic resources such as transportation, education, housing, and employment. In the first decades of the AIDS epidemic, community organizing by groups like ACT UP and the AIDS Treatment Action Group significantly expanded the rights of people living with HIV disease and their access to medical treatments and other basic resources. Community organizing captures the attention of the media and the public, and puts pressure on policymakers to do something about such diverse concerns as accountable policing, environmental health, reproductive justice, and international trade agreements.

At its best, community organizing honors the resources, wisdom, and leadership of local communities and leaves them with a greater capacity to take action on their own to successfully tackle other problems in the future. Just as CHWs can help individual clients develop a greater sense of self-efficacy, they can support communities to enhance their collective efficacy.

23.4 Models of Practice

People have been joining together to organize and advocate for social change throughout human history and across the globe. As a result, there are many different forms and models for community organizing.

In the mid-twentieth century, most approaches to community organizing in the United States, such as those written about by Rothman and Tropman (1987) and Alinsky (1971), were focused on identifying what the community lacked and getting it for them. These approaches included building community capacity to protest and campaign, but largely emphasized the role of the outside organizer or expert to provide communities with needed leadership and assistance.

Rothman's model, rooted in the field of social work, featured the role of outside experts who worked with the community to build its identity, to identify their needs by conducting research, and to propose solutions to these needs or problems. Outside experts also aided in linking communities with existing direct services, such as food programs or housing. This model was need-based, that is, focused on what the community needed or lacked. It used a strategy of building a common agreement to get the community what it needed, and de-emphasized confrontation.

Alinsky's model of social change focused on challenging the existing power relations that contribute to the inequalities facing poor communities. While it moved away from Rothman's use of outsiders to do most of the work for the community, it still assumed that a disadvantaged group must be organized from the outside in order to successfully advocate for increased resources. It assigned a kind of heroic importance to the outside organizer. Alinsky's social action model focused on:

- Addressing issues that a majority of the community would support, such as cleaning up pollution or expanding affordable housing

- Challenging the imbalance of power and privilege between the disadvantaged and the larger community

- Increasing the problem-solving ability of the community through the advice and guidance of an expert

- Supporting goals of social justice, democracy, and the redistribution of power, to grow the community's access to resources and decision making

CONTEMPORARY MODELS OF COMMUNITY ORGANIZING

In recent decades, different models of community organizing have developed, many of them emphasizing an empowerment approach in which the community learns to assume leadership for itself rather than relying on outside experts. These models often include a strength-based or asset-based approach that focuses not only on what communities lack and need, but also on the resources they already have. For example, the process of *community building* emphasizes the positive resources a community has to offer, including its people as community leaders (Walter & Hyde, 2012). By developing connections within and among communities, these approaches often emphasize self-help and collaboration. Cultural humility and the recognition of the unique strengths and needs of each community also play an important role in community organizing efforts in the 21st century.

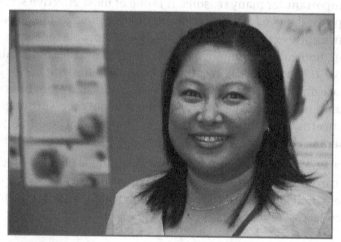

CHWs support and encourage community members to share their experience, skills, and ideas for social change.

Other examples of recent models for organizing include:

- **Community capacity building,** which refers to the ability to develop and sustain strong relationships to work together to identify problems and goals, make group decisions, and take action. This is accomplished by having members of a community share skills, talents, knowledge, and experiences (Mattessich & Monsey, 1997).

- **Collaborative partnerships,** which entail building alliances with people and institutions who share your values and goals. For example, an effort to improve the quality of education in local schools might involve establishing a collaborative partnership among students, parents, teachers, school officials, faith-based and other community-based organizations, and local businesses. Because these partnerships bring people together from all parts of the community, they can build on a diversity of strengths and resources to increase the chances of success.

- **Consensus organizing.** Consensus organizing focuses on cultivating leadership and relationships at various levels to work for change. By building new connections within the community, as well as between the community and the local power structure, it seeks to build a consensus (or broad agreement among a group or community) around goals and policy changes for the good of the community (Ohmer & DeMasi, 2009).

Consensus is a decision-making process that promotes more active participation from all of the members of a group or community. It is different from making decisions by majority vote because it encourages all members to express their opinion, and emphasizes the value of listening to the views of any minority who may have concerns about a particular proposal. People who are strongly opposed to a proposed course of action can prevent a decision from being made until the large group has considered their concerns. Through discussion, the consensus process encourages groups to keep refining their ideas until they are acceptable to all members. While not all members may enthusiastically agree with the final decision, consensus requires that everyone provide their consent to move forward with the decision.

- **Mass mobilization** is not a new approach, but it is a popular one for addressing large social issues at this time. Mass mobilizations engage a large number of people in highly visible protests, sometimes with a single goal and other times with a more diffuse message. For example, the Occupy movement that was highly visible in 2011–2012 drew public attention to the problems of income inequality; yet within any given Occupy site, a wide variety of solutions, some of them contradictory, found support. As a result, Occupy did more to raise important questions than it did to propose specific answers. The Black Lives Matter movement took to the streets in response to the deaths of young Black men at the hands of law enforcement (in particular, the deaths of Michael Brown in Ferguson, MO, and Eric Garner in Staten Island, a borough of New York City, in 2014). This movement put forth common demands in different locations, such as the use of body cameras by police, changes to the grand jury process, practices to overcome conscious and unconscious bias, and new policies regarding the use of force, while also pointing to larger issues of segregation, racism, and lack of opportunity.

Empowerment, as discussed by Wallerstein (1992, 2006), is an essential component of community organizing. Empowerment comes about through the broad participation of people, organizations, and communities, overcoming barriers to increase access to vital resources through engaging with and influencing political structures. Empowerment is achieved through the development of critical consciousness and confidence among community members, as well as through concrete actions that increase community control and improve community conditions.

Four key concepts that are generally incorporated into contemporary approaches to community organizing are:

1. To increase community participation and ownership
2. To build the capacity of the community through leadership and understanding
3. To address the imbalance of power and shift power and local resources back to the community
4. To build a stable power base through coalition building to ensure sustainable social actions and multiple campaigns over time

- *What does empowerment mean to you?*

- *In what ways does your neighborhood or community have power and influence? In what ways does it not?*

- *What different approaches to community organizing have you observed or participated in?*

23.5 Strategies and Tactics of Community Organizing

There are many different kinds of community organizing campaigns. Some campaigns last only a month from start to finish, while others may last for years or even decades. Each campaign uses a mix of tactics (actions or methods) within an overall plan or strategy for how to attain their goals.

When an organizing campaign is fostered through funding and training from a public health department (for example, many of the campaigns mentioned in Chapter 22 were supported in part by the San Francisco Department of Public Health), the institutional ties can open up access to policymakers and other influential sectors of the city. These campaigns tend to adopt a more collaborative strategy for change, compared to campaigns initiated by neighborhood leaders or organizations whose main purpose is organizing (such as ACCE, a California organizing network—see *www.calorganize.org/*).

Community organizing as a field uses a wide range of tactics, from community education and testifying at public hearings, to sit-ins and rent strikes and public demonstrations, and each campaign must decide which techniques best suit their situation. See additional resources listed at the end of this chapter for more examples of organizing strategies, tactics, and campaigns.

POPULAR EDUCATION—A RESOURCE FOR COMMUNITY ORGANIZING

Popular education and the work of Paulo Freire were introduced in Chapter 21 and 22. Popular education is often used in the field of public health to guide the work of CHWs and to support community organizing efforts.

Paulo Freire is frequently seen as the father of popular education. Freire was a Brazilian educator who, in the second half of the twentieth century, fostered new approaches to literacy that went well beyond learning to read; you could say he helped people to read the world around them, not just the words on a page. Freire believed that education should lead to liberation, or freedom from oppression and the creation of social justice. Popular education is the process by which people come together to talk about their social conditions, to analyze the factors that harm their communities, and to take collective action to change these conditions. As people begin to talk about their lives, their values and hopes, and the factors that harm their health and limit the future of their children, they develop a new awareness of the world and their own potential. Freire referred to this process as "conscientization" or the development of critical consciousness.

The process of conscientization must be carried out and defined by the community. Freire wrote about the importance of local communities speaking "their word" or using their own language and concepts to identify and analyze social conditions.

Based on his experience, Freire believed that community action or organizing should first address the issues that the community cares most deeply about. These deep feelings are a key resource for bringing and keeping community members together and motivating them to continue to take action in the face of significant obstacles and challenges.

Popular education, like community organizing, may be initiated and facilitated from outside the community. But the role of outsiders is to facilitate the leadership and decision making of community members rather than to claim such power for themselves. Any process that undermines the leadership, autonomy, and empowerment of the community is not consistent with the principles of popular education.

By posing questions, the facilitator supports community members in analyzing their social reality and in developing a plan of action to advocate for meaningful change (such as improved working conditions, civil rights protections, clean drinking water, or affordable health care). These questions provide community members with a way to speak their own word and to express their identity:

- What are the factors, problems, and institutions that harm the health and well-being of the community?
- What are the community's leading concerns or priorities?
- What are the common values, visions, and goals for social change and a better future?
- What are the key community resources, including knowledge, wisdom, skills, accomplishments, institutions, relationships, and leadership?
- What actions can the community take to reach their goals?
- Who are the key allies who may support the community in advocating for social change?

Popular education informs the Community Action Model (CAM) introduced later in this chapter. Step 1 of the CAM may use popular education approaches to recruit and train the core group of activists. Step 2 of the CAM incorporates popular education concepts and approaches to promote conscientization among community members. The goal is for the community to guide their own analysis of local problems and their root causes.

POLICY 101: BECAUSE HEALTH IS POLITICAL

In order to establish new policies that promote health, we need to learn how to influence the decisions of policy makers. A **policy** is a principle or protocol that guides actions and decisions, often by establishing incentives or penalties. Policies include state and federal laws (legislation), regulations that explain how these laws or decision are to be carried out; local ordinances (municipal decisions); codes of ethics such as those created by professional organizations; and institutional rules and practices. An example of a national policy is the 2010 Affordable Care Act that requires every U.S. citizen (with some exceptions) to have health insurance. The law details who must have insurance and how insurance will be made available, among other things.

Policies are made by the U.S. Congress, state legislatures, municipal governments (city, town, village, or borough), school boards, Tribal governments, professional associations, and other organizations and institutions. We refer to them as policymakers or decision makers because they set the rules and policies that influence our health. As CHWs involved in organizing or advocacy, your job is to help ensure that the voices of the community are heard and their concerns resolved through policy changes.

DEVELOPING A MODEL POLICY RECOMMENDATION

After a community diagnosis has been completed, and the data has been collected and analyzed by the community, the community will have a better understanding of what it needs to become healthier. At this point, the community can decide what "action" it wants to take. For the purpose of this chapter, an action is something that is achievable, sustainable, and compels an entity to make a long-term change for the better of that community, such as a policy. This is the terminology used in the CAM. In other models of organizing, the term "goal" or "policy improvement" may be used instead of "action."

Part of community organizing is to be informed about who are the key political leaders and policymakers (at whatever level you are working—in a city, across a state, or nationwide). It is important to examine the power relationships that exist among them, and to analyze how they may respond to your planned action. One resource that can help you understand these entities is a **power analysis**. Conducting a power analysis will help you to identify who can support you in your efforts and who may oppose you. Once this has been completed, you are in a better position to develop a clear action plan. For the purpose of this chapter, an action is an achievable and sustainable change or policy that benefits a group.

There are many toolkits (see the references and additional resources listed at the end of this chapter) that explain how to conduct a power analysis and provide examples. A power analysis helps to answer the following questions:

- Which policymaker is most approachable and concerned about the issue the community is working on? Who might be a champion for the policy that the community wants enacted?

- Who is in opposition to the community's proposed action and why?

- Who are your allies? Who might support your action?

- Who are the current officials or executives whose jobs will be most changed or affected by this policy? Are they in agreement with or in opposition to the proposed action or policy change?

- Who else is concerned or interested in the issue/concern the community is working on?

- What other policies, laws or rules exist concerning the community's proposed action or policy change?

Phuong An Doan-Billings: [Reflecting on organizing members to meet with Congressional representatives for the Healthy Salons Days of Action in Washington DC (November 11–14, 2014), to discuss community health and environmental health issues for nail salon workers] *We help the members to be aware of their own rights, so eventually they can advocate for themselves, but right now we are right beside them to help them advocate.*

The power analysis technique is used in the CAM approach to organizing, discussed below. Power analysis is especially useful in Steps 2 and 4 of the CAM. It is used to help the community build their base and support, and refine their strategy for influencing policymakers.

MEDIA ADVOCACY

Media advocacy is often important to the success of a community organizing campaign. It is the strategic use of any form of media—newspapers, radio, television, the World Wide Web, advertisements, billboards, and so on—to publicize and raise awareness about the problems that a community is facing and their goals for social change. In particular, media advocacy can shape how an issue or a policy proposal is perceived—and this distinguishes it from other uses of media such as advertising a service or promoting a healthy behavior.

The media are efficient for communicating with a large audience. The media can be used to:

- *Inform* the public about the causes and consequences of a specific issue
- *Recast* these problems as social concerns that affect everyone, not just a distant group
- *Encourage* community members and their leaders to find out more about the problems and to get involved in solving those problems
- *Promote* agencies and services within your community that address the identified problems

Media advocacy can assist community organizing efforts by:

- *Changing* the way key decision makers and the general public look at community issues or problems
- *Creating* a reliable, consistent stream of publicity or media focus for your community's issues and activities
- *Offering possible explanations* of how these problems could and should be solved
- *Motivating* community members and policymakers to get involved

When seeking to influence policymakers, it is important to get into the news. Policymakers look at news media carefully—whether in print, on TV or radio, in blogs or other social media. Even though traditional news media, like newspapers and local television stations, have shrinking audiences, they still influence public policy. Social media, which reach more people than newspapers these days, often repeat and spread stories that originally appeared in the news (the news still "frames" the issues, shaping how readers think about the problem and the solution). If your goal is to recast problems as social concerns that require social solutions, getting your story in the news (told in the way you want it told) is a powerful resource.

Working with the media becomes easier with training and experience. One step that community members and leaders may wish to take is to seek out local opportunities to learn or enhance media advocacy skills. One resource you might consider is the Berkeley Media Studies Group (*http://bmsg.org*), a national leader in media advocacy training.

Chapter 22 described the work of the Queer Youth Action Team (QYAT), a group of youth who successfully advocated for new policies to protect lesbian, gay, bisexual, and transgender youth from discrimination in local schools. The youth did extensive media advocacy, and their work was featured by local and statewide newspapers, radio, and television. The coverage by the media served to change the nature of the debate about student rights and to convince local policymakers to work with the QYAT.

SOCIAL MEDIA

Social media enable people to communicate frequently and broadly using advanced technology, whether on their phones, computers, or other technology. Social media can spread a message or a story quickly and can help you take the pulse of public opinion. Online tools such as Twitter and Facebook have the capacity to reach a greater number of people than ever before. New tools like Thunderclap help organizations concentrate social media messages into a united voice, and websites like Change.org and ColorofChange.org have transformed and accelerated the use of petitions. Social network building allows people who are not in close proximity to each other to work together, share and exchange information, and be part of a larger movement. It is also an opportunity for people across all ethnic groups, social, religious and economic backgrounds to work together where they might otherwise not have such opportunities. And because social media generally link friends, acquaintances, and others who share similar interests, people may have a high level of trust in what they learn about over social media, leading even those who are not active on an issue to support the cause. Good organizing is all about building relationships so that you have a network of supporters who will back you up when you need to get something done. Social media and other online tools can be important additions to your organizing strategy. For more ideas about how to use social media to support advocacy or organizing, see the website of the Nonprofit Technology Network, *http://nten.org*.

- *Which media influence public opinion in your community?*

- *How do you use social media? Have you participated in any advocacy campaigns on social media?*

- *What might help you feel more prepared to use media (of any kind) for organizing or advocacy purposes?*

23.6 The Community Action Model

The CAM is an approach to community organizing developed by the Tobacco Free Project of the San Francisco Department of Public Health (Tobacco Free Project). The CAM (Figure 23.1) is deeply influenced by the theories of Paulo Freire and popular education. It features a five-step process designed to assist community members to further develop their capacity to advocate for social justice by creating changes in social policies.

The goals of the CAM are:

- **Environmental or social change:** To move away from projects that focus only on changing individual lifestyles and behaviors in order to focus on mobilizing community members and agencies to change environmental factors and promote economic, political, and health equality.

- **Empowerment and community leadership:** Through asset-based action research, the CAM provides a framework for community members to acquire the skills and resources to investigate the health of the place where they live and to plan, implement, and evaluate actions that change the environment to promote and improve health.

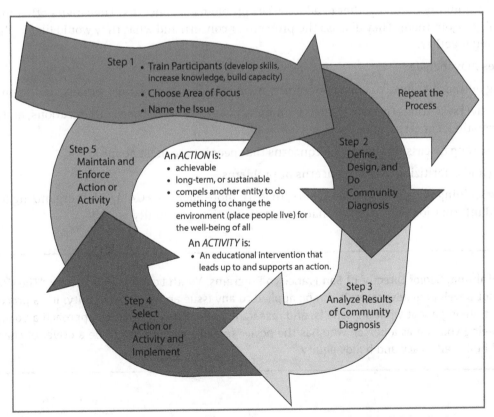

Figure 23.1 The Community Action Model: Creating Change by Building Community Capacity
Source: San Francisco Department of Public Health (n.d., p. 16).

Fundamental to implementing the CAM is the *action* or proposed solution that communities work toward. The selected action should meet three criteria:

1. It must be achievable, meaning that you must be able to complete it within the near future (such as year or two rather than 20 or 50 years).

2. It must be long-lasting or sustainable, meaning that after your project goes away, the actions or the changes achieved will continue.

3. It must compel another entity (person or organization) to do something to change the environment (the place where people live) for the well-being of all. It must benefit a large number of people or a community rather than just one individual.

THE FIVE STEPS OF THE CAM

Below is a summary of the five steps of the CAM, including a list of activities that may take place at each step. (Please note, the CAM makes a distinction between *activities*—things that you do in the course of the campaign—and *actions*—the sustainable policy or environmental change that you hope to achieve. In some other organizing models, the *action* might be called the goal or the policy objective.)

Along with the description of the five steps of the CAM, we have included comments from a community organizer, Patricia Barahona, Senior Director San Francisco Programs for the Youth Leadership Institute (*http://yli.org*). We interviewed Patty about a successful youth-led organizing campaign called TURF, Tobacco Use Reduction Force, that used the CAM to first research the high concentration of stores selling tobacco in low-income neighborhoods and then advocate for a change in a local ordinance, to reduce the density of tobacco outlets and overcome tobacco-related inequalities between neighborhoods. You will also find a case study about the Good Neighbor project and how they used the CAM to improve access to healthy food. The CAM is easily adaptable to any health issue.

Step 1: Identify the Problem

Members of a community come together to address key problems or concerns. They invite other members of their community to join them. They discuss the problem or concern and what they would like to change as a result of working together.

Step 1 activities may include:

- Conducting outreach to involve more community members (flyers, meetings, emails, and so on)
- Meeting at diverse settings (private homes, community centers, faith-based organizations, and so forth) to share information, concerns, and hopes
- Facilitating group discussions about the concerns that people care most about
- Identifying and prioritizing leading concerns or problems
- Facilitating training for community members, to learn more about the CAM, other organizing tools, and/or background information on the issues that most concern the community

> **Patricia Barahona**, Senior Director of San Francisco Programs, Youth Leadership Institute: "The CAM model is really about developing advocates. It can be applied to any issue and any community. It's a process of training for thinking about what an issue is, and researching it in several ways, to approach a policy change. It's about seeing yourself as a person who has the power to make change and to be a driver of change. The CAM model builds advocacy and builds equity."

Step 2: Assess the Problem/Community Diagnosis

Community diagnosis was described in Chapter 22. It is a process of gathering information to better understand the causes and consequences of an issue or problem that the community cares about, such as gun violence, homelessness, or breast cancer. This process takes time and cannot be rushed. It is important for the community to look deeply at the root causes of their concerns, and to discuss and analyze these together. The community diagnosis is vital to the success of the CAM: it provides information that will guide the actions and strategies that the community will take to advocate for social change. This is a step that communities may best be able to take with the support or facilitation of a CHW or other experienced public health provider or community organizer.

Step 2 activities may include:

- Interviewing key opinion leaders in the community
- Conducting surveys or facilitating focus groups with community members
- Making sure that important groups in the community were not left out of the community diagnosis process
- Conducting research to find existing data about the issue at hand, such as the rates of gun violence or breast cancer

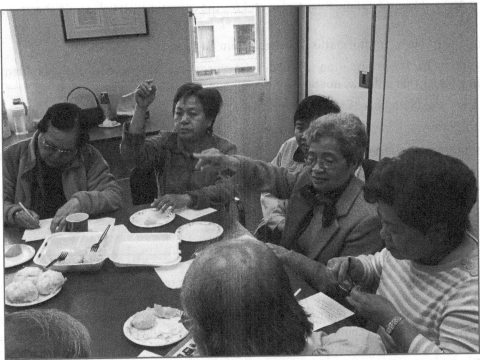

By meeting together, communities can identify the root causes of the problems they face.

- Conducting community-mapping activities
- Researching existing records, laws, and policies
- Looking for examples of actions that other communities have taken to address similar concerns or problems
- Identifying policymaking institutions and individuals
- Identifying potential allies and opponents (people who may support or stand in the way of efforts to create social change)

Chapter 22 gives more detail and explanation about how to conduct the community diagnosis.

Patricia Barahona: "At Youth Leadership Institute, we build community campaigns partnering youth and adults on community change. We employ different approaches to youth-led action research as a way to create change. . . . We feel that young people should be at the forefront of researching an issue and data-driven solutions. Research is a key leadership skill for youth."

Step 3: Analyze Findings

The next step is for the community to meet together to analyze the information that they gathered during the community diagnosis. Again, this is often a step in which the community can benefit from the support of CHWs or other experienced facilitators. Community members will learn how to read and make sense of different types of data, including survey data or epidemiological data from a local health department. Together the community will decide what the information gathered tells them about the problem at hand and what questions remain.

Step 3 activities may include:

- Tallying numbers from a survey
- Discussing the information learned from interviews with key opinion leaders
- Reviewing reports from focus-group discussions
- Reviewing data from existing studies, including public health studies, and arranging this data in ways that make it most accessible, understandable, and useful for the community (such as pie charts, graphs, and picture collages)
- Summarizing the findings or information gathered from all sources
- Deciding together what the information says about the causes and consequences of the problem or concern, and identifying issues that still may not be clear or well understood
- Identifying any outstanding needs to gather more information
- Converting this information into visual resources such as graphs, tables, or facts sheets
- Sharing this information with more members of the community, to foster a common understanding of the issue
- Preparing to share the information (often in visual form) with policymakers, as part of the advocacy action in Step 4

> **Patricia Barahona:** "We use the CAM, because it's really based on research, on data and on driving a policy change, and that's what we are about. We also use the strategy of environmental prevention—moving away from a focus on the individual to understanding the community factors like community norms, media messages, access, and policies in communities—those four factors really interact with the individual and the agent (like tobacco or alcohol). . . . All of those lenses help us think about this work—health equity really being central. Young people having a strong connection to this issue of tobacco density—each youth had a personal connection to the issue."

Step 4: Identify and Implement an Advocacy Action

In this step, community members identify and discuss a list of potential actions to address their identified issue or concern. These actions will include policies that they may want to change. They will analyze these potential actions to see whether they meet the three criteria of the CAM. Together they will analyze the possible choices they identified and select one or more actions that will assist them to create meaningful change and promote the well-being of the community as a whole. Advocates will develop a detailed action plan, including a list of all activities to be undertaken and timelines for completing these activities, and support the community in implementing this plan.

Step 4 activities may include:

A. *Develop the action plan:*

- Coming up with a list or menu of possible actions
- Proposing a model policy around the issue or concern identified
- Developing a timeline for accomplishing tasks

- o Identifying and meeting with stakeholders and decision makers, prioritizing those you think may be important allies in getting your action or policy implemented
- o Developing one to three activities to support your proposed policy and raise awareness, such as a health fair, community forum, media advocacy, or presentations to schools or community groups

B. *Implement the action plan.* The following activities are the building blocks to support the proposed action:

- o Meeting with key stakeholders and policymakers—whether in private or in a public forum
- o Getting media coverage of your work and your proposal for policy change
- o Mobilizing the community to write letters, make calls to policymakers, or participate in public demonstrations
- o Mobilizing the community to testify before policymakers such as the city council, housing authority, or health commission
- o Celebrating your hard work and accomplishments

Patricia Barahona: "At this stage of the CAM, we also use the Midwest Academy strategy chart, once we have a policy solution or proposal. We use that to figure out our target, our allies, opponents, tactics, and different things to implement along the way on the campaign. We try to be really proactive about figuring out who has power in the community, who has influence and how we want to engage with them. How as advocates do we want to engage with power? A lot of self-reflection goes into that. For instance, 'How am I going to engage with this person? This person has too much power, I can't sit across from them!' But if we can personalize the issue, see them as a person, then we are more likely to create change together. That means young people tracking the leaders in the community, the mayor and his office, the Board of Supervisors [like a City Council], investigating who are these people in power, and what do they care about, and what can we do as community to mobilize for what we need, and how can we work with those in power to get it done."

The Midwest Academy: A Resource for Community Organizing

The Midwest Academy strategy chart that Patty Barahona refers to in the textbox is a tool that many community organizers have used and adapted for creating a detailed action plan to achieve their goal (or "action," in the language of the CAM). The strategy chart has five columns: *Goals* (what you want to accomplish); *Organizational Considerations* (for example, resources needed, or limits of your organization); *Constituents, Allies, & Opponents* (those who care most about this issue); *Targets* (the policymakers you want to reach); and *Tactics* (activities). Under each column heading, the chart includes questions to help organizers refine their strategy. The Midwest Academy, one of the top training centers for community organizing in the United States, recommends that groups use three criteria to evaluate an issue or a goal. An organizing goal, if achieved, should (1) win real improvements in people's lives, (2) give people a sense of their own power, and (3) alter the relations of power. To learn more about the Midwest Academy, please see Additional Resources listed at the end of this chapter. Go to *www.midwestacademy.com/*; a guide to using and adapting the Midwest Academy strategy chart (including examples) can also be found at the website of the Greenlining Institute.

What Do YOU Think?

- *What similarities do you see between the three criteria for an organizing goal proposed by the Midwest Academy and the three criteria that distinguish an "action" in the CAM?*

- *What experiences have you had of making a plan to achieve a goal? How did you select tactics or action steps to reach your goal? Did allies, opposition, or other considerations play a part in your plan?*

Step 5: Maintain Actions and Results

This step focuses on ensuring that the action accomplished will be maintained over the long term and enforced by the appropriate bodies.

Step 5 activities may include:

- Continuing to meet with policymakers and groups that enforce public policies
- Gathering new data to see if the situation or problem has changed
- Asking other existing groups, such as a Parent Teacher Organization or Association (PTO) to monitor outcomes
- Continuing to do media advocacy to keep the public informed about community organizing efforts
- Continuing to raise money to support your advocacy work
- Working for greater recognition of the community strengths that led to the success of the action

> **Patricia Barahona:** "As a result we got the most comprehensive tobacco density ordinance led by young people in the country. That's success. . . . We worked with three cohorts of young people over six years—and we won! We went through one process that wasn't successful, we reframed, retooled and kept working on it. There were a lot of lessons learned, to be able to get this win."

The San Francisco Department of Public Health has developed resources to guide community groups in implementing the CAM, including a facilitator's guide or curriculum. These resources are available online at: *www.sfdph.org/dph/comupg/oprograms/CHPP/CAM/default.asp.*

- *What experiences do you have with any of the activities described in the CAM?*

What Do YOU Think?

The CAM in Action: The Good Neighbor Program

Since 1995, the San Francisco Tobacco Free Project, a program of the Department of Public Health, has provided funding to community-based organizations to implement the CAM. The following example illustrates how one project used the model to organize around food security (the extent to which an individual, family, or community has access to regular and sufficient quantities of healthy food to eat).

Food security was identified as a concern by residents of the Bayview Hunters Point Neighborhood in San Francisco. This largely low-income community is home to many public-housing projects, but lacks supermarkets and other places for the community to shop for healthy foods, including fresh fruits and vegetables. Most residents shop at corner liquor stores, and the only other available food outlets in the community are fast-food restaurants. Not surprisingly, the community experiences high rates of diabetes, hypertension, and other chronic conditions.

Literacy for Environmental Justice (LEJ), an urban environmental education and youth empowerment organization, received funding to implement the CAM in the Bayview neighborhood (*www.lejyouth.org*). Their goal was to increase food security and improve the health of local residents.

Step 1: Identify the Problem

This is an example of a community organizing project that was funded to address a problem that had already been identified as a priority by community residents. To begin the project, staff from LEJ recruited youth advocates from the neighborhood high school. The advocates were trained on a variety of issues including health, food security, diversity, the legislative process, and public speaking. As a result, the young people came to understand how the lack of high-quality fresh food contributes to increasing rates of chronic disease and premature death in their community. Together, they decided to focus their work on increasing local access to healthy and affordable food and reducing the availability of processed foods and products such as tobacco.

Step 2: Community Diagnosis

The youth advocates conducted a community diagnosis that included a review of existing research and information gathered by previous projects and the local health department. They mapped the community to identify food sources, interviewed local merchants, and created diagrams of the products available in local stores. They conducted interviews with residents and community agencies to learn where they shop for food products and what they buy. They researched policies around tobacco and alcohol and identified policymakers and local leaders who might have an interest in assisting them to reach their goal. Please refer to Chapter 22 to view the survey and map developed by the LEJ youth advocates.

Step 3: Analyze Findings

When they came together to review and analyze the information they had gathered, the youth advocates found out that most residents shopped in corner liquor stores and ate fast food. To reach a supermarket, they had to take two buses and travel to another neighborhood. The products most available in local stores were tobacco, alcohol, and junk food, especially Kraft and Nabisco products made by tobacco subsidiary companies. Some local merchants said that they were interested in offering healthier choices, but didn't have the economic means to buy refrigeration units or to establish contracts with companies selling healthier foods. The youth advocates then used this information to create diagrams, charts, tables, and maps illustrating the problem of access to healthy food in the community. This information was used to paint a picture of the problem and to work to educate the policymakers.

Step 4: Identify and Implement an Advocacy Action

Based on their findings, LEJ and the youth advocates developed the concept of the Good Neighbor Program (see Figure 23.2). They decided to assist local merchants to sell healthier food and educate the community about the dangers of tobacco, processed food, and fast food, including foods sold by big tobacco companies. They met with local food cooperatives that produce and sell locally grown produce and other healthy foods and established an agreement for them to make their products available to interested stores in the Bayview. They also created posters and stickers to promote what they called the Good Neighbor (GN) Program to provide access to healthy food.

LEJ and the youth advocates conducted media advocacy by writing an article that was published by the local community newspaper, *The Bay View*. They were also successful in getting coverage about their work on local television and radio.

The youth advocates wrote a model policy to promote the Good Neighbor Program and presented it to their district representative on the San Francisco Board of Supervisors (or City Council) and other local policymakers. The City of San Francisco agreed to provide free refrigeration and training to merchants willing to participate in the Good Neighbor Program. They convinced two community agencies and the school district to adopt a policy not to buy Kraft and Nabisco products. A local merchant signed on to become the pilot store for the Good Neighbor Program, selling locally grown produce.

Their work fulfills the three criteria for CAM actions: it was sustainable, achievable, and successful in compelling an entity—in this case a corner store and the city of San Francisco—to change something for the better of the whole community.

(continues)

> ### Step 5: Maintain Actions and Results (*continued*)
>
> Advocates from LEJ and other members of the Bayview Community continue to promote the Good Neighbor idea and monitor and provide assistance to any interested merchants who want to become a Good Neighbor store. Not only did this community organizing project improve food security, it also trained and empowered local youth to become effective advocates for social change. To learn more about the work of LEJ and the Good Neighbor campaign, please go to *www.lejyouth.org/programs/food.html*. The campaign expanded over time to become the "Southeast Food Guardians," or SEFA, a collaboration between the city, community groups, and local merchants to increase access to healthy food. To learn more about SEFA, please visit their website at *http://southeastfoodaccess.org/*.

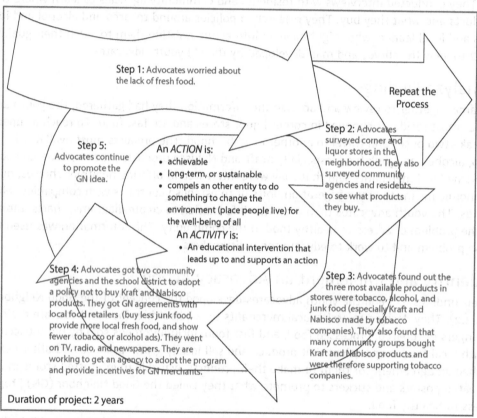

Figure 23.2 The CAM in Action: The Good Neighbor Program
Source: San Francisco Department of Health (n.d., p. 22).

23.7 The Role of CHWs

Have you ever worked with others to plan a meeting, party, or a family reunion? Have you ever spoken out on behalf of a friend or relative? Have your ever spoken to a group to express your opinion about a certain decision or policy? If you have, then chances are you already have experience and skills that are relevant to the task of community organizing.

CHWs have many qualities and skills to support community organizing, including:

- A commitment to social justice
- The ability to develop and maintain trusting relationships with diverse clients and communities
- The ability to listen to the concerns, experiences, and ideas of others with compassion and without judgment
- Information about resources that may be beneficial to the community

- Group facilitation and teamwork skills
- Cultural humility and respect for the experience, wisdom, and skills of others
- Flexibility and the ability to adapt to changing circumstances
- A client- and community-centered approach to their work and a commitment to supporting the self-determination of individuals and communities

- *What other qualities and skills do you and other CHWs have that may be helpful to community organizing efforts?*

Community organizing may take place with or without the participation of a CHW, and the CHW may or may not belong to the community in question. Regardless of whether you are a member of the community, we hope you keep the following suggestions in mind.

When participating in community organizing efforts, we hope that CHWs *will not*:

- **Assume that they know or understand the problems that most affect the community:** Only by listening to the community can you come to understand these problems.
- **Be the leader:** The role of the CHW is to facilitate the leadership of others rather than to assume it themselves.
- **Decide who participates:** All members of the affected community should be invited to take a place at the table and to contribute their knowledge and skills to the community organizing effort.
- **Prioritize tasks and activities or make key decisions:** The community must decide which issues or problems to work on and what actions they will take.
- **Do all the work:** Remember that your role is to assist people to acquire new skills so that they can take ownership of their own community organizing efforts.

We hope that CHWs *will*:

- **Listen to the community:** Your most important job is to listen deeply to the concerns, ideas, aspirations, fears, and accomplishments of the community. You can facilitate this by creating opportunities for people to meet together, and by asking simple open-ended questions that encourage people to speak up and share their knowledge.
- **Learn local history:** Take time to learn about the history of the community, including past community organizing efforts and accomplishments, and any previous attempts to address the same problem or concern.

Phuong An Doan-Billings: Communication is really key. You can use the Vietnamese media, like a magazine or newspaper, to reach the Vietnamese community. Your tool is the ethnic media, and of course your relationships. The basic thing for CHW is you have to establish a relationship with your own community, key stakeholders—like nail salon owners, or groups for seniors or women, the groups where people can gather once in a while—this is how immigrants learn how to survive. CHWs should know how to establish relationships with those people, and at the same time get the idea of how people feel from the ethnic media.

- **Recruit and honor the participation of diverse members of the community:** Drawing upon your existing connections in the community, reach out and invite all members to participate.
- **Provide training to community members:** You may have a role to play in supporting community members in enhancing their skills in areas such as group facilitation, planning, conducting a community diagnosis, or

media advocacy. As always, you need to take direction from the community about which areas, if any, they would like to learn more about. You may provide the training yourself, or identify others who can facilitate workshops for the community.

- **Mentor key people:** Often CHWs play a key role in mentoring community participants and leaders, assisting them to learn new skills and to gain confidence in their own ability to contribute to and to lead a community organizing effort.

- **Aid in facilitating the critical thinking process:** CHWs often support the development of critical consciousness by facilitating meetings and posing open-ended questions designed to provide community members with an opportunity to "speak their word" and arrive at a deeper understanding of the problems they face. As people begin to gain a common understanding of the problems affecting their communities, they will come up with possible actions and strategies to address these problems.

- **Assist the community to build on their strengths:** By supporting community members in conducting a community diagnosis, you can help them to identify existing resources (experience, knowledge, skills, institutions, and leaders).

- **Support communities in shaping strategy:** By facilitating a power analysis (or supporting community members to facilitate it), you can help communities identify the decision makers or policy makers they want to reach. By sharing information and facilitating discussion of strategies and tactics, you can help communities find creative ways to win support for their proposals.

- **Facilitate the implementation process:** Once an action plan has been developed, CHWs can help the community to implement it. Again, you may facilitate group discussions or mentor others to facilitate this process. The community will have a lot of decisions to make: What activities will we undertake? Who will do which activities? How much money do we need? How will we raise these funds? Whom do we need to reach to participate in our efforts? What potential allies do we need to talk with? What additional training and resources do we need?

- *What else do you hope that CHWs who participate in community organizing efforts will and will not do?*

> **Patricia Barahona:** "The youth pitch their policy proposal to the Supervisors [San Francisco's equivalent of a City Council]. They say, 'This is what we have in mind—what do you think?' They impressed the Supervisors on the other side of the table—the youth really had their stuff together, so practiced, so much code switching. They had prepared answers to the questions the Supervisors asked. We ask the youth, in preparing, 'What is the way to present this that will get you what you need? The issue is bigger than you, so it's your responsibility to engage with the policymakers in a powerful way.' And they do. They bring the data. The arguments. They are prepared to push the Supervisors to think more broadly about how they can act as partners. Essentially, the youth push them to join them, and to act in their leadership roles."

A CHECKLIST FOR CHWs ENGAGED IN COMMUNITY ORGANIZING AND ADVOCACY

We have adapted the following checklist from a number of sources, including Institute for Democratic Renewal (1998), the Community Toolbox (n.d.), and from Blackwell and Colmenar's "Principles of Community Building" (2012). As you participate in or develop community organizing and advocacy campaigns, use this checklist to reflect on how your efforts might be made more community-centered and effective.

PROMISING PRACTICE	WHAT DOES IT LOOK LIKE?	FILL IN HERE: HOW CAN YOU USE THIS PRACTICE?
Plan with people, not for them	• Listen to community members • Involve them from the start	
Clarify the focus of your project and its goals	• Facilitate setting a clear purpose or goal for the campaign or program. • State it concisely in a few sentences	
Assess strengths as well as needs	• Identify and celebrate community strengths • Listen for community issues or concerns • Find ways to use the strengths in addressing the needs	
Build local capacity for problem-solving	• Develop leaders • Foster connections between the community and local institutions, agencies, and government	
Practice cultural humility and draw on the strengths of cultural diversity	• Acknowledge complexity—in the community and within each community member • Invite cultural sharing and recognize strengths	
Deal explicitly with health inequalities and discriminatory social conditions, for example, those associated with race, ethnicity, gender, etc.	• Recognize that community issues often have different impacts on different groups • Develop policies and proposals that consider the needs of various populations in the community	
Ensure language access	• Work with interpreters and translators as needed • Partner with bilingual and bicultural (or multilingual and multicultural) CHWs and community residents	
Attend to safety	• Address any physical safety concerns • Use practices like those in Chapter 22 to foster emotional safety in the group	
Connect the community to relevant resources and expertise	• Share contact information • Help form bridges between the community and other resources	
Build partnerships	• Short-term coalitions • Long-term collaborations • Foster the sharing of information and resources	
Develop strategies in an action plan	• Select an overall action or goal that is attainable and significant • Analyze the policymakers who can act on that goal, their interests or influences • Develop activities or tactics to urge policy-makers to take the desired action	
Use the media	• Use media advocacy to influence how the issue is seen or framed • Use social media to develop and mobilize networks	

Figure 23.3 Community Organizing and Advocacy Checklist

PROMISING PRACTICE	WHAT DOES IT LOOK LIKE?	FILL IN HERE: HOW CAN YOU USE THIS PRACTICE?
Build in mechanisms for accountability to the community	• Feedback loops that link community and policymakers • Include community standards and measures of success in the long-term monitoring of the policy implementation	
Stay grounded in the community	• Regularly reach out to new community members to listen to their concerns	
Strengthen commitment—in yourself and in others	• Recognize that making change often takes time • Speak to the deeper motivations for action • Find fun and creative approaches that energize	
Take care of yourself as you take care of others	• Avoid burnout • Celebrate victories, large and small	

Figure 23.3 (*Continued*)

Patricia Barahona: "Community health workers have to have a level of humility in the work they do in partnership with the folks that they serve. Those folks can be defined broadly—and youth have to be a core component in any community health or change effort. Hold your personal experience at your core, but stretch yourself to think about the community's health and wellness."

Chapter Review

1. Review the scenario presented at the beginning of this chapter about the community facing increasing gun violence. Based on the information provided, answer the following questions:

   ○ What are the primary concerns of the community?
   ○ What other challenges does the community face?
   ○ What resources does the community have?
   ○ As a CHW working in the community, how would you bring members together to talk about their concerns and to identify strategies to promote social change? How might you use principles of popular education? Specifically, what would you do? What type of community diagnosis might the community undertake to gather more information about the nature, causes, and consequences of their identified concern?
   ○ What type of key decision and policymakers might be able to influence the issue of concern to the community?
   ○ How might you use media advocacy and social media to support a campaign for change?
   ○ How would you go about identifying possible allies or opponents?
   ○ Once you have picked a desired goal or action to create a sustainable change in the rate of gun violence, what steps would you use to develop a strategy in concert with community members?

2. Consider the following quote from Patricia Barahona of the Youth Leadership Institute, then answer the questions below: "*I think research matters. Interpreting that research from the community is critical. Strategy matters. It's core in terms of anticipating every 'no' you will hear from decision makers. A lot of these campaigns*

started off with a lot of 'nos'—we have to prepare for that, and prepare the young people and families so they can anticipate it, and we can plan what will be our response. <u>How you frame the issue really matters</u>. You have to understand how people can hear or connect to the issue and you have to stay on that message and continuously remind people that that's the framing, because if you let someone else reframe it for you, you stand to lose. Community should drive the framing of the issue, and it's in the community's best interest to be involved in the research and to drive the framing of the issue—that's where a lot of the power lies. If we aren't framing it broadly enough or not framing it in the right way, then we need to figure that out, as a community. . . . <u>Relationships matter</u>—the relationships of young people with us, the relationships we had with other folks, the relationships those people had with others . . . those relationships are key to meeting with merchants, meeting with policymakers. We needed to reach a different level of making a connection to move this work forward."

○ Which of the promising practices included in the Community Organizing and Advocacy Checklist from Section 23.7 do you see reflected in this quote?

○ How might the steps of the CAM help you help the community develop research? Strategy? Framing of the issue? Relationships?

○ The youth-led campaign for a local ordinance to reduce the density of tobacco outlets that Patricia Barahona describes here took six years. What might you do to sustain your commitment and avoid burnout, if you were engaged in a multiyear campaign like this one?

References

Alinsky, S. D. (1971). *Rules for radicals: A pragmatic primer for realistic radicals*. New York, NY: Random House.

Blackwell, A. G., & Colmenar, R. A. (2012). Principles of community building: A policy perspective. In M. Minkler (Ed.), *Community organizing and community building for health and welfare* (3rd ed.) (pp. 423–424). New Brunswick, NJ: Rutgers.

Community Toolbox. (n.d.). *Toolkit 10: Advocating for change*. Retrieved from *http://ctb.ku.edu/en/advocating-change*

Garvin, C. D., & Cox, F. M. (1995). A history of community organizing since the Civil War with special reference to oppressed communities. In J. Rothman, J. L. Erlich, & J. E. Tropman (Eds.), *Strategies of community intervention: Macro practice* (5th ed., pp. 64–99). Itasca, IL: Peacock.

Institute for Democratic Renewal & Project Change Anti-Racism Initiative. (1998). A community builder's toolkit. Retrieved from *www.capd.org/pubfiles/pub-2004-07-03.pdf*

MacQueen, K. M., McLellan, E., Metzger, D. S., Kegeles, S., Strauss, R. P., Scotti, R., Blanchard, L., & Trotter, R. T. (2001). What is community? An evidence-based definition for participatory public health. *American Journal of Public Health, 91*, 1929–1938.

Mattessich, P., & Monsey, B. (1997). *Community building: What makes it work: A review of factors influencing successful community building*. St. Paul, MN: Amherst H. Wilder Foundation.

Ohmer, M. L., & DeMasi, K. (2009). *Consensus organizing: A community development workbook*. Thousand Oaks, CA: Sage.

Rifkin, S. B., Muller, F., & Bichmann, M. (1988). Primary healthcare: On measuring participation. *Social Science and Medicine, 26*, 931–940.

Rothman, J., & Tropman, J. E. (1987). Models of community organization and macro practice perspective: Their mixing and phasing. In J. Rothman, J. L. Erlich, & J. E. Tropman (Eds.), *Strategies of community intervention: Macro practice* (5th ed.) (pp. 3–26). Itasca, IL: Peacock.

San Francisco Department of Public Health. (n.d.). *Community health promotion and prevention: Community Action Model*. Retrieved from *www.sfdph.org/dph/comupg/oprograms/CHPP/CAM/default.asp*

Wallerstein, N. (1992). Powerlessness, empowerment, and health: Implications for health promotion programs. *American Journal of Health Promotion, 6*, 197–205.

Wallerstein, N. (2006). *What is the evidence on effectiveness of empowerment to improve health?* [Report]. Copenhagen, Denmark: WHO Regional Office for Europe. Retrieved from *www.euro.who.int/en/data-and-evidence/evidence-informed-policy-making/publications/pre2009/what-is-the-evidence-on-effectiveness-of-empowerment-to-improve-health*

Walter, C. L., & Hyde, C. A. (2012). Community building practice: An expanded conceptual framework. In M. Minkler (Ed.), *Community organizing and community building for health and welfare* (3rd ed., pp. 78–90). New Brunswick, NJ: Rutgers.

Youth Leadership Institute/Tobacco Use Reduction Force (TURF). (2013). *Where we live, tobacco is everywhere: A case study.* Retrieved from *http://sanfranciscotobaccofreeproject.org/wp-content/uploads/2013-Tobacco-Use-Reduction-Force-YLI-Density.pdf*

Additional Resources

Berkeley Media Studies Group. (n.d.) *Media advocacy 101.* Retrieved from *www.bmsg.org/resources/media-advocacy-101*

Bobo, K. A., Kendall, J., & Max, S. (2010). *Organizing for social change: Midwest Academy manual for activists* (4th ed.). Santa Ana, CA: Forum Press.

Center for Health and Gender Equity. (n.d.). The lobbying process: Basics and how-to guide. Retrieved from *http://genderhealth.org/files/uploads/change/Tools_for_Advocacy/The_Lobbying_Process.pdf*

Center for Tobacco Policy and Organizing. (n.d.) *Organizing tools.* Retrieved from *http://center4tobaccopolicy.org/community-organizing/organizing-tools/*

Community Organizing Toolkit. (n.d.). Retrieved from *http://organizinggame.org/*

Community Tool Box. (n.d.). Retrieved from *http://ctb.ku.edu/en/table-of-contents/*

Freire, P. (1973). *Education for critical consciousness.* New York, NY: Seabury Press.

Greenlining Institute. (n.d.). *Lesson 13: Creating a strategy chart.* Retrieved from *http://greenlining.org/wp-content/uploads/2013/02/HowToCreateaStrategyChart.pdf*

Health Resources in Action. (2013). *Defining healthy communities.* Retrieved from *www.hria.org/uploads/catalogerfiles/defining-healthy-communities/defining_healthy_communities_1113_final_report.pdf*

Lavery, S. H., Smith, M. L., Avila-Esparza, A., Hrushow, A., Moore, M., & Reed, D. F. (2005). The Community Action Model: A community-driven model designed to address disparities in health. *American Journal of Public Health, 95,* 611–616.

McKenzie, J. F., Neiger, B. L., and Thackeray, R. (2013). *Planning, implementing, and evaluating health promotion programs: A primer* (6th ed.). San Francisco, CA: Pearson.

Midwest Academy. (n.d.). Retrieved from *www.midwestacademy.com*

Minkler, M. (2012). *Community organizing and community building for health and welfare* (3rd ed.). New Brunswick, NJ: Rutgers.

National Latino Council on Alcohol and Drug Prevention. (n.d.). *Take action, make change: A community organizing tool kit.* Retrieved from *www.racialequitytools.org/resourcefiles/LCAT_Take_Action_Create_Change_-_Community_Organizing_Toolkit.pdf*

People's Health Movement. (n.d.). Retrieved from *www.phmovement.org/*

Praxis Project. (n.d.). Retrieved from *www.thepraxisproject.org/*

Smith, M. K. (1997, 2002). *Paulo Freire and informal education.* Retrieved from *http://infed.org/mobi/paulo-freire-dialogue-praxis-and-education/*

Youth Leadership Institute. (n.d.). Retrieved from *http://yli.org*

Video Index

CHAPTER	TITLE	DESCRIPTION	URL
Textbook Introduction	CHW Digital Story: Robert's Story	How Robert Scott became a CHW.	*http://youtu.be/Acaf7cKFGyo*
	CHW Digital Story: Luciana's Story	How Luciana Padia became a CHW.	*http://youtu.be/FS9IeOmwACk*
Part 1: Community Health Work: The Big Picture			
Chapter 1: The Role of Community Health Workers	Becoming a CHW: CHW Interview	Two working CHWs share what they value about their profession.	*http://youtu.be/BASkvuq1epw*
	The Emerging Roles of CHWs: Interview	Professor Carl Rush describes the growth of the CHW field.	*http://youtu.be/SnaaAUKK64o*
Part 2: Core Competencies for Providing Direct Services			
Chapter 6: Practicing Cultural Humility	Cultural Humility: Faculty Interview	Instructor Abby Rincon describes the importance of cultural humility for CHW success with clients.	*http://youtu.be/yV3DxgK5pn4*
	Nutrition and Culture: Role Play, Counter	A CHW misses an opportunity to demonstrate cultural humility.	*http://youtu.be/2Ck3V4johPM*
	Depression, Religion, and Cultural Humility: Role Play, Counter	A CHW misses an opportunity to demonstrate cultural humility.	*http://youtu.be/y6d-GdXi8go*
	Depression, Religion and Cultural Humility: Role Play, Demo	A CHW demonstrates cultural humility in working with a client.	*http://youtu.be/Bgr6TXWknQQ*
Chapter 7: Guiding Principles	Confidentiality and Reporting: Faculty Interview	How to inform a client about confidentiality policies and the CHW's obligation to report certain behaviors to authorities.	*http://youtu.be/7oOGAAmQK6o*
	Setting Professional Boundaries: Faculty Interview	The challenges of communicating, establishing, and maintaining boundaries with clients.	*http://youtu.be/WXn-tvVILbY*
	Setting Boundaries with Clients: Role Play, Counter	A CHW has difficulty setting professional boundaries with a client.	*http://youtu.be/kziHCHrwtzo*
	Setting Boundaries with Clients: Role Play, Demo	A CHW sets a professional boundary with a client.	*http://youtu.be/pX9x_w8ME9s*
	Self-Disclosure: Role Play, Counter	A CHW over-discloses personal information.	*http://youtu.be/7CpFvjXO-rs*
	Self-Disclosure: Role Play, Demo	A CHW demonstrates a limited self-disclosure.	*http://youtu.be/12s4zgUUJFs*
	Self-Disclosure: Faculty Interview	The challenges and potential benefits of self-disclosure.	*http://youtu.be/ihcr6GvBAAg*
	Giving Advice: Role Play, Counter	A CHW makes the mistake of giving advice.	*https://youtu.be/Our62-cDogk*
	Giving Advice: Role Play, Demo	A CHW uses client-centered skills rather than giving advice.	*https://youtu.be/J8Jn_okskAM*
	Giving Advice: Faculty Interview	The problem with giving advice to clients.	*http://youtu.be/ffFXsvPAKkA*
	Big Eyes, Big Ears, Small Mouth: Faculty Interview	The value for CHWs of speaking less, and observing and listening more.	*http://youtu.be/jE9uNHRhLA4*
	Talking Too Much: Role Play, Counter	A CHW who talks too much rather than listening.	*http://youtu.be/VhDFNaFow6c*

CHAPTER	TITLE	DESCRIPTION	URL
	Your Approach to Client-Centered Counseling: Faculty Interview	Key aspects for developing your own approach to client-centered counseling.	*http://youtu.be/yHlfoqqkxJI*
Chapter 8: Conducting Initial Client Interviews	Welcoming a Client: Faculty Interview	How a warm welcome helps to build rapport with a new client.	*http://youtu.be/iQrImzhjAIs*
	Confidentiality: Role Play, Demo	A CHW explains confidentiality policies to a client.	*http://youtu.be/odhxp7ILWfc*
	Communicating with Body Language: Role Play, Counter	A CHW shows how negative body language can undermine a relationship with a client.	*http://youtu.be/DbsgG-LObPE*
	Communicating with Body Language: Role Play, Demo	A CHW who incorporates effective body language as they work with a client.	*http://youtu.be/WDV2OPRzfYo*
	Strength-based Practice: Faculty Interview	The advantages of working with clients using a "strength-based" approach.	*http://youtu.be/Cq4PX89tlZE*
	Taking Notes: Role Play, Demo	A CHW demonstrates how to talk with a client about taking notes.	*http://youtu.be/yZ6FiTr3O4o*
Chapter 9: Counseling	Relapse Prevention: Role Play, Demo	A CHW talks with a client about preventing a relapse to prior risk behaviors.	*http://youtu.be/g7UiLRJ-QkE*
	Relapse Prevention: Role Play, Debrief, Faculty Interview	Concepts and skills for relapse prevention, and a discussion of the role play demonstration, "Relapse Prevention."	*http://youtu.be/EaXhsT6B8y8*
	Providing an Affirmation: Role Play, Demo	A CHW provides an affirmation to a client.	*http://youtu.be/FrggzUE7Z_I*
	Safer Sex & Using a Motivation Scale: Role Play, Demo	A CHW uses motivational interviewing and a motivation scale to support a client with behavior change.	*http://youtu.be/h9MP3W4vFFE*
	Rolling with Resistance: Role Play, Counter	A CHW struggles to respond to a client's ambivalence about behavior change.	*http://youtu.be/x_hyIMRMy7A*
	Rolling with Resistance: Role Play, Demo	A CHW demonstrates how to roll with resistance when a client is ambivalent about behavior change.	*http://youtu.be/rgqrusY2MJI*
	Rolling with Resistance: Faculty Interview	The value of rolling with resistance when a client is ambivalent about behavior change.	*http://youtu.be/9vNeWuNUflo*
	The Use of Silence: Role Play, Counter	A CHW who is uncomfortable with silence during a meeting with a client.	*http://youtu.be/e98joohaQwU*
	The Use of Silence: Role Play, Demo	A CHW who is comfortable with silence during a meeting with client.	*http://youtu.be/N5NyZ7OLcMA*
	The Use of Silence: Faculty Interview	Accepting silence as a natural part of conversations with clients.	*http://youtu.be/DZNOeVxZfIs*
	Developing Your Client-Centered Practice: Faculty Interview	Key aspects for developing your own client-centered practice.	*http://youtu.be/A71MPjMuYh8*
Chapter 10: Care Management	Establishing Client Priorities: Faculty Interview	The importance of supporting a client to establish their own priorities.	*http://youtu.be/isOQoAF4kAA*
	Establishing Priorities for an Action Plan, Role Play, Counter	A CHW asserts his own agenda for what a client "should do."	*http://youtu.be/uX65ljyHV6k*
	Developing a List of Referrals: CHW Interview	A CHW describes how to develop a list of reliable and culturally relevant referral resources.	*http://youtu.be/xKJQo6HExq4*
	Providing a Client-Centered Referral: Role Play, Counter	A CHW does not provide a client-centered referral.	*http://youtu.be/SzYoL5tA4DU*
	Providing a Client-Centered Referral: Role Play, Demo	A CHW demonstrates one way of providing a client-centered referral.	*http://youtu.be/2Gol8gJGSZg*

CHAPTER	TITLE	DESCRIPTION	URL
Chapter 11: Home Visiting	Conducting Home Visits: CHW Interview	A CHW shares strategies for conducting successful home visits.	*http://youtu.be/BSgqpdyvZ5w*
Part 3: Enhancing Professional Skills			
Chapter 12: Stress Management and Self Care	Stress Management: Faculty Interview	The value of stress management for clients and CHWs	*http://youtu.be/YH2na2xuuuo*
	Action Planning and Stress Management: Role Play, Demo	A CHW supports a client with stress management.	*http://youtu.be/H_62Cbm5W_c*
Chapter 13: Conflict Resolution Skills	Conflict between Two CHWs: Role Play	A conflict between two CHW co-workers.	*http://youtu.be/8wHwNAnhC1Y*
	Responding to Anger: Role Play, Counter	A CHW does not respond well to a client's anger.	*http://youtu.be/kOZWxisLm5s*
	Responding to Anger: Role Play, Demo	A CHW responds effectively to a client's anger.	*http://youtu.be/IMxXFufpHFc*
	The Art of Apology: Faculty Interview	The value of learning when and how to offer a sincere apology to the clients you work with.	*http://youtu.be/obtQn3fdGOY*
Chapter 14: Professional Skills	Providing & Receiving Constructive Feedback: Faculty Interview	The importance of learning how to provide and receive constructive feedback in a professional manner.	*http://youtu.be/7NqVUo-foEw*
Part 4: Applying Core Competencies to Key Health Issues			
Chapter 15: Promoting the Health of Formerly Incarcerated People	Incarceration as a Public Health Issue: Faculty Interview	Donna Willmott, a teacher at CCSF, talks about why understanding people's incarceration histories is part of promoting their health.	*http://youtu.be/o7AdDUAyu54*
	CHW Digital Story Emory's Story: Hope and Transformation	CHW Emory tells his story.	*http://youtu.be/oSx1OPt6r8M*
	CHW Digital Story Ron's Story: A Grandmother's Love	CHW Ron Sanders tells his story.	*http://youtu.be/ePDOB5OtjzM*
	CHW Digital Story Juanita's Story: Everyone Has Purpose in Life	CHW Juanita Alvarado tells her story.	*http://youtu.be/_AfVE1DCEVc*
	CHW Digital Story Tracy's Story: From Deliverance to Recovery	CHW Tracy Reed tells her story.	*http://youtu.be/KEVRnTTGQlw*
	CHW Digital Story Jermila's Story: A Step Forward	CHW Jermila M. tells her story.	*http://youtu.be/vYOsRcrnZ1M*
	First Meeting between a Patient and a CHW: Interview	A client with a history of incarceration speaks about her first impressions of her CHW and the difficulty of trusting a stranger to help her.	*http://youtu.be/OrfXKN8IgxA*
	A CHW with a History of Incarceration: CHW Interview	A CHW with a history of incarceration talks about the value of his experiences in building relationships with his clients.	*http://youtu.be/PfBJ9GCvkKk*
	CHW Digital Story Ernest's Story	CHW Certificate Program Graduate Ernest tells his story.	*http://youtu.be/2HVB_ZDRs1s*
	CHW Digital Story Lee's Story: Change	Freeman, a patient with the Transitions Clinic in Richmond, CA, tells his story.	*http://youtu.be/VElbOb7BkmQ*
	Listening to a Client's Priorities: Role Play, Counter	A CHW does not do a good job of listening to the client's priorities	*http://youtu.be/n96TZKnnhec*

CHAPTER	TITLE	DESCRIPTION	URL
Chapter 16: Chronic Conditions Management	Self-Management: Finding Reasons to Live Interview	A health coach discusses his approach to supporting clients to uncover their motivation for making changes in their life.	http://youtu.be/nRChT9oHOMM
	Action Planning: Faculty Interview	Strategies for supporting a client to develop an Action Plan.	http://youtu.be/51J58BJeQak
	Action Planning, Diabetes and Exercise: Role Play, Demo	A CHW supports a client with the self-management of diabetes.	http://youtu.be/XCOQyvhX91A
	Medications Management, Part 1: Role Play, Demo	A CHW supports a client with medications management, Part 1 of 4.	http://youtu.be/gleMEwoN72k
	Medications Management, Part 2: Role Play, Demo	A CHW supports a client with medications management, Part 2 of 4.	http://youtu.be/eLRe6wVkLuw
	Medications Management, Part 3: Role Play, Demo	A CHW supports a client with medications management, Part 3 of 4.	http://youtu.be/F2Mndwvfu-c
	Medications Management, Part 4: Role Play, Demo	A CHW supports a client with medications management, Part 4 of 4.	http://youtu.be/SVWbGyEKblk
	Action Planning, Revising an Action Plan: Role Play, Counter	A CHW has difficulty addressing a client's challenges in implementing her Action Plan.	http://youtu.be/g6I5omhDSHU
	Action Planning, Revising an Action Plan: Role Play, Demo	A CHW supports a client to revise their Action Plan.	http://youtu.be/Clr5pcdzo74
	Action Planning, Revising an Action Plan: Faculty Interview	How to support a client to revise an action plan.	http://youtu.be/JUtog9cd29Q
Chapter 17: Promoting Healthy Eating and Active Living (HEAL)	Talking about Weight and Health: Role Play, Counter	A CHW does not do an effective job of talking with a client about weight.	http://youtu.be/FLpx7QHjMRY
	Talking about Weight and Health: Role Play, Demo	A CHW talks with a client about weight and health.	http://youtu.be/83EeBQuXOXo
	Client-Centered Counseling and Nutrition: Role Play, Demo	A CHW supports a client to make changes to her diet.	http://youtu.be/73-ebSBGQUo
	Hypertension and Healthy Eating, Part 1: Role Play, Demo	A CHW provides health education about nutrition to a client with high blood pressure.	http://youtu.be/aGuViTC42G4
	Hypertension and Healthy Eating, Part 2: Role Play, Demo	A CHW provides health education about nutrition to a client with high blood pressure.	http://youtu.be/271pMgUluNg
	Hypertension and Healthy Eating, Part 3: Role Play, Demo	A CHW provides health education about nutrition to a client with high blood pressure.	http://youtu.be/gVlV_8iM_HA
	The Value of Taking Small Steps: Interview	A health coach discusses how he supports clients to initiate realistic but meaningful change in their life.	http://youtu.be/4ILopSTH7lk
	Action Planning and Exercise: Role Play, Demo	A CHW supports a client to develop an Action Plan to manage chronic health conditions.	http://youtu.be/x9kt4EusdwA
Part 5: Working with Groups and Communities			
Chapter 21: Group Facilitation	Group Facilitation: CHW Interview	A CHW describes her work facilitating a support group for Latinas.	http://youtu.be/36IBED_1Nvk

Author Index

Page references followed by *fig* indicate a photograph.

Subject Index

Page references followed by *fig* indicate an illustrated figures and photographs; followed by *t* indicate a table.

reflecting on your practice of, 146

transference of power component of, 145

trauma survivors and use of, 504

video interview with Abby Rincon on, 144

video showing CHW working with, 147

a word of caution on the importance of, 137–138

Cultural self-awareness

building, 144

professional roles of culturally effective CHWs with, 150–151

a word of caution on limitations of our, 137–138

Culture

as barrier to changing our diets, 461

defining and understanding, 142–144

how trauma is influenced by status and, 503–504

influence on our responses to conflict by, 252*fig*, 353

a word of caution on limitations of knowledge of other, 137–138

Culture of individuality, 627

D

Decision making

anticipating consequences of trauma survivors' plans and, 528–529

framework for ethical, 166–167

Deep breathing activity, 339

Deferred Action Childhood Arrivals (DACA) program, 125

Depression

as barrier to changing our diets, 462

videos on working with clients with, 151

Diabetes

as leading cause of death in the U.S. (2011), 67

Pima Indians and rates of type 2 diabetes, 425

Diagnostic and Statistical Manual (DSM) [1982], 494

Diagnostic and Statistical Manual–Fifth Edition (DSM–5), 494–495

Dietary Guidelines Advisory Committee (2015), 460

Diets

benefits of vegetarian and vegan, 469

common barriers to changing our, 461–462

hunger, food insecurity, and our, 460–461

keeping in mind client's life circumstances, 473–476

self-assess your own, 469

See also Healthy eating; Nutrition

Direct services

CHW core role to provide, 13–14

culturally effective CHWs providing, 150

Discharging

challenges related to, 452

reasons for chronic conditions management, 451–452

Discrimination

"Ban the Box" campaign against employment, 408

as barrier to changing our diets, 462

civil rights movement helping to fight, 434

immigrant communities and history of, 140–141

in public health, 141–142

Puerto Rican "population control program" (1937) example of, 141–142

re-entry challenges of stigma and, 405

structural, 141

transgender and gender variant employment, 280

Tuskegee Syphilis Trials example of, 78, 141

WCCUSD school district policy prohibiting LGBT harassment and, 661

Diseases

acute, 68

chronic lower respiratory diseases, 67

heart, 67

infectious, 68

influenza, 67

interactions between different, 68

kidney, 68

multidrug-resistant TB, 398

noninfectious, 68

pneumonia, 67

public health estimation of prevalence of, 69

stroke (cerebrovascular diseases), 67, 557

See also Chronic diseases; Leading causes of death

Disenfranchisement, 404

Documentation

care management, 275*fig*–276*fig*, 279, 292–295

client-centered counseling for behavior change, 251

community health outreach, 571–572

initial client interview forms, 218–219

video on taking notes: role play, 219

when forms don't recognize people's gender identity, 269

Domestic violence survivors. *See* Trauma survivors

Domestic violence training, 587

"Do no harm", 511

Dress code

home visits, 307

job interviews, 378

workplace, 379–381

Drug "mandatory minimums" penalties, 396

Drug Policy Alliance, 396

Drug use, home visits and distraction of, 310

Dual or multiple relationships, 168

Duty of self-awareness, 171–174

E

Ecological models

chronic condition management using, 440

on factors that influence behavior, 183–186

illustrated diagram of ecological model of health, 74*fig*

overcoming health inequalities using the, 96

public health use of, 73–75

Educational groups, 606

Educational level determinant of health, 92–93

Electronic health records (EHRs), 123

Eligibility status determination, 176

Email communication, 382

Emotional responses to stress, 326–327

Emotions

client-centered counseling and anger, 250

home visits when clients are angry, 317

reflection of, 241

trauma and, 496–497

Employment

"Ban the Box" campaign against discrimination in, 408

continued need to eliminate, 126

defining, 84–85

evidence of, 85–86

international comparison of health indicators and, 86t

learning about, 88

negative impact on society by, 878

overcoming, 96–98

policy used to overcome, 96–98

public health concern with, 69–70

race, ethnicity, and, 87–88

the role of CHWs in reducing, 102

in the United States, 86, 87

Unnatural Causes (documentary series) on, 85

See also Social determinants of health; Social justice; Society

Health information

facilitating training or community, 176

mistake of relying only on, 186–187

preparing a release of information, 277

understanding nutrition information, 467

See also Confidentiality

Health insurance

coverage type in the U.S., 112t

employer-based, 116fig–117

health care expenditures paid for by, 115–116

Health Insurance Marketplaces (ACA), 119

Health Insurance Portability and Accountability Act (HIPAA), 163, 206

Health outreach. See Community health outreach

Health practices

alternative medicine, 149

complementary medicine, 149, 507

traditional, 149

Health services

CHW competency for getting people needed, 14–15

CHW competency for providing direct, 13–14

CHW knowledge base on, 16

See also Referrals

Healthy eating

American food policy impacting access to, 460

Carla Moretti's case study on active living and, 458, 471–472, 475, 481–482

common barriers to a, 461–462

hunger, food insecurity, and, 460–461

keeping in mind client's life circumstances, 472–476

practical guidelines for, 470–471

as self-care, 337

videos on hypertension and, 476

See also Diets; Nutrition

Healthy Nutrition Plate, 468–469

Healthy People 2020

achieving health equity as goal of, 85

four overarching health goals by, 65

website on, 645

See also U.S. Department of Health and Human Services (USDHHS)

Healthy Salons Days of Action (November 11–14, 2014), 673

Heart disease, 67

Helping Health Workers Learn (Hesperian Foundation), 46

Henry J. Kaiser Family Foundation, 70

Hepatitis C Virus (HCV), 398, 434

Higher education

CHW educational options including, 46–48

public health practice by institutions of, 71

See also CHW Certificate program (City College of San Francisco)

High school student focus group, 650

Historical trauma, 493

HIV/AIDS epidemic

AIDS Coalition to Unleash Power (ACT UP) focus on, 41

discrimination and stigma associated with, 90

health outreach to men who have sex with men (MSM) to combat, 554

integrating medicine and public health models for treating, 434

jails and prison and spread of, 398

Monterey county AIDS Project's community outreach work on, 564, 570

movements for social change and combatting, 434

social group for Latino men who have sex with men (MSM) and at risk for, 607

social justice and health inequalities related to the, 69–70

spectrum of prevention applied to, 74, 75t

See also Sexual transmitted infections (STIs)

Hoarding or cluttering, 310–311

Homeostasis (balance within family system), 287

Home ownership

"block busting" practice and, 94

FHA and VA financing of, 93

redlining practice and, 93

Home visit challenges

visits to people without traditional homes, 316

when clients are angry, 317

working with clients who are incarcerated, 317

Home visiting

the challenges of, 302

an overview of, 300–302

reasons for, 301–302

Roger's case study on, 300

Home visit process

conducting an assessment, 313–314

conducting an environmental assessment, 314–315

good-bye and thank-you, 316

providing case management, client-centered counseling, and health education, 315

Home visits

common challenges of, 316–317

common courtesies and guidelines during, 306–311

cultural humility practiced during, 308

how to conduct a, 312–316

overcoming distractions during, 310–311

preparing to conduct a, 303–306

respect the client's time during, 306–307

safety guidelines for, 311–312

video on conducting, 309

See also Families; Housing

Honesty, 284–285

Honoring the dead, 510

Hope SF: Sunnydale public housing project case study, 100–101

Hospitals, 120–121fig

Housing

community outreach partnering with public, 555

Hope SF: Sunnydale public housing project case study, 100–101

as re-entry challenge for recently incarcerated people, 403

Veteran's Administration financing of, 93

See also Home visits

Institutional community health outreach, 553, 555
Institutionalized racism, 504
Institutional review boards (IRBs), 638
Instituto Familiar de la Raza, 536
Internal stress management resources, 324–325
Internet
   community health outreach using the, 555–557
   as research tool, 642t, 645
Internship interviews, 377–379
Interpersonal skills competency, 16
Interprofessional Education Collaboration (IPEC), 180
Interviewing
   CHW interviews, 6, 20, 41–42
   dressing for your interview, 378
   follow-up after your interview, 379
   for job, internship, or volunteer positions, 377–379
   preparing for the interview, 377–378
   qualitative interviews as research tool, 643t, 651–652t
   strategies for having a good interview, 378–379
   See also Video interviews/role-playing/demos
"Invisible Punishment" Photovoice project, 655
Iraq health indicators, 86t

J

Japanese health indicators, 86t
Jewish historical trauma, 493
Job application process
   applications for, 373–374
   interviewing, 377–379
   resumes for, 374–377
   sample cover letter for application and resume, 374
Job description, 373
Jobs
   applying for, 373–377
   finding opportunities for, 373
   interviewing for, 377–379
   keeping the, 379–387
   sample description of a, 373
   See also Workplace
Journal of Obesity, 464

K

Key opinion leaders, 554–555, 558
Kidney disease, 68
Kinesthetic (or tactile) learners, 581

Knowledge base
   CHW competency on community, health issues, and available services, 16
   client-centered counseling, 231–235
   harm-reduction, 231–232
   risk-reduction counseling, 232
   Stages of Change theory, 232–233t
   See also Professional skills

L

Lacey, Yvonne, interview with, 41–42
Language
   actions words to include in resumes, 375
   to describe trauma responses, 495–501
   establishing "safe words" to use as safety warning, 568
   formerly incarcerated people and using appropriate, 395–396, 411
   I-messages, 363, 364
   language barriers with clients, 284
   note on language of size and weight, 463
   reflective listening and statements, 240–241t
   to talk about trauma, 493–494
   See also Body language; Communication
Latinos/Latinas
   discrimination against, 140–142
   fear of fighting back following trauma due to undocumented status, 503–504
   health indicators data on, 89
   health inequalities and health expenditures on, 87
   initiating a social group for men, 607
   NCHWAS survey (2014) on, 7
   as percentage of prison population, 396
   Puerto Rican "population control program" (1937) discrimination against, 141–142
   See also Immigrant communities; Racial/ethnicity differences
Lay health advisors (LHAs), 40
Leading causes of death
   chronic diseases as U.S., 68
   infectious diseases (19th/early 20th century), 68
   in the U.S. (2011), 67–68
   See also Diseases
Leading questions and bias, 644

Learners
   "banking" teaching method approach to, 583
   understanding how they learn, 581–582
   visual, kinesthetic or tactile, and auditory, 581
   what is your experience as a, 582
Learning
   conscientization process of, 582
   participatory, 583–584
   popular education for, 582–583, 672
   problem-based, 584–585
Learning zones
   description of, 614
   guiding group participants into the, 614–615fig
LEARN model of Cross Cultural Encounter Guidelines for Health Practitioners, 148
Lethality assessment, 530
Legal issues
   confidentiality, 163–166, 206–207, 631
   ethics and the law, 159
   informed consent, 78, 141, 163, 206–208
   See also Public policy
Legal Services for Prisoners with Children's "Invisible Punishment" Photovoice project, 655
Legislation
   Affordable Care Act (ACA) [2010], 11, 95, 110, 116–117, 119, 123, 125, 178
   Federal Adoption and Safe Families Act, 401
   Federal Migrant Act (1962), 40
   Health Insurance Portability and Accountability Act (HIPAA), 161, 206
   Title VII, 280
LGBT population
   Queer Youth Action Team (QYAT) project to help youth of, 660–661
   sexual orientation and, 89, 261, 270
   WCCUSD school district policy prohibiting harassment and discrimination against youth, 661
   See also Gender identity
Library research tool, 642t, 645
Licensed clinical social workers (LCSW), 223
Lifebooks (or memory boxes), 533
Life expectancy
   definition of, 69
   inequalities between nations, 85–86t